Brief Contents

Brief Content

Advanced Medical Transcription

Critical Thinking in Healthcare Documentation

LAURA BRYAN, MT (ASCP), CMT, AHDI-F

PEARSON

Boston   Columbus   Indianapolis   New York   San Francisco   Upper Saddle River
Amsterdam   Cape Town   Dubai   London   Madrid   Milan   Munich   Paris   Montreal   Toronto
Delhi   Mexico City   Sao Paulo   Sydney   Hong Kong   Seoul   Singapore   Taipei   Tokyo

Publisher: Julie Levin Alexander
Publisher's Assistant: Regina Bruno
Executive Editor: Joan Gill
Development Editor: Alexis Breen Ferraro
Associate Editor: Bronwen Glowacki
Assistant Editor: Nicole Ragonese
Editorial Assistants: Erica Viviani and Stephanie Kiel
Director of Marketing: David Gesell
Executive Marketing Manager: Katrin Beacom
Senior Marketing Coordinator: Alicia Wozniak
Senior Managing Editor: Patrick Walsh
Project Manager: Christina Zingone-Luethje

Senior Operations Supervisor: Ilene Sanford
Operations Specialist: Lisa McDowell
Art Director: Christopher Weigand
Text and Cover Designer: Ilze Lemesis
Media Editor: Amy Peltier
Lead Media Project Manager: Lorena Cerisano
Full-Service Project Management: Michelle Gardner,
    Laserwords Maine
Composition: Laserwords
Printer/Binder: Courier/Kendallville
Cover Printer: Lehigh-Phoenix Color/Hagerstown
Text Font: Goudy 11.5/13.5

Cover Image: Medicine, word collage: Login / Shutterstock.com
Glossy music button set: Ian O'Hanlon / Shutterstock.com

Credits and acknowledgments for content borrowed from other sources and reproduced, with permission, in this textbook appear on appropriate page within text.

Library of Congress Cataloging-in-Publication Data

Cataloging-in-Publication data on file with the Library of Congress

10 9 8 7 6 5 4 3 2 1

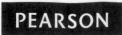

ISBN 10: 0-13-801413-2
ISBN 13: 978-0-13-801413-1

Contents

3 Gastroenterology: The Alimentary Tract 54

4 Gastroenterology: The Organs 90

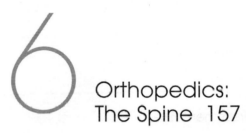

7

Urology and Nephrology 184

8

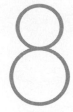

Pulmonology 232

9 Cardiology 278

12 Hematology and Oncology 385

Preface

No doubt, the field of healthcare documentation is in an enormous state of flux. The Health Information Technology for Economic and Clinical Health Act (HITECH Act) passed in February 2009, which incentivized healthcare providers to implement interoperable electronic health records (EHR), is having far-reaching effects on the way medical records are created. While EHR templates, front-end speech recognition, and other forms of point-of-care documentation techniques are replacing traditional dictation and transcription, these methods are best suited for capturing routine, straightforward documentation. Detailed, comprehensive documentation will continue to require a highly skilled transcriptionist to partner with the physician to accurately, efficiently, and completely document the details of patient care. Many believe that a more in-depth knowledge of disease processes, therapeutic procedures, and pharmacology, as well as more technology skills will be needed to accurately document, edit, and verify healthcare data going forward. In addition, it is anticipated that medical transcriptionists can play a vital role in tagging and processing narrative information, thereby transforming the patient's unique story into the type of discrete data that supports the EHR and contributes to clinical decision support, research, and public-health surveillance. In anticipation of these changes, *Advanced Medical Transcription* focuses on critical thinking and research skills that will equip the transcriptionist for a protean career in healthcare documentation that is both professionally and financially rewarding.

This text is aimed at the advanced student who has already completed coursework in medical terminology, anatomy, physiology, and introductory-level transcription practice. It assumes prior knowledge of the structure and function of common document types as well as headings, subheadings, and formats. Issues of style, based on *The Book of Style for Medical Transcription, 3rd Edition* (published by the Association for Healthcare Documentation), are reinforced throughout the text.

Key features of *Advanced Medical Transcription* include:

- A focus on critical thinking, critical listening, and problem solving

- Advanced reading level and graduate-level English vocabulary
- Authentic dictation from acute-care and ambulatory-care settings that correlates to the diseases and conditions described in the text

Advanced Medical Transcription fosters critical thinking and demonstrates how foundational knowledge of physiology and disease processes combined with contextual clues can help decipher difficult dictation, discriminate sound-alike words and phrases, guide research efforts, and efficiently produce accurate documentation. It offers the student a variety of exercises and activities to build cognitive and listening skills. *Advanced Medical Transcription* also takes a unique approach to terminology; an emphasis is placed on medical phrases and medical lingo as opposed to individual terms. Graduate-level English vocabulary words that are commonly encountered in medical reports are incorporated into the explanatory text and reinforced in the end-of-chapter exercises.

Organization

The text is separated into web-based content and printed content. The two chapters housed on the web portal cover technology and health information management. The first chapter available on the web, Using Technology to Increase Productivity, focuses on advanced keyboard-command skills for increasing productivity while working in Windows and Windows-based applications. This chapter also covers editing techniques using shortcut keys, an important skill for editing speech-recognized documents. The second chapter on the web, Working in Health Information Management, covers the electronic medical record, HIPAA, computer security, and industry standards. These chapters can be adapted to any given educational program depending on the depth of coverage already included in the program's course of study.

Chapter 1 of the printed text, Using Critical Thinking to Increase Accuracy, introduces the student to problem solving and listening techniques for deciphering blanks, decoding accents, and using contextual clues to clarify difficult dictation. This chapter also covers electronic search techniques using electronic dictionaries, drug indexes, and the Internet, including contextual searches and search operators.

Chapters 2–12 of the printed text present detailed coverage of eleven medical specialties. Each medical-specialty chapter includes descriptions of diseases and conditions as well as corresponding laboratory tests, diagnostic and therapeutic procedures, and medications sorted by pharmacological class. Content selection is based on data collected by the Centers for Disease Control as the most common medical conditions encountered in the US health system. Each pharmacology section includes the most commonly prescribed drugs, including generic and trade names and dosages. The in-depth coverage of diseases and disorders provides students with foundational knowledge to apply critical thinking while transcribing and researching.

Medical content is written in the "language of dictators" with commonly dictated words and phrases incorporated into the explanatory text and printed in bold type. Examples of dictation using key words and phrases are printed directly in the text to give additional context and to model the use of these words and phrases in actual practice. There is a direct correlation between the bolded phrases in the text and the phrases that will be heard while transcribing. This approach to the language of medicine bridges the gap between "textbook" medical terminology and terminology as it is actually used in dictation. These bolded words and phrases are compiled in the Terms Bank and sorted alphabetically by chapter in Appendix A. In addition, the Terms Bank for each chapter is available in audio form to be transcribed by the student to reinforce learning and to help the student build their own electronic terms bank that can be used as the basis of their personal text expander glossary and on-the-job reference.

A User's Guide to Features of this Text

Features of this book have been specifically designed to encourage critical thinking, enhance understanding, and to bridge the gap between the classroom and employment by demonstrating practical application of the information presented.

Pedagogical Features

Pedagogical features include learning objectives for each chapter, a list of Preview Terms, and several feature boxes.

Objectives

The Learning Objectives focus on terminology and its application to the medical specialty covered in the corresponding chapter. The text itself gives in-depth clinical information that is foundational to understanding the terminology and how it is applied to the art of transcription.

Learning Objectives

After completing this chapter, you should be able to comprehend and correctly transcribe terminology related to:

▶ hypertension

▶ diabetes mellitus

▶ dyslipidemia

▶ overweight and obesity

▶ metabolic syndrome

▶ hypothyroidism

▶ laboratory tests, including reference ranges, used to diagnose and monitor common metabolic disorders

▶ drugs used to treat hypertension and common metabolic disorders

Preview Terms

Each chapter begins with a list of Preview Terms. This list includes terms and concepts that the student should understand before beginning the chapter. Definitions to the Preview Terms are found in Appendix D. Definitions of the Preview Terms for the web-based chapters are included with the online materials.

Preview Terms
Before studying this chapter, make sure you understand the following terms. Definitions can be found in the glossary.

atherosclerosis
cell receptors
electrolytes
extracellular
intracellular
intravascular
metabolism
mole
morbidity and
    mortality
osmosis
solute
transport (carrier)
    proteins

In-Text Features

Feature boxes within each chapter use a theme that has been patterned after the commands on a transcriber: Rewind, Pause, Stop, and Play.

- The yellow Pause icon marks activities and critical-thinking questions designed to increase comprehension and encourage practical application of the concepts and information presented.

Pause 2-6 Describe the role of albumin in the blood. Define albuminuria and hypoalbuminemia. Why do albuminuria and hypoalbuminemia go hand-in-hand?

- The red Stop icon marks information that deserves special attention. These feature boxes highlight particular words and phrases that present auditory discrimination problems or common pitfalls encountered on the job.

Be careful not to confuse creatine and creatinine. Creatinine is a metabolic byproduct found in the blood and excreted by the kidneys. Creatine is a nutritional supplement used by individuals who want to build muscle mass, and creatine kinase is an enzyme found in muscle tissue (see page 149).

- The green Play icon marks excerpts of actual dictation as well as examples of words and phrases associated with imaging studies.

Examination reveals a loud 3/6 pansystolic murmur best heard over the left sternal border and radiating to the axilla.

The Play icon may also mark examples of dictated slang.

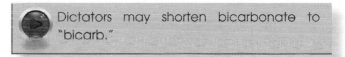

Dictators may shorten bicarbonate to "bicarb."

- The letters T and D indicate Transcribed and Dictated, respectively. Some boxes may use C and I, denoting Correct and Incorrect, respectively.

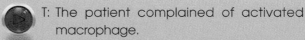

T: The patient complained of activated macrophage.
D: The patient complained of back pain and old age.
T: The patient said she had tryptophan.
D: The patient said she had tripped on a fan.

- The blue Fast Forward icon highlights techniques and approaches that will increase your productivity.

> The strategic application of technology (text expanders, templates, shortcut keys, and electronic references) will allow you to type faster and research more efficiently without compromising the accuracy of the completed transcript. Use software tools to enhance your efficiency so you are not tempted to cut corners on content accuracy.

- Annotations (contained within blue shaded boxes at the bottom of the page) include comments, definitions, and additional explanations to enhance the current topic. References are marked within the text with a corresponding number.

> **(3)** The transvalvular gradient is the change in pressure of the blood as it passes from one side of the valve to the other.

formed along with an echocardiogram provide qualitative estimates of the severity of stenosis and regurgitation by estimating the **transvalvular gradient (3)**. **Transesophageal echocardiogram (TEE)** is also useful for diagnosing valvular disease, especially diseases of the

- The purple Rewind icon marks section summaries that are placed at logical breaks throughout the chapter to recap important points.

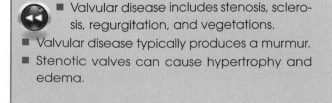

> ■ Valvular disease includes stenosis, sclerosis, regurgitation, and vegetations.
> ■ Valvular disease typically produces a murmur.
> ■ Stenotic valves can cause hypertrophy and edema.

Images

The text includes over 100 full-color images including screen shots, line art, photographs, radiographs, and diagrams to support the text and enhance comprehension of the material.

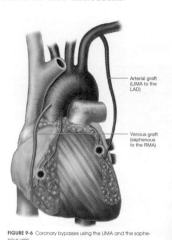

Arterial graft (LIMA to the LAD)

Venous graft (saphenous to the RMA)

FIGURE 9-6 Coronary bypasses using the LIMA and the saphenous vein.

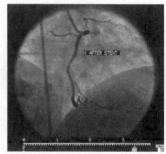

FIGURE 9-11 ST segment, PR interval, and the QRS interval (also called the QRS complex) on a normal EKG tracing.

(b)

FIGURE 9-12 Coronary artery with contrast media (a) before stent placement and (b) after stent placement. *Source:* Courtesy of Dr. Walt Marquardt, Mercy Hospital.

Tables

For easy reference, tables are used to present laboratory and pharmaceutical information. The tabular format of the laboratory information helps the student associate related laboratory tests and laboratory test panels. Medication tables help students to associate drugs with their pharmaceutical class and to compare dosages and dosage forms for related medications.

Table 2-4 Cholesterol and Related Lipoproteins

Test name	Normal Range
total cholesterol	<200 mg/dL
LDL (low-density lipoprotein)	40–130 mg/dL, optimal less than 70 mg/dL
HDL (high-density lipoprotein)	35–80 mg/dL, optimal greater than 40
VLDL (very low density lipoprotein)	5–40 mg/dL
triglycerides	<160 mg/dL
LDL particle size	<255 Å phenotype A >255 Å phenotype B (protective)

Table 2-11 Statins

Generic	Brand Name	Dose
atorvastatin	Lipitor	10 mg, 20 mg, 40 mg, 80 mg
rosuvastatin	Crestor	5 mg, 10 mg, 20 mg, 40 mg
simvastatin	Zocor	5 mg, 10 mg, 20 mg, 40 mg, 80 mg
ezetimibe and simvastatin	Vytorin	10 mg/10 mg, 10 mg/20 mg, 10 mg/40 mg, 10 mg/80 mg

Appendices

Additional resources found in the Appendix include:

- Terminology Bank (Appendix A): An alphabetical listing, sorted by chapter, of all bolded terms and phrases found in the medical-content chapters (Chapters 2–12).
- Sample Reports (Appendix B): A collection of sample reports for each medical specialty covered.
- Resources (Appendix C): A list of recommended web-based resources for clinical medicine, reference, research, and professional development.
- Preview Terms (Appendix D): Definitions of all Preview Terms, sorted alphabetically by chapter.

End-of-Chapter Activities

Each specialty chapter includes end-of-chapter exercises: Using Context to Make Decisions, Terms Checkup, and Look It Up.

Using Context to Make Decisions

These exercises foster critical thinking and problem solving, especially in the area of word search and word discrimination. These questions require the student to use contextual clues to fill in blanks and answer questions.

Terms Checkup

Terms Checkup consists of multiple-choice questions covering terminology and advanced English vocabulary. These questions are delivered electronically and can be found at www.myhealthprofessionskit.com. To access the questions, select the discipline "Medical Transcription," then click on the title of this book, *Advanced Medical Transcription*.

Look It Up

To encourage research and continuing education, each medical specialty chapter includes a research project called Look It Up. This exercise requires the student to research one or two diseases or conditions and list key terminology, related laboratory and imaging studies, and medications used for treatment. Recommended resources for completing research exercises can be found in Appendix C, although the student is not limited to these resources alone. The table below can be used as a guide for students to complete this exercise.

Transcription Practice

Practical experience is gained through transcription exercises included at the end of each medical specialty chapter. Before transcribing the dictated reports, the student is asked to transcribe the Key Terms for each chapter. These bolded terms and phrases have been recorded and can be transcribed from the audio files located on the web portal. The student may choose to import these transcribed terms and phrases into a text-expansion glossary, giving them a reference list and a productivity tool that can be used immediately upon employment.

In addition to transcribing key terms, the transcription exercises include transcribing, proofreading, editing, working with report templates, using sample reports to decipher difficult dictation, and editing normals and standards to match the current dictation. Transcription exercises align with the content presented in the text and are chosen for their difficulty based on the density of terminology, the dictator's accent, and the

Cause	Diagnosis			Treatment	
Pathophysiology	Procedures	Imaging	Laboratory	Medications	Procedures

inherent transcription challenges that require critical thinking. Transcription exercises are accessed through the transcription software module that is available to registered users of this text. This practice module is based on a market-based transcription platform and is designed to introduce the student to an actual working environment. Instructions for downloading and using the transcription software can be found at www.myhealthprofessionskit.com. Select the discipline "Medical Transcription," then click on the title of this book, *Advanced Medical Transcription*.

Ancillary Materials

Instructor materials include PowerPoint presentations for each chapter, answers to Pause questions and multiple-choice questions, and answer keys to the transcription exercises. Instructors have access to transcription management software for easily managing transcription exercises and to aid in grading.

A Note on Style

This text endorses style guidelines described in *The Book of Style for Medical Transcription, 3rd Edition,* published by the Association for Healthcare Documentation Integrity. The instructional text uses a combination of publishing styles and technical-writing styles, but all sample dictation, sample reports, and transcription exercises follow the *The Book of Style for Medical Transcription (BOS)*. The most notable difference between the two styles is in the use of numbers. Instructional text follows the general rule of writing out numbers one through nine, but all transcribed text (excerpts, samples, exercises, and practice transcription) follows the style guidelines for handling numbers as described in the *BOS* and the *AMA Manual of Style*. Another exception is the capitalization of terms in tables and bulleted lists; capitalization is only applied to terms that are always capitalized.

The Development of this Text

The idea for *Advanced Medical Transcription* was born out of conversations with colleagues, both employers and educators, who recognize the cognitive and analytical skills required to work successfully as a medical transcriptionist. These employers and educators noted a need to foster analytical thinking skills and critical listening skills as a part of the educational process. Far from being simply a typing job, transcription is a dynamic and challenging career that involves intensive listening and complex decision-making throughout the transcription process. Physicians rely on transcriptionists to transform conversational speech, normally punctuated with pauses, inflection, and intonation, into the flattened yet structured written word that clearly communicates the dictator's intent. The art of medical transcription requires more than simply typing what is heard; it also requires the transcriptionist to perceive unspoken cues and implied instructions. It is a blending of science and communication that requires an understanding of the medical content, knowledge of the social constructs of healthcare documentation, and mastery of grammar, advanced English vocabulary, medical terminology, and medical lingo. MTs who master this complex dance between the dictator and the listener play a critical role in patient care and risk management.

As a practicing transcriptionist, business owner, and technology consultant, I have found my career in medical transcription to be both interesting and gratifying, and my sincere desire is to see students find meaningful and rewarding work in the field of healthcare documentation. Most of all, I hope the student of medical transcription recognizes and celebrates the unique talents and skills required to produce quality documentation that contributes to patient safety and continuity of care.

Best wishes in your new career,

Laura Bryan, MT (ASCP), CMT, AHDI-F

About the Author

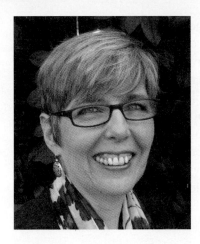

Laura Bryan graduated from the University of Texas at Austin with a degree in Medical Technology. After working ten years in the medical laboratory, she transitioned to a career in medical transcription. As a transcriptionist, Laura has worked as an independent contractor, quality assurance editor, and transcription service manager. As the owner of a transcription software company, she has participated in the development and deployment of a web-based transcription platform. Laura has also worked as an independent technology consultant, focusing on advanced keyboard skills, word-processing tools, and the use of electronic references for increasing efficiency and productivity with accuracy.

Working in a volunteer capacity, Laura has served on the board of the Association for Healthcare Documentation Integrity (AHDI) and has participated in numerous standards-development and credentialing-development programs. Since January 2008, Laura has worked as an editor and subject matter expert with the Health Story Project, a consortium of industry stakeholders working to produce data standards for the flow of information between common types of healthcare documents and electronic health records. She has authored a variety of articles for industry magazines and has edited certification study guides, publications, and continuing education materials for AHDI. Laura has had the opportunity to give presentations focused on technology, clinical medicine, and standards development at numerous local, regional, and national meetings. Laura is the recipient of AHDI's 2009 Advocate of the Year Award and is a Fellow of the Association for Healthcare Documentation Integrity (AHDI-F). She received the Lifetime Achievement Award from AHDI in 2011.

Advanced Medical Transcription is Laura's fourth individually authored book for medical transcription. Previous titles have focused on MS Word and the use of technology to increase productivity and accuracy in transcription.

Laura is married to Bob, who is also her business partner. Together they operate MedEDocs, a transcription technology and services provider, and MTWerks, a technology consulting company. They live just outside of Dallas in Mesquite, Texas, and have three grown children. In addition to her love of medicine and technology, Laura enjoys social networking, reading, and gardening.

Acknowledgments

As always, I must acknowledge the unfailing and unwavering support from Bob, my husband, friend, and business partner. I can't imagine accomplishing anything meaningful in my life without his support, encouragement, and unconditional love.

I would also like to acknowledge my friends and colleagues, especially Georgia Green and Ellen Drake, for their ideas and feedback in the developmental stages of this text. Many thanks to Alexis Breen Ferraro, the developmental editor for this text, for her excellent management, organizational skills, and keen eye. I appreciate her expertise and attention to detail that gives me a level of comfort knowing this text will survive the scrutiny of my peers.

Reviewers, often not recognized by the reader, play an important part in molding and fine-tuning a text. Reviewers give the author a fresh perspective on the writing and contribute to the usability and overall success of the book. I sincerely appreciate the time and effort put forth by the reviewers that offered their candid and constructive criticism as well as their praise for this project.

Reviewers

Judy Anderson, BA, M.Ed.
Department Head/Instructor
Coastal Carolina Community College
Jacksonville, NC

Susan D. Dooley, CMT, AHDI-F
Professor and Program Manager, Medical Transcription
    and Medical Terminology
Seminole State College of Florida
Altamonte Springs, FL

Phyllis Harris, BS
Associate Professor, Program Chair, Office Administration
    Program
Ivy Tech Community College
Kokomo, IN

Karen Milan, CMT
Program Coordinator/Instructor
NH Technical Institute
Concord, NH

Barbara L. Nadolski, CMT
Rend Lake College
Ina, IL

Barbara Riggins, BS, M.Ed.
Instructor
Blinn College
Bryan, TX

Gina Stephens, RN
Program Director, Business Technologies
Georgia Northwestern Technology College
Rome, GA

Using Critical Thinking to Increase Accuracy

Learning Objectives

After completing this chapter, you should be able to:

▶ Use contextual clues, including phrasing, immediate context, interrelated sections of the report, and sample reports to decipher difficult-to-understand dictation.

▶ Use electronic references, including dictionaries, word lists, drug references, and the Internet to research terminology and ensure the accuracy of content and spelling.

▶ Develop strategies for decoding accents based on speech and pronunciation patterns of common native languages.

▶ Implement strategies for proofreading to ensure comprehension and techniques for efficient editing.

Preview Terms

Before studying this chapter, make sure you understand the following terms. Definitions can be found in the glossary.

acronym	English as a second	initialisms	subentry
blank	language (ESL)	keywords	substitutions
bookmarking	entry	phoneme	Universal Resource
browse	filter	query	Locator (URL)
combining form	Find	s/l (sounds like)	vowel insertions
compound modifier	flag	search on definition/	vowel shortening
context	headword	subentry	wild cards
definition	homophones	search on index	
deletions	index	search operators	
devoicing	indications	sound-alikes	

Introduction

Critical thinking is the process of using what you already know to discover what you do not know. Some people might consider medical transcription a "manual" job with an emphasis on the mechanics of typing, but this is a gross misperception. Medical transcriptionists (MTs) are truly critical thinkers and knowledge workers. Accomplished MTs are problem solvers, detectives, and risk managers. Thinking critically in the context of medical transcription requires the MT to be constantly engaged in the content of the report and to continuously question what they hear. Each word transcribed must be assessed carefully, and the entire report must be evaluated for accuracy, consistency, coherency, and reasonableness. The components of critical thinking—analysis, synthesis, and reflection—can be learned and improved with practice. To maximize your critical thinking abilities, you must be your own critic—always questioning and challenging yourself. You must also be deliberate and engaged in your work.

The steps for applying critical thinking to a problem include:

- gathering information
- evaluating that information for relevance
- using that information

Critical thinkers distinguish between fact and opinion, ask questions, make detailed observations, uncover assumptions, define their terms, and make assertions based on sound logic and solid evidence.[1]

A critical thinker:

- asks relevant questions
- sorts out and ignores irrelevant information
- evaluates statements
- values curiosity
- likes finding solutions
- tests assumptions, beliefs, and opinions against facts
- listens intently
- uses critical thinking in all areas of life

- delays decisions until all facts are known or considered
- looks for evidence to support assumptions

Critical Listening

Thinking critically requires listening critically. MTs must be fully engaged in what they are hearing and not simply "typing what they hear." Experienced MTs find it is surprisingly easy to type in "autopilot mode"—a trance-like state in which the fingers seem to have ears. The words go from the headset straight to the fingertips, seemingly bypassing any conscious process. New MTs, however, can become so focused on individual words that they fail to relate each word to the rest of the content. Be careful to avoid both scenarios. Failure to pay close attention to the entire report can result in life-threatening errors that can become a part of the patient's medical record. Errors can originate from the dictator or the transcriptionist, and the transcriptionist is the critical link between what is spoken, what is intended, and what finally becomes a part of the patient's chart.

Speech recognition (SR), the very technology once touted to eliminate the need for MTs, has ironically proven the MT's true value in the documentation process. Interpreting sound in the absence of context with no consideration of intended meaning is a reckless endeavor. Speech recognition engines literally "type based on sound" and have minimal ability to determine meaning or intent.

Paradoxically, MTs must learn to doubt the very thing they must rely upon—their ears. As you gain experience, you will quickly learn that what you initially hear may not necessarily be what was dictated. This is an inevitable consequence of asynchronous communication. Most of us decipher speech by integrating input from both the eyes and the ears, and conversations are synchronous. In normal conversation, we listen contextually, drawing conclusions periodically throughout the conversation. When listening to dictation, however, we tend to listen word by word, because we are responsible for transcribing each word we hear.

When speaking face-to-face, we integrate the person's words with the movement of their lips, their facial expressions, and their body language. These visual cues contribute to our interpretation of what we hear. But these important visual elements are missing in dictation. Sounds that we normally discriminate by unconsciously noting lip movements (eg, the

[1]David Ellis, *Becoming a Master Student* (NY: Houghton Mifflin Co., 1997)

difference between seeing a person say the "s" sound and the "f" sound) cannot be distinguished. The dictator's speed and poor articulation may compound this problem. In addition, dictation often lacks the rhythm and intonations of normal conversation, making the words even more difficult to understand. Transcriptionists must overcome these obstacles using the immediate **context** and sometimes the entire context of the report.

In addition to visual clues, our brains "fill in" missing sounds when hearing familiar words. A working knowledge of thousands of words and phrases contributes greatly to an experienced MTs ability to transcribe, as it is much more difficult to comprehend unfamiliar words. Successful MTs are often voracious readers who constantly "expose" themselves to new words, thereby expanding both their medical and English vocabularies and increasing their auditory word-recognition skills.

Accurate transcription requires the constant application of the "three D's:"

- Doubt—you must always question your ears—they absolutely will fool you.
- Discipline—you must always look up or double-check your work; do not guess.
- Decision making—you must always evaluate the report in its entirety.

MTs must contemplate, investigate, and confirm what they transcribe while maintaining high levels of productivity. Although the two may appear to be mutually exclusive, you will find that being engaged in the content of the report increases both your output and accuracy. Gathering clues from the immediate context as well as from key areas of the report will guide your research efforts and reduce the time you spend searching. You will be less likely to transcribe words and phrases incorrectly and will spend less time proofreading the report. Thinking critically throughout the transcription process will help you develop connections between symptoms, diagnoses, treatments, and outcomes. Thinking critically reduces rote memorization and increases comprehension, which builds a more extensive fund of knowledge, thereby decreasing the time you spend researching. Applying critical thinking will also help you determine when it is reasonable to end your search and leave a **blank**.

As an MT, you must be vigilant in your efforts to maintain concentration. This may be difficult to understand as a student, as you are probably focusing very hard on your studies. The longer you work as an MT, the easier it is to fall into the "zone." To remain alert, build visual images in your mind of what you are hearing. Look for disease associations such as foot ulcers in diabetics. Note prescribing patterns, too, such as the addition of potassium supplements to diuretic regimens. Try to anticipate the diagnosis or the plan based on what you have transcribed so far. Do not simply listen; become engaged with what you are hearing. The more you connect with what you are hearing, the more you will enjoy the work.

The following examples show how easy it is to type what you hear without being fully engaged with the content.

> T: He said that he was unable to do so due to time needed to care for his involute wife.
>
> D: He said he was unable to do so due to time needed to care for his invalid wife.
>
> T: The patient was to continue IV antibiotics and to return every 2 hours.
>
> D: The patient was to continue IV antibiotics and to be turned every 2 hours.
>
> T: Anemia stable after confusion.
>
> D: Anemia stable after transfusion.

> The strategic application of technology (text expanders, templates, shortcut keys, and electronic references) will allow you to type faster and research more efficiently without compromising the accuracy of the completed transcript. Use software tools to enhance your efficiency so you are not tempted to cut corners on content accuracy.

Listening Techniques

When you first encounter a blank, listen two to three times and then move on. It is possible that the word will be repeated later in the report. There is nothing more frustrating than spending ten minutes deciphering a difficult word or phrase only to find that the dictator repeats it very clearly later in the report. If you have heard "nonsense," consider setting the report aside for a short time and give your brain a chance to "forget" the nonsensical phrase. Oftentimes, once you have heard something incorrectly, it is hard to hear anything other than what you think you are hearing. Allowing time to forget will give your brain a fresh start at interpreting what it hears.

When you return to a difficult area of dictation, begin by listening two or three sentences ahead of the blank and continue listening past the blank without pausing or stopping. After listening to several sentences, pause for a moment to let your brain process what you just heard and see if you have that "ah-ha" moment when the brain formulates the sounds into a coherent thought. The first time you encounter the difficult section, you may have been listening piecemeal—starting and stopping the dictation while you transcribed in fragments but not completed thoughts. Listening straight through gives your brain the chance to process the speech more like a normal conversation—something your brain is accustomed to doing.

Do not always assume the difficult word is an obscure medical term; it is just as likely to be an English phrase spoken very quickly. Consider these examples:

> T: The patient complained of activated macrophage.
> D: The patient complained of back pain and old age.
> T: The patient said she had tryptophan.
> D: The patient said she had tripped on a fan.

These transcription errors would most likely not make sense in the context of the remainder of the report; neither are they terms a patient is likely to use.

Also, keep in mind that difficult areas of dictation may be dictated punctuation or an instruction directed at the transcriptionist. Mumbled phrases at the end of a paragraph or just before starting a new section of a report are often directives such as "period, new paragraph" or "next heading" or "exam reveals." Take a moment to consider the location of the difficult phrase in relation to the remainder of the text. If there are

complete thoughts on either side of the mumbled phrase, listen again to see if it is an instruction or punctuation.

> T: There are no other complaints _____. Review of systems is negative.
> D: There are no other complaints. (of uh . . . period paragraph) Review of systems is negative.
> T: She also complains of _____. She otherwise has been well.
> D: She also complains of (strike that). She otherwise has been well.
> T: Hyperlipidemia. Aim for an LDL of less than 70. May need to restart Vytorin and recheck LDL on Vytorin next.
> D: Hyperlipidemia. Aim for an LDL of less than 70. May need to restart Vytorin and recheck LDL on Vytorin. ("next" meant next number)

Isolate the sounds you are most certain of. It can be helpful to focus on a single sound and then build outward to construct several syllables. After isolating several syllables, say the syllables out loud to yourself. Change the stress of the syllables to see if you can "hear" the mystery word. It is not uncommon for dictators to accidentally mispronounce a word, either because they themselves are not familiar with the term or they are speaking quickly and stumbling.

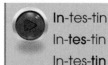
> In-tes-tin
> In-**tes**-tin
> In-tes-**tin**

Using Context to Decipher Difficult Dictation

Using context to decipher difficult dictation will significantly decrease the time you spend trying to make out words by "brute force" as well as the time you spend researching. Using context will also increase the chance of selecting the correct word among many homonyms and sound-alike words. Although there is no perfect formula for making garbled dictation crystal clear, there are techniques you can use to increase your success and decrease your frustration.

Blanks may be caused by transcription errors preceding the actual blank. Listen again and reconsider the words just before and after the blank. If the surrounding text is incorrect, you may actually be hearing the blank correctly but thinking it is incorrect because it makes no sense in the current context.

T: As a result of these findings, he underwent 2-level surgical diskectomy in _____ (s/l fusion) with Dr. Courtney.

D: As a result of these findings, he underwent 2-level surgical diskectomy and fusion with Dr. Courtney.

When reconsidering the surrounding text, try splitting the syllables that fall immediately before and after the blank differently. Part or all of the previous word may be part of the blank.

T: She is to have an MRI performed today. This will help us determine the distance from the apex of the vagina to her _____ (s/l metocolpos).

D: She is to have an MRI performed today. This will help us determine the distance from the apex of the vagina to hematocolpos.

T: Mons pubis ulcer. Skin ulceration may be eczema. I cannot exclude her pediform lesion as well, although patient denies a history of herpes simplex.

D: Mons pubis ulcer. Skin ulceration may be eczema. I cannot exclude herpetiform lesion as well, although patient denies a history of herpes simplex.

T: IMPRESSION: Postop _____ (s/l curative) epigastric pain.

D: IMPRESSION: Postoperative epigastric pain.

Be careful not to misplace or confuse articles such as *a* or *an* with prefixes or suffixes.

T: The infant was noted to have an _____ (s/l alatresia).

D: The infant was noted to have anal atresia.

T: Carotid flow was an _____ (s/l E grade).

D: Carotid flow was antegrade.

T: Despite multiple pain medications, the patient has not had a _____ (s/l bait mint) of her pain.

D: Despite multiple pain medications, the patient has not had abatement of her pain.

Using Contextual Clues

If applying different listening techniques does not reveal the word or phrase, begin gathering contextual clues. Start with clues within the immediate context, then expand your context to the remainder of the paragraph and eventually to the entire report. Use the following techniques for applying critical thinking to the transcription process.

Phrasing

The best approach to applying contextual clues from the immediate vicinity of the blank is to use phrasing. Medical language uses phrases extensively, with two- and three-word phrases being the most common. Medical phrases, often as simple as a noun with an adjective, include terms such as multiple sclerosis, uncontrolled hypertension, and polycystic kidney. The adjective itself is critical and must be chosen correctly.

Pause 1-1 Isolate the phrases in the following transcribed sentences:

1. Echocardiogram showed mitral valve prolapse.
2. Upper endoscopy showed gastric outlet obstruction.
3. Patient was diagnosed with protein losing enteropathy.
4. CBC results are suspicious for iron deficiency anemia.
5. There is pain on palpation of the medial joint line.

Evaluating context in terms of phrases instead of one word at a time is a powerful tool for researching and ensuring accuracy. Often a missing medical term is part of a common medical phrase.

A swift approach to resolving a blank within a phrase is to perform a phrase search instead of an individual word search. Phrase searches are more efficient and more accurate. For example, "left ventricular hypertrophy" is a common phrase used in cardiology, but an MT might easily hear the word "vesicular" instead of "ventricular." Transcribing the word vesicular without regard to the surrounding context would result in an error. Vesicular is the correct part of speech, is spelled correctly, has the same number of syllables, and sounds like ventricular, but "left vesicular hypertrophy" is definitely not the correct phrase.

Examine the words on either side of a blank to see if you can construct a phrase. Use the most unique word in the phrase as the keyword in a medical words-and-phrases index. In this example, *left* is too common and too vague to be of use, but using the keyword *hypertrophy* would reveal a subentry *left ventricular hypertrophy*.

In addition to phrases that describe medical diseases or conditions, there are many general phrases that are used repeatedly by the majority of dictators. The more you listen to dictation, the more you will begin to hear "clusters of words" instead of individual words.

risks and benefits
    clear to auscultation and percussion
bright red blood per rectum
pain on palpation
aspiration and biopsy
return to clinic in 6 weeks
alert and oriented
soft and nontender

Always test new words using a phrase search to make sure that the term fits the context and is used appropriately with the words on either side. The medical specialty chapters in this textbook highlight phrases to help you begin to think in phrases and not single words.

Using a text expander will help you to think in terms of phrases, as you will begin to build your list of shortcuts based on words that are dictated together.

Acronyms

Acronyms (abbreviations pronounced as words) such as GERD (*gurd*), CABG (*cabbage*), MRSA (*mersa*) and ICSI (*ik-see*) can be very tricky to decipher. Acronyms are not usually dictated as part of a phrase, because the acronym (when expanded) is itself a phrase. When you come upon a single-syllable blank (sometimes two syllables as in the case of MRSA) that is not logically a part of a phrase, consider an acronym. Medical dictionaries do not list all acronyms, so you will need to consult a comprehensive reference for acronyms and abbreviations. Once you locate an acronym, make sure the expanded form of the acronym is appropriate to the context in which it is being used. If the acronym appears in the problem list with no surrounding context, refer to the medication list to see if there are any current medications that correspond to the symptoms or disease described by the acronym. You may also find clues to a patient's current or ongoing diagnoses in the History of Present Illness section. If you are still unsure, leave it blank.

Tonia and Jonathan have male factor infertility and have gone through numerous IUI cycles without a pregnancy. In addition, she has recurrent pregnancy loss. I anticipate her IVF cycles should go rather smoothly. They will need ICSI secondary to male factor.

Abbreviations

Abbreviations in the form of **initialisms** (eg, CBC, ANA, C&S, and BMP) are extremely common in medical documentation, but they are rife with difficulty and danger. Initialisms are pronounced one letter at a time, and the individual letters are *extremely difficult if not impossible to distinguish*. Military and police organizations overcome the difficulty in accurately interpreting individual letters by using the phonetic alphabet (eg, Alpha, Bravo, Charlie, etc) to avoid confusion. You will rarely, if ever, hear a dictator make distinctions when dictating initialisms. You must use context to determine what is being dictated. There is no other way to be sure that you have heard and transcribed the correct abbreviation. You cannot rely on your ears to differentiate letters such as /a/ and /h/, /m/ and /n/, /s/ and /f/. You must be able to expand the abbreviation and evaluate the expansion based on the current context. If you do not know what the abbreviation stands for, leave it blank!

> **Pause 1-2** Evaluate the following transcribed sentences and determine whether the abbreviations were transcribed correctly.
>
> 1. The patient's BNP is now 1000, indicating a progression of her congestive heart failure.
> 2. A CVC will be ordered tomorrow to check for further bleeding and to monitor her white count.
> 3. Her most recent CNS showed E coli susceptible to ciprofloxacin.
> 4. The patient returns for her 18-month well-baby checkup and for Hiv and DTaP boosters.
> 5. The patient has had a flu-like illness for the past 2 weeks. EBC titers will be drawn today.
> 6. The patient has a history of a broken arm treated with ORIS.

Using the Entire Context

When the surrounding text does not elucidate the blank, you should begin to gather clues from other sections of the report. Although all areas of the report may provide clues, key areas include the current and past medical history, the assessment, and the plan. Different areas of a report are often interrelated, and you may be able to resolve blanks by comparing content between these interrelated areas, as described in the following sections.

Laboratory Results

Deciphering lab test names and correctly transcribing lab results can be challenging. Many lab values are dictated as abbreviations (eg, CBC, BMP, CMP, H&H, and LFTs) that can be challenging to decipher. More often than not, the results are numerical values that also present auditory discrimination problems. The sheer number of laboratory tests can be daunting, but many are so rare or esoteric that you may never encounter them. However, there are several lab tests and/or panels that are so common you will want to memorize these tests along with their normal ranges. The vast

majority of lab tests fall somewhere in between and can usually be grouped by medical specialty. You will find it helpful to keep categorical lists of lab tests according to medical specialty.

> **Pause 1-3** The following list of lab panels includes the most commonly ordered tests. Review these test panels (including the individual tests that make up the panel) and create your own quick-reference card that includes the individual tests along with their normal values. Use the index to find these tests throughout this text.
>
> 1. Complete blood count (CBC) with differential
> 2. Urinalysis (UA)
> 3. Comprehensive metabolic panel (CMP) (14 individual tests)
> 4. Liver function tests (LFTs)
> 5. Thyroid function tests (TFTs)
> 6. Total cholesterol (and subfractions)

Physicians rarely dictate every lab value drawn; they typically dictate lab values germane to the patient's current condition. Relevant test results include those that are frankly out of range, normal values of tests that were previously out of range, or normal values for those tests that contribute to the differential diagnosis. Concentrate your search on the most common labs (listed in Pause 1-3) and then on those lab tests that relate to the patient's current problem list.

To help decipher lab test names and their values, first look at the Assessment and/or the Plan. Abnormal lab values may be reiterated in the Assessment portion of the report or mentioned again in the Plan with instructions to recheck the value at a later date. Lab values may also be discussed in the Assessment to prove or disprove the diagnosis.

If the Assessment and the Plan do not offer clues, look at the History of Present Illness (HPI) or the Problem List. Think about the tests typically ordered to evaluate or diagnose the patient's current condition(s). Compare this list of diagnosis-related labs with the list of labs that have been clearly dictated. What tests are missing? Listen to the dictation again with a list of test names in front of you. Often, a word that is unclear is easily deciphered when the possibilities are in front of you.

Be sure to compare your transcribed result to the expected reference range or result. Generally speaking, the narrower the reference range, the less tolerance the body has to values outside the range and the less likely that the result is physiologically possible. For example, potassium has a very small reference range of 3.5 to 5 mEq/L. A potassium value of 10 would be physiologically impossible and incompatible with life. An even tighter range exists for arterial blood pH (7.35 to 7.45). Alkaline phosphatase, however, has a range of 20 to 120 units/L, so values well above the reference range would be possible. It is important to compare transcribed lab values to their expected reference range to make sure a dictation or transcription error has not occurred. Of course, not all lab values dictated fall within the normal range, but those values that greatly exceed the range should be researched and/or marked (flagged) for confirmation.

 Pause 1-4 Which of the following transcribed lab values are incorrect?

hematocrit 0.3, hemoglobin 24

sodium 20 mEq/L

bilirubin 1.5 mg/dL

potassium 16 mEq

chloride 108

In addition to comparing lab results to their expected reference ranges, you should also make sure the values are consistent with the patient's condition or diagnosis. For example, if hypokalemia is discussed in the History section, an elevated potassium level may not necessarily make sense.

There is an old saying in Texas: If you hear hoofbeats, look for horses, not zebras (that is, you are more likely to find a horse in Texas and a zebra in Africa). This is good advice for medical transcriptionists. Just because you do not immediately understand the word dictated, do not assume it is an obscure or esoteric term. First look for the most obvious term that fits with the patient's condition and then begin looking for "zebras." Context is important!

Medications

Medications are a perennial challenge for both new and veteran transcriptionists. The number of drugs on the market is enormous, the names are often complex (especially generic drugs which use pharmaceutical nomenclature), and the spelling of brand names do not follow any particular rules. To compound the problem, drug names are often mispronounced and even misspelled. Patients often mispronounce or misspell the names of the drugs they are taking, and if the dictating physician is not familiar with the drug, the misinformation will likely be repeated in the dictation.

There are several strategies MTs can use to decipher medications. The patient's medical history and/or problem list can help you narrow down the list of possible medications. Begin by matching the known drugs to the patient's known problems. For example, a patient with diabetes mellitus will most assuredly be on at least one glucose-lowering medication. If no medication on the list corresponds to the diagnosis of diabetes, try a "reverse lookup" for medications prescribed for diabetics. The Plan section may also provide clues because medication changes are often mentioned in the Plan. Learn more about search techniques on page 11.

Sample Reports

Studying previous reports (sample reports) can be one of the best ways to decipher difficult dictation. A dictator's most common phrases are usually the phrases that are the most difficult to understand because the more often they repeat a phrase, the faster they are able to say it. This repetition and speed leads to sloppy articulation. The Review of Systems and Physical Examination sections are the most common areas of a report to be dictated with such speed and lack of articulation. Dictators often mumble or trail off the opening and closing sentences of a report for the same reason. These areas of the report become monotonous

When you encounter a phrase that has been dictated more quickly than the surrounding text, do not begin your search looking for unusual or obscure words or medical terms. Mumbled and poorly articulated words or phrases are more likely English phrases or medical phrases that the dictator uses all the time.

for dictators, causing them to rush through them unreasonably fast. In fact, some dictators rattle off these sections of the report so quickly, there is simply no way to decipher what they are saying without examining previous reports.

Whenever possible, obtain previous reports, which have had patient information removed, and keep the reports in a specified folder on your computer, or print and store them in a binder. Read through the reports and highlight recurring phrases. Pay close attention to the Review of Systems, the Physical Examination, and the opening and closing sentences.

Searching

The real trick to researching efficiently is knowing where to begin your search. Your three primary sources for searching should be an English language dictionary, a medical dictionary, and a drug reference. Other important resources include the Internet, a medical word glossary, lists of specialty words and phrases, and a compilation of medical abbreviations and acronyms. See Appendix C for a list of recommended resources.

Word Searches

Context can be particularly helpful when searching for a term that you do not know exactly how to spell. Before reaching for the dictionary, analyze the surrounding text and determine the most likely spelling of the prefix or root word. For example, if the surrounding text describes an abdominal complaint, a search starting with *enter(o)* would more likely be successful than one starting with *inter(o)*.

Keep a list of alternative spellings close at hand for those times when you have particular difficulty finding a term. Some of the more challenging words to find in a dictionary include those that start with silent letters such as:

- cn
- gn
- kn
- mn
- ph
- pn
- ps
- pt
- wr

Pause 1-5 Each of the following passages has suggested spellings for starting a word search. Based on the context, choose the spelling that would most likely help you find the missing word in a dictionary or drug reference.

1. The patient has been complaining of abdominal pain since returning from South America. Will order stool analysis to rule out _____ (inter, enter).
2. The patient has significant muscle wasting. The differential diagnosis includes a _____ or nutritional deficiency. (myo, mio)
3. The fungal cultures were positive for _____. (myco, mico)
4. An _____ foreign body was found within the joint cavity. (intra, inter)
5. The patient was found to be hypertensive and _____ with a serum potassium level of 2.0. (hyper+kal, hypo+kal)

To reduce the patient's cholesterol-related risk factors, we will start _____ 625 mg daily. (welcall, welchol)

6. The patient states she has been taking a daily green drink called _____ containing herbs and vitamins. (phyto, fito)
7. A bone marrow biopsy was taken to rule out _____ leukemia. (myelo, myo)
8. The patient was given a prescription for _____ because her insurance will only cover proton-pump inhibitors, not H2 antagonists. (proton, pour)
9. Increase _____ to 600 mg a day for nerve pain. (neuro, uro)

It can also be useful to search for words using the end of the word. Learn more on page 11.

Electronic References

Electronic medical dictionaries, word and phrase indexes, drug references, and medical word glossaries are exceptionally valuable tools for medical transcriptionists. These references, typically sold on CDs or as downloadable files, contain the same content as their corresponding print versions, but they offer many advantages over printed books. Electronic references are stored as databases, so they can be sorted, filtered, and searched in ways that are not possible with traditionally bound materials. Many electronic references also contain appendices with reference tables, sample reports, laboratory reference ranges, and keyword lists.

In addition to the efficiency and accuracy gains achievable with electronic references, many of the practical skills gained through the use of electronic references are applicable to emerging technologies associated with electronic health records and will contribute to your ongoing employability in the healthcare documentation field.

Other notable advantages of electronic references include:

- the ability to search using partial words, sounds, definitions, or concepts
- the ability to copy words directly into the document to prevent typos
- less physical storage space and less desktop space needed
- greater portability when traveling or working from alternate locations

With just a little practice, you will find that searching electronic references is significantly faster than using print materials. To increase your efficiency, place shortcuts to your references on the Windows Start menu for quick access. Read the Help files to learn the shortcut keys used within the electronic reference software so you can quickly access the information you need and return to your document without removing your hands from the keyboard. Using an electronic reference to look up the definition of a word can take as little as 20 seconds, a speed you simply cannot match using print references.

The most common electronic references are dictionaries and word and phrase indexes (eg, Stedman's word book series). Electronic word and phrase indexes are compiled by medical specialty (eg, radiology, obstetrics and gynecology) and only contain indexed words and related phrases; they do not include definitions or pronunciations and therefore do not replace medical dictionaries. You are likely to encounter the following terms when using electronic resources:

Index: An alphabetical list of entries. An electronic index is organized the same way as a traditional printed index. The program displays the definition or other information associated with the highlighted word in a separate pane, usually to the right of the indexed list.

Browse: To move through a list by scrolling. "Browse by index" simply means "scan the indexed list." You can also jump to the word on the list by typing the word in the text box.

Headword/Entry: The primary entry in a word list or dictionary.

Definition/Subentry: The definition associated with the headword or the terms and phrases associated with an indexed word in a word list.

Search or Search Index: To search the index using a partial word and **wild cards** (asterisks and question marks to represent missing letters), also referred to as partial word searches.

Search on Definition/Subentry: To search for a word using words or concepts contained within the definition or within the associated words or phrases in a word list.

Filter: To hide information or eliminate specific information in order to narrow the search results and make it easier to locate the needed information.

Keywords/Indications: A list of words divided by topic, especially lists of drugs categorized by indication.

There are two basic scenarios for using electronic dictionaries: (1) to confirm the meaning of a word you already know how to spell, or (2) to find the correct spelling of a word when you already know the meaning. Electronic dictionaries have two different modes that correspond to these two scenarios. Use the index mode (or browse) to look up the definition or the pronunciation of a word that you already know how to spell (much like you would scan any other list of alphabetized words). Either scroll through the list or type the first few letters of the word into the text box (usually located just above the indexed list) as shown in ■ Figure 1-1.

To search for a word based on a partial spelling, change to *search on index*. Use wild cards to create a

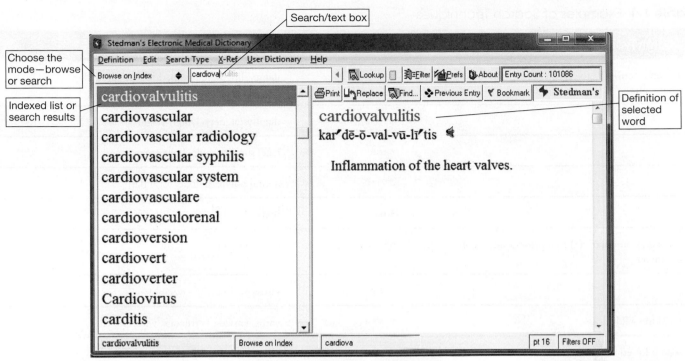

Search/text box

Choose the mode—browse or search

Indexed list or search results

Definition of selected word

FIGURE 1-1 An example of an electronic reference showing the indexed list of entries along with the definition and pronunciation of the selected word. *Source:* Courtesy of Wolters Kluwer Health.

search **query**. An asterisk represents any number of unknown letters and a question mark represents a single unknown letter. Type the partial word into the search box, using asterisks or question marks as appropriate.

To search for a word based on its definition or words contained within the subentry, change to *search/search on definition*. To further refine your search, use the **search operators** AND and NOT. Type either an ampersand or the word AND (in all caps) between two words and the search results will include terms that have both search words in the definition/entry. The word NOT (typed in all caps) or the minus sign can be used to look up words that contain one keyword but exclude the second keyword. **Table 1-1** lists examples of searches and typical results. Refer to the Help files within each electronic reference for more detailed information on search techniques. Some of the search techniques described in Table 1-1 may not be available in all references.

Electronic drug references use many of the same techniques described in Table 1-1 for dictionaries and word lists. Drug references typically have an additional feature, called *Keywords* or *Indications*, that is especially helpful for looking up drug names according to their indication. In addition, electronic drug references allow you to search using dosage information, which is especially helpful for finding less common forms, such as micrograms, milliequivalents, drops, and perles. For example, the physician dictates "_____(s/l salmerol)_____ 50 mcg for COPD." A search using mcg AND COPD or mcg AND pulmonary would return a list of fewer than 100 drugs that could easily be scanned for names beginning with "sal." **Table 1-2** lists other sample drug searches. Constructing queries will get easier with practice. Sometimes an initial simple search returns too many possible answers. By scanning the results, you can often discover terms to include in a second query that will exclude information you do not need and make it easier to find what you do need. You may also have better success searching with dosage information if you place the number first (with no leading spaces).

Be sure to select the correct mode before typing a query. Search types need to correspond to the type of query used. For example, wild cards cannot be used in Browse/Index mode.

Table 1-1 Examples of Search Techniques

Search Type	Sample Search	Sample Results
use an asterisk (*) to represent any number of missing characters	d*p	damp, dip, digital pulp, double pedicle flap
	d*p*l	diaphysial, deep lymph vessel
	*ace	face, surface, midpalmar space
	d*p*p	dental polyp, deltopectoral flap
	*ase	lipase, amylase
use a question mark (?) to represent any single character	b?d	bed, bud, bid
	v?r?s	virus
combine wild cards	v?r*s	varus, varices, verrucous, vertebral ribs
search for entries containing two or more words using ampersand (&) or AND	lipid & arterio*	atherosclerosis, lipochrome
search for entries that contain the first word but not the second word using the minus sign (−) or NOT	thyroid NOT mcg	thyroid medications not dispensed in micrograms
search using a tilde (~) for concepts or "sounds like" (called fuzzy search)	helper~	entries related to the concept of "helper" such as holder, retractor

Table 1-2 Examples of Searches Using Quick Look Electronic Drug Reference

Search Type	Sample Query	Sample Results
partial word search	*pril	Accupril, quinapril, ramipril
	r*il	ramipril, Restoril, Rosanil
fuzzy search (sounds like) using tilde (~)	Xanax~	Vanex-HD, Xopenex, Zantac, Zyrtec
search for drugs whose content contains both words using AND	cholesterol AND niacin	drugs for lowering cholesterol that also contain niacin
search for drugs related to the first word and exclude entries containing the second word using NOT	statin NOT Lipitor	antifungal drugs (Mycostatin, Nilstat, Candistatin) but not drugs related to Lipitor (a statin)
drugs not dispensed in milligrams	150 NOT mg	all drugs dispensed in 150 mcg or mL
search for drugs that include two parameters but do not include the third	40 AND cholesterol NOT Lipitor	drugs dispensed in a dose of 40 (mg, mcg, etc) that include cholesterol in the description but do not contain Lipitor
keyword/indications	dermatitis	drugs used to treat skin rashes

Using the Internet

The Internet is an invaluable tool for the medical transcriptionist. Although the Internet provides a seemingly unlimited amount of information, it is important to remember that not everything on the Internet is accurate. In fact, the vast majority of the information is dubious at best. Using the Internet as a source of information requires the user to be cautious and skeptical. Thinking critically is paramount to the accurate and appropriate use of the Internet.

Evaluating Websites

If you aren't already, begin evaluating reference sites on the Internet and **bookmarking** (ie, saving the website's address in a list of frequently used sites) your favorites for easy access. A list of reputable sites is found in Appendix C. Before using information gleaned from a site, spend a few minutes evaluating the site using the following criteria:

- Author and publisher: Who or what company maintains the website or is responsible for its content? Does the owner have a vested interest or an obvious bias? Is there a lot of advertising on the site that might sway the publisher's opinion? Is the site well organized and free of typos and obvious misinformation?
- Target audience: Is the site directed at laypersons or medical professionals? Has the information been scrutinized by other medical professionals? Peer-reviewed information has been evaluated by individuals with equal or greater experience and knowledge than the author(s). The results of research or medical studies published in medical journals are almost always peer-reviewed and are considered reliable sources of information.
- Date: Is the information up-to-date?

Reliable sites for medical transcriptionists include PubMed, a site maintained by the National Institutes of Health (NIH) and the National Library of Medicine (NLM). The Merck Manual is published online in both professional and home editions and provides helpful information on the pathophysiology of diseases and conditions. Major research centers such as the Mayo Clinic and the Cleveland Clinic are also reliable sites.

There are several types of Internet sites that may seem reliable but should never be used as the source of definitive information. These sites include online pharmacies, patient advocacy sites, a physician's personal website, discussion forums, blogs, and sites maintained by distributors of medical equipment and supplies. Patient support groups often have websites with information on diagnosis and treatment of specific diseases, but these sites are usually managed by laypersons and should never be used as a source of information for medicolegal documents. Forums associated with these sites are especially unreliable. Sites owned by the *actual manufacturer* of a product are considered reliable for spelling purposes. It is important to remember that many websites, especially e-commerce sites, are maintained by information technology professionals, *not* medical professionals.

Internet Searches

No doubt, you have already discovered the value of Internet search engines. Search providers, such as Google, Yahoo!, and Bing, have become an essential part of using the Internet. Medical transcriptionists can use Internet search engines to locate new terms, drugs, and equipment, and to correctly spell the names of referring physicians, hospitals, and clinics, as well as local schools and businesses that are often dictated as part of a medical report. Internet search engines, just like speech recognition engines, *do not evaluate content*. Search engines do not filter inaccurate or outdated information. Evaluating the accuracy, validity, and appropriateness of information gleaned from the Internet is always the user's responsibility.

> Carefully evaluate any information you retrieve from an Internet search engine and then confirm the accuracy of that information using an industry-standard reference. The Internet can be your first stop but never your last!

Before clicking any search result, examine the search results as a whole and then each individual result (often referred to as a "hit"). A well-constructed query should return at least 100 hits—preferably thousands. If your search query is extremely specific and the results are from reliable sources, such as PubMed or the National Library of Medicine, then a few hits (five to ten) would be acceptable. If, however, you searched for the spelling of a medical term and the results listed only 50 sites, none of them peer-reviewed, the spelling is most likely wrong and should not be used.

Next, examine the **Universal Resource Locator (URL)**, which is the unique address that lists the site name, domain name, and page name. The actual site name is discernible from the URL and is located after the two forward slashes (//) and www but *before* any other single forward slash (/). Avoid links that contain the words "message," "forum," or "bulletin board."

In addition to ruling out poor-quality information, being selective about the links you click will protect your computer from malicious activity. The most reputable medical-information sites do not rely on banner ads, pop-up ads, and advertising gimmicks to support the site, so they are the safest sites to visit.

Pause 1-6 Examine the URLs of the following search results. Which would be potentially good sites for retrieving information to be transcribed in a medical report? Explain your answer.

Diabetes mellitus is impaired insulin secretion and variable degrees of peripheral insulin resistance leading to hyperglycemia. Early symptoms are related . . .
www.merckmanuals.com/professional/sec12/. . ./ch158b
.html - Cached - Similar

---

adrenal function in such cases is the **key** and it often. . . . The contents of this **website** are primarily based upon the opinions of **Dr. Lam** unless . . .
www.**drlam**.com/articles/hypothyroidism.asp?page=3
- Cached - Similar

Multiple sclerosis (MS) is a nervous system disease that affects your brain and spinal cord. It damages the myelin sheath, the material that surrounds and . . .
Alternative Therapy - Nutrition - Rehabilitation/Recovery
- Coping
www.**nlm**.nih.gov/medlineplus/**multiplesclerosis**.html
- Cached - Similar

Jul 3, 2008 . . . **healthtalk** Forum Index -> Pull up a chair. . . . study in mice finds caffeine protects mice from a **multiple sclerosis** (MS) like condition. . . .
healthtalk.6.forumer.com/viewtopic.php?t=227&sid . . .
- Cached

Search Engines

Search engines are most useful when you do not already have an appropriate site bookmarked. Gaining usable information from a search engine depends on the quality of the query. You may be able to find the information

you need using a single word in your query, but usually single-word queries return too many results to be useful. As with the search techniques described earlier for electronic references, you can use operators to refine your search and return a more meaningful set of results.

Constructing relevant and fruitful Internet searches truly draws upon critical thinking skills. Use the surrounding context to add additional terms to your search to help filter superfluous results and use operators to further customize your search query. For example, a search for `brace` would return millions of useless results; but a search using `brace postoperative knee replacement` would be far more specific and more likely to display sites that have the information you need. Queries containing a series of related words will return a list of sites that contain *any* of the words but not necessarily *all* of the words.

Google automatically searches for all words when more than one word is included in the query. The order the words are typed into the query will change the search criteria slightly. Type the most significant word into the query first. For example, the search query `heart muscle cholesterol` would build a list of sites that contain all three words and would give slightly different results than the query `muscle cholesterol heart`.

Use the minus sign (−) to exclude sites that contain information you do not need. For example, entering the query `virus -computer` would include a list of sites more likely to contain information about biological viruses as opposed to computer viruses. The minus sign must immediately precede the word to be excluded, without a space in between.

Phrase Searches

Queries containing quotation marks are extremely useful for narrowing the list of results, resolving blanks, and confirming the accuracy of a phrase. Quotation marks keep the words in the search query together, exactly as typed. The search query `"type 2 diabetes mellitus"` would only display sites that contained that exact phrase with that exact spelling. When combined with the asterisk, phrase searches become a powerful tool for deciphering blanks. A search for `"* deficiency anemia"` would quickly reveal the missing word as "iron."

A phrase search using quotation marks will also help distinguish small words such as articles and prepositions (eg, a, an, and, in, on, of, etc) that are rarely articulated yet change the meaning of the phrase or sentence.

> ▶ Incorrect: EKG shows normal sinus rhythm. Low-voltage QRS and the precordial leads.
> Correct: EKG shows normal sinus rhythm. Low-voltage QRS in the precordial leads.

Anytime you encounter a new phrase, confirm the accuracy of every word in the phrase using a phrase index or an Internet search using quotation marks. Be sure to check the source of the information before you type the phrase into your document.

> ⏸ **Pause 1-7** Identify the phrases in the following sentences. Which phrases are transcribed correctly?
>
> 1. We have given her instructions regarding an estrogen climbing protocol and will proceed accordingly.
> 2. Increased left ventricular outflow velocity is seen, most likely secondary to septal hypertrophy.

There are many advanced methods for searching the Internet, and the major search providers publish tips for using various features of their search engines. Look for the Help link on the search provider's home page to learn more ways to customize your searches. The following are examples of queries that can be used with Google:

- `"hepatitis B" "liver enzyme elevation" range` (reference ranges for liver enzymes associated with hepatitis B)
- `"chemotherapy protocol" "chronic lymphocytic leukemia"` (information on treatment protocols for CLL)
- `~cardiac` (sites containing the word cardiac and related words such as heart, cardiology, cardiovascular)
- `"reference range" testosterone female` (normal values for testosterone in females)

Find (On This Page)

Often, your initial search may bring you to an extremely useful Web page with a lot of text. To locate your search word(s) on that page and read the surrounding text, use **Find**. Press CTRL+F and type your keyword into the Find box. Press Enter to highlight the first occurrence of that keyword on the Web page. Press Enter again to highlight the next occurrence.

Image Searches

A clever way to locate the names of muscles, tendons, bones, and other anatomic structures and landmarks is to perform an image search for anatomic diagrams. For example, use Google's image search feature to look for abdominal muscles or blood vessels of the brain. Image searches are especially helpful when transcribing surgical reports as well as radiology and nuclear imaging reports.

Understanding Accents

A significant number of healthcare providers in the United States speak **English as a second language (ESL),** and thus many dictate with an accent. This of course presents many challenges for the MT, as all the usual auditory discrimination problems associated with dictation are compounded by accents and grammatical errors. With practice, it is possible to understand and accurately transcribe dictators with accents. An important part of understanding ESL dictators is having a very basic understanding of how their native language differs from English. As an MT, you may encounter any number of accents, but the most common accents encountered in the medical community include Spanish, Asian, Middle Eastern, and Indian.

A **phoneme** is the smallest sound of speech that has meaning. People acquire the ability to form phonemes early in the language development process, and many individuals are never able to audibly distinguish or pronounce nonnative phonemes. An inability to properly articulate phonemes leads to pronunciation errors such as **substitutions, deletions, vowel shortening, vowel insertions,** and **devoicing** (pronouncing a sound without vibrating the vocal cords that would produce vibration when spoken by a native speaker). There are notable patterns of pronunciation errors common to ESL speakers of a given native language, and understanding these patterns will help tremendously in your efforts to decode foreign-accented speech.

The sentence structure of a person's native language also influences their English syntax and grammar. It is not uncommon for individuals to construct sentences using English words yet follow the word order of their first language. For example, in Spanish, the adjective is placed after the noun, so a native-Spanish speaker may say the *cat brown* instead of the *brown cat*.

Spoken language is marked by rhythm, intonation, inflection, and volume. Some languages are spoken in a soft voice, whereas others are normally loud. Some have a sing-song quality and others sound more staccato. The ups, downs, starts, stops, variations in pitch, and changes in stress contribute to our overall comprehension of language. A lack of any of these voice elements or a change in voice quality diminishes our ability to understand, even when articulation and grammar are correct. When voice quality is vastly different, you must concentrate on sounds even more intently.

English is one of the more challenging languages to master, not only for those learning it as a second language, but also for native speakers. The following characteristics of English make it more difficult to learn:

- Stress patterns: English uses both stressed and non-stressed syllables. Typically, the more important words in a sentence are stressed while the less significant words are brushed over and hardly pronounced. For example, in the sentence, "I can come to your party," *I, come* and *party* would receive more stress than *can, to* and *your*. Generally speaking, native English speakers barely articulate pronouns, articles, auxiliary verbs, prepositions, and conjunctions, and stress is used for contrast or emphasis. Other languages, however, place consistent emphasis on all words.

- Unstressed vowels: Native-English speakers typically replace the vowel sound in an unstressed syllable with /ə/ (uh), also called the schwa. Compare the pronunciation of *the* in the following sentences: "Meet me at the bank" versus "He is the only president to serve eight years." The frequent switch in pronunciation based on the word's location and importance within the sentence may confuse nonnative speakers.

- Unusual phonemes: The /th/ sound (called an interdental fricative because of the apposition of the tongue and the teeth when making this sound) is common in English but is relatively rare in most other languages. This particular phoneme produces substitution errors for many nonnative English speakers.

- Multiple-vowel phonemes: General American English contains more vowel sounds than most languages, making use of monophthongs (single or "pure" vowel sounds such as /ā/), diphthongs (double vowel sounds as in /oi/), and triphthong (triple vowels as in *loyal*). Diphthongs and triphthongs are difficult to hear, and therefore to pronounce, for individuals whose native language uses only pure vowels.

- Dialects: Even within the US, there are dialects that may be difficult for other native English speakers to understand. For example, Boston English is quite different from the Southern drawl. Boston English is characterized by the deletion of the ending /r/ sound ("grammah" vs grammar) and nasalized vowels. Southern English is marked by long, drawn-out words that seem to turn single-syllable words into multiple-syllable words ("ra-ench" versus ranch).

- Large lexicon: The sheer number of words used in the English language adds to its complexity and difficulty for both native and nonnative speakers. Exceptions to spelling rules abound, making rote memorization necessary for the accurate spelling of most words.

Decoding Accents

Although each person who speaks English as a second language will have his or her own idiosyncrasies, there are anomalies of pronunciation and syntax that are common to individuals of the same native language. Understanding the patterns of pronunciation and syntax will help you decipher accented speech.

Dictators of Indian Origin

Dictators whose native language originates on the Indian continent may make the following pronunciation or syntax errors:

- vowel sounds are shortened and the actual time spent pronouncing long vowels is shortened so that the stress is reduced considerably (peas (pēz) = pĕs; cheese (chēz) = chĕs; scoop = scup)

- /r/ is often pronounced with a trill

- final hard consonants are dropped or de-emphasized (dad = dat, things = thinks; frog = fro or frok)

- /th/ may be dropped or substituted with /t/ (that = tat)
- final /th/ may be substituted with /s/ or /z/ (bath = bas, baz, ba)
- /w/ may be substituted for /v/ (vital = wital)

Many ESL dictators from India learn English in grade school. The form of English spoken in India is heavily influenced by British English because of the former colonization of India by Great Britain in the 20th century. Although many Indians have a good grasp of English, Americans often have a difficult time understanding them because they speak considerably faster than the average American. In addition, many are very soft-spoken, as they are accustomed to speaking in a low volume. Common grammatical errors include the omission of the definite article *the*, incorrect use of prepositions, and misuse of the present continuous tense. Phrases such as "I am having" (I have) or "we are not having" (we don't have) are common. You may also hear *since* used in place of *for* ("I have been working since four years" instead of "I have been working for four years.")

Dictators of Asian Origin

Dictators from China, Japan, and other Asian countries may make the following pronunciation or syntax errors:

- final hard consonants are dropped or de-emphasized (dad = dat, things = thin; frog = fro; five = fī)
- /p/ pronounced without puff of air
- /l/ dropped or replaced with /r/ (yellow = yəo; Stella = Stəra)
- /th/ substituted with /f/ or /d/ (they = fay or day)
- /ch/ substituted with /t/
- consonant blends (/pl/, /sk/) changed or pronounced as a single consonant (please = prēs; plastic = pastic, ask = as)
- long, stressed vowel sounds shortened (cheese (chēz) = chēs; peas (pēz) = pēs)

Asian speakers are often quite difficult to understand because of the vast differences in phonemes and syntax. The Chinese language does not conjugate verbs, so you will often hear Chinese speakers use only one verb tense ("I go yesterday" instead of "I went yesterday"). Chinese also does not pluralize nouns, causing Chinese speakers to use only singular forms of nouns ("take three dose" instead of "take three doses"). In addition, the Chinese syntax is the reverse of English, so a native Chinese speaker may say "Store to I go" instead of "I go to the store."

Far Eastern languages do not use gender pronouns, so one of the most noticeable errors you will hear is an inconsistent use of the gender pronouns he/she and his/her. Native Chinese speakers may dictate reports with the opposite gender pronoun used throughout or even both genders in the same report.

Dictators of Hispanic Origin

Dictators from Mexico and South America may make the following pronunciation or syntax errors:

- vowel insertions at the beginning and end of words, especially words beginning with /s/ and ending with a consonant (special = əspecial; spoons = əspoonsə)
- final hard consonants are dropped or de-emphasized (dad = dat, Bob = Bop; frog = frok)
- /th/ substituted with /d/ or /t/ (this = dis; things = tēngs)
- /sh/ substituted with /ch/ (shipping = chipping)
- /v/ substituted with /b/ (vital signs = bital signs)
- vowel shortening these (thēz = dēs)
- vowel substitution, especially with ē (big = bēg)

Native Spanish speakers often use the double negative, as this is used commonly in Spanish. They may say "I don't want nothing" instead of "I don't want anything." Some plural forms in Spanish are treated as singular nouns in English, so English noun-verb pairs may be confused, as in "the people is nice." Spanish also pluralizes adjectives, which may transfer to English as "her greens eyes." In Spanish, once a noun is introduced, the pronoun is inferred, and native Spanish speakers often use this syntax when speaking English. You may hear "Mary came to the office. Complains of pain." When reading English, Spanish speakers often pronounce /i/ as /ē/ and /e/ as /ā/. Spanish only uses pure vowels, so vowel combinations (diphthongs and triphthongs) may be mispronounced or not pronounced at all.

Strategies

Studying previous reports and comparing the transcript with the audio can help you develop an ear for that dictator's pronunciation patterns and other dictators with similar accents. As you work through the accented dictations in this text, create your own list of observations, including sound substitutions, sound deletions, and sentence patterns.

When faced with a difficult word, type the word as you hear it and look for typical substitutions. Hard consonants are the most common sounds to be mispronounced. Replace the consonants with the sounds known to be problematic for that person's native tongue, most commonly the consonant blends of /th/ and /ch/. Vowel sounds are more likely to be pronounced with the correct sound but the incorrect length and stress. Say the word out loud, replacing vowel sounds with a longer and more stressed vowel (chēs → cheeeeze). For words that seem to be more than one syllable, say the word out loud, moving the stress to each of the syllables until you recognize the word.

Pause 1-8 Decode the following words to the most likely medical term or phrase:

Native-Spanish speaker

1. balgus
2. chortness of bret

Native-Indian speaker

1. tecal abces
2. wina cawa

Native-Chinese speaker

1. apastic anima
2. achiry tendon

Editing

Most reports require some editing of dictation simply because spoken English varies from written English. We generally speak with less attention to grammar and sentence construction, but others easily understand us because pauses, inflection, and intonation contribute to meaning. Written communication, however, must follow rules for grammar and punctuation to prevent confusion or loss of meaning. Editing dictation should always be unobtrusive. Changes that clarify meaning are important but MTs must be careful not to change the dictator's style. Common and acceptable edits include:

- repositioning of prepositional phrases and modifiers
- noun-verb agreement
- odd phrasing
- nonsensical comments

D: Father is currently not living.

T: Father is not living.

D: She appears to have 1 tube that is patent, the other tube that may be occluded.

T: She appears to have 1 tube that is patent; the other tube may be occluded.

D: MTHFR gene mutation positive.

T: Positive for the MTHFR gene mutation.

D: We will repeat her TSH, FSH, LH and discuss her abnormal results with her primary care physician at her next visit.

T: At her next visit, we will repeat her TSH, FSH, and LH and discuss her abnormal results with her primary care physician.

D: Her LFT has been steadily worsening, and I would like to perform a liver biopsy.

T: Her LFTs have been steadily worsening, and I would like to perform a liver biopsy.

D: The risks, benefits, and alternatives were discussed in some details.

T: The risks, benefits, and alternatives were discussed in detail.

Dictation Errors—When the Dictator Misspeaks

Medical providers often work in harried, high-pressure, noisy environments. Very few dictators are able to dictate at a leisurely pace or in quiet places. They are often distracted by fatigue, phones, or pagers, and frequently interrupted by staff asking questions. The harried pace and constant interruption can lead to dictation errors. Many of these errors are easily corrected by the MT without the dictator ever knowing they occurred.

It is important that you understand when to make a change and when to flag an error. Thinking critically is of utmost importance when deciding whether to change what was dictated. If in doubt, *do not make the change.* Flag the report for the dictator's review. Be very careful that you do not presume the dictator has made an error and change the text without fully investigating the error. Evaluate the questionable error using related elements throughout the report. Research all terms that are unfamiliar to you. Listen again to make sure you heard the dictation correctly and listen again to the sections that support or refute the problem.

You will find that making corrections is easier and more straightforward after you have worked with a physician for a while and are familiar with his or her habits, common phrases, and idiosyncrasies. However, until you gain confidence and familiarity, you should flag the error instead of making the change yourself.

D: She was at 10 weeks when she lost her pregnancy. Heart tones were visualized at 6 weeks.

T: She was at 10 weeks when she lost her pregnancy. Heart tones were heard at 6 weeks. ("Tones" are heard, not seen.)

D: The patient has 4 siblings—2 sisters and 2 sisters.

T: The patient has 4 siblings—2 sisters and 2 brothers.

D: Her Rh type is O positive.

T: Her blood type is O positive.

D: Compression stockings were placed on the left and right legs bilaterally.

T: Compression stockings were placed on both legs.

D: The patient's last menstrual period was 2/15/11, giving her an EDC of 11/23/10.

T: The patient's last menstrual period was 2/15/11, giving her an EDC of 11/23/11.

D: In 1992, she had a full-term delivery without any problems with her current husband.

T: In 1992, she had a full-term delivery with her current husband, without any problems.

Discrepancies may be caused by the dictator or by a transcription error. Discrepancies are tricky to detect because they usually occur in nonadjacent sentences or in separate sections of the report. The MT must "follow the story" from start to finish in order to catch contradictions. Although these errors may occur anywhere in the report, common trouble spots include the History of Present Illness compared to the Review of Systems, Allergies compared to Current Medications, and the date of birth compared to the dictated age. One of the most common reasons for contradictions is the use of "normals." Physicians often dictate their normals quickly and out of habit, not paying specific attention to the negatives. These "normal negatives" at times contradict the very symptoms the patient reported in the HPI. Right and left are also commonly interchanged. ESL dictators often struggle with the gender pronouns he/she and his/her.

At times, you can resolve a discrepancy by analyzing several clues. If the physician dictates a "normal negative" such as "negative for diabetes," yet the patient is taking two or three diabetic medications, it would be unlikely that the physician dictated several incorrect medications and more likely that the physician dictated "negative diabetes" out of sheer habit. If there is a direct clash between two dictated pieces of information, there may be no way to know which is incorrect. Do not make the mistake of assuming the first instance is correct and change the subsequent discrepancy to match it, especially when right and left are both dictated.

Ultimately, you must refer to the facility's editing policy or the dictator's preference for handling edits. Flagging for clarification is never wrong. If you work in a verbatim environment, you have no choice but to leave the discrepancy in the document and flag the file for dictator review.

She denies dysmenorrhea, galactorrhea, or hirsutism. She has not noted whether she in fact ovulates. She had a hysterosalpingogram in 2001, as mentioned above, and she had a laparoscopy for what appears to be stage II endometriosis. She denies a history of pelvic inflammatory disease, chlamydia, gonorrhea, syphilis, or herpes. Denies uterine fibroids. She admits to severe dysmenorrhea and some dyspareunia.

Height 5 feet 5 inches, weight 210, BMI 21.

Unless there is corroborating information elsewhere in the report to confirm the height or weight, transcribe as dictated and flag for correction.

Proofreading for Accuracy

For a medical transcriptionist, proofreading is a balancing act. You must learn to proofread quickly, as time is always a constraint, yet still catch errors that affect the integrity of the document and impact patient care.

Although some might consider reading and proofreading as the same task, the two actually require different cognitive skills. When we read, we do not focus on every letter of every word; we really do not even focus on every word. Normally, our eyes fixate on three or four words at a time. Our peripheral vision takes in the words on either side. When reading quickly, the brain filters anywhere from 10% to 50% of the *actual* words on the page and fills in the gaps for the remainder. This tendency to "filter and fill" is especially strong when the text is familiar (eg, a document that you have just transcribed). Professional writers overcome the tendency for the brain to "rewrite the page" by proofreading their text hours or days after writing it. Transcriptionists do not have this luxury of time. You must make a concerted effort to change the way your eyes and brain work together to interpret what is *actually on the page* compared with what the brain *assumes* is on the page.

You must re-train your brain to focus on *every word*, not clusters of words. And yet, this approach presents a second challenge. With so much focus on individual words, comprehension is easily lost. This problem is more pronounced when proofreading a transcript with the audio. Some software programs associated with SR editing platforms highlight each word to correspond with the audio playback. As an editor, you can easily become focused on comparing each highlighted word with the audio without actually paying attention to the content. For example, speech-recognized documents have been found to contain nonsensical sentences and even instructions from the dictator—text that should have been deleted during the editing process. In these cases, the words matched the audio perfectly, but the *context* was not evaluated.

Concentration is required at all times. We have all experienced the frustration of having read a paragraph, only to realize we cannot recall anything we just read. This same tendency to read without comprehension creeps into our daily routines as transcriptionists. Physical fatigue and stress can compound the problem. Mental fatigue also sets in when we do not take periodic breaks, get ample sleep and exercise, or eat properly. Muscle and joint pain from poorly designed workstations, hand and wrist pain from overuse or misuse of the mouse and keyboard, as well as headaches from improper lighting and incorrect eyewear affect an MT's ability to concentrate and therefore produce accurate reports. Taking care of yourself is an important part of producing accurately transcribed reports and contributing to patient safety and risk management.

Becoming a better proofreader starts with recognizing the pitfalls and devising strategies to overcome those difficulties. First, recognize that proofreading is a skill to be intentionally developed, not one you likely already possess. Second, proof reports with the expectation that you *will* find errors. Reasonable levels of doubt and skepticism are positive traits for a transcriptionist. Third, identify your weaknesses. Every transcriptionist has strengths and weaknesses, and the best transcriptionists devise strategies for overcoming their weaknesses.

Features built into word processors can be a tremendous help in accurate transcription and proofreading. Consider these proofreading strategies:

- Increase the zoom to the highest setting that still allows the text to fit within the confines of the monitor. Increasing the zoom increases the size of the text (not the font size) and makes it easier to spot mistakes. Spreading out the words across the screen also increases the number of words that are actually *seen* (focused on directly) by reducing the number of words per "visual group."

- Proof with the audio and gradually increase the playback speed as you gain proficiency. Although this may seem to run counter to the earlier discussion about editing SR documents, you will be amazed to discover other errors you may not have noticed, such as numbers that have been keyed incorrectly (eg, 165/80 instead of 132/80 or 145 pounds instead of 155 pounds), missing words, or misunderstood words. You will also gain insight into your transcription weak spots.

- Use the keyboard navigation keys (CTRL+Right arrow) to move the cursor one word at a time to train your eyes to stop on each word. You can also use the mouse to click on each word or every other word to force your eyes to slow down and focus on fewer words at a time.

- Create a macro that increases the page margins and displays the text in narrow paragraphs (like a newspaper column). This reduces the number of words included in a "visual group" and hinders the brain from (erroneously) filling in the gaps. Use a second macro to restore the correct margins after proofreading.

- Read from the end of the word—the most common typos occur at the end of a word (eg, *probably* instead of *probable*, *complains* instead of *complained*).

- Look carefully at verbs such as "was" and "is." These verbs sound very much alike when spoken.

- Use keyboard editing shortcuts (CTRL+Del and CTRL+Backspace) to quickly delete entire words. Deleting whole words reduces the likelihood of leaving stray characters or creating spacing errors between words.

- Create visual images in your mind as you read the report. Imagine the doctor examining the patient as you proof the Physical Examination section of the report. Picture the patient's symptoms as they are described. This keeps your brain engaged in the transcript, lessening the chance of "zoning out." Visual imagery may also help to avoid sound-alike errors such as "near sided" instead of "nearsighted."

- Use your text expander program or AutoCorrect in Microsoft Word to automatically set words in bold that are easily mistyped yet still pass spell check (eg, *from* and *form, of* and *on, of* and *off, an* and *and, in* and *on*). When proofreading, the bold typeface will cause you to slow down and confirm that the correct word was typed.

- Use AutoCorrect or your text expander to automatically correct habitual typos.

- Avoid errors in style, spacing, and format using Auto-Correct or your text expander to insert terms correctly (eg, q46 corrects to q.4-6 h.; her2 corrects to HER-2/ncu; and qday corrects to daily).

- Use fully formatted templates so you can concentrate on content while you are transcribing. This will improve consistency, increase speed, and decrease transcription errors. Anytime you pause to add formatting to your document, you break the rhythm of listening, and you divert your attention away from what is being said. Templates can be created using documents or template files (see page 21 of Chapter 1 on the web). If templates are not an option, use your text expansion program to create report shells that contain headings, standard text, and signature lines.

- Devise strategies to avoid number typos by creating shortcuts for common numbers (eg, t86 or tes or tneps = temperature 98.6; t87 or tev or tnepv = temperature 98.7; rs = respirations 16; and re = respirations 18).

- Use AutoCorrect or your text expansion program to set gender pronouns (he/she, his/her) in bold to draw attention to accidental switches in gender. This can be especially helpful when transcribing ESL dictators who tend to confuse gender pronouns.

- Create shortcuts for quickly inserting a series of asterisks, two question marks, a series of five underscore characters (for a blank line), or highlighting to draw your attention to areas of the report that need to be carefully reviewed during proofreading.

Punctuation

Properly punctuating medical reports can be a challenge. The MT should always consider whether the punctuation changes the meaning or contributes to clarity of meaning. Many times the presence or absence of punctuation does not alter the interpretation. By far, commas and hyphens cause the most difficulty for transcriptionists.

Hyphenating Compound Modifiers

Hyphenation is not so much an element of spelling as it is of grammar. Only a few words include the hyphen as a permanent part of the word's spelling (eg, self-esteem). The most common use of the hyphen in medical transcription, other than indicating range, is to specify a **compound modifier**. If you view hyphenation as a component of spelling, you will definitely remain confused, as the spelling of the word will seem to vary capriciously. But, if you consider hyphens as a component of punctuation, their use becomes far less confusing. The use of the hyphen depends on sentence construction, not the spelling of the words themselves.

In a compound modifier, the hyphen connects the descriptive word to its corresponding noun when two or more descriptive words precede a noun. Often the reader can reread the section of the sentence and determine how the modifiers should be interpreted; so hyphenating the modifiers in many cases is a courtesy to the reader. Other times, the hyphen definitely prevents confusion by connecting the modifier to the actual word it modifies. A simple test for determining placement of a hyphen is to separate the descriptors and see if each descriptor can be applied directly to the final noun without changing the meaning. If both descriptors modify the final noun, no hyphen is needed. If the first descriptor modifies the second descriptor, but not the final noun, a hyphen is required.

Disease entities that contain compound modifiers such as *iron deficiency anemia* (as opposed to *iron-deficiency anemia*) do not typically require a hyphen to prevent confusion because they are already well recognized within the medical community.

Testing compound modifers: compound-modifier test = compound test + modifier test. Splitting the descriptors into two phrases does not convey the same meaning, so *compound* is not describing *test*. In this case, use the hyphen to associate *compound* with *modifier*.

thin, frail female = thin female + frail female. *Thin* and *frail* both modify female and the meaning does not change if you split the modifiers into two phrases, so a comma is used.

5-year history = 5 history + year history. Splitting the descriptors into two phrases changes the meaning and does not make sense. In this example, *5* is modifying *year*, so it is connected to its noun with a hyphen and together the phrase *5-year* modifies the final noun *history*.

low-normal value = low value + normal value. Splitting the descriptors into two phrases changes the meaning. In this example, *low* is modifying *normal*, indicating the value is on the low end of the normal range.

Hyphenating Prefixes

Prefixes are added to the beginning of a word to change the word's meaning without modifying the spelling of its base word. Note that prefixes are not words and cannot stand on their own. For the most part, hyphens are not used to add a prefix to the base word but there are several exceptions:

- Hyphens are used when a double-a or double-i results (eg, anti-insulin). A notable exception to this rule is antiinflammatory, which has become commonly accepted without the hyphen. Double consonants do not require a hyphen (eg, illegal, illegitimate).
- Hyphens may also be used with the prefix *re* to prevent confusion with another word (eg, re-create vs recreate; re-lay vs relay; re-cover vs recover).
- Hyphens are used when a prefix is added to a proper noun (eg, un-American).
- Hyphens are used when the prefix *ex* means former (eg, ex-president, ex-wife)
- Hyphens are used with the prefix *self* (eg, self-assured, self-referred)

The trend is toward dropping hyphens, so you may encounter words that at one time were hyphenated but have since dropped the hyphen. If in doubt, refer to an up-to-date style manual or collegiate dictionary.

 Pause 1-9 Correct the following by adding or removing hyphens.

1. The patient denies a history of abdominal pain, jaundice, clay colored stools, or recent unexplained weight loss.
2. There was no intrahepatic-biliary duct dilatation.
3. It does not involve the bone- or the joint space.
4. He underwent repair of an incarcerated ventral-umbilical hernia with mesh.
5. She is a pleasant 51 year old Hispanic female who complains of recurrent abdominal pain mostly localized to the epigastrium and right upper quadrant areas.
6. She never really followed up post-operatively, but today she is here complaining of mid-epigastric pain.

Commas with Lists

Everyone knows that a comma is used to separate items in a list, but MTs must know where each item ends and the next item begins to properly insert commas in a list. In medical reports, lists are most commonly found under medications and laboratory headings (either lab orders or lab results), and the improper use of commas in these areas can cause confusion. You must know what the items are in order to correctly place the commas. Critical thinking is required, as you cannot depend on the pauses in the dictator's voice to separate items, especially in a complicated list of medications or laboratory tests.

 Incorrect: Aspirin 325 mg a day, clonidine 0.2 mg, patch weekly, Humulin 9 units a day.

Correct: Aspirin 325 mg a day, clonidine 0.2 mg patch weekly, Humulin 9 units a day.

In the previous example, a comma was placed in front of *patch*. This leaves *patch* with no indication of the type of patch or its purpose. Subsequent readers of this document (without benefit of the audio) would not know if clonidine was administered via patch or if a separate medication associated with the patch was omitted.

> Incorrect: PLAN: Will draw C-peptide, HGB, A1c, CBC, hemoglobin, electrophoresis.
>
> Correct: PLAN: Will draw C-peptide, hemoglobin A$_{1c}$, CBC, hemoglobin electrophoresis.

The example above shows the incorrect placement of commas in a series of lab tests. The comma errors indicate two separate errors on the part of the MT: a failure to confirm the meaning of the abbreviation *HGB* and a failure to investigate the term *electrophoresis*. An astute MT would have also recognized that a CBC includes a hemoglobin value and there would be no need to order this test separately. The MT used the dictator's pauses as the basis of comma placement, resulting in significant transcription errors.

Disjoined Sentences

Dictators rarely dictate punctuation, and MTs often use the rise and fall of the dictator's voice to indicate the end of a sentence. There are times, however, when dictators fail to moderate their voice, either because they change their mind midsentence or because they are speaking too fast. ESL dictators who are not accustomed to moderating their voice when speaking in their native language will also run sentences together by either speaking in a staccato rhythm or raising and lowering their voice at the wrong time. MTs must not rely solely on pauses and voice to determine the placement of periods. In the following example, the dictator did not pause after the word *firefighter*, and the MT did not notice the faulty sentence that resulted.

> Incorrect: As you know, Mr. Herron is a firefighter in the process of climbing up ladder steps on the fire truck, he fell.
>
> Correct: As you know, Mr. Herron is a firefighter. In the process of climbing up ladder steps on the fire truck, he fell.

Prepositional phrases may also cause confusion when dictators fail to moderate their voice to indicate

the end of the sentence. MTs may inadvertently tack a phrase intended to start a new sentence onto the end of the preceding sentence. These situations require the MT to evaluate the propositional phrase very carefully to determine the most logical position.

> Incorrect: The patient had been taking Benadryl for her allergies at the time of her fall. She was groggy and didn't notice the toy truck.
>
> Correct: The patient had been taking Benadryl for her allergies. At the time of her fall, she was groggy and didn't notice the toy truck.
>
> Incorrect: The patient is a 28-year-old gravida 1, para 0 with an ectopic pregnancy on 12/03/2009. She had a beta hCG of 3026.
>
> Correct: The patient is a 28-year-old gravida 1, para 0 with an ectopic pregnancy. On 12/03/2009, she had a beta hCG of 3026.

Misplaced phrases may or may not be obvious when you first transcribe the sentences. The faulty construction often becomes obvious as you complete the sentence. Proofreading for comprehension will identify improperly placed prepositional phrases and other problems with sentence construction that do not immediately reveal themselves.

The most common sentence error is the insertion of a comma when a new sentence is indicated. This often creates a run-on sentence and forces the reader to back up and re-sort the sentence.

> Incorrect: Patient had a lysis of adhesions performed, this was performed without difficulty.
>
> Correct: Patient had lysis of adhesions performed. This was performed without difficulty.

Content Errors and Nonsensical Sentences

Transcription errors, whether auditory discrimination errors or typographical errors, can create nonsensical sentences. Careful proofreading will uncover these types of errors.

T: He does not have any unknown medical problems.

D: He does not have any (um) known medical problems.

T: On my manual exam, she is appropriately tender. Transvaginal ultrasound did not show any overt abnormality.

D: On bimanual exam, she is appropriately tender. Transvaginal ultrasound did not show any overt abnormality.

T: HEENT: Near sided.

D: HEENT: Nearsighted.

T: There are no other complaints of papillary stuff.

D: There are no other complaints. (uh, period paragraph)

T: She also complains of a striped back. She otherwise has been well.

D: She also complains of (strike that). She otherwise has been well.

T: Stability testing of both knees is normal with patellofemoral joint track swell.

D: Stability testing of both knees is normal and the patellofemoral joint tracks well.

Homophones

The English and medical lexicons are full of **homophones** and **sound-alikes**, and nothing short of discipline and a commitment to accuracy will ensure that you have used the correct spelling. Electronic spell checkers are of no use in choosing the correct spelling because spell checkers do not evaluate context. You have to know there is more than one spelling of a word, but the catch-22 is that you "don't know what you don't know!" That is to say, until you have looked up every word, even words you think you know, you cannot be sure you have not misused the word. That is where you must be disciplined enough to confirm words using a dictionary. English words are often misused or misspelled because we use the word routinely in conversation, not realizing there are different spellings. You must train yourself to confirm the meaning and spelling of all words, even those words you think you know, until the words are an established part of your vocabulary. You may need to look up any given word several times before you are comfortable with its use.

Reading newsmagazines, medical-related journals, textbooks, and literature will increase your vocabulary and help you recognize homophones and sound-alikes. You may be amazed at the number of words and phrases you have been misusing. Idioms are especially troublesome, as people often use them or pronounce them incorrectly.

discreet, discrete

allude, elude

defuse, diffuse

metal, mettle, medal

Incorrect: Read the right act.

Correct: Read the riot act.

Incorrect: It's a mute point.

Correct: It's a moot point.

Incorrect: Wrecking havoc

Correct: Wreaking havoc

Incorrect: Could of

Correct: Could have

Incorrect: Alright

Correct: All right

Incorrect: Graduated from high school

Correct: Graduated high school

Incorrect: In regards to

Correct: In regard to

MS Word has a built-in English dictionary that makes looking up definitions too easy to forego. Place the cursor anywhere within the word and press CTRL+Shift+O. You can also right-click on the word and choose Look Up. The Research task pane will appear with the definition displayed. The task pane also has a drop-down list of other resources including a thesaurus.

Combining Forms

A **combining form** is a single word created from two words. Examples include anteromedial (anterior and medial), posterolateral (posterior and lateral), postcoital (post and coital), and the oddest one of all, anteroposterior (anterior and posterior). Combining forms are another tricky area for medical transcriptionists because of a lack of consistency in their use. Like homonyms and sound-alikes, you simply must be alert to possible combining forms and look them up. One approach is to type the words together and see how spell check handles the word. Once you have prompted the spell checker, you must follow up with a confirmation step using the dictionary. Do not automatically use suggestions from the spell checker to hyphenate terms, as this is merely a suggestion from the spell-check software and is not based on the current context or actual usage. *Never hyphenate a word simply because the spell checker suggested it.*

In a production-driven work environment, the temptation to cut corners can be intense. You simply must take steps to make research convenient and efficient. Learn to use electronic references and then create shortcuts for accessing them quickly. If using references is quick and easy, you will be more likely to take those few extra seconds to make sure you get it right.

The dictator will err in both directions when it comes to combining forms; they may combine words that should not be combined (eg, *neuroforamen* should be *neural foramen*) and they may dictate separate words when a combining form is available (eg, *anterior medial* should be *anteromedial*). The good news is failure to use a combining form rarely causes confusion or interferes with meaning. Striving to use combining forms correctly adds to the overall integrity of your document and is worth the effort.

Numbers

It is difficult to appreciate all the pitfalls of transcribing numbers until you have worked as a quality assurance editor and have seen the numerous ways numbers can be transcribed incorrectly. Just like abbreviations, every number dictated should send up a red flag. The wrong medication dose, an incorrect blood pressure reading, an erroneous lab value, or an incorrectly recorded age or date of birth can change patient-care decisions that result in serious consequences for the patient.

The teens (13–19) are probably the most difficult numbers to distinguish when dictated. The numbers 15 and 50 are nearly impossible to differentiate when spoken. The /ē/ sound that is the dominate sound at the end of the numbers 13 through 19 sounds just like the /ē/ sound at the end of the tens (30, 40, 50, 60, 70, 80,

and 90). Often, the context will give you confidence in the number you transcribe, but there will be instances where 15 and 50 are both reasonable numbers and you simply cannot determine the actual number dictated. *Never hesitate to flag an ambiguous number.*

Numbers in the 40s, 50s, and 60s also present challenges. The number 55 sounds exactly like 65 when spoken quickly. These two numbers are close enough in value that context will not likely help distinguish them. Comparing the date of birth to the age dictated can resolve issues of age, but the date of birth is not always provided. Listen carefully when these numbers are dictated in the laboratory results section. Always confirm medication doses with the available doses dispensed by the manufacturer. Flag drug dosages that do not match the list of available doses.

Decimals starting with a leading zero present a unique problem. It is important to transcribe the leading zero in a decimal value less than one to ensure that the decimal is not accidentally misread. When the dictator says "zero point five seven," it is quite easy for the fingers to transpose the value and type 5.07 or 0.057. Decimals may also present problems when numbers are dictated in a string without intervening descriptions. For example, numbers dictated as "twenty one point seven" could be interpreted as 21.7, or as separate numbers 20 and 1.7 or even 21 and 0.7. Context may help you determine the correct transcription, but often you need to flag these cases for clarification.

Small Words and Syllables

English is a stress-timed language, which means key words are stressed while smaller words are purposely (yet unconsciously) minimized. This, of course, presents challenges to transcriptionists, who must capture every syllable accurately.

The article *an* and the short words and syllables such as *en*, *in*, *on*, *and*, *end*, and *un* are often pronounced as homophones. Prepositions such as *of*, *out*, *up*, *at*, *from*, and *by* can also be indistinguishable. Often the correct word can be determined by its position within the sentence or by the context. But when transcribing unfamiliar words or phrases, these small words and syllables are especially problematic. Using the phrasing techniques as described on page 5 is often helpful.

And and *or* are distinctly different sounds when spoken slowly, but when spoken quickly, as they usually are in dictation, the two words are surprisingly difficult to differentiate. Sentence structure provides the best clue for properly transcribing these two joining words.

Incorrect: EKG shows normal sinus rhythm. Low-voltage QRS and the precordial leads.

Correct: EKG shows normal sinus rhythm. Low-voltage QRS in the precordial leads.

Incorrect: Left ventricular and systolic dimension.

Correct: Left ventricular end-systolic dimension.

Incorrect: Pertaining to her left axillary hidradenitis, this involves a large area and most likely will require wide excision with attempted primary closure versus a flap.

Correct: Pertaining to her left axillary hidradenitis, this involves a large area and most likely will require wide excision with attempt at primary closure versus a flap.

Incorrect: A 37-year-old G0, P0 with a 4-year history of primary and fertility.

Correct: A 37-year-old G0, P0 with a 4-year history of primary infertility.

The joining word *or* is typically associated with statements using *no* or *none*.

 Incorrect: The patient has no history of hemoptysis, hematemesis, and cough.

Correct: The patient has no history of hemoptysis, hematemesis, or cough.

Incorrect: I recommended either canceling her cycle and moving on to follicular reduction.

Correct: I recommended either canceling her cycle or moving on to follicular reduction.

The joining word *and* is typically used with positive statements.

 Incorrect: The patient has no history of cough, shortness of breath, and 2-pillow orthopnea.

Correct: The patient has a history of cough, shortness of breath, and 2-pillow orthopnea.

Examining common sentence structure can also help with the corollary. The words *no*, *positive*, and *known* are often "swallowed," especially when they begin a sentence. If the word *positive* is brushed over or even shortened to *pos*, only the /o/ sound is heard, and it becomes indistinguishable from the word *no*.

 Incorrect: Positive history of cough, shortness of breath, or 2-pillow orthopnea.

Correct: No history of cough, shortness of breath, or 2-pillow orthopnea.

The types of statements described in these examples are commonly dictated in the History of Present Illness and routinely in the Review of Systems (ROS) and Physical Examination (PE) sections. They are usually dictated at lightning speed because they are dictated so often (as part of the dictator's normal text). Changes to "routine" statements usually require the dictator to slow down or change his or her usual rhythm, providing an important clue for the MT. These tricky areas can often be clarified by comparing statements with the HPI or even the medication list. For example, to verify a statement such as "positive for history of diabetes mellitus," look at the medication list to see if the patient lists insulin or a glucose-lowering medication. Use informed judgment when determining words such as *no*, *positive*, or *negative*, but do not guess.

Several sound-alikes are especially dangerous because they have opposite meanings. MTs must always be alert for these particular words and prefixes. Your ears will absolutely fool you! Almost always, context will help you determine the correct word. For example, the most common, and potentially dangerous, opposite sound-alikes are the phrases *no history* and *known history*.

 Incorrect: No history of heart disease status post 4-vessel bypass in October 2011.

Correct: Known history of heart disease status post 4-vessel bypass in October 2011.

Incorrect: Inadequate amount of fluid was drawn.

Correct: An adequate amount of fluid was drawn.

Other examples include:

- no vs non
- non vs not
- adynamic vs a dynamic
- asystolic vs a systolic
- anovulatory vs an ovulatory

Distinguishing Prefixes

Some of the most common prefixes used in the medical lexicon are also the most easily confused. *Hypo* and *hyper,* because they are opposites, have a significant potential to cause confusion or harm. Dictators rarely enunciate these two prefixes clearly. At times, the correct use is quite clear because the opposite condition is rarely, if ever, encountered (eg, hypertriglyceridemia versus hypotriglyceridemia). Never transcribe these prefixes without confirming the entire word and aligning its meaning with the surrounding context.

The following prefixes are especially troublesome and you should always evaluate them carefully in context:

- hypo vs hyper
- peri vs para
- inter vs intra vs infra
- cata vs ana

Incorrect: We discussed the process of in vitro fertilization including the use of gonadotropins, monitoring, transvaginal oocyte retrieval, intercytoplasmic sperm injection, embryo culture, and embryo transfer.

Correct: We discussed the process of in vitro fertilization including the use of gonadotropins, monitoring, transvaginal oocyte retrieval, intracytoplasmic sperm injection, embryo culture, and embryo transfer.

Incorrect: The patient remains hyperkalemic. We will increase her Kay Ciel and recheck potassium levels in 2 days.

Correct: The patient remains hypokalemic. We will increase her Kay Ciel and recheck potassium levels in 2 days.

Incorrect: Intraventricular conduction delay.

Correct: Interventricular conduction delay.

 Pause 1-10   Correct the following sentences or leave as is if correct.

1. Patient was diagnosed with hyperthyroidism and placed on Synthroid.
2. The patient is status post laparoscopic cholecystectomy secondary to a calculous cholecystitis and biliary dysmotility.
3. The paracardial effusion was confirmed on echocardiogram.
4. She had supernumerary oocytes.
5. The intraumbilical hernia was repaired with mesh.

Proofreading Checklist

Make it a habit to fully proofread the finished transcript from top to bottom. Never assume that a run through the spell checker is the same as proofreading. Use this checklist as a guide for proofreading:

- Is the patient's name spelled correctly and consistently throughout, including the header space?
- Is the age typed correctly? Is it reasonable for the patient's situation (eg, a 7-year-old with prostate cancer)?
- Is the gender consistent throughout and all pronouns typed correctly?
- Is the report coherent? Are there any contradictions?
- Is information reasonable?
- Do diagnostics (lab and imaging) align with assessment (eg, negative diagnostic results should correspond to a negative assessment)?
- Are laboratory values within range, reasonable, and physiologically possible?
- Are there contradictions between allergies and current medications?
- Do any comments in the ROS contradict comments in the HPI?
- Do medications correspond to known medical conditions mentioned in the HPI and past medical history?
- Are all abbreviations and short forms appropriate and accurate? Can you explain the meaning of all abbreviations, initialisms, and acronyms?
- Are numbers typed correctly? Are decimals placed correctly? Do medication dosages match doses dispensed by the manufacturer?

Exercises

Using Context to Make Decisions

1. How does the medication list relate to the Past Medical History section and why should these sections be free of contradictions?

   _____

2. How does the diagnostic section of a report (imaging reports and lab values) relate to the Assessment?

   _____

3. How is the Review of Systems section related to the patient's medical history (past and present)?

   _____

4. How does the Physical Examination section relate to the Assessment?

   _____

5. How can information dictated within the Plan section be relevant for clarifying a medication or medication dose?

   _____

6. Correct the following transcription errors:
   a. The patient was found to have nonobstructed azoospermia.
   b. Endometrial thickness is 13 mm trilaminar fibroid measuring 53 × 53 mm.
   c. Severe atheromatous plaquing of the distal aorta or bilateral iliac arteries.
   d. I will order non-invasive vascular studies and carotid Doppler.
   e. The patient's mother has no heart disease and has undergone angioplasty and stenting twice.
   f. Gallbladder ultrasound from All Saints Medical Center revealed cholecystolithiasis and no ductile dilatation.

Terms Checkup

Complete the multiple-choice questions for Chapter 1 located at www.myhealthprofessionskit.com. To access the questions, select the discipline "Medical Transcription," then click on the title of this book, *Advanced Medical Transcription*.

Look It Up

Research advanced search techniques available on Google and Bing (or two search engines recommended by your instructor). List different ways of performing a search using punctuation marks, symbols, operators, and any other features of the search engine.

Internal Medicine

Introduction

The actual practice of internal medicine encompasses many different body systems and diseases. Internal medicine doctors are often referred to as "doctors for adults." Internists specialize in the diagnosis and treatment of chronic illnesses, especially in patients with multiple chronic diseases. Internists (not interns) also focus on preventive medicine, especially chronic illnesses that can be addressed by lifestyle changes. Internists typically treat patients using medications, as opposed to surgical procedures, and most do not perform invasive diagnostic procedures such as endoscopy or cardiac catheterization.

Diseases most commonly managed by an internist include hypertension, dyslipidemia, peripheral vascular disease, asthma, heartburn, HIV, depression, chronic pain, Alzheimer disease, insomnia, and migraine headaches. Preventive care, also referred to as **health maintenance**, focuses on smoking cessation and risk-factor reduction for cardiovascular and cerebrovascular disease as well as cancer screening (eg, mammography, colonoscopy). When problems escalate and a specialist is needed, the internist serves as a primary care physician to oversee the treatment of the patient by all caregivers.

In the hospital setting, an internal medicine specialist may also be referred to as a "hospitalist." These physicians are part of the hospital's staff and serve as consultants to attending physicians. Hospitalists are often called upon when the patient has many ongoing medical issues that must be evaluated and managed from a larger perspective than that offered by a physician practicing a single medical specialty (eg, orthopedics).

This chapter introduces the most common diseases treated by a doctor of internal medicine. There is much overlap of this chapter with the remainder of the chapters, but it serves as a good starting point for learning the most common medications, diagnoses, and laboratory tests that will be used in the remainder of the book, and more importantly, encountered on the job as a medical transcriptionist.

Hypertension

Hypertension is one of the most prevalent chronic diseases in the United States. Hypertension is defined as a sustained elevation of resting systolic blood pressure greater than 140 mmHg and diastolic blood pressure greater than 90 mmHg, or both. Individuals with hypertension in the gray zone (systolic pressure of 120–139 and a diastolic pressure of 80–89) may be categorized as having prehypertension. Typically, persons with hypertension have few symptoms unless the condition is severe or long-standing. Untreated, hypertension causes **target-organ damage** (heart, brain, retinas, and kidneys) and atherosclerosis. Hypertension can also lead

to thoracic aortic dissection and abdominal aortic aneurysms. Hypertension, although a distinct diagnosis in and of itself, is considered a **modifiable risk factor** for cardiovascular disease (CVD). Hypertension is divided into two main categories: primary and secondary.

> HTN is a common abbreviation for hypertension. Some physicians may dictate the letters "h-t-n" instead of saying the actual word. In this case, transcribe the word hypertension.

> **Pause 2-1** Give the definition of each combining form in the term atherosclerosis and define this word in layman terms.

Primary Hypertension

The most common form of hypertension, accounting for 85% to 95% of cases, is primary hypertension, also called **essential hypertension**. Essential hypertension is rarely attributable to a single cause; rather an interplay of several mechanisms, referred to as the mosaic theory. For this reason, many hypertensive patients require more than one **antihypertensive agent** to adequately control their blood pressure. Increased salt intake and obesity may increase blood pressure in individuals with a genetic predisposition, but salt restriction and weight loss will not lower blood pressure in all individuals. Increased alcohol intake and cigarette smoking are known to increase the risk of hypertension. Age is also a significant factor, as two-thirds of the population over age 65 have hypertension.

Treatment of primary hypertension may include **lifestyle modifications** such as smoking cessation, decreased alcohol intake, weight loss, and increased aerobic activity. The DASH diet (Dietary Approaches to Stop Hypertension) may also be recommended. Drugs used to treat hypertension include diuretics, **beta-blockers**, **angiotensin converting enzyme inhibitors (ACE inhibitors)**, **angiotensin II receptor blockers (ARBs)**, and **calcium channel blockers**.

> ACE inhibitors are dictated as the acronym and should not be confused with the brand name Ace (bandages).

Vascular resistance and **cardiac output** are the two main factors affecting hypertension. Cardiac output refers to the heart's ability to adequately pump blood. Vascular resistance refers to the amount of effort required to push fluid through the circulatory system. Resistance increases when the diameter of the vessels decreases and/or when the vessels lose their elasticity. Vessel diameter may be affected by the tone of the smooth muscle tissue within the wall of the vessels (vasoconstriction) or by accumulation of plaque within the lumen of the vessel (stenosis). An increased volume of fluid in the vascular space can also increase resistance throughout the vascular system because the excess volume pushes against vessel walls, creating resistance.

The ability to constrict and dilate the blood vessels is essential for maintaining oxygen levels under various conditions (rest, exertion, stress, illness, etc). Vasodilation is managed by a complicated interplay of the sympathetic nervous system (epinephrine and norepinephrine), the renin-angiotensin-aldosterone system, and the movement of sodium and calcium across cellular membranes. The variety of antihypertensives used to treat elevated blood pressure is reflective of the many contributing factors. In the most simplistic terms, medications used to treat blood pressure work by either decreasing the plasma volume (diuretics) or lessening the constriction of blood vessels (vasodilators).

The sympathetic nervous system exerts influence on the vascular system through the release of epinephrine. Alpha and beta receptors located on the surface of smooth muscle cells respond to epinephrine by contracting smooth muscle. This system helps the body control blood pressure under situations of stress and is integral to the "fight or flight" reaction when the body senses danger. Hypertension may result when the sympathetic nervous system is overreactive or the alpha and beta receptors become too sensitive. Alpha- and beta-receptor blockers reduce blood pressure by blocking the action of epinephrine.

Because water tends to follow sodium across cellular membranes, controlling the sodium concentration in the extracellular (intravascular) and intracellular spaces is important for controlling total body fluid volume, preventing edema, and maintaining normal blood pressure. For individuals with impaired natriuresis, (1) dietary sodium restriction is an important component of controlling the body's fluid volume and, therefore, blood pressure. These patients may be treated with diuretics and dietary restriction of sodium.

Some patients with essential hypertension have increased concentrations of intracellular sodium and calcium due to abnormal sodium transport across muscle-cell membranes (a different mechanism than natriuresis). This type of hypertension is independent of dietary sodium intake. The tonicity of smooth muscle is affected by the movement of sodium (Na^+) and potassium (K^+) ions across the muscle cell membrane. Increased intracellular sodium is accompanied by increased intracellular calcium, leading to increased tone of the smooth muscle. Blocking calcium from moving into the intracellular space decreases muscle tone and relaxes (dilates) blood vessels (■ Figure 2-1). Calcium channel blockers decrease blood pressure by blocking the movement of calcium, thereby decreasing muscle tone.

> **Pause 2-2** The body has two main "fluid spaces." What are these spaces and how do the electrolytes Na^+ and K^+ influence the flow of water into and out of these spaces?

Blood pressure is also affected by the renin-angiotensin-aldosterone system, a complicated system that controls vasoconstriction through pressure monitors located in the afferent arterioles (2) of the kidneys. This system is designed to detect a drop in blood pressure when there is a decrease in blood volume (eg, in

(1) Natriuresis is the excretion of sodium by the kidneys.

(2) Afferent arterioles are branches of the renal arteries that eventually become the capillaries of the glomerulus.

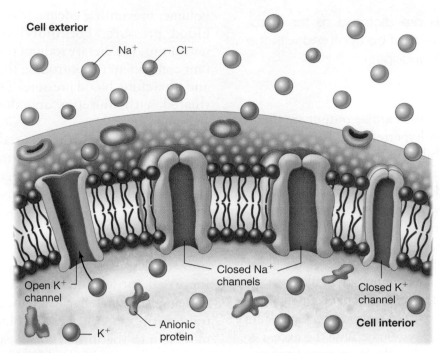

Cell exterior

Na⁺   Cl⁻

Open K⁺
channel

Closed Na⁺
channels

Closed K⁺
channel

K⁺

Anionic
protein

Cell interior

FIGURE 2-1 Movement of sodium, potassium, and calcium across cellular membranes changes the tonicity (dilates or constricts) of blood vessels, thereby affecting blood pressure.

cases of dehydration or hemorrhage). A decrease in pressure releases renin, setting in motion a cascade of reactions to increase blood pressure through vasoconstriction and sodium retention (and therefore water retention). In some patients with hypertension, this system becomes too sensitive and causes the blood pressure to rise under otherwise normal conditions. These patients may be treated with ACE inhibitors and ARBs.

> ACE inhibitors are dictated as the acronym "ace," never as individual letters. Some physicians will dictate ARB as an acronym ("arb" or "arbs") and some will dictate a-r-b. It is generally acceptable to transcribe the abbreviation.

(3) Renovascular refers to the blood vessels of the kidney, especially denoting disease of these vessels.

Secondary Hypertension

Secondary hypertension has a definite cause and is treated by addressing the underlying disorder that secondarily leads to hypertension. Common causes of secondary hypertension include renal disease, renovascular disease, **(3)** primary aldosteronism, Cushing syndrome, and pheochromocytoma. Malformations of the heart or great vessels (congenital abnormalities) may also cause hypertension. Hypertension may also develop during pregnancy or with estrogen use.

Secondary hypertension may also be related to the use of pharmacologic agents and herbs such as sympathomimetics, NSAIDs (nonsteroidal antiinflammatory drugs, pronounced *en-saydz*), corticosteroids, cocaine, or licorice. This type of "curable" hypertension responds to cessation of these agents.

> **Pause 2-3** Why do you think the kidneys contain pressure sensors for monitoring blood pressure? Describe how renovascular disease and renal artery stenosis can lead to hypertension.

- Hypertension may be primary or secondary, the most common being primary, also called essential.
- Hypertension is the result of increased cardiac output and/or increased vascular resistance.
- Blood pressure is controlled by a complicated interplay of the sympathetic nervous system, the renin-angiotensin-aldosterone system, and the kidneys through regulation of electrolytes and fluid volume.

- Hypertension must be controlled to prevent damage to blood vessels and target organs.
- Hypertension is controlled using lifestyle changes, weight loss, and pharmaceutical regimens that lower vascular resistance (vasodilation) and control total body fluid.
- Secondary hypertension is controlled by addressing the underlying condition.

Evaluation and Management of Hypertension

Patients with hypertension are typically asymptomatic but may complain of headache, especially early-morning headaches that subside later in the day. The physical examination is an important component of the diagnosis of hypertension and in the differentiation of primary and secondary hypertension. The physical examination includes measurement of height, weight, and waist circumference; a funduscopic exam for retinopathy and papilledema (**choked disc**); auscultation for bruits in the neck and abdomen; and a full cardiac, respiratory, and neurologic examination. The abdomen is palpated for kidney enlargement and abdominal masses. Diminished peripheral pulses may suggest coarctation of the aorta, especially in individuals under 30 years of age. A fourth heart sound (S4) is one of the earliest signs of **hypertensive heart disease**. Patients may also exhibit a **systolic ejection murmur (SEM)**. Laboratory studies to evaluate hypertension include renal function studies, urinalysis, complete blood count, complete metabolic panel, and thyroid studies.

Hypertension is rarely diagnosed on the basis of a single blood pressure reading. Some patients display hypertension only while in the physician's office, a condition referred to as **white coat syndrome**. To confirm a diagnosis or to monitor **efficacy of treatment**, patients are often asked to keep a **blood pressure diary** and to return to the clinic for **serial blood pressure readings**. Patients with erratic blood pressure readings or blood pressure that is difficult to control are said to have **labile hypertension**.

Note: The phrase is *labile* hypertension, not liable hypertension. Labile means undergoing frequent change.

Hypertensive urgency arises when the systolic blood pressure exceeds 220 mmHg or the diastolic pressure exceeds 125 mmHg. In these situations, the blood pressure must be reduced within a few hours. A **hypertensive emergency**, however, must be controlled within one hour to avoid the risk of serious morbidity and mortality. Emergencies occur when the diastolic pressure reaches 130 mmHg or higher. **Malignant hypertension** is characterized by encephalopathy, papilledema, and nephropathy with ensuing renal failure.

Clonidine (Catapres) and nifedipine are often given orally for the treatment of an acute hypertensive event. More severe or life-threatening events may be treated with parenteral (IV) medications such as nitroprusside sodium, nitroglycerin, labetalol, and enalapril.

Diabetes Mellitus

Diabetes mellitus (DM) is a syndrome of disordered metabolism characterized by hyperglycemia. The inappropriate level of blood glucose may be the result of insulin deficiency or it may result from **insulin resistance** in the setting of adequate insulin. Glucose is the essential form of energy consumed by all cells in the body. Insulin receptors bind insulin, which in turn open membrane channels that allow glucose to enter cells. Insulin also plays a role in the regulation of lipids as well as the utilization of protein and fat. Altered insulin levels, with its attendant changes in glucose and lipid control, have profound effects on metabolism, leading to myriad complications, including dyslipidemia and atherosclerosis, heart disease, neuropathies, nephropathies, and retinopathies.

The term **osmolality** describes the concentration of a solute. Osmolality of blood is determined by the concentration of electrolytes, protein, and glucose. When glucose is blocked from entering cells, it accumulates in the blood, resulting in hyperosmolality. Water tends to follow sodium and glucose across a cell membrane, so controlling the concentration of these elements in the blood is imperative to controlling fluid volumes in the various fluid spaces. Hallmark symptoms of DM are increased urination (**polyuria**) and increased thirst (**polydipsia**). These symptoms are a direct consequence of the **hyperosmolality** of urine—the kidneys excrete the excess glucose and water "follows" the glucose into the urine in a process called **osmotic diuresis**. As the body excretes more water, it increases thirst to replace the lost water, and the cycle continues. The hyperosmolar fluids also cause the lenses of the eyes to dehydrate, resulting in blurry vision, a common presenting symptom of DM.

Because insulin is also involved in the regulation of lipids, inappropriate insulin levels can lead to diabetic dyslipidemia and increased triglyceride levels. This accounts for the increased incidence of atherosclerosis, **peripheral vascular disease (PVD)**, and **coronary heart disease (CHD)** in patients with DM. Learn more about dyslipidemia on page 38.

Diabetes is divided into two major classifications: type 1 and type 2 (**4**). Diabetes mellitus is on the increase worldwide; according to the Centers for Disease Control, diabetes is increasing in the United States in epidemic proportions. Although the exact mechanism is not understood, the sharp rise is related to increasing obesity rates and sedentary lifestyles.

Diabetes Mellitus Type 1

Type 1 diabetes mellitus results from the destruction of pancreatic islet B cells that are responsible for the production of insulin. Onset is often in early childhood or around puberty but may occur at any age. The destruction of islet B cells in the pancreas diminishes or eliminates endogenous insulin, so these patients are

---

(4) Use arabic numbers 1 and 2 to designate diabetes (not roman numerals).

(5) Idiopathic means the cause is unknown.

(6) Nocturnal enuresis is the involuntary release of urine during sleep.

---

dependent upon exogenous insulin. Up to 90% of cases of type 1 diabetes are thought to be immune-related, wherein the immune system misinterprets islet cells as "foreign" and destroys them. The remaining 10% of cases are considered idiopathic (**5**) and are designated type 1B. Physicians may use the terms **juvenile-onset diabetes** or **insulin-dependent diabetes mellitus (IDDM)**, but these references are falling out of use in favor of type 1 diabetes mellitus.

 Pause 2-4 Describe endogenous and exogenous insulin and give examples.

Initial symptoms of type 1 diabetes include polyuria and polydipsia. Patients may also have **polyphagia** (increased appetite) yet still lose weight. When glucose levels are high, patients may complain of burning or tingling sensations in the arms and/or legs (**peripheral paresthesia**) or **neuropathy**. As the disease progresses, patients may complain of weakness, fatigue, decreased muscle mass, orthostatic hypotension, and **nocturnal enuresis (6)**. Symptoms may develop slowly with subacute DM. Acute-onset DM will cause anorexia, nausea, and vomiting.

Because patients with type 1 DM do not produce insulin, they lack the normal feedback mechanisms that stimulate the release of insulin in response to carbohydrate intake. Patients must monitor their carbohydrate, fat, and protein intake; routinely measure **capillary blood glucose (CBG)** levels; and adjust their insulin levels throughout the day. Typically, patients monitor blood glucose using the fingerstick method in which a small lancet is used to prick the finger for a small droplet of capillary blood. The droplet is placed on a test strip that reacts with glucose. A pocket-size glucometer measures the glucose concentration on the test strip and reports a numeric value. Common names of fingerstick glucose meters include **OneTouch**, **Glucometer Elite**, **Accu-Chek**, and **FreeStyle**. Depending on the methodology used to calculate the glucose level, meter readings may vary as much as 10% when compared to venous glucose levels measured by venipuncture. Self-monitoring is especially important in patients requiring **tight metabolic control** and also in **brittle diabetics** (also called **labile diabetics**). Brittle diabetics have erratic and unpredictable fluctuations in blood glucose levels.

Patients must be educated in all aspects of diabetes in order to control their diet, manage insulin and glucose levels, and prevent life-threatening emergencies. Patients are instructed to eat according to the **ADA diet**, as prescribed by the American Diabetic Association. To prevent severe elevations in blood sugar, diabetics are encouraged to use nonnutritive sweeteners such as saccharin, sucralose (Splenda), and acesulfame potassium, as well as nutritive sweeteners such as sorbitol and fructose.

Diabetic patients may suffer both acute and chronic complications as a result of their diabetes. Acute complications include hyperglycemia and hypoglycemia, both of which may result in **diabetic coma**. Hypoglycemia due to accidental insulin overdose may cause the patient to become sleepy at first and then progress to coma. Patients are advised to carry packets of table sugar or candy to quickly raise blood sugar levels and counteract the effects of hyperinsulinism.

Hypoinsulinemia can result in **diabetic ketoacidosis (DKA)**, an acute, life-threatening emergency. Without insulin, glucose metabolism stops, and the body switches to metabolizing fats and proteins. **Ketones** are byproducts of fat metabolism, and the accumulation of ketones in the blood lowers the blood pH (**acidosis**), producing electrolyte imbalances and hyperosmolality. Hyperglycemia and elevated **ketone bodies (ketonemia)** cause osmotic diuresis, further exacerbating dehydration and electrolyte imbalances. Symptoms of DKA include polydipsia and polyuria (typically the day before the onset of acute symptoms), nausea, vomiting, fatigue, muscle stiffness, dehydration, tachycardia, mental status changes, and a "fruity," ketone-like odor (similar to nail polish remover) to the breath. Untreated, patients become comatose. Patients taking insulin (especially in the form of insulin pumps) are advised to monitor urine for ketones (**ketonuria**) using simple test strips (**Acetest, Ketostix**) to detect rising levels of ketones.

Diabetes Mellitus Type 2

Type 2 diabetes mellitus has traditionally been referred to as **non-insulin-dependent diabetes mellitus (NIDDM)**, (7) but there are a significant number of patients who require exogenous insulin even though they still produce normal amounts of insulin. Because insulin treatment is not always the distinguishing factor, the term type 2 diabetes mellitus is preferred. Up to 90% of all diabetics in the United States are classified as type 2.

Patients with type 2 diabetes continue to produce insulin, but their cells have developed resistance to the effects of insulin; therefore, type 2 diabetics require higher levels of insulin to maintain blood sugar levels in the normal range. Known risk factors for type 2 diabetes include family history of diabetes, age, sedentary lifestyle, and obesity, especially **abdominal-visceral obesity** with a **high waist-to-hip ratio** (greater than 0.9 in men and 0.8 in women).

Like patients with type 1 diabetes, type 2 patients may present with polyuria, polydipsia, weakness, fatigue, blurred vision, and/or peripheral neuropathy. Many patients are asymptomatic and are discovered to have elevated glucose on routine blood and urine laboratory studies. Often, a presenting symptom for women is recurrent **candidal vaginitis**.

A diagnosis of type 2 diabetes is based on elevated **fasting blood glucose** levels of greater than or equal to 126 g/dL or a postprandial glucose level of greater than or equal to 200 g/dL. Fasting blood glucose may also be called **fasting blood sugar (FBS)**. Patients may be classified as prediabetic when fasting glucose levels are between 100 and 125 g/dL. When diabetes is suspected, an **oral glucose tolerance test (OGTT or GTT)** may be performed. To perform this test, a patient who is fasting drinks a solution of concentrated glucose (1.75 mg of glucose per kilogram of body weight), and blood glucose levels are measured at baseline (before drinking the glucose) and again after two hours. Sometimes several levels are drawn at 30-minute intervals. The rise and fall of postprandial plasma glucose levels indicates the body's response to a glucose load.

Be aware that the abbreviation DKA (diabetic ketoacidosis) sounds very much like BKA (below-knee amputation). Both of these abbreviations are common in reports involving diabetic patients. Use context, not sound, to determine which abbreviation is being dictated.

(7) Although the prefix *non* is typically joined without a hyphen, the disease non-insulin-dependent diabetes mellitus includes a hyphen after *non* because *non* modifies the phrase "insulin-dependent." The word "noninsulin" (without a hyphen) infers the wrong meaning.

Treatment of type 2 diabetes starts with lifestyle changes, including increased exercise, weight loss in obese patients, and dietary changes. Dietary changes include a reduction in simple carbohydrate intake (white sugar, white flour, simple sugars). Because diabetic patients typically have **concomitant (8)** dyslipidemia, patients should consume less saturated fats in favor of essential fatty acids such as those found in olive oil, canola oil, nuts, and avocados. Increasing dietary fiber to 25–30 g daily is also recommended. Unfortunately, as many as 50% of patients fail to comply with dietary and lifestyle changes.

When diet and lifestyle changes are unsuccessful, medications are used to reduce hyperglycemia and decrease insulin resistance. Insulin may be used when the patient demonstrates severe insulin resistance and other **oral hypoglycemic agents** are not sufficient to achieve normal glucose levels (**euglycemia**). Medications used to control type 2 diabetes include sulfonylureas, thiazolidinediones, and alpha-glucosidase inhibitors.

Patients must be monitored carefully to assess the efficacy (9) of their diet and medication regimen and to forestall the many complications of diabetes. **Glycosylated hemoglobin**, also called **hemoglobin A$_{1c}$**, (10) is measured to assess average plasma glucose levels over the preceding 90 days. Under normal circumstances, 4% to 6% of circulating hemoglobin becomes glycosylated (11). In the presence of high plasma glucose, more hemoglobin becomes glycosylated and the hemoglobin A$_{1c}$ level rises above 6%. Because red cells have a typical lifespan of 90–120 days, the hemoglobin A$_{1c}$ value gives an indication of overall glucose control over the previous 8–12 weeks. Glucose may also bind to albumin to form **fructosamine**, which can also be measured to assess glucose control. Because albumin molecules have a much shorter half-life (12) than red blood cells, serum fructosamine levels are indicative of glucose control over the previous one to two weeks. Normal fructosamine levels are 1.5 to 2.4 mmol/L (when the albumin level is normal).

Complications of Diabetes

Chronic diabetes leads to a number of complications involving the small and large blood vessels, cranial and peripheral nerves, skin, and eyes. Hypertension, renal failure, blindness, neuropathies, myocardial infarction, and cerebrovascular accidents are common in diabetic patients of both types, although to varying degrees. Routine care of diabetic patients include annual eye examinations and podiatric examinations as well as neurological evaluations and cardiac testing. Blood pressure and peripheral pulses are monitored carefully. Pertinent laboratory studies include **renal function studies** (BUN, creatinine), total cholesterol, and triglyceride levels.

Mononeuropathies, polyneuropathies, as well as autonomic neuropathies such as **gastroparesis** are common in diabetics. **Peripheral neuropathy**, typically in the **stocking-glove distribution** (ie, feet and hands), is common in diabetics of both types. Patients have decreased perception to pain and temperature changes as well as decreased **vibratory sensation**. Decreased sensation in the feet often causes changes in gait, putting diabetic patients at risk for pressure sores on the feet and joint changes such as **Charcot arthropathy**. (13) Patients must pay particular attention to **foot care**, wear properly fitted shoes, and routinely examine their feet for sores (■ Figure 2-2). Foot sores are particularly problematic in diabetics who also have peripheral vascular disease because the decreased vascular supply hinders healing and leads to ulceration. **Refractory (14)** ulcers may progress to gangrene, osteomyelitis, and amputations of the toes or feet, or **below-knee amputation (BKA).** To detect changes in sensation, patients may be evaluated by pressing a **5.07 Semmes-Weinstein monofilament** on the plantar surface of the foot (■ Figure 2-3).

---

(8) Concomitant means occurring together, especially in a subordinate or incidental way.

(9) Hemoglobin A$_{1c}$ is written with 1c formatted as subscripts. It may be transcribed on the line (A1c) if subscripts are not compatible with the electronic record system. This form of hemoglobin may also be called glycated hemoglobin, glycosylated hemoglobin, or HbA1c.

(10) Efficacy describes the ability of something to produce an effect. Drugs and other treatments are often described in terms of their efficacy and safety.

(11) Glycosylated means a glucose molecule has been attached. Glycosylated hemoglobin refers to hemoglobin within red blood cells that has molecules of glucose attached.

(12) Half-life is the time it takes for half the amount of a substance to disintegrate or be eliminated from the body.

(13) Charcot is pronounced *shahr-kō*.

(14) Refractory means resistant to treatment or cure.

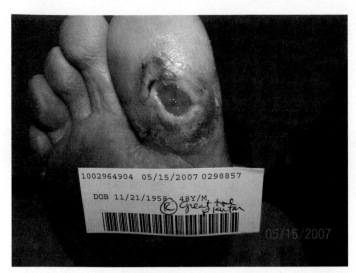

FIGURE 2-2 Diabetic plantar ulcer. *Source:* Courtesy of Harold Engle.

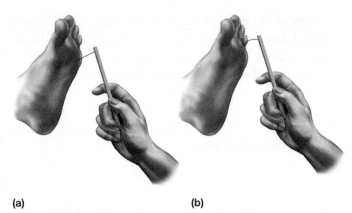

(a)   **(b)**

FIGURE 2-3 A Semmes-Weinstein monofilament is used to screen diabetic patients for loss of protective sensation.

Pause 2-5 Describe the three types of neuropathy mentioned in the previous section. Describe gastroparesis and its symptoms.

Listen carefully for the difference between diabetic neuropathy and diabetic nephropathy. These words are difficult to distinguish, so you must listen in context.

Diabetic nephropathy, which is a significant cause of morbidity and mortality in both types of diabetics, typically appears 10–15 years after onset of disease. The first sign of nephropathy is **microalbuminuria, (15)** which subsequently progresses to **albuminuria** and **hypoalbuminemia.** Close attention to blood pressure control and the use of ACE inhibitors and angiotensin receptor blockers have been shown to slow the progression of diabetic nephropathy, although many patients still eventually proceed to end-stage renal disease (ESRD), requiring dialysis and kidney transplant.

Pause 2-6 Describe the role of albumin in the blood. Define albuminuria and hypoalbuminemia. Why do albuminuria and hypoalbuminemia go hand-in-hand?

(15) Microalbuminuria refers to small amounts of albumin in the urine (not "small" albumin molecules).

- Diabetes is a disease of disordered metabolism that affects insulin levels and/or the ability of insulin to affect insulin receptors.
- Insulin regulates glucose and lipid metabolism.
- Type 1 diabetics require exogenous insulin. Type 2 diabetics may or may not require insulin.
- Blood glucose levels must be within the normal range to properly supply cells with energy. Extremely high glucose levels can cause fluid shifts due to osmosis. Extremely low levels of blood glucose can lead to coma.

- When glucose is unavailable, the body shifts to fat and protein as sources of energy. Sustained fat metabolism produces ketone bodies that lower blood pH (acidosis) and increase the osmolality of plasma and urine.
- Diabetic patients are at risk for developing atherosclerosis, coronary, cerebrovascular, and peripheral vascular disease, nephropathy, retinopathy, and neuropathies.
- Treatment involves management of insulin and glucose levels, lipids, and blood pressure to prevent vascular disease and end-organ damage.

Myocardial infarction is the leading cause of death in type 2 diabetics, so control of hypertension and dyslipidemia are essential to the long-term care of the diabetic patient. In addition to oral hypoglycemics, the type 2 diabetic's medication regimen often includes cholesterol-lowering medications, blood pressure medications, and possibly **low-dose aspirin** (81 mg per day) to reduce the risk of thrombosis.

Dyslipidemia

The two main lipids in the blood are cholesterol and triglycerides. Cholesterol is essential to cellular membranes and is the building block for many hormones as well as the **bile acids**. Triglycerides are molecules consisting of fat and sugar that serve as a source of energy. Lipids are not water soluble; to keep them suspended in the blood, they must be attached to transport proteins to render them water soluble. Proteins that transport lipids are called apoproteins, and the combined molecules of lipids and proteins are called lipoproteins. Lipoproteins are described in terms of the density of the apoproteins. **High-density lipoproteins (HDL)** and **low-density lipoproteins (LDL)** carry cholesterol, while **very low density lipoproteins (VLDL)** carry mostly triglycerides but also small amounts of cholesterol. Total cholesterol is the sum of these three forms of lipoproteins.

Hypercholesterolemia has long been implicated in atherosclerosis, a pathologic process characterized by deposition of lipids and inflammatory cells in the intimal layer of arterial vessels, creating atheromatous **plaques**. A local inflammatory reaction occurs with remodeling (16) of the vessel wall. These plaques cause the vessel walls to become hardened and stiff. The plaques continue to build up, eventually causing narrowing or complete occlusion of the vessel. Calcium is also deposited in the plaques, which can be detected on **EBCT (electron beam CT scan)**. Studies of cholesterol and its effect on the vascular system have shown that the relative amount of each cholesterol fraction is more indicative of risk than the total cholesterol value. For unknown reasons, LDL cholesterol is more atherogenic than HDL. **Dyslipidemia** is defined as an increase in LDL cholesterol and a decrease in HDL cholesterol. Elevated levels of LDL and VLDL

are associated with a higher risk of atherosclerosis, and HDL cholesterol is associated with a lower risk.

Atherosclerotic changes occur in arteries throughout the body, resulting in coronary heart disease, peripheral vascular disease, cerebrovascular disease, renovascular disease, erectile dysfunction, and aneurysms, especially **abdominal aortic aneurysms (AAA)**. Diabetics are particularly prone to atherosclerosis because insulin regulates circulating lipoproteins.

> Dictators often refer to an abdominal aortic aneurysm as a "triple A," but you should transcribe the phrase, or where appropriate, the abbreviation AAA.

Screening for dyslipidemia in individuals age 45 and older is recommended because lowering LDL cholesterol is known to slow the progression of atherosclerosis and may prevent or forestall a life-threatening event such as a myocardial infarction or stroke.

Dyslipidemia, in and of itself, has no particular signs or symptoms. Often patients are diagnosed on routine laboratory screening tests or after an acute vascular event such as a heart attack or stroke. Primary lipid disorders are hereditary, but many patients have dyslipidemia secondary to obesity, sedentary lifestyle, and/or increased alcohol intake. Hypothyroidism and diabetes mellitus can also cause lipid abnormalities. Medications such as oral contraceptives, diuretics, and some beta-blockers may also increase total cholesterol. Hyperthyroidism and malignancy are known to *decrease* total cholesterol.

Treatment of dyslipidemia includes lifestyle changes such as increased exercise, weight loss, and dietary changes. A diet high in soluble fiber (eg, oat bran, **psyllium**), monounsaturated fats (olive oil, canola oil, avocados, nuts), and antioxidant-rich fruits and vegetables has been shown to have positive effects on total cholesterol and lipoprotein ratios in some but not all individuals.

When lifestyle changes are not sufficient, medications are used to bind cholesterol (**bile acid binding resins**, also called **sequestrants**), block cholesterol from being absorbed in the intestinal tract, or interfere with cholesterol production in the liver (**statins**). **Fibrates** (fibric acids) are prescribed to lower triglyceride levels. **High-dose niacin** is very effective at

---

(16) Remodeling refers to structural changes in the vessel walls that alter their shape and possibly their function.

- Dyslipidemia is characterized by altered ratios of LDL and HDL cholesterol.
- Increased LDL cholesterol is atherogenic and leads to arteriosclerosis, coronary heart disease, peripheral vascular disease, renal artery disease, and hypertension.
- Dyslipidemia is managed with diet and lifestyle changes and medications to lower total cholesterol and raise the HDL-to-LDL ratio.

increasing HDL cholesterol while lowering LDL cholesterol. **Omega-3 oils,** (17) now available in prescription form, are also used to correct dyslipidemia. Dietary supplements such as garlic, vitamin C, and plant sterols may also be helpful.

Risk factors for atherosclerosis are cumulative, so target values for total cholesterol, HDL, and LDL depend on the presence of other risk factors. Patients with known coronary, carotid, or peripheral vascular disease, or those at high risk for vascular disease should aim for an LDL value of less than 70 g/dL. Patients at moderate risk for disease should aim for an LDL value of less than 100 g/dL. Optimal values of HDL are 40–70 g/dL with values above 70 considered more protective. Patients taking statins and high-dose niacin should be monitored routinely with liver function studies to detect **myositis** or **transaminitis.** (18)

Obesity

Obesity is defined as an excess of adipose (fat) tissue. Obesity is one of the most common medical disorders in the United States and accounts for a considerable amount of morbidity and mortality. Obesity is on the rise and is considered by some to be increasing in epidemic proportions. Upwards of 60% of Americans are overweight and 30% are obese. Obesity is associated with both metabolic and structural disorders as well as psychosocial disability. The majority of obese patients also have metabolic syndrome (see page 40). Bariatrics is the medical specialty concerned with the treatment of obesity.

The **body mass index (BMI)** is commonly used to classify patients as to the extent of overweight and obesity based on the patient's height and weight. BMI is calculated by dividing the patient's weight in kilograms by the patient's height in meters squared (weight/height²). Normal weight corresponds to a BMI of 18.5 to 24.9. (19) Overweight corresponds to a BMI of 25 to 29.9. Patients with a BMI of 30 or greater are considered to have **morbid obesity.**

Obesity is known to increase the risk of diabetes mellitus, hypertension, hyperlipidemia, and structural disorders such as degenerative joint disease (DJD). Obesity may also cause **obstructive sleep apnea (OSA).** The distribution of fat also plays a significant role in the consequences of overweight and obesity. Increased **abdominal circumference** (greater than 102 cm in men and 88 cm in women) and increased waist-to-hip ratio are associated with greater risk for diabetes, stroke, coronary artery disease, and early death when compared to patients of equal BMI and lower waist-to-hip ratios. Visceral fat within the abdominal cavity appears to carry greater health risks than fat carried predominantly in the buttocks and thighs.

A sedentary lifestyle and increased caloric intake are the most common causes of obesity, but there is also a strong genetic component. Collectively, genes, environment, and behavior play significant roles in overweight and obesity. Treatment involves a hypocaloric diet, behavior modification, aerobic exercise, and social support. A **very low calorie diet** (less than 800 kcal per day) may be prescribed but must be administered under a physician's care. **Anorexiants** may also be prescribed, although there are relatively few approved by the FDA for the treatment of overweight. Phentermine (Adipex and Ionamin) may be prescribed for short-term use only. Sibutramine (Meridia) blocks uptake of serotonin

(17) Omega-3 oils, commonly found in cold-water fish, flax, and nuts, are essential fatty acids that must be obtained through diet because, unlike other fatty acids, they cannot be manufactured by the body.

(18) Transaminitis is an emerging term that describes an elevation in the transaminases (ALT and AST), often as a result of statin therapy.

(19) BMI is an index, not a percentage, and is written without any units.

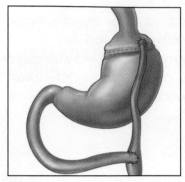

FIGURE 2-4 A Roux-en-Y bypass decreases the size of the stomach and bypasses a significant portion of the small intestine. *Source:* National Institutes of Health (2000). *The Practical Guide: Identification, Evaluation, and Treatment of Overweight and Obesity in Adults.* Retrieved December 10, 2008 from http://www.nhibi/nih.gov/guidelines/obesity/prctgd_c.pdf.

and norepinephrine in the central nervous system and helps to control appetite. Orlistat (Alli and Xenical) does not affect appetite, but reduces caloric intake by decreasing fat absorption in the gastrointestinal tract.

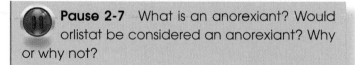

Pause 2-7 What is an anorexiant? Would orlistat be considered an anorexiant? Why or why not?

Bariatric surgery may also be used in individuals with a BMI greater than 40 or greater than 35 with comorbidities. A common bariatric surgical procedure is **laparoscopic Roux-en-Y gastric bypass** (■ Figure 2-4). (20) This surgery reduces the size of the stomach by stapling the upper portion of the stomach to form a small pouch. A portion of the small intestine is sectioned off and the remaining segment is attached (anastomosed) to the stomach pouch, bypassing the pyloric

(20) Roux-en-Y is pronounced *rū-en-wī.*

(21) Early satiety is the feeling of being full after eating a small portion of food.

(22) Lap band is short for laparoscopic banding and LAP-BAND is the trademarked name for a device used to perform this procedure. It can be difficult to determine from the context if the physician intends the brand name or the name of the procedure (lap band). When in doubt, type the procedure name, not the trademarked name.

sphincter. Patients lose weight because the smaller stomach causes **early satiety**. (21) Calorie absorption is also reduced because of the decreased length of the small intestine. Because the pyloric sphincter no longer regulates the passage of food into the small intestine, patients may experience a physiologic reaction after ingesting sugary foods, called **dumping syndrome**. The patient may experience a rapid heart rate, sweating, nausea, and a feeling of panic that subsides after 30 minutes to an hour. Although bariatric surgery is very effective at achieving weight loss, it also has a high rate of complications.

Laparoscopic gastric banding is another form of bariatric surgery. This procedure places a removable, adjustable, silastic band around the upper part of the stomach, creating a small pouch. Like the Roux-en-Y procedure, the stomach is limited in the amount of food it can hold, creating a feeling of satiety after eating small amounts of food. The band is connected to an easily accessible port placed just under the skin that allows fluid to be added or removed, thus adjusting the stricture of the band postoperatively. As opposed to the Roux-en-Y procedure, the band is removable and does not permanently alter the gastric anatomy. The most common band is marketed under the brand name LAP-BAND. (22)

Metabolic Syndrome

Metabolic syndrome is a collection of metabolic disturbances that increases the risk of atherosclerotic heart disease. Patients are characterized as having metabolic syndrome (also called **syndrome X**) if they display three or more of the following metabolic disturbances:

- increased triglycerides (greater than 150 mg/dL)
- decreased low-density lipoproteins with high-density lipoproteins less than 40 in males and less than 50 in females
- increased blood pressure (greater than 130/85 mmHg)
- fasting blood sugar greater than 110 mg/dL
- hyperuricemia (increased uric acid in the blood)
- abdominal obesity (waist circumference greater than 102 cm in males and 88 cm in females)
- prothrombotic state with increased plasminogen activator inhibitor–1 (PAI-1) and increased fibrinogen
- proinflammatory state (increased C-reactive protein)
- hyperinsulinemia with insulin resistance

- Obesity, especially abdominal visceral obesity, increases the risk of metabolic and structural disorders which cause a significant amount of morbidity and mortality.
- The degree of overweight and obesity are measured using the BMI.
- Medications may be prescribed to control appetite or to reduce absorption of fat.

- Bariatric surgery to reduce the size of the stomach may be used to reduce weight in patients with a BMI greater than 35.
- Metabolic syndrome has no particular symptoms but should be recognized and treated to reduce the risk of developing diabetes and heart disease.

The dominant, underlying characteristics of metabolic syndrome are abdominal obesity and insulin resistance. There are no particular symptoms of metabolic syndrome. Its significance lies in the recognition that patients with three or more of these criteria are at imminent risk of diabetes and atherosclerosis, and therefore, these patients should be managed aggressively to control as many of these risk factors as possible.

Hypothyroidism

The endocrine system controls body functions by releasing hormones directly into the blood. Hormones act on cells that possess the corresponding hormone receptors on their surface. The endocrine system uses a negative feedback system for communicating among the various endocrine glands and cells throughout the body. The thyroid gland, under the direction of the pituitary gland, is responsible for maintaining the body's temperature by raising and lowering the metabolic rate. When body temperature drops, a negative condition, the pituitary releases **thyroid stimulating hormone (TSH)**, the feedback, causing the thyroid to release more thyroid hormone.

Primary hypothyroidism is underactivity of the thyroid gland, causing inadequate production of the thyroid hormones triiodothyronine (T_3) and thyroxine (T_4). The most common form of hypothyroidism is **Hashimoto thyroiditis**, which is thought to be an autoimmune disorder. Antibodies (called anti-TPO) attack the thyroid gland, causing the gland to at first become enlarged (goiter) but later to recede, becoming shrunken and fibrotic.

Symptoms of hypothyroidism, also called **myxedema**, include a dull expression, hoarse speech, dry skin, cold intolerance, constipation, forgetfulness, weight gain, paresthesias in the hands and feet, bradycardia, fatigue, and depression. Women may have menorrhagia or amenorrhea. Hypothyroidism is diagnosed on the basis of laboratory studies, usually referred to as **thyroid function tests (TFTs)**. (23) Patients with hypothyroidism have increased TSH and decreased T_3 and T_4. Treatment requires replacement of thyroxine, usually for the remainder of the patient's life.

Hypothyroidism and hyperthyroidism are extremely difficult to differentiate when dictated. The medication list often provides the best clue as to which one to transcribe. Patients on thyroid replacement therapy are usually hypothyroid unless they have had a thyroidectomy due to hyperthyroidism.

(23) There are several tests that are collectively referred to as thyroid function tests, so the phrase/abbreviation should always be written as a plural.

- The thyroid gland, under control of the pituitary gland, controls the metabolic rate in order to control body temperature.
- A common cause of primary hypothyroidism is Hashimoto thyroiditis.

- Hypothyroidism is usually diagnosed by blood tests showing decreased T_3 and T_4 levels and increased TSH levels.
- Hypothyroidism is treated using thyroid hormone replacement.

> **Pause 2-8** Describe how the negative feedback system of the endocrine system is like a thermostat that controls the temperature of your home. Why are TSH levels inversely related to circulating thyroid hormone levels?

Laboratory Studies

Internal Medicine addresses many of the most common metabolic disorders and relies heavily on laboratory studies of blood and urine to diagnose and manage metabolic diseases. It is imperative that laboratory values be transcribed accurately, because laboratory tests are used to develop a diagnosis and form the basis of medical decisions. When dictating, physicians often read laboratory results directly from a laboratory report, which enables them to dictate incredibly fast, and consequently, not very clearly. Often lab values are dictated together in related groups or panels; therefore, knowing which tests are grouped together will help tremendously in deciphering lab test names and values.

Keep a reference list of laboratory values, grouped by panels and related tests, easily accessible while you transcribe. When having difficulty deciphering lab test names, look at the patient's symptoms or the diagnosis. Consider which tests are typically ordered to evaluate or manage the patient's known medical conditions and compare what you are hearing to the tests that are related to the patient's situation.

It is important to be familiar with the normal values (reference ranges) of the most common laboratory tests. *Always compare the values you have transcribed to the reference range to make sure the values are reasonable and physiologically possible.* Generally, laboratory values that have a small reference range are tightly controlled by the body, so values that fall far outside these ranges are often physiologically impossible. For example, the blood pH is maintained within an extremely narrow range of 7.35 to 7.45. Even a slight change in pH (eg, 7.7) is incompatible with life.

Basic Metabolic Profile

The **basic metabolic panel (BMP)** is one of the most common sets of tests ordered. It is not specific to any disease or disorder but nonetheless gives physicians valuable information about critical metabolic components. The BMP consists of eight tests that are fundamental to metabolic functions (**Table 2-1**). The BMP typically includes glucose, electrolytes (sodium, potassium, chloride, and CO_2), calcium, and kidney function tests (BUN and creatinine). Sodium, potassium, chloride, and bicarbonate interact to help the body maintain normal fluid levels in the intracellular and extracellular spaces, maintain acid-base balance (pH), and muscle contractility. The **anion gap** is sometimes reported with the BMP. This particular value is not actually measured but rather is calculated using the electrolyte values. The anion gap is the difference between the negatively charged and positively charged ions and molecules in the blood. A high anion gap is indicative of **metabolic acidosis (24)**, such as diabetic ketoacidosis. Low anion gap values are rare.

> It is important to transcribe the decimal in the potassium value, even when the decimal is zero. Typically, a zero trailing a decimal would not be transcribed, but the potassium value is maintained in such a tight range that the decimal point is always significant.

Blood urea nitrogen (BUN) and **creatinine** are screening tests to evaluate kidney function. BUN, a byproduct of protein metabolism, is excreted by the kidneys, and elevated levels of BUN are indicative of renal impairment or decreased blood flow to the kidneys. BUN may also be decreased in cases of severe protein deficiency. Creatinine is a normal byproduct of muscle breakdown and is produced at a constant rate; highly muscular individuals such as body builders may have normal creatinine values as high as 2 mg/dL. Creatinine is excreted through the kidneys, so a rise in *serum* creatinine is indicative of renal impairment or decreased blood volume passing through the kidney. The normal range for creatinine is very small. Very slight changes (two- or three-tenths above the reference range) are indicative of kidney disease, so always confirm that the dictated value fits the patient's clinical picture.

> **(24)** Metabolic acidosis is a decrease in pH of the body fluids. It may be caused by an accumulation of acid or the excess excretion of bases.

> You may hear dictators pronounce BUN as separate letters (b-u-n) or as the acronym "bun."

Table 2-1 Basic Metabolic Profile

Test name	Normal Range
Na+ (sodium)	136–145 mEq/L
K+ (potassium)	3.5 to 5 mEq/L
Cl⁻ (chloride)	100–106 mEq/L
HCO_3^- (bicarbonate)	24–30 mEq/L
CO_2	22–26 mEq/L
anion Gap	8–12 mEq/L*
Ca (calcium)	8.2 to 10.2 mg/dL
BUN (blood urea nitrogen)	5–20 mg/dL
creatinine	0.6 to 1.2 mg/dL
glucose (fasting)	60–115 mg/dL

* Anion gap reference ranges are highly dependent upon the method used by the lab to calculate the gap. Normal values may vary and the range reported by the laboratory should always be used when it differs from published reference ranges.

Be careful not to confuse creatine and creatinine. Creatinine is a metabolic byproduct found in the blood and excreted by the kidneys. Creatine is a nutritional supplement used by individuals who want to build muscle mass, and creatine kinase is an enzyme found in muscle tissue (see page 303).

Dictators may shorten bicarbonate to "bicarb."

Serum Glucose and Insulin

A blood glucose level may be ordered as a single test or as part of a panel of tests. Glucose levels may be elevated in diabetes, metabolic syndrome, or chronic states of stress. Glucose may be decreased for many reasons, but most notably during a diabetic crisis, insulin overdose, or as a result of fasting or starvation. Insulin levels may be evaluated, especially in patients suspected of insulin resistance. Hemoglobin A_{1c} is used to monitor average glucose levels over the preceding

90 days and to assess the efficacy of treatment or the patient's **noncompliance** with their prescribed diet and medication regimen. **Table 2-2** lists the normal ranges for glucose, insulin, and hemoglobin A_{1c}.

Table 2-2 Glucose and Related Tests

Test name	Normal Range
glucose (fasting)	60–115 mg/dL
insulin	5–25 microunits/mL
hemoglobin A_{1c}	4% to 6%

Osmolality

Urine osmolality and **serum osmolality** (**Table 2-3**) measure the concentration of all solutes (dissolved solids) in urine or serum, reported in milliosmoles per kilogram of water (mOsm/kg H_2O). Major solutes contributing to osmolality include glucose, albumin and other carrier proteins, electrolytes, and ketone bodies. Osmolality is important in the management of diabetic ketoacidosis and other metabolic disorders involving fluid balance. Also see Chapter 7 for a more detailed discussion of osmolality.

Table 2-3 Osmolality

Test name	Normal Range
osmolality, urine	50–1200 mOsm/kg H_2O
osmolality, serum	275–301 mOsm/kg H_2O

Cholesterol and Triglycerides

Physicians typically order a **fasting lipid panel** to determine cholesterol and triglyceride levels. Cholesterol values are reported as total cholesterol as well as the cholesterol fractions high-density lipoprotein (HDL) and low-density lipoprotein (LDL). You may also hear these values reported as **HDL-C** and **LDL-C**. Very low density lipoproteins (VLDL) may or may not be dictated. When the VLDL is not reported, the total cholesterol value should be slightly higher than the sum of the HDL and LDL values. You may also hear physicians dictate a **cholesterol ratio**. The ratio may be reported as total cholesterol to HDL cholesterol (calculated by dividing the total cholesterol value by the HDL value). A target value for this ratio is less than 5:1 with an optimal value of 3.5:1. When transcribing a ratio, the words are always written out using "to" and connecting hyphens to describe the ratio; numerical values are written with a colon.

D: The cholesterol to HDL ratio is five to one.
T: The cholesterol-to-HDL ratio is 5:1.

Further studies may be performed to more fully characterize the LDL cholesterol using nuclear magnetic resonance (NMR) spectroscopy. This test is marketed under the brand name **NMR LipoProfile**. Smaller, denser **LDL particles (LDL-P)** are considered more atherogenic than larger, more buoyant molecules. Patients with an LDL particle size of less than 255 (measured in ångströms) are classified as phenotype A (or type A), and patients with larger particles (above 255 ångströms) are classified as phenotype B (or type B). (See page 499 for the definition of phenotype). In addition to reporting particle size, the NMR LipoProfile reports the concentration of LDL-P in nanomoles per liter (nmol/L). An LDL-P concentration of less than 1000 is considered optimal and associated with a lower risk of atherosclerosis.

Triglycerides are considered an **independent risk factor** for the development of coronary heart disease. Normal levels are less than 160 mg/dL. Elevated levels are also associated with type 2 diabetes, obesity, and metabolic syndrome. Very high levels, above 1000 mg/dL, are associated with **familial hypertriglyceridemia**. Since triglyceride levels are normally high immediately following a meal, patients should be fasting to obtain baseline levels. **Table 2-4** lists the normal values for total cholesterol and related lipoproteins.

Thyroid Function Tests

Patients with suspected hyperthyroidism or hypothyroidism are first evaluated with standard thyroid function tests (TFTs). Although there are many tests available to evaluate thyroid function, the most common tests included in a thyroid function panel are T_3, T_4, and TSH. Additional thyroid studies may be ordered if these three values fail to provide a definitive diagnosis.

Table 2-4 Cholesterol and Related Lipoproteins

Test name	Normal Range
total cholesterol	<200 mg/dL
LDL (low-density lipoprotein)	40–130 mg/dL, optimal less than 70 mg/dL
HDL (high-density lipoprotein)	35–80 mg/dL, optimal greater than 40
VLDL (very low density lipoprotein)	5–40 mg/dL
triglycerides	<160 mg/dL
LDL particle size	<255 Å phenotype A >255 Å phenotype B (protective)
LDL-P concentration	<1000 nmol/L (optimal)
total LDL particle concentration (LDL-P)	<1000 nmol/L (optimal)
small LDL particle concentration	<600 nmol/L (optimal)
total HDL particle concentration	<23 mcmol/L (low)
large HDL particle concentration	<4.0 mcmol/L (low)

As with many hormones, the thyroid hormones T_3 and T_4 are attached to transport proteins in the blood. Only a very small fraction (less than 1%) of T_3 and T_4 are found in the blood not bound to either **thyroxine binding globulin (TBG)** or albumin. Only the free, unbound molecules, referred to as **free T3 (FT3)** and **free T4 (FT4)**, are metabolically active. The most common thyroid studies are listed in **Table 2-5**, although there are many other thyroid tests that may be ordered by an endocrinologist, a physician who specializes in interpreting these highly complex tests.

Listen carefully for *free T_3*. This test name can be tricky to hear correctly because each syllable has the long e sound and the beginning sounds are very similar.

Table 2-5 Thyroid Function Tests

Test Name	Normal Range
T_4 (thyroxine)	4.5 to 12 mcg/dL
free T_4 (FT$_4$)	0.8 to 2.7 ng/dL
T_3 (triiodothyronine)	70–190 ng/dL
free T_3 (FT$_3$)	260–480 pg/dL
TSH (thyroid stimulating hormone)	0.4 to 4.2 mcU/mL
TBG (thyroxine binding globulin)	1.25 to 2.5 mg/dL
resin T_3 uptake (RT$_3$U) (an indirect measure of TBG)	25% to 38%
antithyroid antibodies (also called anti-TPO or thyroid peroxidase antibodies)	None

Pharmacology

Diseases treated by the internal medicine physician are primarily treated pharmacologically. The list of medications you will encounter in this specialty is extensive but very important. These drugs are some of the most common prescriptions and will undoubtedly become part of your routine pharmacology vocabulary.

Insulin

Insulin is available as biosynthetic human insulin marketed under the names Humulin and Novolin. Insulin is dispensed as either regular (R) or (NPH) insulin and commonly as combinations of the two. Insulin is also available in several forms, called analogs, (25) which have very slight changes in the amino acid chains that make up the insulin molecule. These amino acid substitutions change the insulin molecule's biologic action. Some analogs are designed to be slowly absorbed and therefore have a long duration of action, while others are absorbed quickly after injection and are short-acting. **Table 2-6** lists various insulin preparations.

It is important to understand how insulin preparations are dispensed so you can accurately transcribe the type and amount of insulin prescribed. Insulin preparations are dispensed in concentrations of 100 units of insulin per milliliter (100 U/mL, also written U100) and 500 units of insulin per milliliter (U500). Many patients take a mixture of regular insulin and NPH insulin, so pharmaceutical companies premix insulins in set ratios. A common mixture is 70% NPH and 30% regular insulin, written 70/30 insulin. Since these numbers are percentages, they must always add up to 100 (eg, 70/35 would not be possible).

Patients requiring insulin self-inject insulin on average twice a day into areas of loose skin (abdomen, thighs, upper arms, flanks, and buttocks). Insulin is drawn into insulin syringes that are marked in 0.1 mL increments. Drawing the syringe to 0.3 would deliver 30 units of insulin U100 (ie, 1 mL contains 100 units of insulin, so three-tenths of 100 equals 30). Patients may also inject insulin based on their body weight and current blood sugar reading. The amount to be injected is calculated using a **sliding scale**.

(25) An analog is a molecule that is structurally very similar to the original molecule and has similar but not identical biologic activity.

Table 2-6 Insulin Preparations

Rapid-Acting Analogs	Short-Acting Analogs	Intermediate-Acting	Long-Acting	Premixed Insulins
insulin lispro (Humalog)	regular insulin (Humulin R, Novolin R)	NPH insulin (Humulin N, Novolin N)	insulin glargine (Lantus)	70/30 insulin 50/50 insulin (consisting of NPH and regular)
insulin aspart (NovoLog)			insulin detemir (Levemir)	NovoLog 70/30 (consisting of insulin aspart protamine and insulin aspart)
insulin glulisine (Apidra)				Humalog 70/30 Humalog 50/50 (consisting of insulin lispro protamine [NPL] and insulin lispro)

MEDICATIONS: Aspirin 325 mg a day, Humulin 70/30 as 50 units in the morning and 30 units in the evening, and sliding-scale insulin as needed.

Insulin may also be delivered using **continuous subcutaneous insulin infusion (CSII)**. Pumps, about the size of a pager, can be programmed to deliver an insulin **bolus** at specific times throughout a 24-hour period. Insulin pumps are marketed under brand names such as Medtronic MiniMed, MiniMed Paradigm, Animas, and Deltec Cozmo.

Antidiabetic Agents

Antidiabetic agents and oral hypoglycemic agents are medications (other than insulin) designed to reduce blood glucose levels. These drugs act by increasing insulin secretion, altering insulin action, or reducing glucose absorption. Often, patients take more than one hypoglycemic/antidiabetic agent.

Sulfonylureas

Sulfonylureas (**Table 2-7**) act directly on pancreatic B cells to increase insulin secretion. This particular class of drug is not helpful in type 1 diabetics. Note that the generic names in this class end in *–ide*.

Table 2-7 Sulfonylureas

Generic	Brand Name	Dose
glyburide	DiaBeta Glynase	1.25 mg, 2.5 mg, 5 mg 1.5 mg, 3 mg, 6 mg
glipizide	Glucotrol and Glucotrol XL	5 mg, 10 mg
glimepiride	Amaryl	1 mg, 2 mg, 4 mg

Thiazolidinediones

The thiazolidinedione class of antidiabetic medications (**Table 2-8**) sensitizes peripheral tissues to insulin. The generic names of drugs in this class end with *–glitazone*. These medications can be combined with insulin for treatment of type 2 diabetics with severe insulin resistance. They may also be combined with sulfonylureas and metformin.

Table 2-8 Thiazolidinediones

Generic	Brand Name	Dose
rosiglitazone	Avandia	2 mg, 4 mg
pioglitazone	Actos	15 mg, 30 mg, 45 mg
rosiglitazone and glimepiride	Avandaryl	4 mg/1 mg, 4 mg/2 mg, 4 mg/4 mg, 8 mg/2 mg, 8 mg/4 mg

Biguanides

Metformin (**Table 2-9**) is the only drug in the biguanide class. Its primary action is to alter insulin action. It can be used alone or in combination with other oral medications to lower blood glucose levels.

Table 2-9 Metformin

Generic	Brand Name	Dose
metformin	Glucophage and Glucophage XR	500 mg, 850 mg, 1000 mg
rosiglitazone and metformin	Avandamet	2 mg/500 mg, 2 mg/1000 mg, 4 mg/500 mg, and 4 mg/1000 mg
glipizide and metformin	Metaglip	2.5 mg/250 mg, 2.5 mg/500 mg, 5 mg/500 mg

Miscellaneous Antidiabetic Drugs

Exenatide (Byetta) is an injectable drug called an incretin. This medication amplifies the release of insulin. One other drug that has a similar action is sitagliptin (Januvia). Combinations of these drugs are also available (**Table 2-10**).

Table 2-10 Miscellaneous Antidiabetic Drugs

Generic	Brand Name	Dose
exenatide	Byetta	1.2 mg, 2.4 mL
sitagliptin	Januvia	25 mg, 50 mg, 100 mg
sitagliptin and metformin	Janumet	50 mg/500 mg, 50 mg/1000 mg

The drug name Byetta is difficult to distinguish at times, but it is one of the few drugs that contains a decimal in the dose. This can be a helpful clue when deciphering what you hear.

Antilipemic Medications

This group of medications lowers cholesterol and triglyceride levels or alters the ratio of LDL and HDL cholesterol.

Statins

Statins (**Table 2-11**) are used to lower total cholesterol values, and they derive their name from the ending applied to generic drugs in this class. These drugs inhibit HMG-CoA reductase, an enzyme that participates in the production of cholesterol. These medications may cause liver and muscle damage, so liver function studies are monitored routinely.

Table 2-11 Statins

Generic	Brand Name	Dose
atorvastatin	Lipitor	10 mg, 20 mg, 40 mg, 80 mg
rosuvastatin	Crestor	5 mg, 10 mg, 20 mg, 40 mg
simvastatin	Zocor	5 mg, 10 mg, 20 mg, 40 mg, 80 mg
ezetimibe and simvastatin	Vytorin	10 mg/10 mg, 10 mg/20 mg, 10 mg/40 mg, 10 mg/80 mg

Bile Acid Binding Resins (Sequestrants)

The bile acid binding resins (**Table 2-12**) are also called sequestrants because they bind bile acids in the intestine and prevent the reabsorption and recycling of cholesterol through the portal circulation. Side effects include constipation and gas. Note that resins are dispensed in grams, not milligrams.

Table 2-12 Sequestrants

Generic	Brand Name	Dose
cholestyramine	Questran	4 g

Fibrates

Fibrates (fibric acids), listed in **Table 2-13**, are used to reduce triglyceride levels and VLDL. Note that the names of the drugs include the syllable *fib*.

Table 2-13 Fibrates

Generic	Brand Name	Dose
fenofibrate	TriCor	48 mg, 145 mg
gemfibrozil	Lopid	600 mg

Nutritional Derivatives

Pharmaceutical-grade niacin dispensed in high doses is used to lower LDL cholesterol. Niacin is known to cause facial flushing, which may discourage patients from taking their medicine regularly. Doses may be **titrated (26)** to help alleviate the side effects. Niacin may be given alone or combined with a statin drug (**Table 2-14**). Omega-3 oils (often in the form of fish oil) are used to lower triglyceride levels. These drugs are given in high doses and may be dictated in milligrams or grams (1000 mg equals 1 g).

Table 2-14 Nutritional Derivatives

Generic	Brand Name	Dose
niacin	Niaspan	500 mg, 750 mg, 1000 mg
lovastatin and niacin	Advicor	500 mg/20 mg, 750 mg/20 mg, 1000 mg/20 mg, 1000 mg/40 mg
omega-3 oils (as omega-3 acid ethyl esters)	Lovaza	1 g

(26) Titrated doses are either increased or decreased incrementally over the course of several days or weeks. Titrating medication doses helps the body adjust and lessens the side effects of starting or suddenly stopping a drug.

Antihypertensives

Antihypertensives are used to treat hypertension. There are many classes of antihypertensives that address the many causes of hypertension. Generally, antihypertensive medications either decrease vascular resistance or decrease overall fluid volume, but there are many ways in which these drugs approach these goals.

Receptor Blockers

Alpha-receptor blockers (**Table 2-15**) and beta-receptor blockers (**Table 2-16**) act by blocking the action of epinephrine on various types of smooth muscle cells in the heart, blood vessels, and bronchi. Alpha receptors are found on the surface of smooth muscle cells in the heart. Beta 1-receptors are also found on the surface of smooth muscle cells in the heart, and beta 2-receptors are found on smooth muscle cells in the peripheral blood vessels and bronchioles. Generic names for the alpha-blockers end in *–zosin*. Generic names for the beta-blockers end in *–olol*.

Table 2-15 Alpha-Receptor Blockers

Generic	Brand Name	Dose
doxazosin	Cardura	1 mg, 2 mg, 4 mg, 8 mg
prazosin	Minipress	1 mg, 2 mg, 5 mg
terazosin	Hytrin	1 mg, 2 mg, 5 mg, 10 mg

Table 2-16 Beta-Receptor Blockers

Generic	Brand Name	Dose
atenolol	Tenormin	24 mg, 50 mg, 100 mg
metoprolol	Toprol	25 mg, 50 mg, 100 mg
	Toprol XL	25 mg, 50 mg, 100 mg, 200 mg
	Lopressor	50 mg, 100 mg
propranolol	Inderal LA	60 mg, 80 mg, 120 mg, 160 mg
	Inderal	10 mg, 20 mg, 40 mg, 80 mg
sotalol	Betapace	80 mg, 120 mg, 160 mg, 240 mg
carvedilol	Coreg	3.125 mg, 6.25 mg, 12.5 mg, 25 mg

ACE Inhibitors

ACE inhibitors (**Table 2-17**) interfere with angiotensin-converting enzyme. ACE inhibitors limit the body's ability to constrict blood vessels, thereby lowering blood pressure. The medications in this class end in *–pril*. The most common side effect of ACE inhibitors is a dry cough.

Table 2-17 ACE Inhibitors

Generic	Brand Name	Dose
fosinopril	Monopril	40 mg
captopril	Capoten	12.5 mg, 25 mg, 50 mg, 100 mg
enalapril	Vasotec	2.5 mg, 5 mg, 10 mg, 20 mg
lisinopril	Prinivil	5 mg, 10 mg, 20 mg
	Zestril	2.5 mg, 5 mg, 10 mg, 20 mg, 30 mg, 40 mg

Angiotensin II Receptor Blockers

This class of drug blocks angiotensin II receptors, thereby preventing vasoconstriction of blood vessels. Generic drugs in this class (**Table 2-18**) end in *–sartan*.

Table 2-18 ARBs

Generic	Brand Name	Dose
candesartan	Atacand	4 mg, 8 mg, 16 mg, and 32 mg
losartan	Cozaar	25 mg, 50 mg, and 100 mg
valsartan	Diovan	40 mg, 80 mg, 160 mg, and 320 mg

Hydrochlorothiazide

Hydrochlorothiazide is a diuretic that acts on the kidney to increase sodium and potassium excretion, and because water follows sodium, water excretion is also increased. Decreasing total body fluid volume results in decreased blood pressure. Diuretics that cause the increased excretion of potassium are usually prescribed with a potassium supplement to prevent hypokalemia. The most common diuretic used to treat hypertension is **hydrochlorothiazide (HCT** or **HCTZ)**. Although commonly prescribed as a single agent, many antihypertensives are prescribed in combination with hydrochlorothiazide (**Table 2-19**). Other types of diuretics are described on page 224.

Table 2-19 Drugs Containing Hydrochlorothiazide

Generic	Brand Name	Dose
hydrochlorothiazide		12.5 mg, 25 mg
metoprolol and hydrochlorothiazide	Lopressor HCT	50 mg/25 mg, 100 mg/25 mg, 100 mg/50 mg
benazepril and hydrochlorothiazide	Lotensin HCT	5 mg/6.25 mg, 10 mg/12.5 mg, 20 mg/12.5 mg, 20 mg/25 mg
lisinopril and hydrochlorothiazide	Prinzide	10 mg/12.5 mg, 20 mg/25 mg
lisinopril and hydrochlorothiazide	Zestoretic	10 mg/12.5 mg, 20 mg/12.5 mg, 20 mg/25 mg
captopril and hydrochlorothiazide	Capozide	25 mg/15 mg, 25 mg/25 mg, 50 mg/15 mg, 50 mg/25 mg
losartan and hydrochlorothiazide	Hyzaar	50 mg/12.5 mg, 100 mg/12.5 mg, 100 mg/25 mg

Although you will often hear the abbreviation HCTZ dictated, it is on the list of dangerous abbreviations and should be spelled out. Some drug manufacturers use the abbreviation HCT as part of the brand name in combination drugs that contain hydrochlorothiazide (eg, Atacand HCT, Benicar HCT). When dictated as part of the brand name, it is acceptable to use the abbreviation HCT. Be sure you do not confuse HCT (uppercase) with Hct, the abbreviation for hematocrit.

Potassium Supplements

Patients taking potassium-losing diuretics such as hydrochlorothiazide typically require concomitant potassium supplementation to prevent hypokalemia. Potassium supplements (**Table 2-20**) come in a variety of forms including effervescent tablets, powders, liquid, and capsules. A common side effect of potassium supplementation is gastric upset. It is important to note that potassium is dispensed in **milliequivalents (mEq)**.

Table 2-20 Potassium Supplements

Generic	Brand Name	Dose
potassium chloride (KCl)	Kay Ciel	20 mEq
	K-Dur	10 mEq, 20 mEq
	Klor-Con	8 mEq, 10 mEq, 10 mEq, 15 mEq, 20 mEq
	microK	8 mEq, 10 mEq

Listen carefully for Micro-K vs Micronase. The largest dose of Micronase is 5 mg and MicroK is dispensed in milliequivalents, the lowest of which is 8 mEq. The dose should help distinguish the two medications.

The brand name Kay Ciel sounds exactly like the chemical name KCl, making it impossible to know which is intended. When in doubt, transcribe the generic name instead of the brand name.

Thyroid Replacement

Thyroid replacement (**Table 2-21**) comes in two major forms: synthetic T_3 and T_4 or as a thyroid extract (desiccant). It is important to note that Synthroid and the other synthetic forms of T_4 are dispensed in micrograms. The thyroxine dose must be matched to the patient's exact needs, so thyroid replacement is available in many dosages with small increments to more easily customize the patient's dose. Armour Thyroid (note the spelling of Arm*our*) is a naturally derived preparation from desiccated thyroid tissue and contains both levothyroxine (T_4) and L-triiodothyronine (T_3). Also note that Armour Thyroid is dispensed in milligrams, not micrograms.

Table 2-21 Thyroid Replacement

Generic	Brand Name	Dose
T_4 (levothyroxine)	Synthroid, Levoxyl, Levothroid	from 25 to 300 mcg
desiccated thyroid extract (levothyroxine [T_4] and L-triiodothyronine [T_3])	Armour Thyroid	from 15 to 300 mg

Carefully consider the thyroid dose and units when dictated. Physicians are so accustomed to dictating dosages in milligrams that they often misspeak and dictate thyroid replacement medications in milligrams instead of micrograms. Always double-check the dose and the units to make sure they correspond.

Hypnotics and Anxiolytics

Hypnotics and anxiolytics are commonly prescribed by internal medicine physicians and are among the most widely used prescription medications. **Table 2-22** lists two commonly prescribed hypnotics (sleep aids) used to treat insomnia.

Table 2-22 Hypnotics

Generic	Brand Name	Dose
zolpidem tartrate	Ambien Ambien CR	5 mg, 10 mg 6.25 mg, 12.5 mg
eszopiclone	Lunesta	1 mg, 2 mg, 3 mg

The benzodiazepine class of medications is used to treat anxiety and sleep disorders. They may also be used as a sedative or amnesiac given prior to diagnostic procedures. **Table 2-23** lists the most common benzodiazepines. Note that most of the generic names in this class end in *–pam*.

Table 2-23 Benzodiazepines

Generic	Brand Name	Dose
alprazolam	Xanax	0.25 mg, 0.5 mg, 1 mg, 2 mg
clonazepam	Klonopin	0.5 mg, 1 mg, 2 mg
lorazepam	Ativan	0.5 mg, 1 mg, 2 mg
temazepam	Restoril	7.5 mg, 15 mg, 22.5 mg, 30 mg
diazepam	Valium	2 mg, 5 mg, 10 mg

Exercises

Using Context to Make Decisions

Use the following dictated lab values to answer questions 1 and 2.

TSH 6.0, T_3 50, anti-TPO positive, cholesterol 200, sodium 136, potassium 3.5, chloride 102, BUN 30, creatinine 2.0.

1. Which of the following assessments is consistent with these lab values?

    a. Hypothyroidism and renal impairment

    b. Hyperthyroidism and renal impairment

    c. Hypothyroidism and hyperkalemia

    d. Hyperthyroidism and hyperkalemia

2. Which of the following would not be possible?

    a. LDL-P 255

    b. VLDL 30

    c. LDL 150, HDL 50

    d. Triglycerides 130

Use the sample report on page 461 in Appendix B to answer questions 3–5:

3. Has the patient been able to control his/her blood glucose levels over the preceding weeks? Explain your answer. _____

_____

4. What does CPAP stand for? _____

_____

5. What evidence is there that the patient's dyslipidemia is controlled? _____

_____

Use the excerpt on page 53 to answer questions 6–15.

6. Review the rules in the *Book of Style* for transcribing a zero trailing, a decimal point, and a zero leading a decimal point. Assuming a zero is not dictated, which of the following are transcribed correctly?

potassium 3.0	calcium 9.30
chloride 103.0	free T_4 .8
glucose 250.0	Metaglip 2.5/250.0 mg
creatinine 0.9	

7. Blank #1 sounds like "h*lin.". What word would be transcribed in blank #1? _____

8. What number would be transcribed in blank #2?

_____

9. How would you expand the abbreviation DKA? _____. Could the physician have actually dictated BKA? Why or why not?

_____

10. What word would be transcribed in blank #3?

_____

11. Blank #4 sounds like "ach-tee-en.". What would you transcribe here? _____

12. What prefix (hypo or hyper) would be transcribed in blank #5? _____

13. In Plan #2, CBG stands for _____

_____.

14. Blank #6 sounds like "sly* ale.". What would you transcribe here? _____

15. Which item under Plan contains a transcription error (hint: the error is not a punctuation error)?

_____

Terms Checkup

Complete the multiple choice questions for Chapter 2 located at www.myhealthprofessionskit.com. To access the questions, select the discipline "Medical

Transcription," then click on the title of this book, *Advanced Medical Transcription*.

Look It Up

Using the guidelines described on page xvii, complete a research project on hyperthyroidism.

Antidepressants are among the most commonly prescribed medications and will be encountered in reports from all specialties. Perform an Internet search for the most commonly prescribed drugs (the most recent year available) and extract from the list the most commonly prescribed selective serotonin reuptake inhibitors (SSRIs) and serotonin-norepinephrine reuptake inhibitors (SNRIs).

Transcription Practice

1. Transcribe the key terms and phrases for Chapter 2.
2. Complete the proofing and transcription practice exercises for Chapter 2.

HISTORY OF PRESENT ILLNESS: The patient was admitted to Memorial Hospital on September 23 by her urologist, Dr. Carter, and stayed for 3 days. She was treated for a urinary tract infection with E coli sepsis and a newly diagnosed neurogenic bladder that was felt to be due to long-standing diabetes. During that hospital stay, Internal Medicine was consulted and increased her insulin and took her off Avandamet, which she had been taking along with insulin at home. They noted that her hemoglobin A_{1c} was very high at 12.6. The patient apparently was not checking her sugar very often at home prior to that hospital stay but now is checking it at least 3 times a day. When she first went in the hospital, her sugar was over 434, but she says this morning it is down to 119. She is currently on _____(1)_____ 70/30 insulin 50 units in the morning and 30 units in the evening and is on an 1800-calorie ADA diet. She is also trying to walk more. Incidentally, the patient states she has been cold lately and has very dry skin. She sounds a bit hoarse today.

IMPRESSION

1. Insulin-dependent diabetes mellitus with recent poor control. It sounds like she has type _____(2)_____ insulin-requiring diabetes mellitus. She does not report a history of DKA.
2. Neurogenic _____(3)_____ due to #1.
3. Recent urinary tract infection with sepsis, treated.
4. _____(4)_____ , well controlled on metoprolol.
5. Obesity.
6. Elevated lipids.
7. Probable stress urinary incontinence by history.
8. Depression and insomnia.
9. Need to rule out _____(5)_____ thyroidism.

PLAN

1. Continue current medications except try to wean off the Elavil because of the neurogenic bladder. She was given 10 mg tabs to take 1–2 at bedtime as needed and taper off.
2. Continue to check CBGs 3–4 times a day until her blood sugars are controlled and add _____(6)_____ Humulin R if needed.
3. ProSom 2 mg at bedtime as needed, #30, with 5 refills.
4. Continue weight loss efforts and 1500- to 1800-calorie ADA diet. She was given an order for a dietitian and diabetic education.
5. Celexa 20 mg ½ tab a day for 1 week and then 1 a day.
6. Labs: BNP for kidney function, CBC, lipid profile, free T_4, TSH, hemoglobin A_{1c}, and UA.
7. Exercise more. Continue weight loss efforts.

3

Gastroenterology: The Alimentary Tract

Learning Objectives

After completing this chapter, you should be able to comprehend and correctly transcribe terminology related to:

▶ diseases of the upper gastrointestinal tract, including esophageal disorders and diseases of the stomach and duodenum

▶ diseases of the lower gastrointestinal tract including gastroenteritis, acute abdomen, mesenteric ischemia, bleeding, and obstruction

▶ diseases of the small intestine, colon, and rectum

▶ laboratory and imaging tests used to diagnose and monitor diseases of the upper and lower gastrointestinal tract

▶ drugs used in the treatment of upper and lower gastrointestinal disorders

Introduction

Gastroenterology is the medical specialty that is concerned with diseases of the alimentary tract (also called the digestive tract), biliary tree, and organs that contribute to digestion and elimination. The most common gastrointestinal (GI) complaints include dyspepsia, indigestion, nausea, vomiting, regurgitation, belching, flatus, hematemesis, hematochezia, jaundice, diarrhea, constipation, acute or chronic abdominal pain, and tenesmus.

Often, no physiologic cause for a patient's GI complaints can be found, even after extensive evaluation, and these patients are said to have functional illness. **Functional abdominal pain syndrome (FAPS)** is pain that persists longer than six months without evidence of physiologic disease. The pain is significant enough to interfere with daily functioning. This syndrome shows no relationship to eating, bowel movements, menses, or other normal physiologic events. It is thought that some patients have visceral hypersensitivity in which they experience discomfort caused by luminal distention and peristalsis, sensations that other people do not find uncomfortable. Psychological conditions such as anxiety, conversion disorder, and somatization in depression may also cause GI symptoms. **Nonulcer (functional) dyspepsia** is defined as dyspeptic symptoms in a patient who has no abnormalities on physical examination or on upper GI endoscopy.

Disorders of the Upper Gastrointestinal Tract

The upper gastrointestinal tract (UGI) is the source of much discomfort, and many patient complaints result from disorders of the esophagus and stomach. Patients may have symptoms associated with a specific disorder or may suffer from pain and discomfort due to lifestyle choices and diet. Upper GI complaints include chest pain, dysphagia, odynophagia, dyspepsia, lump in the throat, halitosis, hiccups, nausea, and vomiting. One particular symptom with no known etiology is **globus sensation**, also called **globus hystericus**, which is the sensation of a lump or mass in the throat unrelated to swallowing. Patients with this complaint do not actually have a lump or mass, and typically no reason can be found for the globus sensation.

Esophageal Disorders

Primary disorders of the esophagus are characterized by heartburn, odynophagia, and dysphagia. Heartburn is a feeling of substernal burning that often radiates to the neck. Odynophagia is sharp, substernal pain on swallowing that is indicative of severe erosive disease or infectious esophagitis caused by candida infection, herpesvirus, cytomegalovirus, injury due to ingestion of corrosive substances, or from pill-induced ulcers. Dysphagia (difficulty swallowing) may be the result of difficulty transferring the **bolus of food** from the oropharynx to the esophagus (**oropharyngeal dysphasia**). Dysphagia may also be caused by impaired transport of the bolus through the esophagus (**esophageal dysphagia**) due to a motility disorder or a mechanical lesion obstructing the esophagus.

> **Pause 3-1** Compare and contrast the combining forms *-phagia* and *-phasia*. Give examples of contextual clues that will help you distinguish between the use of dysphagia and dysphasia. Give an example of a condition that causes dysphasia.

Normally, food moves through the alimentary canal by a mechanism referred to as **peristalsis**, which is characterized by alternating waves of circular contractions and relaxations of a tubular structure. **Achalasia** is an esophageal motility disorder caused by uncoordinated contractions of the esophagus and a failure of the **lower esophageal sphincter (LES)** to relax. Symptoms of achalasia include slowly progressive dysphagia, **nocturnal regurgitation** of undigested food, halitosis, and chest discomfort. Patients with esophageal motility disorders (also called **dysmotility**) have dysphasia for both liquids and solids. Motility disorders may be caused by upper esophageal sphincter dysfunction, diffuse esophageal spasm, or scleroderma. **Disordered motility** may also have a neurologic origin (eg, cerebrovascular accident). Motility disorders may be treated with a **prokinetic**, which is a drug that increases contractile force and accelerates intraluminal transit. Surgical treatment may include a **Heller myotomy**, which cuts the muscle of the LES and allows food to pass more easily. A myotomy may also be combined with a **Dor fundoplication** (a partial anterior plication).

Patients with mechanical obstruction typically have **dysphagia for solids** but not liquids. Mechanical obstruction may be caused by a **Schatzki ring**, which is a smooth, benign, circumferential ring of tissue that forms in the esophagus just above the stomach. The ring narrows the esophagus, preventing solid food from passing easily. Rings are almost always associated with hiatal hernia and reflux symptoms. Rings over 20 mm in diameter are typically asymptomatic. Rings less than 13 mm in diameter typically cause solid-food dysphagia. Large boluses of poorly chewed food are most likely to become "stuck" and can often be dislodged by drinking fluids.

Impacted boluses must be removed endoscopically. Rings are diagnosed using a barium esophagogram and are effectively treated with a large **bougie dilator**. (1)

Mechanical obstructions may also be caused by **peptic stricture**, esophageal cancer, or **eosinophilic esophagitis**. Peptic stricture causes a gradually progressive dysphagia for solid foods. Structural disorders leading to dysphagia include Zenker diverticulum, cervical osteophytes, cricopharyngeal bar, proximal esophageal webs, postsurgical, and radiation changes.

> The patient is a 63-year-old fit gentleman who has had severe dysphagia and was noted to have peristalsis of the antral body with failure to relax the LES on manometry. He also had an upper GI series with a classic bird's beak deformity and a dilated esophagus with retained food, all consistent with classic achalasia.

> **Pause 3-2** Using Google, perform an image search for Schatzki ring. Copy/paste into your notes both a diagram and an x-ray image of a Schatzki ring.

Upper endoscopy can be used to diagnose and simultaneously treat dysphagia. Strictures may be successfully dilated using **flexible weighted bougies**, catheters, or balloons. Dilation of 13 to 17 mm typically relieves dysphagia due to narrowing of the esophagus. Barium swallow, also called barium esophagography, is often used to diagnose dysphasia and odynophagia. **Esophageal manometry** (also called **esophageal motility studies** or **esophageal function studies**) may be used to assess esophageal contractions, esophageal motility, and LES pressure.

Zenker diverticulum is a protrusion of the pharyngeal mucosa at the pharyngoesophageal junction. Symptoms tend to develop slowly and insidiously and include oropharyngeal dysphagia, coughing, and throat discomfort. As the diverticulum enlarges, food may become trapped, and patients complain of halitosis, regurgitation of undigested food, nocturnal choking, gurgling, or a protrusion in the neck. Complications include aspiration pneumonia, bronchiectasis, and lung abscess. Diagnosis requires a barium esophagogram, and treatment consists of diverticulectomy.

Heartburn

Heartburn, also called **pyrosis** and acid indigestion, is characterized by substernal burning that often radiates to the neck. The burning sensation is caused by the reflux of acidic stomach contents into the esophagus. Rarely, heartburn may be caused by an alkaline reflux into the esophagus. Occasional heartburn may result from eating a spicy meal or a large meal, causing gastric distention and upward pressure on the LES. Chronic heartburn is pathognomonic (2) for gastroesophageal reflux disease. Occasional episodes of heartburn are easily treated with antacids containing calcium carbonate or magnesium hydroxide (eg, Tums and Rolaids). Overuse of these antacids can cause constipation, diarrhea, or more serious problems such as alkalosis, kidney stones, and hypermagnesemia.

Gastroesophageal Reflux Disease (GERD)

Gastroesophageal reflux disease (GERD) affects 20% of adults who report at least weekly episodes of heartburn and up to 10% of individuals who report daily symptoms. The lower esophageal sphincter normally closes to retain the stomach's contents, preventing the churning motion of the stomach from pushing gastric juices upward into the esophagus. The ability of the sphincter to retain gastric contents depends on intrinsic LES pressure, the location of the sphincter, and the extrinsic compression of the sphincter by the diaphragm. A common cause of GERD is an incompetent

(1) A bougie (*boo zhē*) is a cylindrical instrument used to calibrate or dilate a tubular structure such as the esophagus or urethra. Bougies may be used to guide the insertion of other instruments. Some are equipped with pressure sensors and some have balloons for dilating strictures or removing obstructions. These instruments get their name from the French word bougie (candle), because they resemble the shape of a candle.

(2) A pathognomonic symptom or sign is a characteristic observation so closely associated with a disease that its presence is almost sufficient to make a diagnosis.

lower esophageal sphincter. Normal baseline pressure is 10–30 mmHg. Some patients have a chronically incompetent sphincter, causing free reflux. Decreased sphincter competence can also cause stress reflux, which occurs during lifting, bending, or abdominal straining.

> ▶ Gastroesophageal reflux disease (GERD) is almost always referred to by its acronym, pronounced "gurd."

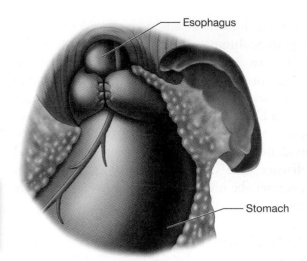

Esophagus

Stomach

FIGURE 3-1 A Nissen fundoplication wraps the upper fundus around the lower esophagus and is used to treat refractory GERD and hiatus hernia.

Although increased reflux episodes occur while eating, the swallowing reflex causes increased peristalsis and concomitant relaxation of the LES, allowing reflux to quickly return to the stomach. Also, acid in the esophagus is neutralized by bicarbonate in the saliva. During sleep, swallowing is decreased, thereby decreasing peristalsis and exposing the esophagus to acid for longer periods of time. Impaired salivation, resulting from Sjögren syndrome, anticholinergic medications, and other oral medications, can exacerbate GERD because of decreased bicarbonate and fewer swallowing episodes. Delayed gastric emptying due to gastroparesis (3) or partial **gastric outlet obstruction** also worsens GERD. A hiatus hernia, or hiatal hernia, can worsen reflux or be the primary cause of reflux due to the displacement of the LES by the hiatal sac pushing through the diaphragm.

Atypical symptoms of GERD include asthma, chronic cough, chronic laryngitis, sore throat, and **noncardiac chest pain**. GERD may be the primary cause of these symptoms or it may exacerbate these problems when they already exist. Untreated, GERD can lead to esophageal mucosal damage (**reflux esophagitis**) and other more serious complications such as Barrett esophagus (see page 58) or peptic stricture. (4)

The goal of treatment is to provide symptomatic relief, heal esophagitis, and prevent complications. Treatment includes **H₂-receptor antagonists**, **proton pump inhibitors (PPIs)**, and lifestyle modifications. Raising the head of the bed six inches, avoiding lying down within two to three hours of eating, and avoiding foods and habits that relax the LES or delay gastric emptying (eg, high-fat meals, peppermint, chocolate, alcohol, and smoking) all help to retain food in the

stomach and discourage reflux. Also, weight loss, avoiding bending after meals, and reducing meal size may be helpful. Relapse occurs in 80% of patients that discontinue antacid therapy. Refractory cases may be treated surgically with a **Nissen fundoplication** (■ Figure 3-1). Endoscopic treatment may include a **Stretta procedure** that uses radiofrequency energy to heat the target tissues. This intentional tissue damage causes the tissue to constrict and the muscle wall to thicken. These changes decrease the frequency of **transient lower esophageal sphincter relaxations (tLESRs)**, a major contributor to GERD.

Esophagitis

Esophagitis is inflammation of the esophageal mucosa. About 10% of patients with chronic esophagitis develop esophageal (peptic) stricture. Severe esophagitis may lead to esophageal erosion and esophageal hemorrhage. Upper endoscopy will demonstrate single

(3) Gastroparesis is a weakness in the peristaltic action of the stomach, causing delayed emptying of the stomach's contents.

(4) A peptic stricture is a narrowing of the esophagus, usually in the area of the squamocolumnar junction, caused by esophageal damage from acid reflux.

or multiple erosions or ulcers in the distal esophagus at the **squamocolumnar junction**, also known as the **Z line**. The Los Angeles classification grades esophageal abnormalities on a scale of A to D, with A being one or more isolated mucosal breaks of less than or equal to 5 mm and D denoting lesions that extend to 75% of the esophageal circumference. Patients without endoscopic evidence of disease have **nonerosive esophageal reflux disease (NERD)**. Ambulatory esophageal pH monitoring may be used to assess NERD but is usually not necessary.

Barrett Esophagus

A long-term complication of untreated or undertreated GERD is **Barrett esophagus**. In the setting of chronic irritation, squamous epithelium of the esophagus is replaced by metaplastic tissue. On endoscopy, Barrett's appears orange with gastric-type epithelium that extends upward from the stomach into the distal tubular esophagus in a tongue-like or circumferential fashion. Barrett's is confirmed on biopsy. Barrett esophagus carries an increased risk of adenocarcinoma, and patients with known Barrett esophagus should have routine endoscopic surveillance. The first line of treatment for Barrett's is PPI therapy, and if this is unsuccessful, endoscopic mucosal resection,

photodynamic therapy, cryotherapy, or laser ablation may be used. In extreme cases, patients may undergo fundoplication.

> **Pause 3-3** In the previous section, Barrett is written both with and without the apostrophe s. Using the *Book of Style* as a reference, explain why both are correct.

Hiatal Hernia

The esophagus passes through a hiatus in the crural area (5) of the diaphragm. **Hiatal hernia** (also called **hiatus hernia**) is a protrusion of the stomach through an opening in the diaphragm. Most hernias are asymptomatic and typically do not cause problems. While there is no causal relationship between hiatal hernia and GERD, patients who have a hernia as well as GERD have more severe symptoms of esophagitis and are more likely to develop Barrett esophagus. A **sliding hiatal hernia**, where the gastroesophageal (GE) junction and a portion of the stomach are above the diaphragm, rarely needs treatment other than treating symptoms of GERD if present. A **paraesophageal hiatal hernia**, where the GE junction is in the normal location but a portion of the stomach lies adjacent to the esophagus, may incarcerate and strangulate (■ Figure 3-2). Paraesophageal hernias should be **surgically reduced** to prevent strangulation and infarction of the affected tissue. Larger hernias are often diagnosed incidentally on chest x-ray, and smaller hernias are typically noted on barium swallow.

> **(5)** Crural comes from the Latin word *crus*, meaning leg. The crura of the diaphragm are leg-shaped structures made of tendinous material that extend from the diaphragm to the vertebral column.

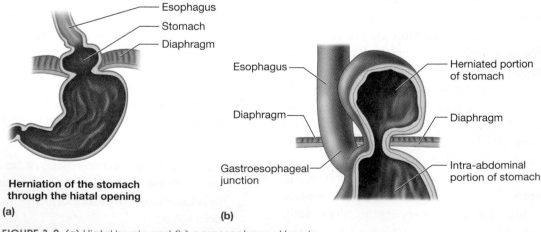

Herniation of the stomach through the hiatal opening

(a)

(b)

FIGURE 3-2 (a) Hiatal hernia and (b) paraesophageal hernia.

- Esophageal disorders are characterized by heartburn, dysphagia, and odynophagia.
- Chronic heartburn is pathognomonic for GERD.
- Heartburn, GERD, and esophagitis are treated with acid-suppression therapy.

- Hiatal hernia may exacerbate GERD. Para-esophageal hernias should be reduced to prevent strangulation.
- Untreated disorders of the esophagus may lead to strictures, rings, obstruction, or malignancy.

ASSESSMENT: Cervical esophageal dysphagia concerning for primary esophageal or posterior pharyngeal pathology. Differential diagnosis includes reflux esophagitis, esophageal stricture, Schatzki ring, Barrett esophagus, and/or underlying obstructive esophageal lesion.

Pause 3-4 Describe strangulation and incarceration as these terms relate to parts of the body.

Stomach and Duodenum

Stomach acid in the form of **hydrochloric acid (HCl)** plays a central role in digestion. Acid is secreted by parietal cells in the body of the stomach (■ Figure 3-3). Acid secreted during digestion lowers the pH for optimal functioning of pepsin and gastric lipase. The acid also stimulates pancreatic bicarbonate secretion to neutralize the acid using a negative feedback loop. The stomach mucosa is protected from the damaging effects of acid (low pH) by a layer of mucus as well as the neutralizing effects of bicarbonate (HCO_3^-). While stomach acid plays a critical role in digestion, it is also implicated in many disorders of the esophagus, stomach, and duodenum.

Gastritis

Gastritis (not to be confused with gastroenteritis) is inflammation of the gastric mucosa. Factors that interfere with mucosal defenses lead to damage of the gastric mucosa with ensuing erosion and/or inflammation. Common causes of gastritis include bacterial infection, drugs (most commonly NSAIDs and alcohol), acute stress, and autoimmune phenomena. Gastritis may be described as erosive or nonerosive.

An inherited cause of nonerosive gastritis is **autoimmune metaplastic atrophic gastritis (AMAG)**. In this disease, antibodies attack the fundic glands, causing **achlorhydria** (too little hydrochloric acid) and loss of **intrinsic factor**. Without intrinsic factor, B_{12} is not absorbed. Vitamin B_{12} is required for the production of red blood cells, and the lack of B_{12} results in pernicious anemia. Gastrectomy and chronic treatment with proton pump inhibitors also cause a deficiency of intrinsic factor and resultant anemia.

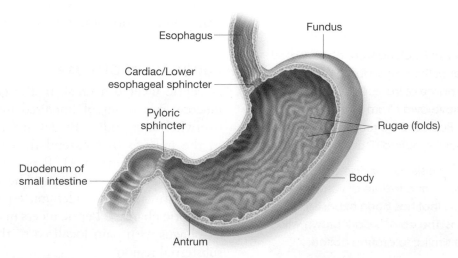

Esophagus

Cardiac/Lower esophageal sphincter

Pyloric sphincter

Duodenum of small intestine

Antrum

Fundus

Rugae (folds)

Body

FIGURE 3-3 Longitudinal view of the stomach showing regions and internal rugae.

The most common cause of nonerosive gastritis is a bacterial infection with **Helicobacter pylori (H pylori),** (6) a gram-negative, spiral-shaped rod that infects the mucosal layer of the stomach. The infection typically begins as an acute illness with nausea and abdominal pain, but the infection often becomes chronic. The infection may be asymptomatic but often leads to dyspepsia and peptic ulcer disease. Untreated, a chronic infection may progress to adenocarcinoma of the stomach. The organism secretes urease that protects it from the acid environment of the stomach. A positive **urea breath test** is diagnostic for H pylori infection. Biopsies may also be taken if endoscopy is being performed for other reasons, but rarely is it necessary to perform a biopsy solely to diagnose H pylori. Biopsy specimens may be tested for the enzyme urease as opposed to culturing, because it is difficult to grow H pylori in a laboratory setting. A **fecal antigen test** is also available to aid in the diagnosis. Treatment consists of combination therapy including antibiotics, proton pump inhibitors, and bismuth. Combination therapy is marketed under specific brand names such as Helidac and Prevpac (see more in the Pharmacology section of this chapter).

Erosive gastritis causes dyspepsia and upper GI bleed. Symptoms include anorexia, epigastric pain, nausea, and vomiting. The most common cause of erosive gastritis is NSAID use, but it may also be caused by alcohol, stress due to severe medical or surgical illness, and portal hypertension. Endoscopy shows epithelial hemorrhage, petechiae, and erosions. Presenting symptoms include hematemesis or **coffee grounds emesis.** (7) Patients with a **nasogastric tube (NG tube)** placed will have blood in the NG tube or NG aspirate.

The most significant contributing factor to erosive gastritis is the use of **nonsteroidal antiinflammatory drugs (NSAIDs).** Prostaglandins are important components of the body's pain, inflammatory, and healing mechanisms. Reducing prostaglandins that promote pain and inflammation is the principal mechanism of NSAIDs. Prostaglandins also play an important role in protecting and repairing the stomach lining from the harmful effects of low pH. Cyclooxygenase is an enzyme involved in the production of prostaglandins. The body actually produces two types of cyclooxygenase, referred to as COX-1 and COX-2. COX-1 is the principle enzyme involved in the production of the stomach's protective prostaglandins. Many NSAIDs block both COX-1 and COX-2, thereby reducing the amount of both protective and inflammatory prostaglandins. A subgroup of NSAIDs, referred to as the "coxibs," are **selective COX-2 inhibitors.** Because coxibs do not affect COX-1, they have proven to be less ulcerogenic and are associated with far fewer clinically significant events compared to nonselective NSAIDs.

Symptoms of NSAID-induced gastritis include pain, weight loss, vomiting, and low-grade GI bleeding with subsequent anemia. The first line of treatment is to discontinue treatment with the offending agent and then help heal the mucosal damage with antisecretory agents such as proton pump inhibitors.

A significant number of cases of gastritis occur in patients in acute stress following severe trauma, burns, and surgery. Patients on mechanical ventilators and those with coagulopathy, sepsis, CNS injury, or organ failure are also at increased risk of acute gastritis. Stress gastritis can occur within 72 hours in the critically ill. Patients at risk of stress-induced gastritis are typically given prophylactic H_2-receptor antagonists by IV, an oral proton pump inhibitor, or sucralfate.

Peptic Ulcer Disease

A peptic ulcer is a break in the gastric or duodenal mucosa as a result of impaired mucosal defenses or overwhelming acidity. By definition, ulcers are breaks in the mucosa that extend through the **muscularis mucosae** (■ Figure 3-4). Peptic ulcers are typically 5 mm in diameter or larger. The majority of peptic ulcers form in the duodenum, especially in the bulb or pyloric channel. Peptic ulcers may also occur in the esophagus with pain localized to the xiphoid or high substernal region.

(6) Previously, names of bacteria were abbreviated with the first letter of the genus and a period followed by the name of the species (eg, E. coli). The trend is to move away from inserting the period, and the *Book of Style* recommends writing the name without the period (E coli).

(7) Coffee grounds emesis gets its name from the characteristic color and texture of vomitus containing blood that has been exposed to gastric secretions. The color is dark brown with a granular texture similar to ground coffee.

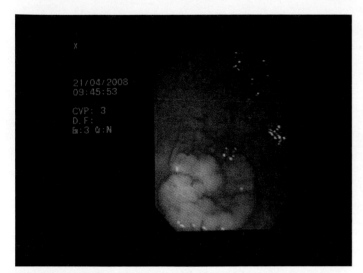

FIGURE 3-4 Peptic ulcers extend through the mucosa into the muscularis mucosa. *Source:* Photolibrary.

The three main causes of **peptic ulcer disease (PUD)** are NSAID use, chronic infection with H pylori, and acid hypersecretory states such as Zollinger-Ellison syndrome. Cigarette smoking also increases the risk of ulcers. Aspirin is the most ulcerogenic NSAID. Localized epigastric pain is the hallmark of PUD, and is often described as gnawing, dull, or aching. Patients may get relief with food but the pain recurs two to four hours later. Patients may also complain of nausea and anorexia. A change in the pain intensity or radiation of the pain may indicate perforation of an ulcer or penetration into a contiguous organ such as the pancreas, liver, or biliary tree. A **fecal occult blood test (FOBT)** is positive in approximately one-third of patients with PUD. Patients may also have a positive urea breath test or positive fecal antigen, providing evidence of H pylori infection. Definitive diagnosis of PUD is made on endoscopy. The mainstay of treatment is antisecretory agents (proton pump inhibitors, H$_2$-receptor antagonists). Diet modification may also be helpful.

 Pause 3-5 What is fecal occult blood?

Complications of PUD result when bleeding or perforation occur. Approximately half of all episodes of upper GI bleeding are caused by peptic ulcers. In addition, ulcer perforations may cause **chemical peritonitis** in which the patient suffers acute, severe, sudden-onset abdominal pain. Physical examination of the patient may reveal a very ill-appearing patient with a rigid, **quiet abdomen** and **rebound tenderness**. Upright or decubitus films of the abdomen show **free intraperitoneal air**. Bacterial peritonitis may follow as contamination from the bowel seeds the peritoneum with bacteria. Until recently, treatment included surgical closure of the omentum with a Graham patch, but conservative (ie, nonsurgical) treatment is now preferred. Patients are given antisecretory agents (ie, medications to reduce secretion of acid) to encourage healing of the ulcers and the stomach mucosa.

An additional complication of PUD is gastric outlet obstruction due to edema or cicatricial (8) narrowing of the pylorus or duodenal bulb. Symptoms of obstruction include early satiety, vomiting, weight loss, epigastric fullness, or heaviness after meals.

Surgical treatment for refractory PUD or PUD with complications includes a parietal cell vagotomy or resection of part of the stomach (antrectomy, hemigastrectomy, partial gastrectomy, or subtotal gastrectomy). Procedures requiring removal of part of the stomach (■ Figure 3-5) also require gastric drainage via a gastroduodenostomy (**Billroth I** procedure) or gastrojejunostomy (**Billroth II** procedure).

Upper GI Bleed

Upper GI bleeding is a common cause for hospitalization in the United States. The mortality rate is 7% to 10%, with the majority of deaths being in patients over age 60. Patients typically present with hematemesis, as either **bright red blood** or coffee grounds. A massive upper GI bleed or rapid GI transit time may result in hematochezia or melena, although hematochezia is far more common with lower GI bleeds. Bleeding in the esophagus may be due to varices, esophageal tears, or erosions. Bleeding may also originate from the stomach due to

(8) A cicatrix is a scar. Cicatricial narrowing is a reduction in the diameter of a lumen or passageway due to scar tissue.

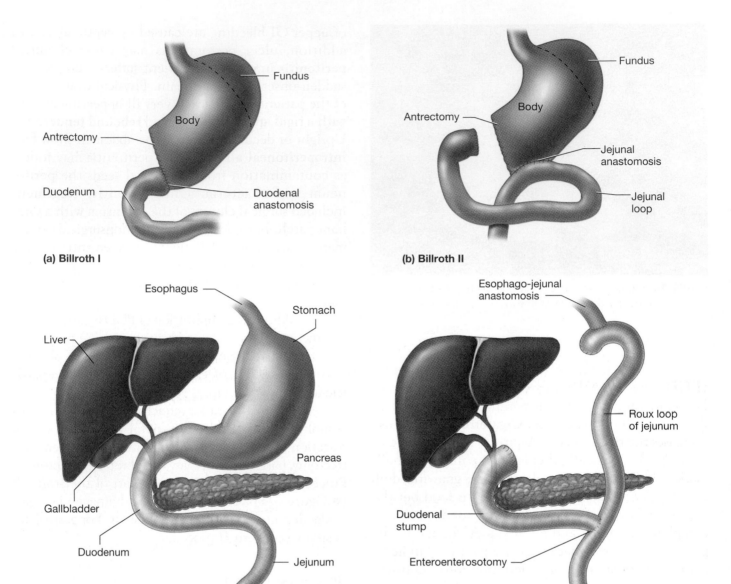

(a) Billroth I

(b) Billroth II

(c) Total Gastrectomy

FIGURE 3-5 (a) Billroth I, (b) Billroth II, and (c) total gastrectomy.

peptic ulcers. Other causes of upper GI bleeding include vascular ectasias and a **Dieulafoy lesion**. (9) On rare occasions, esophageal erosions due to gastroesophageal reflux can cause bleeding.

Pause 3-6 Compare and contrast hematemesis, hematochezia, and melena. Explain how the color gives the investigator clues as to the location of the bleed. Why would a rapid GI transit time produce hematochezia?

(9) Ectasia is dilation of a tubular structure. A Dieulafoy lesion, an example of an ectasia, is an aberrant, large-caliber artery typically found in the proximal stomach. Note the spelling and pronunciation of the French term Dieulafoy (*dyū-lah-fwah'*).

There has been no hematemesis or coffee grounds emesis. There is no melena or bright red blood per rectum. The patient reports that prior to her gastric bypass in 2011 she did undergo endoscopy, which was normal.

- Acid plays a central role in digestion as well as the pathogenesis of gastric and duodenal disorders.
- Gastritis may lead to pernicious anemia due to loss of intrinsic factor and decreased B$_{12}$ absorption.

- H pylori infection is a major cause of nonerosive gastritis and PUD.
- NSAID use is a major contributor to nonerosive gastritis and PUD.
- The most common cause of upper GI bleeding is PUD. Bleeding may also be caused by tears or varices resulting from portal hypertension.

Patients with a known or suspected upper GI bleed will typically have an NG tube placed. A **Levin** or **Salem sump** tube may be used for gastric decompression or analysis. Aspiration or lavage through the NG tube showing bright red blood or coffee grounds confirms an upper-tract source of the blood. Treatment includes transfusion with packed red blood cells (pRBCs or packed RBCs) to restore lost red blood cells and then stabilization of the underlying cause of the bleed. Endoscopy is typically used to both diagnose and treat the bleed. Patients with upper GI bleed are at risk for **rebleeding**.

Varices

Varices (10) may appear in the distal esophagus or proximal stomach due to an elevated pressure in the portal venous system, typically from cirrhosis. Varices are usually asymptomatic other than they tend to bleed. Patients with bleeding varices typically present to the emergency department with sudden, painless, yet massive upper GI bleeding. Varices in the distal esophagus are more prone to acute bouts of bleeding. Varices in the gastric fundus tend to be subacute and chronic. Patients with massive bleeding may also present with shock from sudden volume depletion.

When acute bleeding occurs, the first line of treatment is **fluid resuscitation** to correct or prevent hypovolemia and shock. Varices may be treated with **sclerotherapy** using a sclerosant such as ethanolamine or tetradecyl sulfate. Epinephrine may also be used to control bleeding. Using upper endoscopy, varices may be ligated with rubber bands. Octreotide can be used to reduce splanchnic blood flow and portal blood pressure

and is useful in the initial control of bleeding due to portal hypertension.

Patients with portal hypertension and bleeding varices who have failed other treatment modalities may be treated with **transvenous intrahepatic portosystemic shunt (TIPS)**. This procedure uses a wire stent running from the hepatic vein through the liver to the portal vein to decompress the portal venous system. Yet another approach to controlling bleeding is balloon tube tamponade using a specially designed nasogastric tube containing large gastric and esophageal balloons (Minnesota or Sengstaken-Blakemore tubes).

Tears

A significant number of upper GI bleeds are due to **Mallory-Weiss syndrome**, which is characterized by a mucosal tear (laceration) at the gastroesophageal (GE) junction. It is thought that these tears result from events that raise transabdominal pressure such as lifting, retching, or vomiting. Alcoholism is a strong predisposing factor for Mallory-Weiss tears. Tears may spontaneously stop bleeding and require no therapy. When therapy is required, bleeding may be stopped using epinephrine, cautery, or compression of the artery using a band or **Endoclip**.

Disorders of the Lower Gastrointestinal Tract

Lower GI complaints include constipation, obstipation, diarrhea, gas and bloating, abdominal pain, rectal pain, and bleeding. As with upper GI complaints,

Pause 3-7 Look up the term splanchnic. How does it relate to viscus (*pl* viscera)? Describe in layman terms the sentence, "Octreotide can be used to reduce splanchnic blood flow."

(10) Varices (singular varix) are enlarged, dilated, and possibly tortuous blood vessels. They may be found in the esophagus, lower extremities, and other places affected by increased venous pressure.

lower GI complaints may be the result of physiologic illness or represent a functional disorder.

 Pause 3-8 Compare the terms constipation and obstipation.

Gastroenteritis

Gastroenteritis is inflammation of the lining of the stomach as well as the small and large intestines. Symptoms include anorexia, nausea, vomiting, diarrhea, and abdominal discomfort. Treatment is usually symptomatic, as most cases are brief and self-limited. Healthy adults typically recover quickly, but dehydration caused by gastroenteritis may have serious implications for the very young, elderly, or seriously ill patient.

Common causative agents of gastroenteritis include viruses (Rotavirus and Norovirus, formerly the Norwalk virus), bacteria (Salmonella, Shigella, Campylobacter, and various pathogenic subtypes of Escherichia coli), and parasites (Giardia lamblia and Cryptosporidium). Symptomatic treatment includes antidiarrheals and antiemetics. Parasitic gastroenteritis may be treated with antimicrobials such as metronidazole (Flagyl).

Acute Abdomen

Acute abdomen refers to abdominal symptoms of such severity as to warrant immediate consideration for surgical attention. The predominant presenting complaint of patients with acute abdomen is severe pain of sudden onset. Acute and severe abdominal pain should be attended to swiftly. Gangrene and perforation of the gut can occur in as little as six hours from the onset of pain, especially in cases of arterial embolus or other causes of loss of intestinal blood supply. Situations requiring immediate surgical attention include ruptured abdominal aortic aneurysm (AAA), perforated viscus, mesenteric ischemia, and ruptured ectopic pregnancy. Other situations that are only slightly less urgent include intestinal obstruction, appendicitis, and severe acute pancreatitis.

On physical exam, the clinician looks for the presence of guarding, rigidity, and rebound (ie, **peritoneal signs**) as well as distention and the presence of surgical scars. Guarding is an involuntary contraction of abdominal muscles that is slightly slower and more sustained than the rapid, voluntary flinch exhibited by sensitive or anxious patients. The clinician should also palpate the abdomen for masses, organomegaly, and hernias. Examination should also include auscultation for the presence or absence of bowel sounds and percussion for tympany (**tympanitic abdomen**). (11)

There are several types of abdominal pain: visceral, somatic, and referred. Visceral pain is usually vague, dull, and nauseating. Pain may be located in the foregut (stomach, duodenum, liver, and pancreas), midgut (small bowel, proximal colon, and appendix), or hindgut (distal colon and GU tract). Somatic pain, which is typically sharp and well localized, arises from irritation from infectious, chemical, or other inflammatory processes. Referred pain is perceived in a location away from the actual source of the pain due to convergence of nerve fibers at the spinal cord. For example, biliary pain may refer pain to the scapular area, renal colic may refer pain to the groin, and irritation of the diaphragm may be felt in the shoulder.

Perforation

Perforation within the GI tract is a serious, life-threatening situation. A perforation releases gastric and/or intestinal contents into the peritoneal space with sudden onset of severe pain and quickly ensuing systemic shock. Esophageal, gastric, and duodenal perforation usually present acutely with catastrophic results.

Patients with suspected GI tract perforation or obstruction should be evaluated with an **abdominal series** consisting of **flat and upright abdominal x-rays** and chest x-rays. Patients unable to stand may be evaluated with **left lateral recumbent x-rays** and anteroposterior (AP) chest x-rays. These may be followed with an abdominal CT with contrast if x-rays are nondiagnostic. On x-rays, patients with perforation will typically show free air under the diaphragm.

Abdominal x-ray showed free peritoneal and retroperitoneal air. CT abdomen was performed with intravenous contrast and showed mottled air and feces in the extraluminal space in the pelvis close to the rectosigmoid, along with extensive free air in the retroperitoneum, extending into the mediastinum. A diagnosis of sigmoid perforation with possible fecal peritonitis was made on CT.

(11) Tympany (*tĭm′ pă nē*) is a low-pitched, drum-like sound heard on percussion of an air-filled space such as the abdomen or thorax.

Peritonitis

Peritonitis is inflammation of the peritoneal cavity. Peritonitis has several causes, the most serious of which is perforation within the GI tract. Peritonitis may also be caused by appendicitis, diverticulitis, strangulating intestinal obstruction, pancreatitis, pelvic inflammatory disease, or mesenteric ischemia. Peritonitis causes fluid to shift into the peritoneal cavity and bowel, resulting in dehydration and electrolyte imbalances. The ensuing complications of peritonitis are life-threatening; death can occur within days.

Ascites refers to the pathologic accumulation of fluid in the peritoneal cavity. Normally males do not have any peritoneal fluid, but females may have up to 20 mL depending on the phase of their menstrual cycle. The most common cause of ascites is portal hypertension secondary to liver disease. Other causes include intraabdominal malignancy, inflammatory disorders of the peritoneum, or biliary obstruction.

> Peritoneal fluid may be referred to as ascitic fluid, the adjectival form of the word ascites. It sounds the same as acidic, so be sure to use context to distinguish between ascitic and acidic.

Patients with ascites typically present with **increasing abdominal girth** and abdominal pain. A large accumulation of fluid that causes the abdomen to be tight and distended is referred to as **tense ascites**. Abdominal ultrasound is the most reliable way to detect ascites. Abdominal paracentesis is performed to remove the fluid and also to analyze the fluid for diagnostic purposes. Cell counts (for red and white blood cells) are performed to assess for intraabdominal infection. Albumin is also measured to determine the **serum-ascites-albumin gradient (SAAG)**, which is the most reliable way to determine if the ascites is due to portal hypertension. A SAAG value greater than or equal to one suggests portal hypertension. Fluid is also sent for **aerobic and anaerobic culture (12)** and Gram stain.

Spontaneous **bacterial peritonitis** may be caused by enteric gram-negative bacteria (Escherichia coli, Klebsiella pneumoniae, enterococcus species) or gram-positive bacteria such as Streptococcus pneumoniae and viridans streptococci.

Mesenteric Ischemia and Infarction

The abdomen receives its blood supply by way of three major arteries: the **celiac trunk**, the **superior mesenteric artery (SMA)**, and the **inferior mesenteric artery (IMA)**. In addition to these major arteries, the stomach, duodenum, and rectum have a large number of collateral arteries that reduce the chance of frank infarction in these particular areas of the GI tract (see Figure 4-1). The splenic flexure, however, is at particular risk of ischemia and infarction.

Mesenteric ischemia is caused by interrupted intestinal blood flow due to an embolism, thrombosis, or decreased perfusion resulting from decreased hemodynamic volume. Because of its high metabolic rate, the intestinal mucosa has a high blood-flow requirement (normally receiving up to 25% of total cardiac output). It is therefore quite sensitive to decreased perfusion. Ischemia quickly disrupts the integrity of the mucosal barrier, leading to the release of bacteria, toxins, and vasoactive mediators. Sepsis due to bacterial dissemination as well as shock from leakage of vasoactive mediators further complicates an already critical situation. Multiorgan failure may ensue due to a further decrease in systemic blood pressure. Ischemia quickly progresses to complete infarction; necrosis can occur in as little as 10–12 hours after the onset of symptoms.

 Pause 3-9 Describe the relationship between perfusion, ischemia, infarction, and necrosis.

(12) Microorganisms vary in their oxygen requirements; aerobic microorganisms require oxygen, anaerobic organisms can tolerate oxygen but do not require it, and obligate anaerobes cannot tolerate any oxygen at all. An aerobic culture is incubated with oxygen and an anaerobic culture is incubated without oxygen. Blood and body fluids from abscesses and body cavities are usually tested for both aerobic and anaerobic bacteria.

Lower Gastrointestinal Bleed

A **lower GI bleed (LGIB)** is defined as bleeding that occurs below the **ligament of Treitz**. The majority of cases occur in the colon. Hemorrhoids are the most common cause of lower GI bleeding in younger patients, but the bleeding is typically minor. The leading causes of significant LGIB in older patients are diverticulosis and angiodysplasia. The majority of angiodysplastic vessels are located in the cecum and proximal ascending colon, but they may occur anywhere within the alimentary tract. Radiation therapy can cause radiation-induced colitis and mucosal telangiectasias that bleed. (13) Bleeding may also originate in the anus or rectum due to hemorrhoids, fistulas, and fissures.

The stool color may provide clues to the location of the bleed, but not reliably enough to depend solely on this information. A bleed from the right side of the colon often manifests as **maroon-colored stools**, and a left-sided bleed appears as **bright red blood per rectum**. A bleed higher in the GI tract often presents as melena due to the effect of digestive enzymes on blood cells. But a brisk bleed from anywhere within the tract can also present as bright red blood due to fast transit times and minimal exposure to digestive enzymes. Patients with chronic, intermittent bleeding may present with Hemoccult-positive stools, iron deficiency anemia, and syncope. Hemorrhoidal bleeding typically coats the stool during defecation and patients may note **bright red blood on the toilet paper**.

Severe bleeds can become **hemodynamically significant**, (14) requiring immediate treatment. Several modalities are employed to determine the source of a lower GI bleed and to stop the bleeding. Colonoscopy is the most common, but radionuclide scans and angiography may also be used. Endoscopic procedures used to diagnose upper and lower GI bleeds include **esophagogastroduodenoscopy (EGD)**, **wireless capsule endoscopy (WCE)**, **push enteroscopy**, and double-balloon enteroscopy.

Obstruction

Intestinal obstruction is a serious, life-threatening emergency. An obstruction can occur anywhere along the alimentary tract, but a **small bowel obstruction (SBO)** develops acutely and represents the most serious threat to life. Untreated, an obstruction leads to perforation, peritonitis, and death. SBO is the cause of 20% of acute surgical admissions. The most common causes of mechanical obstruction are adhesions, hernias, and tumors. Other causes include diverticulitis, foreign bodies (including gallstones), volvulus, and intussusception. **Volvulus** is an intestinal obstruction caused by the twisting of the intestine on the mesentery (■Figure 3-6). A contrast enema easily shows the site of volvulus with a typical **bird-beak deformity** at the site of the twist.

> **(13)** Angiodysplasia is a structural abnormality in a blood vessel that makes the vessel prone to bleeding. Telangiectasia is the dilation of a small, terminal vessel.
>
> **(14)** A hemodynamically significant bleed is a bleed that is extensive enough to affect the patient's vital signs.

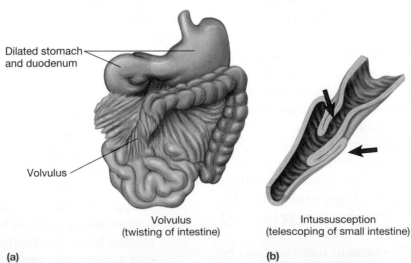

Dilated stomach and duodenum

Volvulus

Volvulus
(twisting of intestine)

Intussusception
(telescoping of small intestine)

(a)

(b)

FIGURE 3-6 Intestinal obstruction: (a) volvulus (a twist of the intestinal lumen on the mesentery) and (b) intussusception (telescoping of the small intestine).

Intussusception, which most commonly occurs at the terminal ilium, results when a portion of bowel telescopes on the adjacent portion. The portion which invaginates is called the **intussusceptum** and the adjacent bowel is called the **intussuscipiens**. Intussusception is more common in infants and toddlers and has no known cause. Patients with intussusception may have the classic **currant-jelly stool** consisting of blood and mucus. Barium contrast studies are both diagnostic and therapeutic, as the majority of intussusceptions can be reduced (ie, reversed) with contrast media.

When blockage occurs, ingested food, digestive secretions, and gas (swallowed air) accumulate up to the point of the obstruction. The bowel located proximal to the obstruction becomes distended, and the bowel distal to the obstruction collapses. The bowel wall becomes edematous. The absorptive functions of the intestine are depressed while the secretory functions are increased, leading to more fluid accumulation, more peristalsis, and a progressively worsening situation. Complications of obstruction include dehydration, electrolyte imbalances, and strangulation of the bowel. The increased hydrostatic pressure in the capillary beds produced from the edema results in massive **third spacing (15)** of fluid, electrolytes, and proteins into the intestinal lumen. A strangulating obstruction compromises blood flow, progressing to infarction and gangrene in as little as six hours. Strangulation is less common in the large bowel.

Symptoms of small bowel obstruction include abdominal cramps in the periumbilical area or epigastrium. Vomiting and obstipation are common. Hyperactive, **high-pitched peristalsis with rushes** can be heard on auscultation. Dilated loops of bowel may be detected on palpation. When infarction occurs, the abdomen becomes tender with no bowel sounds (**silent abdomen**).

Obstruction of the large bowel is less acute and produces milder symptoms than small bowel obstruction. Initial symptoms include constipation progressing to obstipation and abdominal distention. Vomiting is less common. The abdomen becomes distended and auscultation reveals loud **borborygmi**.

Obstructions are treated with a laparotomy to remove the obstructed area of bowel. Gallstones may be removed through an **enterotomy**. Fecal impaction, typically within the rectum, can be removed digitally (ie, with the fingers) or with the use of enemas. Fecal concretion, typically located in the sigmoid colon, requires laparotomy. Incomplete obstructions, such as strictures, may be treated with **strictureplasty** (also spelled **stricturoplasty**). This surgical procedure widens the narrowed segment of intestine.

Pause 3-10 Based on what you know about the combing form *entero-* and *-tomy*, write a definition for the word enterotomy.

Two of the most commonly misheard words are "thecal" and "fecal." Although hearing the difference between these two words is difficult, context will enable you to determine the correct term quite easily. Thecal refers to a sheath, especially a sheath around a tendon.

---

(15) Third spacing is based on the concept of "fluid spaces" in the body. Normally, fluids are retained in the intravascular and interstitial spaces (the "first" and "second" spaces). Third-spacing occurs when fluid moves into a space that normally does not contain fluid, depleting the first and second spaces of normal fluid volumes and essentially creating dehydration.

- Gastroenteritis is typically a self-limited disease caused by an infectious agent.
- An acute abdomen is a potentially life-threatening emergency most likely requiring surgical intervention.
- Because of its high metabolic activity, the abdomen receives as much as 25% of total cardiac output, and conditions that reduce flow to the abdomen have serious consequences.
- Mesenteric ischemia can quickly advance to infarction and death.
- Lower GI bleeds may be acute or chronic. Acute bleeds may lead to hypovolemia and shock. Chronic bleeds lead to iron deficiency anemia.

Disorders of the Small Intestine

The small intestine is comprised of the duodenum, jejunum, and ileum. The small intestine is responsible for digestion and absorption of the nutrients contained within food. The duodenum digests food using pancreatic enzymes and bile acids to break proteins, fats, and carbohydrates into smaller molecules capable of moving across the intestinal membrane. Digestive enzymes and bile are secreted into the duodenum through the **sphincter of Oddi.** Peristalsis mixes the food with the digestive fluids and moves the chyme through the small intestine. The jejunum absorbs the majority of the food molecules and the remainder is absorbed through the ileum. The lining of the small intestine is made up of many tiny folds call villi that dramatically increase the surface area of the intestine and magnify its absorptive power. The villi themselves are made of cells with microvilli, which are projections of the cell membrane. Among the villi are lacteals, which are collections of lymphatic vessels that carry food particles, especially fats, to the liver. The small intestine has a dense supply of blood vessels to provide the energy required for digestion and the "trucking capacity" to carry food particles to the remainder of the body.

Celiac Disease

Celiac disease, also known as **nontropical sprue, celiac sprue,** or **gluten enteropathy,** involves an immune response to gluten, a protein component of wheat, rye, and barley. Patients, who are genetically predisposed to the disorder, form antibodies against gliadin, a protein moiety (16) of gluten. Ingestion of gluten causes mucosal inflammation, mucosal villus atrophy, malabsorption, diarrhea, and abdominal discomfort. Patients often go undiagnosed for ten years or more because of celiac disease's protean (17) manifestations. **Dermatitis herpetiformis** is the cutaneous form of the disease that causes a pruritic, papulovesicular rash over the extensor surfaces of the arms and legs, the trunk and scalp.

Diagnosis of celiac disease is most easily made using serologic markers—circulating antibodies directed at gluten and connective tissue proteins. Treatment is a gluten-free diet, avoiding all foods containing gluten or traces of gluten. Patients typically respond to a gluten-free diet in as little as one to two weeks and remain symptom-free as long as they are compliant with the diet. Patients who have advanced to malabsorption and malnutrition may need vitamin and mineral supplementation, especially hematinics (18) such as iron and B_{12}.

Ileus

Ileus, also referred to as **adynamic ileus,** is a temporary paralysis of intestinal peristalsis without mechanical obstruction. It occurs commonly following abdominal surgery and is also associated with intraperitoneal or retroperitoneal inflammation, intraabdominal hematomas, metabolic disturbances, and drugs. Critically ill patients, especially patients on respiratory support and patients with electrolyte imbalance, are also vulnerable to ileus. The stomach and intestines commonly show motility disturbances following abdominal surgery, but the small intestine typically returns to normal within a few hours. Stomach emptying may be impaired for up to 24 hours following surgery. The colon is most affected by abdominal surgery, sometimes requiring 48–72 hours to return to normal motility and function.

> Pay close attention when transcribing "adynamic ileus." It could easily sound like "a dynamic ileus," which has the opposite meaning.

Symptoms of ileus include abdominal distention, nausea, vomiting, and possibly obstipation. Auscultation reveals a silent abdomen or minimal peristalsis. Plain films of the abdomen show distended, gas-filled loops and possibly **air-fluid levels.** Patients are **kept n.p.o.,** and given IV fluids with electrolytes. Continuous suction is applied to a nasogastric tube to remove fluids and secretions.

(16) A moiety is a part of something, often referring to a distinct part or area of a larger molecule. You may hear it pronounced *moy'i tē* or *mo ī' i tē.*

(17) Protean (*prō' tē an*) refers to something that is highly changeable in form.

(18) A hematinic promotes the formation of red blood cells.

> He was found to have ileus with question of volvulus. He was kept n.p.o. and treated conservatively. He continued to have problems with distension and pain and was taken to the operating room today. He was found to have a sigmoid volvulus and underwent a sigmoid colectomy with colocolostomy.

Appendicitis

Appendicitis is acute inflammation of the vermiform (19) appendix. Patients presenting with acute appendicitis complain of vague, often colicky, periumbilical or epigastric abdominal pain that shifts to the right lower quadrant. Patients may also complain of anorexia, nausea, vomiting, abdominal tenderness, and low-grade fever. The most common cause of appendicitis is obstruction of the appendiceal lumen, typically by lymphoid hyperplasia, but the appendix may also be affected by a fecalith, (20) foreign body, or even worms. Other conditions that may affect the appendix include diverticulosis, Crohn disease, or ulcerative colitis. Obstruction of the lumen causes the appendix to become distended, creating an environment prone to bacterial overgrowth, inflammation, and ischemia. Complications of untreated appendicitis include necrosis, gangrene, and perforation. An appendiceal abscess may form if the perforation is contained within the omentum.

 Pause 3-11 Explain how distention of the appendix can lead to ischemia.

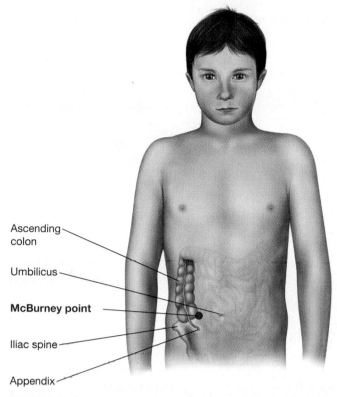

FIGURE 3-7 Tenderness at the McBurney point is indicative of appendicitis.

Physical examination may reveal a positive **psoas sign** (pain with passive extension of the right hip) and a positive **obturator sign** (pain on passive flexion and internal rotation of the right hip). Patients may also exhibit tenderness or localized rigidity at the **McBurney point** (■ Figure 3-7). **Retrocecal** or **retroileal appendicitis** may be confused with ureteral colic or pyelonephritis.

Treatment of appendicitis is appendectomy via laparotomy or laparoscopy. An abscess may be treated with CT-guided drainage of the abscess and antibiotic therapy.

Disorders of the Colon

The colon is the last major segment of the digestive tract. It is divided into four sections: the ascending colon, transverse colon, descending colon, and sigmoid colon. The turn from the ascending colon to the

(19) Vermiform means resembling a worm or worm-shaped.

(20) A fecalith is a hard, stone-like mass made of feces.

- Celiac disease is caused by an immune reaction to gluten, resulting in mucosal inflammation in the small intestine. Left untreated, celiac disease results in malabsorption of nutrients.
- Ileus is temporary paralysis of intestinal peristalsis. It most commonly occurs following abdominal surgery but can occur following trauma or in the critically ill.
- Appendicitis is acute inflammation of the vermiform appendix and is associated with rigidity at the McBurney point.

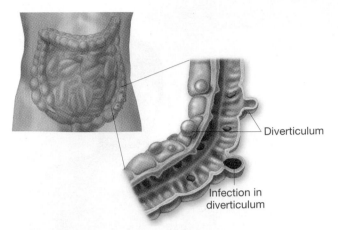

FIGURE 3-8 Diverticula are outpouchings of intestinal mucosa.

transverse colon is just below the liver and is referred to as the **hepatic flexure**. The corresponding curve on the left, where the transverse colon turns downward to the descending colon, is just below the spleen and is referred to as the **splenic flexure**. The last curve from the descending colon to the rectum is referred to as the sigmoid colon (because it resembles the curve of the Greek letter sigma). The colon's primary responsibility is to reabsorb water and electrolytes from the feces and prepare the feces for expulsion (defecation).

Diverticular Disease

Diverticula are outpouchings that form along the alimentary tract, most commonly in the duodenum near the ampulla of Vater (periampullary) or the sigmoid colon. Duodenal and jejunal diverticula are usually asymptomatic and are discovered incidentally during radiologic or endoscopic evaluation for an unrelated condition. Diverticula may occur anywhere within the large bowel, but they are typically found in the sigmoid colon and only rarely below the **peritoneal reflection** of the rectum. **Diverticulosis** is the presence of multiple diverticula in the colon. The exact etiology is not known, but diverticulosis is associated with a history of a low-fiber diet (■ Figure 3-8).

Diverticulitis results when a diverticulum perforates and becomes inflamed. Intestinal bacteria (**normal flora**) are released, and localized inflammation ensues.

(21) Empiric means based on observation and experience but not necessarily directly proven. Treatments are often given "empirically" before tests have confirmed the diagnosis.

About one-quarter of perforated diverticula develop complications such as abscesses, intraperitoneal perforation, bowel obstruction, or fistulas. Patients with acute diverticulitis complain of left lower quadrant pain and low-grade fever. CBC reveals leukocytosis, and a palpable mass may be detected on physical exam. Peritoneal signs may be present if there is an abscess or free peritoneal perforation. FOBT is often positive, but frank hematochezia is rare. Fistulas may cause **pneumaturia** (air bubbles in the urine), feculent vaginal discharge, or a cutaneous or myofascial infection in the abdomen or groin.

Pause 3-12 Research the term fistula. Give a definition, a list of types of fistulas, examples of where they can occur, and reasons for fistula formation. Translate the following into layman's terms: "Fistulas may cause pneumaturia, feculent vaginal discharge, or a cutaneous or myofascial infection in the abdomen or groin."

For a mild case of suspected diverticulitis, patients are treated **empirically (21)** with antibiotics, typically ciprofloxacin, amoxicillin with clavulanate, or metronidazole, along with a liquid diet. Abdominal CT with oral contrast is preferred over endoscopy during the acute phase, but CT is not always definitive. After resolution of symptoms, colonoscopy or barium enema may be performed to confirm the diagnosis of colonic diverticular disease. A high-fiber diet helps to prevent diverticulosis and reduce flare-ups. Patients are advised to supplement their diet with psyllium fiber, bran, or methylcellulose to increase stool bulk and reduce **straining at stool**.

Polyps

Polyps are discrete mass lesions that arise from the bowel wall and protrude into the intestinal lumen. Polyps may be described as **pedunculated** (having a stalk) as in ■ **Figure 3-9**, **sessile** (having a broad base), or flat. Polyps are most often found in the rectum and sigmoid colon, but may be located anywhere within the digestive tract. Most polyps are asymptomatic but may cause occult bleeding. Chronic occult bleeding may eventually lead to iron deficiency anemia. A large, ulcerated polyp may cause intermittent hematochezia.

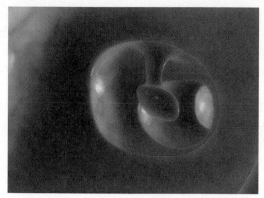

FIGURE 3-9 A pedunculated polyp in the colon. Note the polyp is growing on a stalk. *Source:* Sebastian Kaulitzki/Shutterstock.com.

A small polyp was identified in the left colon, and it was removed with forceps. However, a larger polyp was identified in the rectosigmoid area, which required removal with snare cautery.

Pathologically, polyps are classified as neoplastic (adenomatous) or nonneoplastic. **Adenomatous polyps** have malignant potential and are of greatest clinical concern. Nonneoplastic polyps may be classified as hyperplastic juvenile polyps, hamartomas, inflammatory polyps, submucosal lesions, or lipomas. The vast majority of polyps removed are classified as adenomatous, but a significant number are hyperplastic. Histologic studies are required to reliably distinguish adenomatous from hyperplastic polyps.

Histologic examination of biopsied polypoid tissue further classifies adenomas as **tubular**, **villous**, or **tubulovillous** (also called **villoglandular polyps**). The larger the polyp, the higher the likelihood the polyp contains cancerous cells. Polyps with villous features or high-grade dysplasia are considered advanced and are believed to have a higher risk of progressing to adenocarcinoma. A polyp that extends through the muscularis mucosae into the submucosa is considered malignant. Aspirin and NSAID use is thought to decrease the risk of adenomas and colorectal cancer.

Diagnosis is typically made by colonoscopy. Polyps may also be seen on barium enema, but a colonoscopy can be both diagnostic and therapeutic, so it is the preferred test when polyps are suspected. Polypectomy can be performed during colonoscopy using biopsy forceps or **snare cautery**. Polyps may also be found on flexible sigmoidoscopy, but if polyps are found in the sigmoid colon, this should be followed with a colonoscopy that extends to the cecum. Patients with multiple polyps, often in the tens or hundreds, may have **familial adenomatous polyposis (FAP)**. For these patients, prophylactic colectomy is advised, as colon cancer is inevitable by age 50.

Irritable Bowel Syndrome

Irritable bowel syndrome (IBS) is characterized by abdominal pain that is relieved by defecation. IBS is considered a functional disorder, unlike Crohn disease and ulcerative colitis, which are inflammatory, cell-mediated disorders. (22) The cause of IBS is unknown, and there is no specific laboratory or imaging study to diagnose this syndrome; it is a diagnosis of exclusion. It is thought that emotional states, diet, drugs, or hormones precipitate or exacerbate episodes of pain.

Patients complain of abdominal pain that is usually relieved by defecation. Patients typically have a change in bowel-movement frequency or stool consistency. Either diarrhea or constipation may predominate, but some patients have alternating bouts of both. Symptoms typically do not wake the patient from sleep. Because there is no specific test to definitively diagnose IBS, other etiologies for abdominal pain must be ruled out before presuming IBS. Physical examination may reveal tenderness in the left lower quadrant and/or a palpably tender sigmoid colon, but with no other physical findings. Overall, patients appear to be healthy.

When other gastrointestinal disorders have been ruled out, the diagnosis may be appropriately made using the **Rome criteria**. To qualify using these criteria, patients should have abdominal pain or discomfort for at least three days per month over the previous three months and at least two of the following: improvement with defecation, onset of episodes associated with a change in bowel-movement frequency, and a change in the consistency of the stool.

Treatment is symptomatic, consisting of medications, diet, and management of psychological factors. Anticholinergics (eg, hyoscyamine, dicyclomine, methscopolamine) are used to decrease spasm, and loperamide

(22) A cell-mediated disorder is an immune system disorder that involves the cellular arm of the immune system (as opposed to antibodies).

is used to treat diarrhea. Antidepressants with serotonin-receptor activity, such as the tricyclic antidepressants (TCAs), are also helpful for controlling abdominal discomfort. Patients with constipation find relief with osmotic laxatives such as milk of magnesia and polyethylene glycol. The probiotic Bifidobacterium infantis has been found to reduce bloating and improve overall symptoms. Carminatives, such as oil of peppermint, have been found to relax smooth muscle and relieve crampy pain in some patients.

Infectious Colitis

Infectious colitis is caused by a variety of bacterial, viral, parasitic, and amoebic agents. The most common causes of infectious colitis are Salmonella, Shigella, Campylobacter jejuni, **Escherichia coli O157:H7**, and Entamoeba histolytica. Patients typically present with fever, bloody diarrhea, dehydration, and abdominal pain. Salmonella and Shigella cause colonic tissue damage, leading to characteristic symptomatology, but E coli O157:H7 produces an enterotoxin that in some cases causes **hemolytic uremic syndrome** with hemolysis, thrombocytopenia, uremia, and possibly death.

> Escherichia coli is almost always dictated as E coli (*ē kō' lī*). The specific serotype E coli O157:H7 will be dictated with the serotype designation when applicable (not all E coli have this particular designation). The serotype is dictated as "oh-one-fifty-seven-ach-seven."

Pseudomembranous Colitis

Pseudomembranous colitis, also referred to as **antibiotic-associated colitis**, is caused by an anaerobic, gram-positive rod named Clostridium difficile. The bacteria is found commonly in hospitals, nursing homes, and even soil, water, and household pets. It is the most common form of hospital-acquired diarrhea. Although 3% to 8% of healthy adults carry C difficile

> **(23)** A cytotoxin is a chemical that is detrimental to cells. An enterotoxin is a chemical that is active in the intestinal tract and is detrimental to the intestinal mucosa.

in their intestinal tract, the bacterium typically only causes disease following treatment with antibiotics (for any other medical condition). Antibiotics affect the normal flora of the bowel and upset the normal balance of pathogenic and nonpathogenic bacteria, allowing C difficile to get the upper hand. C difficile secretes a cytotoxin (toxin B) and an enterotoxin (toxin A). **(23)**

> Clostridium difficile is almost always dictated as "see dif" but should be transcribed C difficile.

Symptoms usually begin five to ten days after starting antibiotic therapy, but patients may present as early as the first day or as late as two months following completion of antibiotic therapy. Patients complain of mild to moderate, greenish, foul-smelling, watery diarrhea with lower abdominal cramps. Nausea and vomiting are rare. There is usually mucus but rarely frank blood. Patients with severe disease may have profuse, watery diarrhea.

The most common diagnostic test is a rapid enzyme immunoassay (EIA) for toxins A and B that gives results in two to four hours. Sigmoidoscopy is usually not necessary, but when performed shows discrete, yellow-white, plaque-like pseudomembranes scattered along the colonic mucosa.

The first line of treatment is metronidazole for ten days. Patients sensitive to metronidazole may be given vancomycin. Concomitant treatment with probiotics to help restore the normal flora may also be recommended.

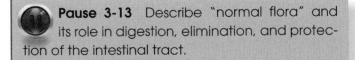

> **Pause 3-13** Describe "normal flora" and its role in digestion, elimination, and protection of the intestinal tract.

Inflammatory Diseases

Inflammatory bowel disease (IBD), which includes Crohn disease and ulcerative colitis (UC), is a relapsing and remitting condition characterized by chronic inflammation at various sites in the GI tract that results in diarrhea and abdominal pain. Ulcerative colitis is limited to the colon while Crohn disease may affect any portion of the GI tract from the mouth to the anus. Both forms of IBD are associated with **extraintestinal manifestations** in approximately 25% of patients. Patients may suffer intermittent bouts of oligoarticular or polyarticular arthritis, spondylitis, or sacroiliitis. Arthritis associated with IBD tends to involve the large joints and is migratory and transient. In addition to joint complications, patients may also experience episcleritis, uveitis, erythema nodosum, pyoderma gangrenosum, sclerosing cholangitis, and thromboembolic events. Patients positive for the **HLA-B27 antigen** also show a higher incidence of ankylosing spondylitis.

Although Crohn disease and ulcerative colitis are distinctly different diseases, they are both treated with the same pharmacologic agents. The mainstay of treatment is 5-aminosalicylic acid (5-ASA). Because both diseases are immune mediated, patients are also treated with corticosteroids and immunomodulating agents such as methotrexate and infliximab.

Crohn Disease Crohn disease (CD) is a chronic, transmural (24) inflammatory disease that mostly affects the colon and the distal ileum (**ileocecal Crohn's**) but may affect any part of the gastrointestinal tract. CD is a lifelong disease characterized by periods of exacerbation and remission. Crohn disease is noted to affect a higher proportion of persons of Northern European and Anglo-Saxon origin, and it is even more common in **Ashkenazi Jews. (25)**

The initial inflammatory lesions begin with small abscesses that progress to aphthoid ulcers. The lesions may progress to deep longitudinal and transverse ulcers. The inflammation extends through the bowel mucosa. Areas of ulceration alternating with mucosal edema create the characteristic **cobblestone** appearance. Areas of involvement are easily distinguished from areas of normal bowel, and imaging studies often describe the presence of **skip lesions**. The mesenteric lymph nodes enlarge in response to the extensive inflammation, and the muscularis mucosa becomes fibrotic, leading to stricture formation and bowel obstruction. Fistula formation (fistulization) is also common in CD, creating passages between adjacent loops of bowel, the bladder, and even the psoas muscle. Perianal fistulas are also quite common in CD. Enterocutaneous fistulas usually develop at the site of surgical scars. Patients with an enterovesical fistula may produce air bubbles in the urine (pneumaturia).

Patients typically present with chronic diarrhea and abdominal pain, fever, anorexia, and weight loss. Approximately one-third of patients present with perianal disease in the form of fissures or fistulas. Bowel obstruction is not uncommon in CD patients, leading to colicky pain, distention, obstipation, and vomiting. Diagnosis is made through endoscopy with an **upper GI series with small bowel followthrough** and **spot films of the terminal ileum**. CT enterography with high-resolution CT and ingested contrast are becoming more popular. Capsule imaging may also be used to visualize the entire digestive tract. Patients may also be positive for **anti-Saccharomyces cerevisiae antibodies (ASCA)**. A minority of patients are also positive for **antineutrophil cytoplasmic antibodies with perinuclear staining (pANCA)**.

Day-to-day management of CD is primarily pharmaceutical with diet modifications. Cramps and diarrhea can be relieved with loperamide on a p.r.n. basis. Fiber in the form of methylcellulose or psyllium adds bulk and firmness to the stool. Mild to moderate disease is managed with 5-ASA (Pentasa and Asacol). Severe exacerbations of disease are treated with corticosteroids to dampen the cellular immune response. If steroid treatment is unsuccessful, patients may be treated with azathioprine, 6-mercaptopurine, or possibly methotrexate. The immune-modulating drug infliximab is also used. Surgical removal of sections of diseased bowel is required at some point in approximately 70% of chronic CD patients (■ **Figure 3-10**).

Patients with a history of eight or more years of CD are at increased risk of dysplasia and colon carcinoma. Screening colonoscopy is recommended. Patients are also at risk of bacterial overgrowth and resultant malabsorption.

Stricture formation from chronic inflammation and scarring is a significant complication of long-term CD. Extensive resection of the small bowel causes malabsorption syndrome, but a newer procedure, called **side-to-side isoperistaltic strictureplasty (SSIS)**, repairs long segments of strictures without resulting loss of absorption.

Ulcerative Colitis Like Crohn disease, ulcerative colitis (UC) is an idiopathic inflammatory disease that causes ulcers in the colonic mucosa. Unlike CD, ulcerative

---

(24) Transmural means it affects the full thickness of the bowel wall.

(25) Ashkenazi (*ăsh kə nah zē*) is an ethnic group that has been studied extensively for genetically linked diseases.

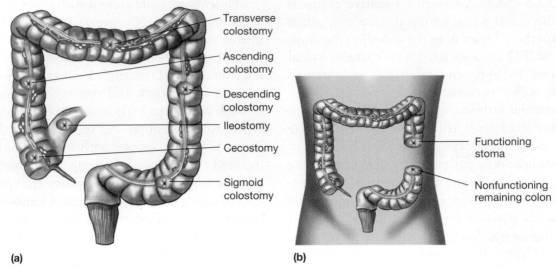

FIGURE 3-10 (a) Various ostomy sites and (b) descending colostomy with nonfunctioning sigmoid colon, rectum, and anus.

colitis is confined to the colonic tissue, affecting the mucosa and the submucosa. Part or all of the colon (**pancolitis**) may be involved. Typically the muscularis is not involved unless the disease is severe. The mucous membrane becomes erythematous, finely granular, and friable **(26)** with scattered hemorrhagic areas. Bloody diarrhea is the hallmark of the disease. Rectal inflammation causes fecal urgency and tenesmus. Patients with severe disease may have greater than ten bloody stools per day, leading to anemia, hypovolemia, and impaired nutrition with hypoalbuminemia. In severe exacerbations, ulcers produce copious, purulent exudate. Toxic or fulminant colitis occurs when transmural ulceration leads to ileus and peritonitis. In these situations, the colon loses muscular tone and begins to dilate. Dilation of the transverse colon greater than 6 cm in diameter is referred to as **megacolon**. Severe dilation can be life-threatening as the colon is liable to perforate. Unlike CD, fistulas and abscesses do not occur.

Patients with UC suffer intermittent bouts of abdominal cramps with blood and mucus in the stool. Episodes may begin insidiously with an increased urgency to defecate.

UC must be distinguished from CD, and infectious etiologies should be ruled out. Plain x-rays are typically not diagnostic for UC but may show mucosal edema and **loss of haustration**. **(27)** Sigmoidoscopy with biopsy is the most useful diagnostic test. A shortened, rigid colon with an atrophic or pseudopolypoid mucosa is often seen after several years of illness.

Nearly one-third of patients with extensive UC require surgery at some point. A total proctocolectomy is curative since UC is limited to the colon. A proctocolectomy with ileoanal anastomosis creates a pelvic reservoir (pouch) using the distal ileum. A recurring inflammatory reaction called **pouchitis** occurs in about half of all patients undergoing this procedure. Pouchitis may be controlled with the use of **probiotics** containing nonpathogenic strains of lactobacillus, bifidobacteria, and streptococci (VSL#3). When pouchitis cannot be controlled, the pouch can be converted to a conventional ileostomy (**Brooke ileostomy**). When surgery is on an emergent basis, as in the case of a massive hemorrhage, fulminating toxic colitis, or perforation, a **subtotal colectomy with ileostomy** and rectosigmoid closure or mucous fistula is performed. This procedure leaves a rectosigmoid stump that later can be revised to an ileoanal anastomosis with a pouch, or it can be completely removed.

Anorectal Disease

The most common affliction of the anorectal area is hemorrhoids. Hemorrhoid veins are a normal part of the anal anatomy and help to retain stool in the anal vault, but chronic straining or pressure (for example from obesity, pregnancy, or prolonged sitting) can cause

(26) Friable means easily broken down, crumbly.

(27) Haustra are sac-like pouches of the colon. Loss of haustration may be described as a lead-pipe appearance of the colon on x-ray imaging.

- Diverticular disease is characterized by outpouchings of the intestinal mucosa. Multiple diverticula constitute diverticulosis, and an infection involving one or more diverticulum is diverticulitis.
- Polyps are typically benign mass lesions that may progress to adenocarcinoma.
- Irritable bowel syndrome is a functional disorder characterized by pain, diarrhea, and/or constipation.
- The most common causes of infectious colitis are Salmonella, Shigella, Campylobacter jejuni, Escherichia coli O157:H7, and Entamoeba histolytica.

- The most common hospital-acquired colitis is pseudomembranous colitis caused by Clostridium difficile and typically develops during or following antibiotic treatment.
- Inflammatory bowel diseases, including Crohn disease and ulcerative colitis, are immune-mediated disorders that often have extraintestinal manifestations.
- Crohn disease is a relapsing disease that mostly affects the ileum and colon, but may cause lesions anywhere in the intestinal tract. Ulcerative colitis is a relapsing disease confined to the colon.
- Hemorrhoids are the most common form of anorectal disease.

the veins to become engorged and symptomatic. Hemorrhoids may be external or internal. External hemorrhoids arise from inferior hemorrhoidal veins located below the **dentate line**. Symptoms include bleeding, prolapse, and mucoid discharge. Internal hemorrhoids occur above the dentate line. Internal hemorrhoids are typically less painful than **thrombosed external hemorrhoids**, and symptoms may include irritation, mucus, and a feeling of **incomplete evacuation**.

Hemorrhoids are divided into stages based on their progression. Stage I hemorrhoids are confined to the anal canal. Stage II hemorrhoids protrude from the anal opening during straining and then spontaneously reduce. Stage III hemorrhoids prolapse during defecation and require manual reduction. Stage IV hemorrhoids are chronically prolapsed and produce a mucoid perianal discharge. Pain mainly occurs when hemorrhoids thrombose.

The most common symptom of hemorrhoids is rectal bleeding. Bright red blood may be seen on the stool itself, on the toilet paper, or drip into the bowl following a bowel movement. Rectal bleeding should always be evaluated to rule out a more serious cause for bleeding. Anoscopy in the **prone jackknife position** and sigmoidoscopy are used to examine the anus, **rectal vault**, and sigmoid colon and to rule out other sources of bleeding. A **digital rectal exam (DRE)** can also be performed. Treatment of stage I through stage III hemorrhoids is conservative and focused on reducing symptoms. Patients are encouraged to eat a high-fiber, low-fat diet to increase stool bulk and

reduce straining. Stool softeners may also be used. Pads soaked with witch hazel or **sitz baths** can soothe discomfort. Hemorrhoidectomy is performed for stage IV hemorrhoids that have thrombosed. Hemorrhoids may also be treated with **endoscopic banding** or injection sclerotherapy.

Pause 3-14 What is a digital rectal exam?

The scope was withdrawn from the colon into the patient's rectum. Upon retroflexion, internal hemorrhoids were noted. The scope was withdrawn completely. She tolerated the procedure well and will be sent back to the recovery area in stable condition.

Abdominal Surgery

Abdominal surgeries are very common, and although the terminology and equipment used is vast, many abdominal procedures share common approaches and terminology. Surgical procedures on the abdomen fall into two major categories: laparotomy and laparoscopy. A laparotomy is an incision into the abdomen. Laparoscopy uses scopes inserted through small abdominal incisions to perform **minimally invasive surgery**. **(28)** Surgeons may perform an **exploratory laparotomy** or **exploratory laparoscopy** to make a diagnosis when imaging techniques have failed to provide sufficient information.

Most abdominal procedures require general anesthesia administered by **endotracheal intubation**. Sequential compression devices (SCDs) are also commonly used (see page 143). Before surgery begins, the patient is given prophylactic antibiotics, oftentimes Ancef, and is placed in the proper position for the given surgery. The most common positions for abdominal surgery include prone, Trendelenburg, and modified lithotomy. The patient is then prepped with antiseptic cleansers and covered with sterile surgical drapes to isolate the surgical field.

> Following adequate endotracheal anesthesia, SCD boots were applied and IV Ancef was given. The abdomen was prepped with ChloraPrep and draped sterilely. The patient was placed in the modified lithotomy position on a beanbag and carefully padded stIrrups.

Laparotomy

To access the surgical site, incisions are made through the skin, muscle, and fascia. The peritoneum and mesentery are also dissected. Abdominal structures located behind the peritoneum are referred to as **retroperitoneal**. The incision site is often described relative to the umbilicus: **supraumbilical**, **periumbilical**, **infraumbilical**. Cutting can be accomplished using a scalpel, ultrasonic scalpel (**harmonic scalpel**), blade, or electrocautery. A common cutting technique is **blunt and sharp dissection**. **Retractors** are used to keep the wound open and to move structures out of the operative field. Retractors commonly used during abdominal procedures include

(28) Minimally invasive surgery describes various techniques used to perform surgical procedures using very small surgical incisions that decrease intraoperative bleeding and reduce postoperative pain and recovery time.

(29) The Iron Intern is a mounted retractor with articulating arms. It replaces the (human) surgical intern who is often tasked with holding retractors throughout the surgical procedure.

Alexis, Iron Intern **(29)**, self-retaining, and atraumatic triangular liver retractor. Transcribing abdominal surgical procedures requires a working knowledge of abdominal anatomy including muscles, ligaments, and blood vessels. A helpful way to search for anatomical structures is to perform a Google *image* search using a keyword phrase such as "abdominal ligaments" to view detailed anatomical charts.

Surgical procedures use a variety of sutures and suture materials to **approximate** tissues. Tissues may also be **held in apposition** using surgical clips (eg, Endoclip). Common suture materials include catgut, Ethibond, Prolene, PDS, Vicryl, and Monocryl. Sutures are either absorbable or nonabsorbable; **absorbable sutures** will dissolve over time and do not require removal. Sutures are always described by their size, with a size #7 being the largest in diameter and #0 (dictated as either zero, oh, or **aught**) indicating a smaller diameter. Suture sizes continue to get smaller and smaller, so the smallest suture sizes are described in multiples of zero. For example, a #0000 (4-0) suture is smaller than a #00 (2-0) suture. Different stitches are used depending on the tissue and type of closure. Common stitches include **pursestring**, **interrupted**, **mattress**, **running**, and **figure-of-eight**. At the end of the procedure, the incision is closed stepwise in layers, including the **fascial** and **subcuticular** layers. A **field block** (local anesthesia) using 0.25% Marcaine may be created just before closing the skin. **Dermabond** may also be applied to the skin to seal the incision.

> Do not confuse Monocryl, a suture material, with Monopril, an antihypertensive medication.

> The right lower quadrant fascia was closed with a #0 Vicryl figure-of-eight stitch. The midline fascia was closed with a #1 PDS running suture. The subcutaneous tissue was irrigated well with saline and then a 4-0 Vicryl subcuticular suture was used to close the skin. Steri-Strips and sterile dressings were applied.

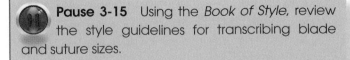

> **Pause 3-15** Using the *Book of Style*, review the style guidelines for transcribing blade and suture sizes.

Surgical staples are commonly used in place of sutures to approximate tissues and close skin wounds. Staple guns (eg, Endo GIA) are used to place the staples. Some staple guns are used to both cut (divide or excise) and suture simultaneously. Staples are especially useful for bowel anastomoses, including **side-to-side anastomoses** and **end-to-end anastomoses**. Staple guns are loaded with cartridges containing titanium staples ranging from 2.0 to 4.8 mm wide. Staple cartridges are color coded to indicate the staple size or purpose, so the color or the type of staple may be dictated instead of the actual staple size. The guns are said to be **fired** (to apply the staple) and reloaded (with new blades and staples). An anastomosis can be checked for adequate closure using a **saline leak test**.

In the postoperative period, both serous and serosanguineous fluid may accumulate in the surgical area, so surgical drains are often placed to allow the fluid to drain outside the body. Commonly used drains include Drake, Penrose, and Jackson-Pratt (JP). At the end of the procedure, **needle, instrument, and sponge counts** are performed to confirm that no sponges (strips of gauze) or other surgical items have been left inside the patient. The **estimated blood loss** is also assessed and recorded in the operative note. Patients are transported to the **postanesthesia care unit (PACU)** to be monitored during the immediate postsurgical period.

> The subcutaneous tissue was irrigated with saline and then a 4-0 Vicryl subcuticular suture was used to close the skin. Steri-Strips and sterile dressings were applied. The patient was extubated and taken to the PACU in stable condition. All sponge, needle, and instrument counts were correct. Estimated blood loss was less than 100 mL.

> The abbreviation PACU may be dictated as the initials p-a-c-u or as the acronym (pāc´ ū).

Laparoscopy

A laparoscopic procedure begins with the creation of a **pneumoperitoneum** using a **Hasson trocar (30)** or a **Veress needle** to **insufflate** the abdomen with CO_2 to about 15 mmHg. Insufflation lifts the abdominal wall and separates it from the viscera, making it easier to visualize the abdominal contents and maneuver the laparoscopic instruments. Following insufflation, small incisions, called ports or **trocar sites**, are made at three to five points around the abdomen to accommodate trocars ranging from 5 to 12 mm in diameter. After insertion into the abdomen, the trocar is removed, leaving the cannula in place to pass surgical instruments through to the surgical site.

> A #15 blade was used to make a 10 mm incision at the umbilicus. A Hasson trocar was secured to the fascia and the abdomen was insufflated to 15 mmHg. Under direct vision, the 5 mm ports were placed in the right and left midabdomen and the right and left lower quadrant.

> The following are terms you may hear in relation to abdominal surgery:
>
> antimesenteric anastomosis
> white line of Toldt (colectomy)
> mesoappendix (appendectomy)
> the triangle of Calot (cholecystectomy)
> Morison pouch (hepatorenal recess)

Diagnostic Studies

The gastroenterologist has an extensive array of diagnostic and therapeutic tests to evaluate and treat patients with gastrointestinal disorders. Studies can be divided into several categories including acid-related tests, manometry, endoscopy, x-ray imaging, and nuclear imaging studies.

Acid-Related Studies

Acid-related studies are used to assess the effectiveness of acid-reducing therapies, also called antisecretory therapies. Probes that measure pH are inserted into

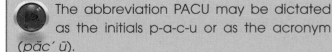

(30) A trocar is a removable plug with a sharp cutting tip inside a cannula. The trocar cuts a path through the tissues to allow placement of the cannula.

the esophagus or stomach. The pH may also be determined by aspirating a sample of the stomach contents using an NG tube. In an **ambulatory pH monitoring test**, the pH probe is positioned in the esophagus for 24–48 hours while the patient carries out normal daily activities. The patient maintains a journal of symptoms to be compared to the data obtained by the pH probe. Measured pH values below 3.5 are considered abnormal. The Bravo Capsule pH test is an example of an ambulatory pH monitoring system. A test capsule, which is attached to the esophageal wall, sends data via radio signals to a receiver worn on the patient's belt.

Manometry

Esophageal manometric motility studies are used to measure the pressure in the upper and lower esophageal sphincters and the coordination of peristaltic movements of the esophagus. This test is performed with the patient awake. Measurements are taken while the patient swallows. The test may be performed to evaluate disorders such as achalasia, **nutcracker esophagus**, esophageal spasm, or noncardiac chest pain. New technology, called **high-resolution manometry (HRM)**, allows the procedure to be completed in less time and with less patient discomfort.

Endoscopy

Endoscopic procedures are among the most common diagnostic tools for the gastroenterologist. Endoscopy allows for direct visual examination of the gastrointestinal tract by means of a flexible, fiberoptic endoscope. Endoscopic procedures may be simultaneously diagnostic and therapeutic, which gives them an advantage over imaging procedures alone (such as x-ray, CT scan, and MRI). Endoscopes are equipped with additional devices such as biopsy forceps, polyp snare, cytology brush, cautery or laser device, and suction. Therapeutic procedures that may be accomplished during a diagnostic endoscopic procedure include removal of foreign bodies, hemostasis by thermal coagulation, laser photocoagulation, variceal banding or sclerotherapy, debulking of tumors, dilation of webs or strictures, stent placement, reduction

> **(31)** To insufflate is to inject air or gas (eg, CO_2) under pressure into a body cavity, lumen, or space.

of volvulus or intussusception, and decompression of acute or subacute colonic dilatation.

Endoscopic equipment may also be fitted with ultrasound transducers, allowing ultrasound images to be taken from within the intestinal tract (as opposed to applying the transducer externally). Endoscopic ultrasound can measure the depth and extent of lesions and evaluate blood flow in the given region—information that cannot be obtained with conventional endoscopy.

Upper Endoscopy

Upper GI endoscopy (UGIE) includes a group of endoscopic procedures with names corresponding to the actual structures examined: esophagoscopy, gastroscopy, esophagogastroscopy, esophagogastroduodenoscopy (EGD), and upper GI with small bowel followthrough.

> **Pause 3-16** List each of the anatomical structures examined in the following procedures:
>
> 1. esophagoscopy
> 2. gastroscopy
> 3. esophagogastroscopy
> 4. esophagogastroduodenoscopy (EGD)
> 5. upper GI with small bowel followthrough

During an endoscopic procedure, the endoscope is advanced down the esophagus and passed into the stomach and possibly through the pyloric sphincter into the duodenum (in the case of an EGD). After examining the duodenum, the endoscope is then withdrawn into the stomach for a closer look at the cardia, fundus, greater and lesser curvature, and antrum. Insufflation (31) is used to distend the stomach. The tip of the scope is retroflexed in the shape of a letter J (called a **J maneuver**) in order to examine the fundus and gastroesophageal junction. Although the scope is flexible and can be retroflexed, there are still several areas that are difficult to fully visualize, referred to as blind spots. Areas that are difficult to examine include the duodenal bulb, portions of the fundus, and the lesser curvature below the incisura.

> The esophagus was intubated under direct visualization without difficulty. The scope was passed down to the Z line at 40 cm. The esophageal mucosa appeared normal. There was no evidence of Barrett esophagus. The scope passed through this into the stomach and duodenum. The duodenal bulb and second portion were normal. Multiple small-bowel biopsies were taken to rule out celiac disease, though the mucosa appeared normal endoscopically. The gastric mucosa was unremarkable, including retroflex exam of the cardia and fundus. The patient tolerated the procedure very well. There were no complications.

When necessary, the examiner can perform a **push endoscopy**, which is capable of advancing farther into the duodenum than standard endoscopy procedures. The push endoscope is approximately 200 cm long and has a rigid overtube to prevent the scope from coiling in the stomach, thereby extending its reach.

In addition to traditional endoscopic procedures, patients may undergo wireless capsule endoscopy (also called **video capsule endoscopy**) that allows visualization of the upper GI tract all the way through to the small bowel—obtaining information much farther into the small intestine than a tethered endoscope. A camera encapsulated into a swallowable device the size of a large pill transmits photographic data to a receiver worn on the patient's belt. Over seven to eight hours, the camera travels the length of the GI tract, taking snapshots at the rate of two images per second. The "pill" is eventually expelled and discarded. The videotape is reviewed by a gastroenterologist. This procedure is particularly useful for diagnosing obscure GI bleeding in the small bowel. Brand names include PillCam and Olympus Endo Capsule. The most significant complication of capsule endoscopy is capsule retention. In cases of proven retention (using abdominal radiographs), **double-balloon enteroscopy** may be used to remove the capsule.

Lower Endoscopy

Lower endoscopy includes procedures that visualize the terminal ileum, colon, rectum, and anus.

Anoscopy   The anoscope is used to view the anus, anal canal, internal sphincter, and distal rectum using a 7 cm scope. The test is typically preceded by a visual inspection of the outer anus and a digital rectal exam. Anoscopy, also called proctoscopy, is used to diagnose internal hemorrhoids and anal fissures.

Flexible Sigmoidoscopy   A flexible sigmoidoscopy uses a flexible endoscope to examine the sigmoid colon. Patients are placed in the jackknife position during the procedure. The instrument is either 35 cm or 60 cm long, limiting the procedure to visualization of the sigmoid colon. A flexible sigmoidoscopy requires less bowel prep, no sedation, and is more comfortable for the patient than a full colonoscopy. Instrumentation also allows for biopsy, fulguration, and stool sampling. The rectum is visualized during withdrawal of the scope by retroflexing the tip 180 degrees.

> A flexible sigmoidoscopy is typically dictated as a "flex sig." This short form should be spelled out.

Colonoscopy   Colonoscopy allows for the direct visual examination of the entire colon, ileocecal valve, and portions of the terminal ileum and is the preferred screening method for cancers of the colon and rectum. Mucosal surfaces are examined for ulcerations, polyps, friable areas, hemorrhagic sites, neoplasms, and strictures. Biopsies for histopathology and cultures may also be taken during the procedure, and therapeutic procedures such as electrocoagulation of bleeding sites, polypectomy, and fulguration of tumors may also be accomplished.

Thorough bowel prep is critical to obtaining a **technically adequate study**. Colonoscopes range in length from 135–185 cm. Specific landmarks are noted as the scope is **advanced under direct visualization**. The rectum is highly vascular with bluish vessels. The sigmoid colon is distinguished by ring-like valves. The descending colon is narrow and tubular, and the transverse colon shows triangular folds. The hepatic flexure is noted to have a dark blue hue from the adjacent liver, and the ascending colon is notable for a large lumen. The ileocecal valve and the terminal ileum are also visualized.

A colonoscopy report typically includes comments pertaining to the adequacy of the bowel prep, the type of instrument used, medications administered, the most proximal segment of the bowel examined, and mucosal abnormalities. The examiner comments on the size and appearance of polyps and pseudopolyps, the presence of hemorrhagic areas, ulcers, neoplastic or obstructing lesions, diverticula, friable areas, telangiectasias, and lipomas. The examiner may also include comments on the competence of the ileocecal valve and the presence of spasms.

> With the patient in the left lateral decubitus position, the Olympus pediatric colonoscope was inserted into the rectum and advanced under direct visualization to the cecum. The quality of the bowel prep was extremely poor. There were no large, fungating tumors, but I could have easily missed smaller polyps and vascular anomalies. Mild, left-sided diverticulosis was noted. The rectum showed normal mucosa in antegrade, retrograde, and retroflexed views.

> The patient was placed in the left lateral decubitus position. After she was adequately sedated, a diagnostic adult colonoscope was inserted into the patient's rectum under direct visualization. The scope was easily advanced to the base of the cecum. The ileocecal valve was identified and intubated. The terminal ileum was normal. Careful retrograde examination revealed diffuse diverticular disease primarily involving the left colon. The patient had multiple wide-mouth diverticula present.

Pause 3-17 Explain the use of the terms antegrade, retrograde, and retroflexed views as mentioned in the excerpt of a colonoscopy report above.

X-Ray Imaging

X-ray imaging techniques are very useful in gastroenterology, especially for diagnosing mass lesions, structural abnormalities, and motility disorders. X-ray studies may be used to visualize the entire GI tract from pharynx to rectum. Plain films as well as studies using video and contrast are used. A **double-contrast study** refers to the use of both positive and negative contrast agents to increase the sensitivity of the examination. Barium and Gastrografin are examples of positive contrast media, and air and CO_2 are examples of negative contrast media. The gas may be intrinsic gas (already present in the bowel), or the bowel may be insufflated by the examiner. Barium is a radiopaque substance, which means x-rays do not pass through. Structures coated with barium appear white on the x-ray images. Both still images and video images may be obtained. Video is especially helpful for diagnosing motility disorders.

Barium Swallow

A barium swallow, also called barium esophagography or an upper GI series, uses barium as a contrast media. Patients drink a barium solution, also called a **small-bowel meal**, before the test is performed. Gas may be injected into the alimentary tract by the examiner to obtain a double-contrast study. A barium swallow allows visualization of the esophagus, stomach, and small intestine (■ **Figure 3-11**).

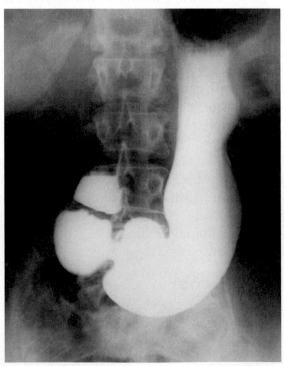

FIGURE 3-11 Upper GI series (barium swallow). *Source:* Biophoto Associates/Photo Researchers, Inc.

Enteroclysis

Enteroclysis, also referred to as a small-bowel enema, provides even better visualization of the small bowel. Instead of the patient swallowing the barium contrast, a balloon-tipped catheter is inserted into the nose and threaded down to the duodenum. Barium and methylcellulose are injected directly into the duodenum. Double-contrast x-ray images are obtained.

Barium Enema

A barium enema, also referred to as a lower GI series, is used to examine the colon for lesions such as polyps or tumors, obstructions, fistulas, diverticulosis, abscesses, dilation of the colon, or abnormal colonic motility. Barium is placed in the colon using a catheter inserted through the anus. X-rays are taken to examine the colon anatomy (■ Figure 3-12). Depending on the distribution of the barium, the distal end of the small intestine may also be visualized.

CT Scans

CT scanning for diagnosis of abdominal pathology is increasing in use, especially in the detection of colon polyps and masses. Also referred to as a virtual colonoscopy and CT enterography (when the small bowel is studied), CT scanning is a noninvasive method of detecting pathology within the lumen of the intestinal tract. CT colonography and enterography use a **multidetector CT (MDCT)** scanner (also called a multidetector helical CT scanner) to generate 3-dimensional images of the intestine using a combination of oral contrast and gas distention. Thorough bowel prep is still necessary, as residual stool may mimic the appearance of polyps on the CT images. For certain indications, such as obscure GI bleeding, small-bowel tumors, and chronic ischemia, a biphasic, contrast-enhanced MDCT study is done. Multiphase MDCT scans are performed by taking multiple images at specific intervals, specifically timed to the injection of the IV contrast.

> CT scan of the abdomen and pelvis revealed an inflammatory process around the cecum. Findings represent nonspecific typhlitis or colitis. Cecal diverticulitis cannot be excluded. The appendix and terminal ileum appeared grossly normal.

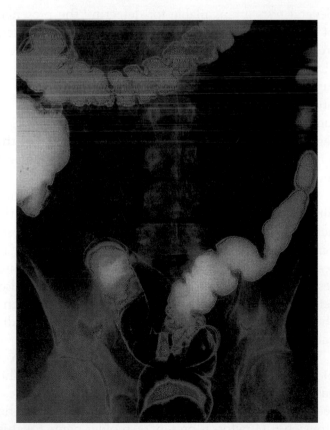

FIGURE 3-12 A color-enhanced radiograph following a barium enema. *Source:* © Picade LLC/Alamy.

Nuclear Imaging Studies

Nuclear imaging studies use radiolabeled tracers that can be detected using a gamma detector. **Nuclear bleeding scans** are used to detect sites of bleeding within the gastrointestinal tract. Patients are given RBCs labeled with technetium (Tc99m), or occasionally Tc99m-labeled colloid, and examined using a gamma camera. Active bleeding sites are identified by focal areas of tracer that correspond to peristaltic movements and increase with time.

Gastric emptying may also be evaluated using nuclear imaging techniques. Patients ingest a radiolabeled meal and are then examined with a gamma detector. The tracer can be seen entering and leaving the stomach, indicating the rate of gastric emptying. This test is helpful in the diagnosis of gastroparesis and gastric obstruction and to evaluate response to prokinetic drugs such as metoclopramide (Reglan).

Terms and phrases heard on GI diagnostic imaging studies:

scalloping and atrophy of duodenal folds

blunting of intestinal villi

hypertrophy of intestinal crypts

infiltration of lamina propria with lymphocytes and plasma cells

duodenal ulcer with a clean base

clean-based ulcer

haustral folds (colon)

loss of haustral markings

rugae (stomach)

valvulae conniventes (mucosal folds of the small intestine)

coffee-bean sign

bird-beak sign

apple-core sign, also known as a napkin ring sign

antral nipple sign (refers to redundant pyloric mucosa protruding into the gastric antrum as seen in pyloric stenosis)

inflammatory phlegmon

appendicolith

thumbprinting

accordion sign

pericolic stranding

fat halo sign

gastrointestinal string sign

lead-pipe appearance of colon

fluid-filled, dilated small-bowel loops

Laboratory Studies

Gastroenterology takes advantage of the clinical laboratory for a range of diagnostic studies but also uses tests at the point of care, especially in the case of suspected Helicobacter pylori infection. Stool samples are commonly collected to test for blood and microorganisms.

Fecal Occult Blood Test

A fecal occult blood test (FOBT) is a standard screening test used to detect small amounts of blood in the stool. The blood may originate from any point within the GI tract, so a positive test should be followed by a more extensive evaluation to determine the source of the blood. The test is usually performed on three separate days in case the bleeding is intermittent. The test detects the heme portion of hemoglobin, so even blood that has passed through the digestive tract and destroyed by acid and enzymes can be detected. Other names used to reference the test include stool occult blood, Hemoccult, guaiac test, and gFOBT (guaiac fecal occult blood test).

 Typical phrases used to describe an FOBT result include:

negative FOBT, positive FOBT

heme-positive stool, heme-negative stool

Hemoccult-positive stool, Hemoccult-negative stool

guaiac-positive stool, guaiac-negative stool

Helicobacter Pylori

Several tests are available for detecting the presence of Helicobacter pylori. A test that can be performed in the physician's office includes the urea breath test (UBT). Patients swallow a capsule containing urea tagged with a radioisotope of carbon. If H pylori is present in the stomach, the urea will be converted to ammonia and radio-tagged carbon dioxide. The radio-tagged carbon can be detected in the patient's breath. The breath test is useful for diagnosing H pylori and monitoring the efficacy of treatment.

A blood test is also available to detect antibodies directed at H pylori. Patients with recent or currently active infection will have a positive antibody test. Since antibodies can persist after the infection is resolved, the antibody test is not ideal for monitoring response to treatment. The H pylori antigen test, also referred to as the fecal antigen test, looks for antigens shed in the stool. A negative fecal antigen test indicates there is no current infection.

The rapid urease test (RUT) is performed on a biopsy specimen at the time of gastric endoscopy. The gastric mucosa is sampled and combined with the test reagents to detect urease, which only occurs in the stomach if H pylori is present. An older name for this test is the CLO (*klō*) test, which stands for Campylo-bacter-like organism.

Celiac Antibodies

Patients intolerant to gluten (celiac disease) will be positive for IgA or IgG **antigliadin antibodies (AGA)**. Other antibodies which may be detectable in the blood of patients with celiac disease include antireticulin antibody (ARA), anti-transglutaminase antibody (TGA), and antiendomysial antibody (EMA). These tests have greater than 90% sensitivity and specificity for celiac disease.

> **Pause 3-18** Diagnostics tests are often described by their sensitivity and specificity for a specific disease or disorder, which indicate how likely a test is able to detect a particular disease without producing an erroneous result. Research the terms *sensitivity* and *specificity* and explain which one refers to the ability to detect a disease and which refers to the ability to distinguish a disease.

Clostridium Toxin

Clostridium difficile is difficult to culture, so the most effective method of diagnosing C difficile infection is to test for the presence of toxin A and/or toxin B in the stool of the infected patient. Patients suspected of having antibiotic-associated diarrhea will be asked to provide a stool sample to be tested for C difficile toxin.

Microbiology

Patients suspected of having a parasitic intestinal infection typically undergo a test for **ova and parasites (O&P)**. This test involves the direct examination of a stool sample under a microscope. Laboratory personnel place a sample of the patient's stool on a microscope slide and carefully scan the slide for ova (eggs) and parasites that are known to be pathologic to humans. Parasites go through lifecycles and will intermittently shed either ova or the mature form of the parasite in the stool, so three samples taken over a ten-day period are usually obtained to ensure that at least one sample contains evidence of infection. Common parasitic infections include Giardia lamblia and Cryptosporidium. Other infections might include Entamoeba histolytica, helminths (worms) such as Strongyloides stercoralis, Ascaris lumbricoides, hookworms, tapeworms, and trematodes such as Schistosoma species.

Stool culture may be performed to detect Salmonella, Shigella species, Entamoeba histolytica, Campylobacter jejuni, and E coli subtypes, especially E coli O157:H7. A stool sample is collected by the patient and a small portion of the stool is cultured in specially prepared petri dishes. Stool culture results typically take 24–48 hours. Physicians often order **stool for culture and sensitivity**, which means the stool sample will be cultured, and if positive for a known pathogen will be tested against a range of antibiotics to determine which drug will be most effective in treating the infection.

Pharmacology

Gastroenterology uses a wide range of pharmacological treatments to manage diseases of the gastrointestinal tract.

Antispasmodics

Antispasmodic drugs (**Table 3-1**), also known as anticholinergics, reduce intestinal spasms caused by intestinal disorders such as irritable bowel syndrome, inflammatory bowel disease, spastic colon, diverticulitis, and peptic ulcers. The neurotransmitter acetylcholine causes the release of gastric acid and promotes peristalsis. Antispasmodics block the action of acetylcholine by blocking the acetylcholine receptors. Anticholinergic drugs may also be given to treat diarrhea by decreasing peristalsis. The most common drug used for this purpose is Imodium (loperamide).

Table 3-1 Gastrointestinal Antispasmodics

Generic	Brand Name	Dose
dicyclomine	Bentyl	10 mg, 20 mg
hyoscyamine	Levsin	0.125 mg
	Levbid	0.375 mg
	Levsinex	0.375 mg
loperamide	Imodium	2 mg

Antimicrobials

Many gastrointestinal infections are self-limited and resolve without treatment, but when treatment is required, antimicrobial therapy may be used (**Table 3-2**). Conditions commonly requiring antiinfective treatment include Clostridium difficile, Giardia lamblia, Vibrio cholerae, Campylobacter jejuni, Shigella, and Entamoeba histolytica. Patients with diverticulitis and appendicitis may also be treated with antibiotics.

Table 3-2 Antimicrobials Used for Gastrointestinal Infection

Generic	Brand Name	Dose
ciprofloxacin	Cipro	100 mg, 200 mg, 250 mg, 400 mg, 500 mg, 750 mg, 1000 mg
doxycycline	Doryx	75 mg, 100 mg, 150 mg
	Vibramycin	100 mg 50 mg per 5 mL
metronidazole	Flagyl	250 mg, 375 mg, 500 mg
	Flagyl ER	750 mg
sulfamethoxazole and trimethoprim (SMX and TMP in a 5:1 ratio)	Sulfatrim	200 mg/40 mg per 5 mL
	Bactrim, Septra	400 mg/80 mg
	Bactrim DS, Septra DS	800 mg/160 mg
nitazoxanide	Alinia	500 mg
azithromycin	Zithromax	250 mg, 500 mg, 600 mg
bismuth	Pepto-Bismol	

Cytoprotective Agents

The cytoprotective agents (**Table 3-3**) act by coating or promoting healing of the gastric mucosa. Sucralfate specifically coats ulcerated areas in the gastric mucosa, forming a protective layer over the wound while it heals.

Table 3-3 Cytoprotective Agents

Generic	Brand Name	Dose
sucralfate	Carafate	1 g
misoprostol	Cytotec	100 mcg, 200 mcg

Antacids

Antacids can be divided into several categories based on their mode of action. Some neutralize acid while others inhibit the production or the secretion of acid.

Acid Neutralizers

Acid neutralizers are weak bases that are capable of neutralizing hydrochloric acid. These drugs are used to treat occasional heartburn and acid indigestion but are no longer used to treat peptic ulcer disease or GERD. The active ingredients in these agents are usually aluminum, magnesium, calcium, sodium, or a combination of these. Examples include milk of magnesia (MOM), Tums, Maalox, Alka-Seltzer, and Rolaids.

Simethicone, an antigas medication, is often added to antacids to help relieve the pressure of gas that often accompanies acid indigestion. Simethicone alone is found in products such as Mylicon and Phazyme.

Proton Pump Inhibitors

Proton pump inhibitors (**Table 3-4**) decrease acid production by interfering with the secretion of acid within the parietal cells of the stomach. The proton pump is responsible for secreting H^+ ions into the stomach, and this class of drug inhibits the action of the proton pump. Because the drug irreversibly inhibits a key enzyme involved in proton secretion, the effects of a single dose of a proton pump inhibitor (PPI) is long lasting—up to two to three days. PPIs are currently the most effective means of inhibiting gastric acid; they reduce acid secretion up to 99%. The generic names of this class share the common ending –prazole.

Table 3-4 Proton Pump Inhibitors

Generic	Brand Name	Dose
esomeprazole	Nexium	40 mg
lansoprazole	Prevacid	15 mg, 30 mg
omeprazole	Prilosec	10 mg, 20 mg, 40 mg
pantoprazole	Protonix	40 mg
rabeprazole	Aciphex	20 mg
omeprazole and sodium bicarbonate	Zegerid	20 mg, 40 mg

Be very careful when spelling Protonix. A sound-alike word *Protonics* will spell check but is the wrong spelling for the drug.

H$_2$-Receptor Antagonists

Histamine activates histamine 2 (H$_2$) receptors on the parietal cells of the stomach, causing the cells to release hydrochloric acid (HCl). H$_2$-receptor antagonists, called **H$_2$-blockers**, interfere with the action of histamine on the parietal cells and reduce the amount of acid released. The H$_2$-receptor blockers (**Table 3-5**) may also be referred to as H$_2$-receptor antagonists. This class of drug is used to treat heartburn, gastroesophageal reflux disease, and peptic ulcers. Generic drugs in this class end in *–tidine*.

Table 3-5 H$_2$-Receptor Antagonists

Generic	Brand Name	Dose
cimetidine	Tagamet	300 mg, 400 mg, 800 mg
	Tagamet HB	200 mg
famotidine	Pepcid	20 mg, 40 mg
	Pepcid AC	10 mg, 20 mg
nizatidine	Axid	150 mg, 300 mg
	Axid AR	75 mg
ranitidine	Zantac	150 mg, 300 mg
	Zantac (OTC)	75 mg, 150 mg

Helicobacter Pylori

Treatment of Helicobacter pylori requires combination therapy (**Table 3-6**) to decrease gastric acid and to eliminate the infectious organism. Combination drugs typically contain combinations of an antacid, an antibiotic, and an antiprotozoal drug.

Table 3-6 Combination Drugs to Treat H Pylori

Generic	Brand Name
bismuth, metronidazole, tetracycline	Helidac Pylera
amoxicillin, clarithromycin, lansoprazole	Prevpac

Antidiarrheals

Antidiarrheal medications (**Table 3-7**) are used to control diarrhea. Diphenoxylate is used to slow peristalsis, thereby reducing diarrhea. Loperamide increases the tone of circular smooth muscles, slowing down the transit time and allowing more water to be absorbed.

Table 3-7 Antidiarrheals

Generic	Brand Name	Dose
diphenoxylate and atropine	Lomotil	2.5 mg/0.025 mg
loperamide	Imodium A-D	1 mg/5 mL, 1 mg/7.5 mL, 2 mg

Laxatives

Laxatives are used for the short-term treatment of constipation and can be categorized as to their mode of action.

Osmotic Laxatives

Osmotic laxatives (**Table 3-8**) work by drawing water into the bowel lumen to soften the stool and allow it to pass more easily. Magnesium and glycerin are the most common active ingredients in osmotic laxatives. Lactulose, available only by prescription, is a synthetic sugar whose metabolites have an osmotic effect on the bowel.

Table 3-8 Osmotic Laxatives

Generic	Brand Name
magnesium sulfate	Epsom salt
glycerin	
milk of magnesia (MOM)	Phillip's Milk of Magnesia
lactulose	Enulose
polyethylene glycol (PEG)	MiraLax

Bulking Laxatives (Fiber)

Bulk-producing laxatives are primarily indigestible fiber that add mass, absorb water, and soften the stool. Fiber may be naturally occurring, as in psyllium, or synthetic, as in methylcellulose. These laxatives are sold over the counter under brand names such as Citrucel, FiberCon, and Perdiem.

Stool Softener

Stool softeners (**Table 3-9**) work by emulsifying the fat and water in the stool, which retains more water in the stool.

Table 3-9 Stool Softener

Generic	Brand Name	Dose
docusate	Colace	50 mg, 100 mg

Mucosal Irritants

Irritants (**Table 3-10**) work by stimulating the intestinal mucosa to promote peristalsis. The sennosides are derived from the senna plant and are available in a variety of forms including teas, capsules, and liquids.

Table 3-10 Sennosides

Generic	Brand Name	Dose
sennosides	Senokot	8.6 mg
docusate and sennosides	Peri-Colace	50 mg/8.6 mg

Evacuants

Evacuants (**Table 3-11**) are used to prepare the bowel for endoscopy or surgery. The most common evacuant is a solution of polyethylene glycol and electrolytes (PEG-ES). Patients typically must consume 2–4 L to complete the bowel prep.

Table 3-11 Bowel Evacuants

Generic	Brand Name
PEG with electrolytes	Colyte, GoLYTELY, NuLYTELY

Note: The manufacturer has trademarked these names using mixed case (with mostly uppercase letters). The use of idiosyncratic capitalization in drug names is optional; you may need to follow facility/employer preference.

Polyethylene glycol (PEG) is a common ingredient used in medications and medical procedures. You may hear it referenced as the acronym "peg."

Antiemetics

Antiemetics are used to control nausea and vomiting. Antiemetics may be administered orally, by IV, or by rectal suppository. Antiemetics fall into several classes: antimuscarinics, antihistamines, and phenothiazines. The antiemetics that are derived from phenothiazine share a common ending –*azine* (**Table 3-12**). This class of antiemetic is an H_1 (histamine) -receptor antagonist and also has strong sedative effects.

Table 3-12 H_1-Receptor Antagonists

Generic	Brand Name	Dose
promethazine	Phenergan	12.5 mg, 25 mg, 50 mg
prochlorperazine	Compazine	5 mg, 10 mg, 25 mg suppository

The selective 5-HT_3 receptor antagonists (a class of serotonin-receptor antagonists) act centrally on the vomiting center and are the most effective drugs for preventing nausea and vomiting, but they are also the most expensive. This class of drug can be recognized by the common ending –*setron* (**Table 3-13**). These drugs are very safe and may even be prescribed in the first trimester of pregnancy. They are most commonly used in patients undergoing chemotherapy.

Table 3-13 Selective 5-HT_3 Receptor Antagonists

Generic	Brand Name	Dose
ondansetron HCL	Zofran	4 mg, 8 mg
palonosetron	Aloxi	injection only

The prokinetic class of antiemetics (**Table 3-14**), represented by Reglan, is commonly used before and after surgery to restore bowel peristalsis and relieve nausea associated with an "akinetic" bowel.

Table 3-14 Prokinetic Antiemetic

Generic	Brand Name	Dose
metoclopramide	Reglan	5 mg, 10 mg

Antiinflammatories

A select group of antiinflammatory medications are used to target the inflammatory response in the gastrointestinal tract by reducing the production of prostaglandins. The most common class of drugs used for inflammatory bowel disorders is the aminosalicylic acid (ASA) drugs (**Table 3-15**). These drugs may be administered orally or rectally.

Table 3-15 Gastrointestinal Antiinflammatory Medications

Generic	Brand Name	Dose
Mesalamine	Asacol	400 mg
	Canasa	1000 mg (suppository)
	Pentasa	250 mg, 500 mg
	Rowasa	4 g/60 mL (rectal suspension)
	Lialda	1.2 g
Sulfasalazine	Azulfidine	500 mg

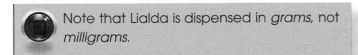 Note that Lialda is dispensed in *grams,* not *milligrams.*

Cortisone (**Table 3-16**) may also be used rectally as an antiinflammatory.

Table 3-16 Rectal Cortisone

Generic	Brand Name
hydrocortisone	Cortenema, Cortifoam

Antimetabolites

Antimetabolites (**Table 3-17**) may be used to downregulate the immune system in autoimmune disorders such as Crohn disease and ulcerative colitis. Drugs in this category interfere with metabolic processes, especially in rapidly dividing cells, by interfering with DNA and RNA synthesis. See also page 433 in Chapter 12.

Table 3-17 Antimetabolites

Generic	Brand Name	Dose
azathioprine	Imuran	50 mg
methotrexate (MTX)	Rheumatrex	2.5 mg, 5 mg, 7.5 mg, 10 mg, 15 mg
mercaptopurine	Purinethol	50 mg

Anticytokine Monoclonal Antibodies

Crohn disease may be treated with a class of drugs called monoclonal antibodies directed against cytokines (see also page 339). This class is distinguished by the suffix –*mab* (for *m*onoclonal *a*nti*b*ody). Monoclonal antibodies are commonly used to treat autoimmune diseases, including Crohn disease and ulcerative colitis. These drugs (**Table 3-18**) are administered on a weekly or monthly basis by IV.

Table 3-18 Anticytokine Monoclonal Antibodies

Generic	Brand Name
infliximab	Remicade
certolizumab pegol	Cimzia
adalimumab	Humira

Exercises

Using Context to Make Decisions

Use the sample report 3B on page 465 in Appendix B to answer the following questions 1–4.

1. Based on information in the History of Present Illness, which of the following medications could the patient have been taking previously for her acid reflux?
   a. Tums
   c. Milk of magnesia
   b. Prevacid
   d. Tagamet

2. Where is the patient's dysphagia?
   a. At the level of the thyroid.
   b. At the back of the throat.
   c. Near the LES.
   d. In the right lower quadrant.

3. The patient is noted to have abdominal distention. Does the examiner believe this is due to peritoneal fluid? Why or why not? _____
   _____

4. Match the patient's medications to items listed in the Past Medical History. Which medical problem is not being treated pharmacologically?
   Exforge _____
   Singulair _____
   Advil _____
   Nexium _____

5. How do the following drug names relate to their pharmaceutical class and active ingredient? Asacol, Canasa, Pentasa, Rowasa _____
   _____

6. Read the following excerpt and explain the meaning of the phrase "treat empirically." _____
   _____

   ASSESSMENT AND PLAN: Patient with 2-week history of epigastric and retrosternal pain. She will have a stress test next week, but in the meantime, we will treat empirically with Nexium.

7. Nissen and Dor fundoplications are used to treat GERD and achalasia. What is a plication? What is a fundoplication? _____
   _____

8. Explain the use of the term *purchase* in the following excerpt: _____

   The clips were in place on the cystic duct and cystic artery with good purchase.

9. Given the following excerpt, what does *manual reduction* mean in this context? _____
   _____

   Stage III hemorrhoids prolapse during defecation and require manual reduction.

Use the sample report on page 89 to answer questions 10–15.

10. What word should be transcribed in blank #1?
    _____

11. What word should be transcribed in blank #2?
    _____

12. What word should be transcribed in blank #3?
    _____

13. What word was transcribed incorrectly in the third paragraph that starts "Of note . . . "? _____
    _____

14. Identify the discrepancy in the History of Present Illness and the Plan. _____
    _____

15. Identify the transcription error that occurred in the second paragraph (that starts "Due to her presentation . . . ")? _____
    _____

Terms Checkup

Complete the multiple-choice questions for Chapter 3 located at www.myhealthprofessionskit.com. To access the questions, select the discipline "Medical

Transcription," then click on the title of this book, *Advanced Medical Transcription*.

Look It Up

Using the guidelines described on page xvii, complete a research project on small bowel bacterial overgrowth.

Transcription Practice

1. Transcribe the key terms and phrases for Chapter 3.
2. Complete the proofing and transcription practice exercises for Chapter 3.

HISTORY OF PRESENT ILLNESS: The patient is a very pleasant 74-year-old female referred by Dr. Callejas for GI consultation. Currently the patient states she feels well except for _____(1)_____, which began fairly recently with a resultant 15-pound weight loss. There has been no concurrent nausea, vomiting, difficulty with swallowing, or evidence of active gastrointestinal bleeding.

Due to her presentation, laboratory data was collected on March 19, 20XX, documenting iron _____(2)_____ anemia with hemoglobin 32.0, hematocrit 10.9, and MCV 80.1. In addition, ferritin was evaluated and is markedly _____(3)_____ at 4 ng/mL.

Of note, the patient has no prior history of bile malignancy, GI bleed, nor has she undergone previous endoscopic inspection of the gastrointestinal tract. Otherwise, there are no additional comments or medical complaints.

ASSESSMENT
1.   Iron-deficiency anemia of unclear etiology. Rule out primary gastrointestinal origin.
2.   Progressive weight loss related to anorexia, concerning for possible occult neoplasm.
3.   High blood pressure.
4.   Seasonal allergies.

PLAN: The patient will be scheduled for a diagnostic colonoscopy and EGD. If the aforementioned studies are inconclusive, then we may need to consider a small-bowel capsule endoscopy. During the interim, I have recommended that she continue iron supplementation and obtain repeat CBC in approximately 4 weeks. Need to obtain previous records of upper GI series.

4

Gastroenterology: The Organs

Learning Objectives

After completing this chapter, you should be able to comprehend and correctly transcribe terminology related to:

▶ diseases of the liver, including portal hypertension, jaundice, hepatitis, hepatic failure, fatty liver disease, cirrhosis, and alcoholic liver disease

▶ the gallbladder and biliary tract, including cholecystitis, choledocholithiasis, and cholangitis

▶ pancreatitis

▶ laboratory and imaging tests used to diagnose and monitor diseases of the liver, biliary tract, and pancreas

▶ drugs used in the treatment of jaundice, cholelithiasis, pancreatitis, and hepatitis

Introduction

The organs of the gastrointestinal system include the liver, gallbladder, and pancreas. These vital structures play a role in digestion, elimination, metabolism, and detoxification. These three organs are connected to one another through the biliary ducts and often disease of one structure leads to secondary disease in one or both of the other organs.

The Liver

The liver is the most metabolically complex organ in the body and receives approximately 30% of resting cardiac output. The liver plays such a vital role in detoxification, excretion, protein production, lipid and glucose metabolism that disruption of the liver's functional capacity has widespread and profound effects on the body with a high rate of morbidity and mortality.

Hepatocytes, which make up the liver parenchyma, carry out the majority of the work of the liver. Major functions of the liver include:

- production of bile
- regulation of carbohydrate metabolism
- storage of glycogen and iron
- regulation of lipid metabolism
- production of clotting factors and enzymes
- production and regulation of albumin and other carrier proteins
- detoxification of endogenous waste (metabolic byproducts) and exogenous toxins (drugs, chemicals)

An important function of the liver is to deaminate amino acids so they can be converted to glucose or fats as needed. Deamination involves the removal of the nitrogen-containing group NH_2 that quickly changes to ammonia (NH_3). Ammonia is very toxic and must be immediately converted to urea that is easily excreted by the kidneys.

Another critical role of the liver is the management of plasma albumin, one of the most important forms of protein in the body. Albumin is the main contributor to osmotic pressure and therefore plays a key role in the fluid distribution between the intravascular and extravascular spaces. Albumin also acts as a carrier protein in the blood by binding (chemically attaching to) hormones, drugs, and electrolytes. Substances that are not water soluble ordinarily do not stay in the solution within the plasma and cannot be adequately transported through the water-based circulatory system. Albumin acts as a carrier to keep these molecules suspended in the plasma.

The liver receives blood from two major vessels; it receives oxygenated blood via the **hepatic artery** and deoxygenated venous blood by way of the **hepatic portal vein**. The hepatic portal vein receives blood from the small and large intestines by way of the **superior and inferior mesenteric veins** (■ Figure 4-1). The hepatic portal vein also receives blood from the stomach, spleen, pancreas, and gallbladder.

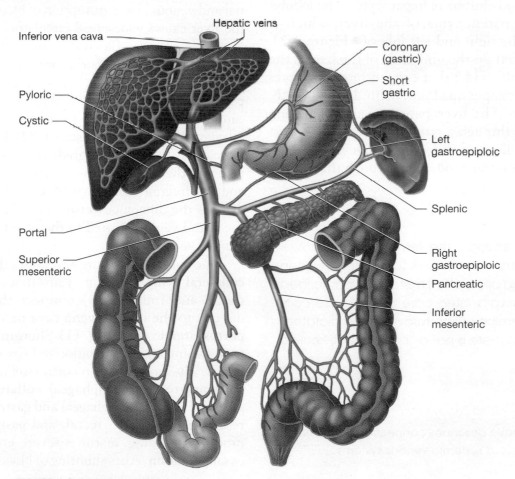

FIGURE 4-1 Portal circulation.

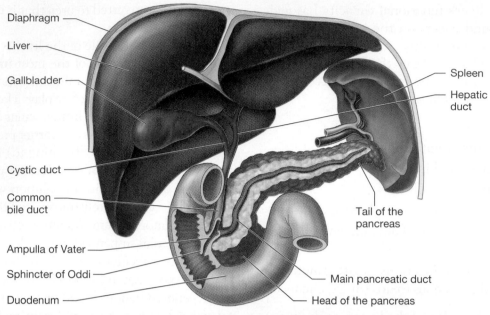

FIGURE 4-2 Anatomy of the liver, gallbladder, pancreas, and spleen.

At the cellular level, the liver is organized into lobules that consist of a terminal branch of the hepatic vein and clusters of hepatocytes. The lobules make up the parenchyma of the liver, which is divided into the right and left lobes (■ **Figure 4-2**). Nestled in a cleft on the underside of the liver is the pear-shaped gallbladder that concentrates and stores bile. In the left upper quadrant, behind the stomach, is the pancreas. The liver, pancreas, and duodenum are connected through a system of ducts that join at the **common bile duct**. Bile and pancreatic enzymes are secreted into the duodenum through the sphincter of Oddi.

> Oddly enough, the terms *bile* and *bowel* are extremely difficult to distinguish when dictated, and bile is often mistakenly transcribed as *bowel*. Always listen carefully and use context to determine which term is being dictated. Keep in mind there is not a "bowel duct," only a "bile duct."

(1) Portosystemic describes connections between the portal and systemic venous systems.

Portal Hypertension

Because the liver receives a large volume of both arterial and venous blood, disruption of blood flow through the liver causes widespread circulatory problems with dire consequences. Blood flow may be restricted due to a **portal thrombus**, portal obstruction, or impaired blood flow through the liver due to cirrhosis. The excessive backpressure created by the restricted flow causes the blood pressure to rise in the hepatic portal vein. **Portal hypertension (PH)** is defined as an increase in the **pressure gradient** between the portal vein and the hepatic veins or between the portal vein and the inferior vena cava (IVC). The pressure gradient is the difference between the blood pressure in the portal vein compared to the blood pressure in the hepatic veins or IVC.

The increased pressure also causes the formation of **collateral veins,** which are veins that create alternate routes and (mistakenly) connect the portal vein directly to the inferior vena cava in a process called **portosystemic shunting**. (1) Shunting causes blood from the intestinal circulation to bypass the liver altogether. The most common portosystemic shunt creates **coronary-to-gastroesophageal collateral veins** and gives rise to **lower esophageal and gastric varices**. The resulting esophageal, rectal, and gastric varices are prone to bleeding, at times severe enough to cause **exsanguination**. Also, shunting of blood away from the liver causes absorbed products that would otherwise be detoxified by the liver to enter the systemic circulation and pass to the brain with ensuing **portosystemic encephalopathy**. Symptoms include impaired concentration, confusion, drowsiness, flapping tremor, and eventually coma. Encephalopathy can also follow surgically created anastomoses that connect the portal vein and vena cava (**portacaval shunts** or transjugular intrahepatic portosystemic shunting.

> The patient returns for a followup evaluation of chronic GI blood loss secondary to gastric and small-bowel angiodysplasia. She has cirrhosis and portal hypertensive gastropathy. She continues to have chronic blood loss requiring frequent blood transfusions.

> **Pause 4-1** Read the previous section on portal hypertension again. As you read, use Figure 4-1 to trace the flow of blood. Indicate points on the figure that could represent areas of obstruction or decreased blood flow. Put an H on the figure to mark a high-pressure point and put an L on the figure to mark a low-pressure point for the purpose of comparing pressure gradients. Add collateral veins to the figure.

Restricted blood flow within the liver also causes hypertension in the hepatic artery, causing blood flowing from the lungs toward the liver to put back pressure on the lungs' circulatory system. Hypertension in the hepatic artery results in **intrapulmonary right-to-left shunting** and ventilation/perfusion mismatch (**hepatopulmonary syndrome**).

Jaundice

The majority of bilirubin is produced by the conversion of the heme component of hemoglobin following red-cell breakdown. **Jaundice (icterus)** is yellowing of the skin, sclerae, and mucous membranes caused by the accumulation of bilirubin (**hyperbilirubinemia**). Normally, total bilirubin in the blood is 0.2 to 1.2 mg/dL. Jaundice develops when the bilirubin reaches 2–3 mg/dL.

Hyperbilirubinemia may be due to abnormalities in the formation, transport, metabolism, or excretion of bilirubin.

> **Pause 4-2** Explain why intravascular hemolysis increases bilirubin.

Until the bilirubin is processed by the liver, it is **unconjugated**, also referred to as **indirect bilirubin**. Bilirubin attaches to albumin to be transported to the liver and then is conjugated with glucuronic acid, which makes it soluble in water and more easily excreted. **Conjugated bilirubin** (also called **direct bilirubin**) is excreted into the bile and therefore excreted into the duodenum during normal digestion. In the intestine, bacteria convert indirect bilirubin to **urobilinogen**, which is partially eliminated in the feces. Some of the urobilinogen is reabsorbed by the intestines and returned to the liver where it is again excreted in the bile.

Accumulation of bilirubin may be due to intrahepatic or extrahepatic causes. In the presence of hepatic inflammation or damage, the hepatocytes may not be capable of completely conjugating bilirubin, leading to increased indirect bilirubin. In the face of overwhelming hemolysis, even a healthy liver is not able to adequately conjugate and excrete the excess bilirubin.

Cholestasis refers to any condition in which the flow of bile from the liver is blocked. **Cholestatic jaundice** refers to the accumulation of conjugated bilirubin due to impaired bile flow. A blockage within the biliary system (**obstructive jaundice**) may result from bile duct tumors, cysts, bile duct strictures, stones, pancreatitis, pancreatic tumors, or **primary sclerosing cholangitis**. Evaluation of obstructive jaundice begins with ultrasound and is usually followed by **cholangiography**.

Intrahepatic cholestasis (impaired bile formation and secretion) occurs when damage within the liver prevents the proper excretion of bilirubin. There are many causes for intrahepatic cholestasis including alcoholic liver disease, amyloidosis, liver abscess, **total parenteral nutrition (TPN)**, pregnancy, primary biliary cirrhosis, primary sclerosing cholangitis, and viral hepatitis.

Patients typically complain of pruritus that accompanies hyperbilirubinemia. Stools may be light in color (**clay-colored stools**) or urine may be darker than usual.

- The liver is the most metabolically complex organ in the body and is responsible for regulation of bile, carbohydrate, protein, and lipid metabolism, and the production of albumin, carrier proteins, and clotting factors as well as detoxification of endogenous and exogenous toxins.
- Disorders of hepatic circulation caused by cirrhosis, portal hypertension, and portal thrombosis produce widespread systemic effects including portosystemic shunting, varices, encephalopathy, and hepatopulmonary syndrome.
- Jaundice is a symptom of either intrahepatic or extrahepatic disorders and is evaluated by measuring total, direct, and indirect bilirubin levels.

Patients may also complain of abdominal pain, nausea, vomiting, fever, malaise, and myalgias. Treatment of jaundice is dependent upon the etiology, as jaundice is typically a symptom, not a disorder in and of itself.

Pause 4-3 What is total parenteral nutrition (TPN)?

Hepatitis

Hepatitis refers to inflammation of the liver. Inflammation can be due to a number of causative agents, but the most common causes are viral infection and alcohol consumption.

Viral Hepatitis

Viral hepatitis refers to infection by a diverse group of hepatotropic viruses. These viruses vary taxonomically, have different modes of transmission, and have different clinical courses, but they all cause diffuse liver inflammation and liver necrosis. Although other viruses may also infect the liver, such as Epstein-Barr virus, yellow fever virus, and cytomegalovirus, acute viral hepatitis typically refers to the hepatotropic viruses designated hepatitis A, B, C, D, and E. Viruses are not complete organisms because they lack an independent metabolism. They consist of nucleic acid, either DNA or RNA, and a protective envelope, also called a capsid. Viruses infect cells and incorporate their nucleic acid into the host cell and take advantage of the host's cellular processes to replicate. The hepatitis viruses A, C, and E consist of RNA, and hepatitis B virus consists of DNA. Hepatitis D, also referred to as delta agent, is a defective RNA virus that can only replicate in the presence of the hepatitis B virus.

Symptoms of hepatitis are similar across the various types. Each has an **incubation period**, which is the time between exposure and the first signs or symptoms of infection. The incubation period may be as short as two weeks or as long as six months. Onset of symptoms may be abrupt or **insidious**. The prodromal, or **preicteric phase**, produces nonspecific symptoms such as profound anorexia, malaise, **easy fatigability**, myalgia, nausea, vomiting, fever, and right upper quadrant abdominal pain. Patients may also complain of urticaria and arthralgias. The **icteric phase** is marked by dark urine, jaundice, and **acholic stools**. The jaundice actually peaks as the appetite returns and the patient begins to feel better.

(2) Atypical lymphocytes are white blood cells that have been activated and are involved in fighting an infection. They are often seen in viral infections. They are referred to as atypical because of their changed appearance when viewed under a microscope.

(3) Aminotransferases are a group of enzymes, including AST and ALT, used to remove amino groups (NH_2) from amino acids as part of normal protein metabolism.

 Listen carefully for the phrase acholic stools. This phrase sounds like colic stools, which is incorrect. Acholic means there is no bile (*chole-*) in the stool.

Examination may reveal mild hepatomegaly and possibly splenomegaly. A CBC drawn during the preicteric phase may show a decreased or normal white blood cell count with large, **atypical lymphocytes**. (2) **Aminotransferase levels** (3) may "roller coaster,"

intermittently spiking and returning to normal throughout the course of the disease. An increased prothrombin time (PT) is indicative of **fulminant hepatitis** and has an ominous prognosis.

Acute hepatitis typically resolves four to eight weeks after onset of symptoms. Some cases of hepatitis may evolve to a chronic state. Hepatitis A and C viruses may cause an **anicteric hepatitis** that presents as a minor flu-like illness but never results in jaundice. **Recrudescent hepatitis (4)** occurs in a small percentage of patients and is characterized by recurrent symptoms during the recovery phase. In rare cases, acute viral hepatitis progresses to fulminant hepatitis and acute hepatic failure.

Fulminant hepatitis is marked by massive liver necrosis and an actual decrease in liver size, referred to as acute yellow atrophy or **Rokitansky disease**. The patient develops portosystemic encephalopathy with ensuing coma in a matter of hours or days. Complications include bleeding, disseminated intravascular coagulation, and **hepatorenal syndrome**. Emergency liver transplantation provides the best hope for survival.

There is no definitive treatment for *acute* viral hepatitis. Supportive treatment is given in the form of IV glucose when indicated. Cholestyramine (Questran) may be given to ameliorate pruritus if cholestasis is present. Strenuous exertion, alcohol, and hepatotoxic drugs should be avoided. Most patients recover in three to six weeks.

Hepatitis A Virus

Hepatitis A virus (HAV) is the most common cause of acute viral hepatitis worldwide. HAV spreads primarily through the fecal-oral route but may also be waterborne or food-borne. People are contagious before the onset of symptoms, so the virus is easily spread. Unlike hepatitis B and C, HAV is not known to evolve to chronic hepatitis or cirrhosis. HAV infection may be subclinical or mild and may not necessarily produce jaundice. Since the introduction of the vaccine for hepatitis A in 1995, the incidence of acute viral hepatitis from HAV has dropped over 75% in the US.

Currently there are no tests available to detect the hepatitis A *virus* in infected patients. Diagnosis is made indirectly using serological tests for the detection of IgM and IgG antibodies directed against HAV. **Anti-HAV IgM (5)** appears early in the infection and is a marker of current infection. **Anti-HAV IgG**

appears during convalescence and is a marker of past infection.

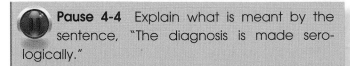

Pause 4-4 Explain what is meant by the sentence, "The diagnosis is made serologically."

Immune globulin should be given to family members and close contacts of patients for postexposure prophylaxis. Immune globulin administration may prevent or attenuate infection. Individuals at risk of HAV infection (eg, travelers to endemic areas, military personnel, daycare workers, healthcare personnel) can be vaccinated against HAV (Havrix and Vaqta). Twinrix is a combination vaccine against hepatitis A and hepatitis B viruses. Patients with other chronic liver diseases should be vaccinated to prevent fulminant hepatitis caused by concomitant HAV infection.

Hepatitis B Virus

The **hepatitis B virus (HBV)** is a DNA virus that has a viral core, inner envelope, and a viral coat containing a surface antigen. It is the second most common cause of acute viral hepatitis. It produces a wide range of clinical presentations from a subclinical carrier state to severe or fulminant hepatitis. **Defervescence** (an elevated temperature returning to normal) and a fall in pulse rate often coincide with the onset of jaundice. Hepatitis B is primarily transmitted through contact with blood and body fluids. Screening tests performed on donor blood by blood banks have nearly eliminated transmission through contaminated blood transfusions and other blood products, but parenteral transmission through needles shared by IV drug users is still common. Infants born to infected mothers may also become infected during delivery.

Infection with HBV is sometimes associated with extrahepatic manifestations such as polyarteritis nodosa, membranous glomerulonephritis, and

(4) Recrudescent means becoming active again; waxing and waning.

(5) Antibodies are identified by combining the prefix *anti-* with the name of the antigen (eg, anti-HAV).

cryoglobulinemia, possibly through an autoimmune mechanism. Infected individuals may become chronic carriers of HBV and are at significant risk of developing cirrhosis and **hepatocellular carcinoma**. Coinfection with human immunodeficiency virus (HIV) is common. HBV is known to have a **chronic carrier state**.

Hepatitis B is diagnosed using serological tests. Laboratory studies test for the presence and concentration (**titer**) (6) of three distinct antigen-antibody systems (Ag-Ab systems) (7) related to HBV: the **core antigen (c)**, the **surface antigen (s)**, and the **envelope antigen (e)**. The **hepatitis B surface antigen (HBsAg)** is detectable early in the disease but generally subsides during convalescence. Its corresponding antibody (**anti-HBs**, also written **HBsAb**) is usually detectable after clinical recovery and confers lifetime immunity. Anti-HBs titers are used to determine **seroconversion**. The core antigen itself is difficult to detect, but antibodies directed against the core antigen (**anti-HBc**, also written **HBcAb**) *are* detectable. **Anti-HBc IgM** is a sensitive marker of acute HBV infection and **anti-HBc IgG** indicates a recent recovery or remote infection.

> **Pause 4-5** Research the term seroconversion. Explain in layman terms the statement, "Anti-HBs titers are used to determine seroconversion."

(6) The term titer is used to describe the relative concentration of a substance that is difficult to measure in precise units. To determine a titer, serial dilutions (a series of successively higher dilutions) of patient serum are made. Serial dilutions dilute the antigen or antibody until the concentration is too small to detect. The higher the initial concentration, the more dilutions are required to reduce the concentration to undetectable levels. Results expressed as a titer represent the highest dilution of patient serum that still gives a positive result.

(7) Ag is the abbreviation for antigen and Ab is used to abbreviate antibody.

(8) A genotype is a variation in the chromosomal makeup of an organism that gives it distinctly different qualities, yet not enough variation to create a separate genus.

Vaccination against HBV is recommended for all US residents beginning at birth. Twinrix is a combination vaccine against HAV and HBV. Other HBV vaccines are marketed under the names Engerix-B and Recombivax HB. Individuals with known exposure to HBV may be given prophylactic treatment by combining the hepatitis vaccine with **hepatitis B immune globulin (HBIG)**, a product with high titers of anti-HBs. The combination treatment does not always prevent infection but may attenuate the severity of the illness if given within seven days of exposure. Chronic hepatitis B infection may be treated with **interferon** or with **nucleoside** and **nucleotide analogs** (see page 111).

Hepatitis C Virus

Hepatitis C virus (HCV) is a single-stranded RNA virus with six major genotypes. (8) The genotypes are designated with arabic numbers (eg, **genotype 1, genotype 2**, etc). HCV is primarily transferred by dirty needles shared between IV drug users or by needles used for tattoos and body piercing. HCV is noted to occur concomitantly with essential mixed cryoglobulinemia, porphyria cutanea tarda, and glomerulonephritis. The reasons for these associations are not known. Infection rates are also high among alcoholics and patients with HIV.

Of all the hepatotropic viruses, HCV is the most likely to become chronic. Chronic infection is defined as elevated aminotransferase levels for greater than six months. Chronic hepatitis C is an **indolent**, often **subclinical** disease. Even though the patient may be asymptomatic, cirrhosis develops in 20% to 30% of patients with chronic HCV infection. These patients are also at higher risk of hepatocellular carcinoma. Patients who have not yet received treatment are described as **treatment naïve**.

HCV may be diagnosed serologically by testing for anti-HCV. Patients positive for anti-HCV are further tested for the actual presence of the virus's RNA in the blood (**viremia**) as well as the virus's genotype.

Genotyping is important for determining treatment and prognosis. HCV genotypes 2 and 3 have a better prognosis than patients infected with genotypes 1 and 4. When deemed appropriate, HCV is treated with interferon alfa-2a or **pegylated interferon** for 6–24 weeks. Ribavirin (Rebetol) may be added if HCV RNA fails to clear after three months of interferon or pegylated interferon. This regimen reduces the chance of the disease progressing to chronic hepatitis and subsequent cirrhosis.

- The most common cause of hepatitis is infection with one of the hepatotropic viruses.
- HAV is the most common hepatitis virus worldwide, is transmitted through the fecal-oral route, and is not known to have a chronic state.
- HBV is the second most common cause of acute viral hepatitis with a wide range of clinical presentations from subclinical infection to fulminant hepatitis. HBV has a carrier state and may become chronic, leading to cirrhosis and possibly hepatocarcinoma. Chronic HBV is treated with interferon and antiviral medications.
- HCV has six major genotypes and is transferred primarily through shared needles. HCV is the most likely hepatotropic virus to become chronic and increases the patient's risk of cirrhosis and hepatocarcinoma. Chronic HCV is treated with interferon and antiviral medications.
- Hepatitis D virus is a defective virus and is only found in patients with hepatitis B coinfection. There are no known outbreaks of hepatitis E in the United States.

Patients with an initially low **viral load** tend to respond better than patients with higher viral loads (greater than 400,000 copies of viral RNA per milliliter of blood). The long-term prognosis is less favorable if treatment with pegylated interferon and ribavirin does not produce at least a **2-log reduction in viral load**. (9) Patients with chronic hepatitis infection are known to develop autoimmune disorders and are monitored for autoimmune antibodies (see page 318 in Chapter 10 for a list of autoimmune antibodies).

The patient was previously seen for initial consultation on March 25, 20XX, for hepatitis C. Laboratory data was obtained, confirming a chronic viral infection with HCV PCR assay equal to 265,510 units/mL. Liver function parameters remain abnormal with AST and ALT of 73 and 97, respectively. In addition, antinuclear antibody and actin smooth muscle antibody are both elevated to 175 and 48, respectively.

Other Hepatitis Viruses

Hepatitis D virus (HDV), also called delta agent, is a defective RNA virus. It can only replicate in the presence of hepatitis B and most commonly occurs as a **superinfection** (10) in chronic hepatitis B. HDV is passed parenterally, especially through dirty needles shared between IV drug users. Hepatitis E virus has a similar mode of transmission and clinical course as hepatitis A, but there have been no known outbreaks of hepatitis E in the United States.

Hepatic Failure

Hepatic failure is characterized by the development of **hepatic encephalopathy** and coagulopathy (defined as an INR value greater than or equal to 1.5). **Acute liver failure (ALF)** may be described as fulminant or subfulminant. **Fulminant hepatic failure** occurs within eight weeks of the onset of acute liver disease, and **subfulminant disease** occurs between eight weeks and six months of the onset of liver disease. The most common cause of hepatic failure is **drug-induced liver injury (DILI)**, with acetaminophen being the most common culprit. Suicide attempts using acetaminophen account for 40% of acetaminophen-related liver failure, the remaining being accidental overdose. Other causes of hepatic failure include **idiosyncratic drug reactions**, (11) viral hepatitis, poisonous mushrooms, shock, hyperthermia or hypothermia, **Budd-Chiari syndrome**, and malignancy.

Acetaminophen overdose is treated with an **antidote**, specifically **N-acetylcysteine (NAC)** given intravenously. In general, treatment of hepatic failure focuses on correcting the metabolic abnormalities that result

(9) Viral loads are measured in very large numbers and often reported in exponential notation (eg, 10,000 units/mL is written as 1×10^5 units/mL). A 2-log reduction would be a decrease by a logarithmic factor of 2 (eg, from 10^5 to 10^3 or 1000).

(10) A superinfection is a second infection in addition to an initial infection.

(11) An idiosyncratic drug reaction is an abnormal reaction to a drug; it may have a genetic basis.

from impaired or absent liver function. Coagulation defects are corrected using blood products to replace missing coagulation factors. Electrolyte and acid-base disturbances must also be managed. **Extradural sensors** are placed to monitor for cerebral edema, which is treated with **mannitol** or hypothermia to 33.1 degrees Celsius. **Lactulose**, which inhibits intestinal ammonia production, is given to treat encephalopathy. Liver failure carries a poor prognosis, and transplantation may offer the patient the highest chance of survival.

Fatty Liver Disease

The most common response to liver injury is inflammation and accumulation of fat within the liver itself. Alcoholism is a common cause. **Fatty liver disease** that is not a result of excess alcohol intake is called **nonalcoholic fatty liver disease (NAFLD)**. It is typically a benign disease, marked by excess lipids in the hepatocytes. There are many causes of NAFLD, including obesity, diabetes, and dyslipidemia as well as an adverse reaction to a drug or injury caused by chemotherapy or a toxin. Patients on long-term total parenteral nutrition (TPN) may also have NAFLD. A variant of NAFLD is **nonalcoholic steatohepatitis (NASH)** in which patients develop liver disease that is histologically indistinguishable from alcoholic hepatitis. NASH is thought to be linked to insulin resistance because many affected patients have obesity, type 2 diabetes mellitus, or dyslipidemia.

Most patients with NASH are asymptomatic, but they may have right upper quadrant discomfort. Hepatomegaly is palpable on examination in the majority of patients. Other **stigmata of liver disease** are uncommon. Laboratory evaluation shows a mild elevation in the aminotransferases and **alkaline phosphatase** levels in about 20% of patients with NASH. Left untreated, NASH may progress to cirrhosis.

> **Pause 4-6** Explain the phrase "stigmata of liver disease." Give some examples of stigmata.

A **percutaneous liver biopsy** typically provides a definitive diagnosis. Treatment focuses on eliminating or reducing causative factors. Patients are encouraged to lose weight, exercise, and limit dietary fat. Medication may be given to treat dyslipidemia, and metformin may be prescribed to treat insulin resistance.

Cirrhosis

Chronic liver inflammation and injury cause excessive connective tissue to form in a process called **fibrosis**. Fibrotic tissue is not functional. Left unchecked, fibrosis progresses to **cirrhosis**, an end-stage liver disorder with a high mortality rate. The most common causes of cirrhosis are chronic infection with hepatitis B and C viruses and excessive alcohol consumption. Many cases are cryptogenic (ie, the cause is never determined). The fibrotic tissue of cirrhosis distorts the liver's cellular architecture and restricts the flow of blood through the liver. Symptoms of cirrhosis result from both hepatic cell dysfunction and narrowing of the intrahepatic circulatory pathways (see earlier discussion of portal hypertension). Cirrhosis is among the top ten causes of death in the United States. **Table 4-1** lists common symptoms of cirrhosis.

Two models are used to assess the severity of liver disease. The **Child-Pugh scale** classifies patients into class A, B, or C, with class C having the lowest two-year survival rate. The scale is based on serum bilirubin, INR value, serum albumin, the degree of ascites, and the grade of hepatic encephalopathy. The **model for end-stage liver disease score (MELD score)** is used to assess the risk of mortality from liver disease and also to prioritize patients on liver transplant waiting lists. The MELD score is calculated using serum bilirubin, creatinine, and INR values. MELD scores range from a low of 6 (less ill) to 40 (gravely ill). MELD scores are divided into four levels:

- ≥ 25
- 24-19
- 18-11
- ≤ 10

> MELD is pronounced as the acronym "meld."

Alcoholic Liver Disease

Alcohol (ethanol) is a significant contributor to liver disease. Alcohol use is high in Western countries where up to 10% of the population uses or abuses alcohol regularly. Chronic alcohol intake first manifests as fatty liver, also called **steatohepatitis**, and progresses to alcoholic hepatitis and eventually cirrhosis. Patients with excess alcohol consumption are also at increased risk of hepatocellular carcinoma. Although the amount of

Table 4-1 Symptoms of Cirrhosis

Symptom	Cause	Comments
abdominal pain and distention	ascites	Increased hydrostatic pressure in the portal venous system forces fluid out of the vessels and into the peritoneal space.
edema	hypoalbuminemia	Albumin passes from the blood into the ascitic fluid in the peritoneal space, reducing the albumin in the circulating blood. Reduced albumin in the peripheral circulation causes fluid to move into the interstitial spaces.
shortness of breath, hypoxia	hepatic hydrothorax	Ascites moves across the diaphragm into the pleural space.
abdominal pain and fever	spontaneous bacterial peritonitis	Irritation from ascitic fluid promotes bacterial infection in the peritoneal space.
fluid overload	azotemia (elevated urea in the blood), hyponatremia, low urinary sodium, oliguria, renal failure	Hepatorenal syndrome occurs in up to 10% of patients with advanced cirrhosis and ascites.
disordered CNS function, confusion, lethargy	hepatic encephalopathy	Neurotoxicity is caused by noxious agents not cleared by liver.
anemia	microcytic anemia, macrocytic anemia, or mixed anemia with high RDW	Decreased blood cells may be due to chronic bleeding (varices, coagulopathies), hypersplenism, undernutrition with deficiency of folate, iron, or vitamin B_{12}, chronic disease, or effects of alcohol.
clubbing	hepatopulmonary syndrome	Chronic hypoxia leads to clubbing of the fingers.
fragility fractures	osteoporosis	Malabsorption of fat-soluble vitamin D and malnutrition lead to osteoporotic bone that breaks easily.
icterus	hyperbilirubinemia	Disordered bilirubin metabolism increases bilirubin in the circulatory system with deposition in the tissues.
petechiae, purpura, bleeding	coagulopathies and thrombocytopenia	Malabsorption of fat-soluble vitamin K causes bleeding disorders; platelets are sequestered in the enlarged spleen causing thrombocytopenia.
pruritus, xanthelasmas	hyperbilirubinemia	Disordered bilirubin metabolism increases bilirubin in the circulatory system with deposition in the tissues.
splenomegaly	portal hypertension	Increased portal hypertension causes spleen to enlarge.
clay-colored stool	steatorrhea	Lack of bile for fat absorption increases fat in the stool.
stomach pain	gastropathy	Increased blood pressure in the portal system leads to gastric varices and stomach disorders.
hematochezia	bleeding from rectal varices	Increased blood pressure in the portal system leads to rectal varices.
hematemesis	bleeding from esophageal and gastric varices	Increased blood pressure in the portal system causes esophageal and gastric varices that bleed.

alcohol required to cause hepatic damage varies, generally an intake of 80 g or more of alcohol per day in males and 30–40 g or more in females results in liver inflammation. The majority of the damage is believed to be caused by the oxidative metabolite acetaldehyde and **tumor necrosis factor alpha (TNF alpha)**.

> Dictators commonly use the abbreviation for ethanol, which is EtOH (pronounced *ee-tee-oh-ach*). All alcohols (methanol, ethanol, propanol, butanol, etc) share the *–ol* suffix and chemically share a hydroxyl group (OH, one oxygen and one hydrogen). The abbreviation EtOH is derived from the combining form "ethyl" and the common chemical group "OH." Transcribe the full term ethyl alcohol or ethanol, not the abbreviation.

Patients suffering from chronic alcohol intake typically present with anorexia, nausea, hepatomegaly, and jaundice. They may also complain of abdominal pain and tenderness. Examination may reveal splenomegaly, ascites, fever, and encephalopathy. Often alcoholics are undernourished and have signs and symptoms of protein and vitamin deficiencies. Patients presenting with suspicious symptoms should be questioned about their alcohol intake and may be evaluated using the **CAGE questionnaire** (need to *c*ut down, *a*nnoyed by criticism, guilty about drinking, and need for a morning *e*ye-opener).

> **(12)** A shift to the left (or a left shift) refers to the presence of less mature white cells in the peripheral blood. The term originates from lab reports that listed white cells in order of maturation, with the most immature cells listed on the left side of the page.

One of the first changes to occur in the liver as a result of alcohol intake is the accumulation of fat in the form of triglycerides. The liver regulates fat metabolism and normally converts dietary fat to energy and prepares the excess dietary fat for storage in lipocytes throughout the body. In the presence of increased alcohol, fat metabolism is altered; triglycerides accumulate within the hepatocytes, and lipids increase in the blood (hyperlipidemia). Increased fat storage in the liver causes more damage, leading to even more fat accumulation. Eventually, the damage advances to nodular cirrhosis, also called **Laennec cirrhosis**.

Laboratory evaluation will show abnormalities in **liver function tests (LFTs)**. The aminotransferases are usually elevated but typically not above 300 units/L. Gamma glutamyl transpeptidase (GGT), alkaline phosphatase, and bilirubin are also increased. Serum albumin is often low, which may be a consequence of malnutrition or may result from decreased synthesis due to liver damage. A complete blood count (CBC) shows macrocytic red cells (MCV greater than 100 fL) due to the effect of alcohol on the bone marrow as well as a deficiency of folate. CBC may also show leukocytosis with a **shift to the left. (12)** Alcohol is toxic to the bone marrow, causing decreased platelet production (**thrombocytopenia**). Platelets may also be **sequestered** in the spleen due to splenomegaly, further reducing the platelet count. Patients with severe disease have a marked prolongation of the prothrombin time.

Liver biopsy will definitively diagnose alcoholic liver disease. Fibrillar protein forms in the cytoplasm of the hepatocytes, and histologic examination shows **Mallory bodies**, also called **alcoholic hyaline bodies**.

Treatment for alcoholic liver disease is mostly supportive. Abstinence from alcohol is imperative, and patients who abstain may improve significantly. Restoring nutrition and supplementing with vitamins, especially B vitamins, is also necessary. Severe, acute alcoholic hepatitis typically requires treatment in an

---

> ◄◄ ■ Hepatic failure is characterized by hepatic encephalopathy and an INR greater than or equal to 1.5. The most common cause of hepatic failure is drug-induced toxicity, most commonly acetaminophen.
> ■ Accumulation of fat (fatty liver) is the most common response to liver inflammation and injury.
>
> ■ Cirrhosis is the end result of long-term liver inflammation and scarring and results in intrahepatic and extrahepatic circulatory disturbances. The most common causes of cirrhosis are chronic hepatitis B and C infection and alcoholism.
> ■ Long-term, excessive alcohol intake leads to steatohepatitis and cirrhosis with increased risk of hepatocellular carcinoma.

intensive care unit to manage complications such as infection, bleeding, **Wernicke encephalopathy**, **Korsakoff psychosis**, electrolyte imbalances, portal hypertension, ascites, and portosystemic encephalopathy. Patients with severe disease may be candidates for liver transplantation. Pentoxifylline, an inhibitor of tumor necrosis factor, may reduce the mortality rates in patients with severe alcoholic liver disease.

Biliary Tract

The biliary tract refers to the gallbladder and ductwork involved in the transport and storage of bile. Bile consists of water, bile salts, cholesterol, phospholipids (mostly lecithin), electrolytes, and bilirubin, which gives it its typical yellow-green color. The liver synthesizes 500–600 mL of bile per day. Bile is secreted from hepatocytes into the canaliculi of the liver and flows into the intrahepatic collecting system toward the right and left hepatic duct. The left and right hepatic ducts join to form the **common hepatic duct**. Bile flows from there to the **cystic duct** into the gallbladder for concentration and storage (see Figure 4-2).

Ingestion of dietary fat stimulates the gallbladder to contract, forcing bile back through the cystic duct to the common bile duct and into the **ampulla of Vater**, the point where the common bile duct and the **pancreatic duct** join. Both bile and pancreatic fluids are excreted into the duodenum through the sphincter of Oddi. Before joining with the pancreatic duct, the common bile duct tapers to a diameter of less than or equal to 6 mm. In the duodenum, bile emulsifies fats so they can then be broken down by lipases. Bile also acts as a "biologic detergent" to facilitate the elimination of fat-soluble, endogenous metabolites and exogenous toxins such as drug metabolites. Bile is taken up by the small intestine at the terminal ileus and returned to the liver for recycling. Bile circulates through this intrahepatic pathway 10–12 times a day.

 Pause 4-7 What are endogenous metabolites and exogenous toxins?

Cholecystitis

Cholecystitis is inflammation of the gallbladder. It is marked by thickening of the bladder wall, **pericholecystic fluid**, and a **sonographic Murphy sign**. It is almost always due to gallstones (**cholelithiasis**) becoming lodged in the cystic duct. The obstruction causes an infiltrate of inflammatory cells and fluid to accumulate in the gallbladder. Repeated episodes of cholecystitis result in chronic cholecystitis with extensive fibrosis and shrinkage of the gallbladder. A shrunken, calcified gallbladder is referred to as a **porcelain gallbladder**.

An acute attack of cholecystitis is often precipitated by a high-fat meal. Patients complain of sudden-onset pain in the epigastrium and right hypochondrium. Pain may be accompanied by vomiting and low-grade fever. Physical examination reveals right upper quadrant pain on palpation during inspiration as well as muscle guarding and rebound pain. Laboratory evaluation often shows a moderately elevated white blood count (12,000 to 15,000), elevated liver function tests, and elevated amylase. Plain films of the abdomen and **transabdominal ultrasound** studies reveal gallstones in the bladder. **Hepatobiliary iminodiacetic acid (HIDA scan)** is useful for demonstrating an obstructed cystic duct.

 HIDA is pronounced as an acronym (hī'də).

Definitive treatment for recurrent cholecystitis is **cholecystectomy**. Most operations are performed laparoscopically (often referred to as a **lap choley**). Surgeons may convert a laparoscopic procedure to an open procedure (**open cholecystectomy**) during the procedure if intraoperative complications prevent a laparoscopic approach. Untreated, cholecystitis and cholelithiasis may cause a localized perforation or a free perforation with subsequent peritonitis. **Empyema** (puss in the gallbladder) is marked by increasing abdominal pain, high fever, rigors, and rebound tenderness.

Acalculous Cholecystitis

While the majority of cases of cholecystitis are caused by gallstones, **acalculous cholecystitis** accounts for 5% to 10% of cases of acute cholecystitis resulting in cholecystectomy. Ultrasound studies of patients with acalculous cholecystitis demonstrate a sonographic Murphy sign, a distended gallbladder, **biliary sludge**, or a thickened gallbladder wall without pericholecystic fluid.

 Use context to differentiate acalculous (no stone) and a calculous (with a stone).

Choledocholithiasis

Choledocholithiasis is the presence of gallstones in the gallbladder as well as in the common bile duct and/or the ampulla of Vater, causing biliary obstruction, biliary colic, gallstone pancreatitis, or cholangitis (see below). Inflammation and infection of the bile ducts produce strictures and cholestasis. Laboratory studies reveal markedly elevated aminotransferase levels with elevated bilirubin. Amylase may be elevated if secondary pancreatitis is present. **Endoscopic retrograde cholangiopancreatography (ERCP), magnetic resonance cholangiopancreatography (MRCP)**, or endoscopic ultrasound may be used to confirm a diagnosis of choledocholithiasis. The ducts may be decompressed endoscopically or surgically with stone extraction, sphincterotomy, and stent placement.

Cholangitis

Cholangitis is an infection within the bile ducts, especially the common bile duct. Obstruction of the common bile duct with resulting inflammation may cause the sphincter of Oddi to malfunction and allow microorganisms to migrate from the intestinal tract into the biliary tract. Obstruction may be due to biliary stones, strictures, or tumors. The increased pressure within the biliary tree allows further **retrograde ascent** of bacteria into the hepatic circulatory system and eventually the general circulatory system (bacteremia). Common infecting organisms include gram-negative bacteria (eg, Escherichia coli, **Klebsiella** and **Enterobacter** species). Less commonly, gram–positive bacteria (eg, **Enterococcus** species) or **mixed anaerobes** (eg, **Bacteroides** and **Clostridia** species) may be the causative agents. Symptoms include abdominal pain, jaundice, and fever with chills. These three symptoms are collectively referred to as **Charcot triad**.

Physical examination reveals abdominal tenderness and hepatomegaly. Patients who also show confusion and hypotension (**Reynold pentad**) require emergency endoscopy to remove the obstruction and débride the infected ducts. Mortality can be as high as 50%.

 Pause 4-8 Explain the phrase "retrograde ascent."

Pancreas

The pancreas, a glandular organ approximately six inches long, is located behind the stomach in the left upper quadrant. It is divided into three major sections: the head, body, and tail, with the head lying adjacent to the first curve of the duodenum (Figure 4-2). The pancreas is both an endocrine gland and an exocrine gland. As an endocrine gland, the pancreas releases insulin and glucagon; as an exocrine gland, the pancreas secretes the digestive enzymes **chymotrypsin**, **pancreatic lipase**, and **pancreatic amylase**. The digestive enzymes are produced in the acinar cells and collected by the **main pancreatic duct (MPD)**. The MPD joins the common bile duct at the ampulla of Vater (see Figure 4-2).

Pancreatitis is inflammation of the pancreas caused by the release of activated pancreatic enzymes. Inappropriate release of these enzymes causes severe pain, typically severe enough to require opioid pain medication. Pain typically develops suddenly in **gallstone pancreatitis**. When alcoholic pancreatitis is implicated, the pain crescendos over a period of days. Nausea and vomiting are common. A single episode is considered acute pancreatitis, but recurrent, intermittent episodes define chronic pancreatitis. Chronic pancreatitis may be classified as **chronic calcifying pancreatitis**, **chronic obstructive pancreatitis**, or **chronic inflammatory pancreatitis**.

The pancreas typically fully recovers from a single episode of pancreatitis, but chronic exacerbation leads to functional and structural changes in the gland.

- The biliary tree refers to the gallbladder and the ducts that transport bile.
- Cholecystitis is inflammation of the gallbladder, most often caused by gallstones.
- Acalculous cystitis is marked by inflammation of the gallbladder with a thickened gallbladder wall but no gallstones.
- Choledocholithiasis is the presence of gallstones in the gallbladder, common bile duct, and/or the ampulla of Vater, causing biliary obstruction, biliary colic, gallstone pancreatitis, or cholangitis.
- Cholangitis is a life-threatening infection within the bile ducts, especially the common bile duct, caused by retrograde ascent of bacteria from the ileus into the biliary system.

Severe bouts of pancreatitis activate the immune system's complement cascade (see page 314) and the inflammatory process, leading to systemic inflammation and edema. Acute respiratory distress syndrome and renal failure may ensue. Activated enzymes and cytokines in the peritoneal cavity cause a chemical burn and third spacing of fluid.

The vast majority of pancreatitis cases are brought on by alcohol, especially binge drinking, but also chronic alcoholism. Gallstones in the common duct may also initiate pancreatitis. Extremely elevated levels of triglycerides (hypertriglyceridemia exceeding 1000 mg/dL) may also cause pancreatitis.

Patients often present to the emergency department acutely ill. Examination reveals tachycardia, shallow but rapid respirations with **limited diaphragmatic excursion**, postural hypotension, and normal or even subnormal temperature. Abdominal exam reveals tenderness, distension, guarding, and rigidity, with diminished or absent bowel sounds. Patients may display a **blunted sensorium**. Jaundice may be evident. Severe cases may reveal a **Grey Turner sign** (bluish discoloration of the flanks) and **Cullen sign** (bluish discoloration of the periumbilical area) due to **hemorrhagic pancreatitis**.

A significant number of patients will form collections of pancreatic fluid and tissue debris in and around the pancreas, some of which will form **pseudocysts** and abscesses (**necrotizing pancreatitis**). Pseudocysts form when granulation tissue walls off the irritating fluid. These cysts are at risk of hemorrhage, rupture, or infection.

Chronic inflammation also causes fibrosis and calcification of the parenchyma, replacing functional cells with nonfunctioning scar tissue. The loss of pancreatic exocrine and endocrine function causes steatorrhea (from loss of digestive enzymes) and diabetes mellitus (from loss of insulin). Eventually, the pain of chronic pancreatitis subsides as the pancreas ceases production of digestive enzymes. When enzyme secretions drop below 10% of normal, steatorrhea develops; patients may even pass oil droplets. **Creatorrhea** may also be present, which is the presence of undigested muscle fibers in the feces. The lack of insulin and glucagon production causes brittle diabetes.

Laboratory studies to evaluate pancreatitis include liver function studies, lipase, amylase, and **trypsin**. A CBC may show an elevated white count. The hematocrit may be increased due to hemoconcentration if third spacing has occurred.

Pause 4-9 Explain the sentence, "The hematocrit may be increased due to hemoconcentration if third spacing has occurred."

ERCP with **brush cytology** is helpful to rule out biliary or pancreatic cancer. Plain radiographs can also aid in the diagnosis. Abdominal x-rays may show gallstones, a **sentinel loop** (a segment of air-filled small intestine in the left upper quadrant), or the **colon cutoff sign**, which is a gas-filled segment of transverse colon abruptly ending at the area of pancreatic inflammation. Pancreatic calcification is pathognomonic for chronic pancreatitis. CT is the most helpful diagnostic imaging tool. CT scans of the pancreas are graded using the **Balthazar grading system:**

- grade A—normal pancreas
- grade B—focal or diffuse gland enlargement
- grade C—intrinsic gland abnormality recognized by haziness on the scan
- grade D—single, ill-defined collection or phlegmon
- grade E—two or more ill-defined collections or the presence of gas in or near the pancreas

The first line of treatment in an acute attack often involves fluid resuscitation with both crystalline and colloid solutions because third spacing of fluid produces severe dehydration and electrolyte imbalances. A central line and a **Swan-Ganz catheter** are placed to administer fluids and monitor hemodynamic pressures. Often antibiotic coverage is given, especially when a pancreatic **phlegmon (13)** is seen on CT scan. Ceftriaxone (Rocephin), a third-generation cephalosporin with broad-spectrum gram-negative activity, or ampicillin (Marcillin, Omnipen) are given until **culture and sensitivity (C&S)** results are completed. Administration of an H_2 blocker or PPI decreases gastric acid and thereby decreases secretin and the subsequent release of pancreatic enzymes.

The abbreviation C&S (culture and sensitivity) and CNS (central nervous system) sound exactly alike when dictated.

(13) A phlegmon is an acute, suppurative (pus-forming) inflammation that may progress to an abscess.

- The pancreas is both an endocrine and an exocrine gland that secretes insulin and glucagon and the digestive enzymes trypsin, pancreatic lipase, and pancreatic amylase.
- Pancreatitis is inflammation of the pancreas caused by the release of activated pancreatic enzymes, resulting in severe pain. The most common causes of pancreatitis are alcohol intake and gallstones in the biliary tract.
- Chronic pancreatitis leads to functional and structural changes of the pancreas, eventually resulting in diabetes mellitus, steatorrhea, and nutritional deficiencies.

Patients with chronic pancreatitis should follow a low-fat diet to prevent steatorrhea. Patients are also prescribed pancreatic enzymes (pancrelipase) and supplemental fat-soluble vitamins (A, D, K, and E). Patients with **refractory steatorrhea** can be given **medium-chain triglycerides (MCTs)** as a source of dietary fat because they do not require pancreatic enzymes for absorption. Patients should be monitored for the development of pancreatic cancer using brush biopsy of biliary strictures and measurement of **CA 19-9** and **carcinoembryonic antigen (CEA)**.

Surgical treatment may be required for pain relief of pancreatitis. A **lateral pancreaticojejunostomy (Puestow procedure) (14)** provides significant relief of pain when the main pancreatic duct is dilated in the 5–8 mm range. A partial resection of the pancreas may also be effective. A **distal pancreatectomy** (removal of the tail) or a **Whipple procedure**, also called a **pancreatoduodenectomy** (removal of the head of the pancreas and part of the duodenum), may be performed.

The **Ranson score** is used to assess the severity of pancreatitis and to evaluate the prognosis. At the time of admission, the score is based on the patient's age, white blood count, glucose level, LDH, and AST values. After 48 hours, the score is based on the hematocrit, BUN, calcium, oxygen saturation, electrolytes, and fluid sequestration. A Ranson score of 0–2 has a minimal mortality rate. A Ranson score of 3–5 has a 10% to 20% mortality rate. A Ranson score higher than 5 has a mortality rate above 50% and is associated with more systemic complications. Other scoring systems include **Glasgow, Imrie,** and **APACHE II**.

(14) A lateral pancreaticojejunostomy involves a side-to-side anastomosis of the pancreatic duct and the jejunum. The duct is split longitudinally and attached to a section of the jejunum, allowing pancreatic enzymes to flow directly from the gland into the jejunum.

Diagnostic Imaging

Imaging tests play a critical role in the diagnosis and management of liver and biliary disease. Ultrasonography, endoscopy, and nuclear medicine techniques are used.

Ultrasound

A transabdominal ultrasound study is a safe, cost-effective method of diagnosing disorders of the liver, gallbladder, and pancreas, but most importantly the gallbladder. Ultrasound can detect gallstones as small as 2 mm in diameter. Endoscopic ultrasound can detect stones as small as 0.5 mm (**microlithiasis**).

Ultrasound elastography is used to measure liver stiffness to determine the extent of hepatic fibrosis. A transducer emits a vibration and the rate of propagation is measured. Fibrosis increases liver stiffness, which in turn increases the rate at which the vibrations propagate.

Ultrasound studies with Doppler are used to assess the direction of blood flow and the patency of vessels leading into and out of the liver, especially the hepatic portal vein. This method is useful for evaluating portal hypertension, portal thrombosis, patency of liver shunts and stents, as well as detection of collateral blood flow.

Phrases heard on liver and biliary ultrasound studies:

biliary sludge

sludge in the gallbladder

thickened gallbladder wall (greater than 3 mm)

tenderness on palpation of the gallbladder with the ultrasound probe

echogenic lesion suspicious for tumor

acoustic shadowing

intense echoes with distal acoustic shadowing that move with gravity

Nuclear Medicine

Nuclear medicine techniques use radioactive isotopes, also called radionuclides, for assessment and diagnosis. A radioactive particle is combined with a physiologically active substance and administered to the patient either orally or by IV. The physiologically active material is taken up preferentially by the target organ or structure to be studied. Radioactive decay, emitted by the isotope, is measured by an external gamma camera. Nuclear medicine techniques not only provide information about anatomy but also physiologic activity and metabolism. The amount of scintigraphic activity detected can be quantified, so nuclear medicine results are not only diagnostic but also quantitative (ie, can measure the amount of a given fluid, an ejection fraction, or the extent of impairment). Another term used in reference to nuclear medicine techniques is scintigraphy.

Cholescintigraphy is a nuclear medicine technique used to diagnose calculous and acalculous cholecystitis. Patients are given a technetium-labeled iminodiacetic compound (eg, hydroxy or diisopropyl iminodiacetic acid [HIDA or DISIDA]) by IV. These substances are taken up by the liver and passed into the gallbladder. The abdomen is scanned for scintigraphic activity in the gallbladder and biliary ducts. Cholecystokinin, which causes the gallbladder to contract, may be administered before and/or after the nuclear agent. Scintigraphic counts are used to calculate the gallbladder ejection fraction, which is the amount of bile that flows from the gallbladder when it contracts. Acalculous cholecystitis will cause a decreased ejection fraction. A lack of scintigraphic activity in the gallbladder indicates blockage of the cystic duct because the radionuclide cannot reach the gallbladder.

Endoscopy

Endoscopic retrograde cholangiopancreatography (ERCP) uses a combination of endoscopy and x-ray to diagnose and treat disorders of the biliary tract. An endoscope is inserted into the esophagus and passed through the stomach into the duodenum. The scope is then threaded in a retrograde direction (15) through the sphincter of Oddi into the ampulla of Vater and further into the pancreatic duct or the common bile duct. This test can detect and often simultaneously treat gallstones and strictures. Brush cytology for histopathology studies may also be performed to rule out

carcinoma. In this procedure, a brush is attached to the endoscope and cells are gathered by moving the brush across the surface of strictures or masses. The scope procedure can also be used to inject dyes into the biliary tree and pancreas to improve visualization on x-ray. Risks and complications of ERCP include pancreatitis and perforation of any of the structures through which the endoscope travels.

ERCP can be both diagnostic and therapeutic, meaning treatment (such as placing stents and removing stones) can take place at the same time as the diagnostic procedure. MRCP, a noninvasive study, carries much less risk than ERCP and has mostly replaced ERCP (see below) except when a therapeutic procedure is also anticipated.

> The patient will be scheduled for an MRCP to determine if there is underlying retained common bile duct stone. If normal, I anticipate he may require an ERCP with manometry study to evaluate for sphincter of Oddi dysfunction.

MRCP (MRI)

Magnetic resonance cholangiopancreatography (MRCP) is a noninvasive and therefore safer method of detecting bile-duct stones, strictures, dilatations, and obstructions but less reliable for distinguishing malignant causes from nonmalignant ones. MRCP is more sensitive than CT or ultrasonography in diagnosing common bile duct abnormalities, particularly stones. A **filling defect (16)** is seen within the biliary tree on thin, cross-sectional T2-weighted imaging. Because it is noninvasive, MRCP is a useful screening tool when biliary obstruction is suspected.

(15) Retrograde direction refers to a direction that is opposite the normal flow of fluids or substances through a canal, orifice, or lumen.

(16) The phrase "filling defect" is used in many imaging studies involving structures that normally fill with fluid. Filling defects are indicative of strictures and obstructions.

X-Ray

Percutaneous transhepatic cholangiography (PTC) may be used to identify the cause, location, and extent of biliary obstruction. A needle is inserted through the skin and directly into a bile duct within the liver itself. X-ray dye is injected through the needle into the ducts, and the distribution of the dye throughout the biliary tree is detected on x-ray. An **intraoperative cholangiography**, performed during laparoscopy, laparotomy, or other surgical procedure, may also be performed.

CT scans are commonly used to identify hepatic masses (**hepatocarcinoma**), particularly small metastases, as well as **cavernous hemangiomas**. It is also helpful in diagnosing masses of the pancreas (pancreatic carcinoma) and pancreatitis.

 Words and phrases that may be heard on diagnostic imaging of the biliary tree:

pearl-necklace sign

pseudocalculus sign

pneumobilia (air in the biliary tree)

emphysematous cholecystitis (gas in the gallbladder)

Laboratory Studies

Laboratory evaluations play a major role in the diagnosis and monitoring of liver, biliary, and pancreatic disorders. The majority of tests are performed on serum, which is obtained by drawing a sample of blood, allowing the sample to clot, and then centrifuging the sample to separate the watery portion of the blood from the cellular components. Coagulation studies, however, are performed on **plasma**, which is obtained by drawing a sample of blood into a tube containing an anticoagulant that prevents the sample from clotting. This preserves the clotting factors so they can be measured in the laboratory.

Liver Function Tests

The liver function tests (LFTs) are a group of blood tests used to diagnose and monitor liver disorders. The standard panel of tests typically referred to as "LFTs" includes the aminotransferases, alkaline phosphatase, total protein, albumin, and bilirubin. Extended evaluations include coagulation studies, lactate dehydrogenase, and ammonia.

The phrase "liver function tests" is always plural since it refers to a group of tests used to assess liver function. There is no *single* test that adequately evaluates liver function (ie, there is not a singular "liver function test").

Aminotransferases

Aminotransferases, also referred to as **transaminases**, are enzymes that transfer amino groups away from amino acids (**Table 4-2**). This is an important chemical step in the metabolism of protein, especially in the process of converting amino acids to energy. The term usually refers to a group of enzymes associated with the liver and biliary system, including alanine aminotransferase (ALT), aspartate aminotransferase (AST), and gamma glutamyltransferase (GGT). These enzymes are normally contained within the cells of the liver, biliary system, and to a lesser degree the pancreas. Cellular damage causes the enzymes to be released from the cells and to spill into the circulatory system, so the presence of transaminases in the peripheral blood indicates hepatic, biliary, or pancreatic cell damage. Elevated levels of GGT are most indicative of biliary obstruction.

ALT was formerly known as serum glutamic pyruvic transaminase (SGPT), and AST was formerly known as serum glutamic oxaloacetic transaminase (SGOT). Occasionally, dictators will refer to these enzymes by these older abbreviations.

Table 4-2 Aminotransferases

Test Name	Normal Range
ALT (SGPT)	8–45 units/L
AST (SGOT)	<35 units/L
GGT	<65 units/L

Alkaline Phosphatase

Alkaline phosphatase (**Table 4-3**) is used to remove phosphate groups from molecules as part of normal metabolism. It is found in the liver, biliary tract, pancreas, and bone. Like the aminotransferases, damaged cells cause alkaline phosphatase to spill into the blood stream. Elevated levels in the peripheral blood may indicate liver damage, biliary obstruction, or pancreatic disorder. Bone growth in children or bone remodeling after bone injury will also cause elevated alkaline phosphatase, so this test alone is not specific for liver disease.

Table 4-3 Alkaline Phosphatase

Test Name	Normal Range
alkaline phosphatase	20–120 units/L

> Dictators often refer to alkaline phosphatase using the short form "alk phos," but this term should be spelled out when transcribed.

Total Protein and Albumin

Protein levels (**Table 4-4**), especially serum albumin, are an important measure of liver function since many proteins are synthesized in the liver. Decreased albumin levels may indicate decreased production capacity of the liver. Total protein may also be measured in addition to albumin. Total protein includes albumin, carrier proteins (eg, transferrin and ceruloplasmin), clotting factors, and immunoglobulins. The total protein value should always be greater than the albumin value, since albumin is a fraction of the total protein.

Table 4-4 Serum Protein

Test Name	Normal Range
total protein	6.4 to 8.3 g/dL
albumin	3.5 to 5.0 g/dL
globulin	1.5 to 3.0 g/dL
A/G ratio (albumin/globulin ratio)	1.5 to 3.0

Coagulation Studies

Because the liver synthesizes fibrinogen and the vitamin K–dependent clotting factors (prothrombin, factors V, VII, and X), coagulation studies are an important assessment tool for the liver. Decreased coagulation factors are indicative of diminishing liver synthetic capacity and progression toward hepatic failure. Malabsorption of fat and the fat-soluble vitamin K also leads to decreased production of coagulation factors and resulting coagulopathies. See page 430 in Chapter 12 for a detailed explanation and list of normal coagulation study values.

Bilirubin

Bilirubin levels (**Table 4-5**) are an important indicator of both liver function and liver damage. Bilirubin is measured in two forms: direct and indirect. The sum of direct and indirect bilirubin equals the total bilirubin value. The liver conjugates (ie, attaches) bilirubin to glucuronic acid to make bilirubin water soluble, allowing bilirubin to dissolve in the bile. Direct bilirubin is the measure of bilirubin that has been conjugated (ie, processed) by the liver. Indirect bilirubin represents bilirubin that has not been conjugated (ie, not processed) by the liver. Increased levels of unconjugated bilirubin are the result of liver impairment with an inability to cope with normal levels of bilirubin or overwhelming hemolysis that causes bilirubin to rise faster than the liver can process it.

Table 4-5 Bilirubin

Test Name	Normal Range
total bilirubin	0.2 to 1.3 mg/dL
direct bilirubin	0.1 to 0.4 mg/dL
indirect bilirubin	0.1 to 0.9 mg/dL

> Dictators often refer to bilirubin simply as "bili," but the complete term should be transcribed.

Lactate Dehydrogenase

Lactate dehydrogenase (**Table 4-6**) is normally contained within liver cells and red blood cells. Damage to either type of cell will increase levels in the plasma, indicating liver damage or red cell hemolysis.

Table 4-6 Lactate Dehydrogenase

Test Name	Normal Range
lactate dehydrogenase (LD or LDH)	100–190 units/L (newborn values are much higher)

Ammonia

Ammonia (**Table 4-7**) is a normal byproduct of protein metabolism and is normally converted to urea to be excreted by the kidneys. Ammonia may be produced within the liver as well as in the intestinal tract by the action of normal flora on amino acids. Ammonia levels become elevated in the blood stream due to portosystemic shunting as ammonia produced within the intestinal tract bypasses the liver and enters the general circulation. An elevated ammonia level may also be indicative of hepatic failure and is a contributing factor in hepatic encephalopathy.

Table 4-7 Ammonia

Test Name	Normal Range
ammonia (NH_3)	10–40 mmol/L

Viral Hepatitis

Viral cultures are not routinely performed in a medical laboratory because they are time-consuming and expensive. Instead of cultures, serological studies are used to diagnose remote, recent, or current infection and to monitor efficacy of treatment. Serology tests detect either components of the virus itself (antigens or nucleic acid) or antibodies formed in response to the virus. Although there are five classes of immunoglobulins (IgA, IgD, IgE, IgG, and IgM), IgG and IgM are most relevant to the diagnosis of infection. (See Chapter 10 for more information on antibody classes). The IgM class of antibody appears early in the immune process and is considered the immune system's "first responder." Eventually, IgM titers give way to IgG, considered the immune system's "memory" immunoglobulin. IgG antibodies against a given organism are considered protective because IgG can be recalled from the immune system's memory on short notice to quickly squelch a subsequent invasion before the organism produces symptoms.

HAV

Tests for hepatitis A virus include:

- anti-HAV IgM: antibodies of the IgM class directed against the hepatitis A virus, detected during active infection
- anti-HAV IgG: antibodies of the IgG class directed against the hepatitis A virus in the convalescent or postrecovery stage

HBV

Hepatitis B has the most extensive set of serological tests and is the only hepatitis virus with a detectable core antigen (c) and a detectable surface antigen (s). Tests used in the diagnosis and management of hepatitis B include:

- HBsAg: hepatitis B surface antigen detectable during active infection
- anti-HBs (HBsAb): antibodies directed against the hepatitis B surface antigen detectable in the postrecovery phase and in individuals vaccinated against HBV
- IgM anti-HBc (HBcAb): IgM class antibodies directed against the hepatitis B core antigen detectable early in the infection
- IgG anti-HBc (HBcAb): IgG class antibodies directed against the hepatitis B core antigen detectable late in the infection or in a recovered patient
- HBeAg: hepatitis B "e" antigen that is contained within the hepatitis B viral core and detectable during active infection; used as a prognostic indicator
- anti-HBe: antibodies directed against the hepatitis B "e" antigen that is contained within the viral core; used as a prognostic indicator
- anti-HDV: antibody to hepatitis D virus; only measured if serologic tests indicate a severe HBV infection (HDV is only active in the presence of HBV infection)

The abbreviations used to describe the viral hepatitis studies are very difficult to distinguish because the letters sound so much alike. The letter /h/ can sound like the letter /a/; the letters /b/ and /v/ are very difficult to distinguish, and /c/ and /e/ are easily misheard. Listen carefully to the entire abbreviation and make sure that what you transcribe matches a known serological test (eg, there is no serological marker named HCVcAg because the hepatitis C virus does not have a core). Test names and results should also correlate with the patient's history and assessment.

HCV

Tests used to diagnose and monitor hepatitis C include:

- anti-HCV: When hepatitis C is suspected, an enzyme immunosorbent assay (EIA) is used to test for antibodies against hepatitis C. A positive EIA test is confirmed using a **recombinant immunoblot assay (RIBA)** for anti-HCV. (17)

- HCV-RNA: Patients with known HCV infection can be monitored using testing methods that detect the actual viral nucleic acid and indicate the viral load. The higher the quantity of nucleic acid, the more viral particles. Methods include **polymerase chain reaction (PCR)**, **transcription mediated amplification (TMA)**, and **branched DNA (bDNA)**.

Pancreatic Enzymes

The pancreas manufactures and releases lipase and amylase (**Table 4-8**) into the duodenum to aid in digestion. Cellular damage causes these enzymes to escape the pancreas and spill into the circulation. Amylase has two isoenzymes—pancreatic-type amylase (p-type isoamylase) and salivary-type amylase (s-type isoamylase). (18) An amylase level elevated three times the normal range is highly suspicious for pancreatitis. Lipase levels usually increase from 7 to 11 times the upper limit of normal in acute pancreatitis, although lipase may be elevated in any number of disorders—not just pancreatitis.

Table 4-8 Pancreatic Enzymes

Test Name	Normal Range
lipase	23–300 units/L
amylase	30–100 units/L

Alpha Fetoprotein

Alpha fetoprotein (**Table 4-9**) is normally found in higher concentrations in fetuses and pregnant women. Even slight elevations in a nonpregnant adult should prompt a workup for primary hepatocellular carcinoma.

Table 4-9 Alpha Fetoprotein

Test Name	Normal Range
alpha fetoprotein (AFP)	10–20 ng/mL (10–20 mg/L)

Ascitic (Peritoneal) Fluid

Normally only a small amount of fluid is present in the abdominal cavity. When large amounts of fluid accumulate in the peritoneal cavity, the fluid is analyzed to determine the cause of the fluid accumulation (eg, infection, cirrhosis, pancreatitis, cancer, nephrotic syndrome). A differential count (similar to the CBC differential) can be performed on fluid with a high white count to determine the relative number of each type of white cell. The fluid is often cultured by placing a sample of fluid into **blood culture bottles**. Since the presence of ascites is not normal, there are no normal reference ranges. **Table 4-10** outlines the interpretation of results.

Table 4-10 Ascitic Fluid Analysis

Test Name	Result	Interpretation
amylase	>3× serum amylase	indicative of pancreatitis
RBC	<10,000 cells/mcL	higher values indicate bleeding into peritoneal cavity
WBC	<500 cells/mcL	higher values with increased neutrophils indicative of spontaneous bacterial peritonitis
SAAG (serum-to-ascites albumin gradient)	>1.1 g/dL	ascites due to portal hypertension
	<1.1 g/dL	ascites due to cancer or nephrotic syndrome

Pharmacology

Medication plays a significant role in the long-term treatment of liver disease and pancreatic disease.

Sequestrants

Sequestrants (**Table 4-11**) are drugs that bind substances and prevent their normal absorption or metabolism. This class of drugs binds bile acids in the digestive tract and prevents their reabsorption at the terminal ileus, thereby reducing bile acid levels. This class is also used in the same way to reduce cholesterol levels (see page 47).

(17) The acronym RIBA is pronounced *rē´ bə*.

(18) Isoenzymes are molecules with the same function but vary slightly in structure and chemical properties.

Table 4-11 Sequestrants

Generic	Brand Name	Dose
cholestyramine	Questran, Questran Light, Prevalite	4 g
colestipol	Colestid	multiples of 1 g

Gallstone Dissolution Agents

For patients unable to undergo surgical removal of gallstones, medications are available to slowly dissolve stones (**Table 4-12**).

Table 4-12 Gallstone Dissolution Agents

Generic	Brand Name	Dose
ursodiol	Actigall	300 mg
	Urso 250	250 mg
	Urso Forte	500 mg

Pancreatic Enzymes

Orally administered pancreatic enzymes (**Table 4-13**) are given to patients with chronic pancreatitis, obstruction, or other causes for decreased enzymes. Pancrelipase is a mixture of amylase, trypsin, and lipase.

Table 4-13 Pancreatic Enzymes

Generic	Brand Name
pancrelipase	Creon, Ultrase

(19) Naturally occurring immune substances that include the Greek letter alpha in their name take the usual spelling of alpha. Pharmaceutical preparations such as interferon alpha created by recombinant gene technology are spelled with the non-Greek spelling alfa (with an f).

Immune Globulins

Individuals with known exposure to hepatitis B may receive hepatitis B immune globulin (HBIG) to provide passive immunity and attenuate the infection. HBIG (**Table 4-14**) should be given as soon after exposure as possible (within seven days). It is not effective against active hepatitis or chronic hepatitis. Infants born to mothers with an active infection of hepatitis B are also given HBIG.

Table 4-14 HBIG

Generic	Brand Name
HBIG	HepaGam B, HyperHEP B S/D

Biological Response Modulators

Interferon (IFN) is normally produced by the immune system to fight viral infections. It is induced early in the infectious process before the humoral arm of the immune system has time to respond with specific antibodies directed at the invading organism (see also Chapter 10). Interferon alpha (**19**) is a family of approximately 20 related proteins that act as antiviral agents. Interferon is referred to as a biological response modulator because it stimulates, or up-regulates, the activity of the immune system. Common side effects of interferon are fatigue, fever, malaise, and muscle aches. Patients with chronic viral hepatitis B and C are treated with interferon (**Table 4-15**) to prevent long-term infection and progression to cirrhosis and liver failure.

Table 4-15 Biological Response Modulators

Generic	Brand Name
interferon alfa-2a (PEG conjugate) pegylated interferon alfa-2a	Pegasys
interferon alfa-2b	Intron A
peginterferon alfa-2b	PegIntron
pegylated interferon alfa-2b	PegIntron Redipen
interferon alfa-2b and ribavirin (antiviral agent and biological response modulator)	Rebetron

Hepatitis may be treated with pegylated interferon, which is interferon combined with polyethylene glycol (PEG). This formulation allows for once-weekly injections instead of the three weekly injections required for conventional interferon.

Antiviral Treatments

Nucleoside and nucleotide analogs (**Table 4-16**), also called nucleoside and nucleotide reverse transcription inhibitors (NRTIs and NtRTIs), are molecules that mimic the naturally occurring deoxyribonucleic acid molecules that make up DNA. They compete with the naturally occurring molecules for incorporation into the DNA chain during DNA synthesis, but the analogs are slightly modified so that additional DNA molecules cannot attach to the analog once incorporated into the

growing DNA chain. Once an analog is incorporated into a chain of DNA, synthesis of that chain ceases. To replicate, viruses must be able to synthesize DNA, so NRTIs and NtRTIs are effective antiviral agents.

Table 4-16 Nucleoside and Nucleotide Analogs

Generic	Brand Name	Dose
entecavir (NRTI)	Baraclude	0.5 mg, 1 mg
lamivudine (NRTI)	Epivir-HBV	100 mg
tenofovir (NtRTI)	Viread	300 mg
adefovir (NtRTI)	Hepsera	10 mg

Exercises

Using Context to Make Decisions

Use the excerpt on page 114 to answer questions 1–5.

1. Which of the following would complete blank #1?

    a. CBC
    b. LFTs
    c. serology
    d. coagulation

2. According to the information given in the report, which of the following serology tests would have been negative?

    a. IgM anti-HAV
    b. IgG anti-HBV
    c. IgG anti-HBc (HBcAb)
    d. All of these

3. Which of the following would complete blank #2?

    a. hepatic
    b. bile
    c. pancreatic
    d. bowel

4. What term would complete blank #3? _____

5. Which of the following would complete blank #4?

    a. cholescintigraphy
    b. transabdominal ultrasound
    c. MRI
    d. ERCP

Use the following excerpt to answer questions 6 and 7.

LABORATORY STUDIES

Hepatitis C antibody was positive. Hepatitis B surface antigen was negative, as was the hepatitis B core antibody. Hepatitis A total antibody was positive, consistent with remote hepatitis A. Hepatitis C RIBA was positive.

6. Write the abbreviations for the four antigens and antibodies described in the excerpt. _____
_____

7. What type of hepatitis does this patient currently have? _____

Use the following excerpt to answer questions 8 and 9.

SUBJECTIVE

The patient was previously seen for initial consultation on March 25 with a positive antibody for hepatitis C. Laboratory data was obtained, confirming a chronic viral infection with HCV TCR assay equal to 265,510 units/mL. Liver function studies remain abnormal with AST and ALT equal to 33 and 97, respectively. In addition, antinuclear antibody and F actin smooth muscle antibody are both elevated and equal to 175 and 48, respectively.

8. Which laboratory result is transcribed in error?
_____

9. Which laboratory test name is transcribed in error?
_____

10. Are any of the results in the following panel associated with chronic liver disease?

LABORATORY DATA

AST 19, ALT 34, alkaline phosphatase of 60, WBC of 13.5, hemoglobin of 14.4, hematocrit of 43.3, and platelets of 206. PT 10.2 and INR 0.98. Blood cultures were negative.

11. Explain why a patient's social history is pertinent to the diagnosis of liver disease. _____
_____

12. Given the following statement, what is the meaning of recrudescent? _____
_____

Recrudescent hepatitis occurs in a small percentage of patients and is characterized by recurrent symptoms during the recovery phase.

13. Given the following statement, what is the meaning of attenuate? _____

_____

Standard immune globulin should be given to family members and close contacts of patients for postexposure prophylaxis. Immune globulin administration may prevent or attenuate an infection.

14. Which word in the following excerpt is transcribed in error? What do you think is the correct word to fit this context? _____

_____

The patient has opted to proceed with therapy. The risks of therapy have been explained in detail. She understands and wants to proceed with treatment. She states that if side effects are significant, she will stop treatment but would like to attempt viral ratification if at all possible. The patient will be treated with Pegasys and ribavirin.

15. Given the following excerpt, what is meant by sequestered? How is this term used in reference to pharmacology? Write at least three other forms (conjugations) of the word sequester. _____

_____

Platelets may also be sequestered in the spleen due to splenomegaly, further reducing the platelet count.

Terms Checkup

Complete the multiple choice questions for Chapter 4 located at www.myhealthprofessionskit.com. To access the questions, select the discipline "Medical Transcription," then click on the title of this book, *Advanced Medical Transcription*.

Look It Up

Using the guidelines described on page xvii, complete a research project on autoimmune hepatitis and Budd-Chiari syndrome.

Transcription Practice

1. Transcribe the key terms and phrases for Chapter 4.
2. Complete the proofing and transcription practice exercises for Chapter 4.

SUBJECTIVE

The patient was previously seen on April 28, 20XX, for evaluation of refractory nausea, vomiting, and abdominal pain. During the interim, laboratory data was obtained, confirming improved ____(1)____ with alkaline phosphatase 443, total bilirubin 1.4, AST 36, and ALT 113.

Of note, an acute viral hepatitis profile was obtained, documenting no evidence of viral hepatitis. In addition, the iron index was normal, thus refuting hemochromatosis, and prothrombin time was within reference range, suggesting adequate hepatic synthetic protein function.

Currently the patient states that the nausea, vomiting, and pain are improved, although there have been 2 episodes since he was last seen. Reglan controls the nausea, but his appetite remains suppressed.

ASSESSMENT

Refractory nausea, vomiting, and abdominal pain with elevated LFTs. Features appear concerning for cholestatic disease, potentially retained common ____(2)____ duct gallstone, sphincter of ____(3)____ dysfunction, or other obstructive disease. Drug-induced hepatitis is also a possibility.

PLAN

The patient will be scheduled for an MRCP to determine if there is a retained common bile duct stone. If normal, then I anticipate he may require ____(4)____ with manometry study to evaluate for sphincter of Oddi dysfunction. Repeat LFTs will be obtained in 1–2 weeks. Further recommendations will follow.

Orthopedics: The Appendicular Skeleton

Preview Terms

Before studying this chapter, make sure you understand the following terms. Definitions can be found in the glossary.

appendicular skeleton
articulation
chondral
condyle
immobilization

Learning Objectives

After completing this chapter, you should be able to comprehend and correctly transcribe terminology related to:

▶ the orthopedic physical examination

▶ disorders of the joints

▶ common orthopedic injuries including fractures, sprains, strains, dislocations, and tendinopathy

▶ carpal tunnel syndrome and plantar fasciitis

▶ metabolic and infectious diseases of bones

▶ deep venous thrombosis

▶ laboratory and imaging tests used to diagnose and monitor musculoskeletal diseases and injuries

▶ therapeutic procedures used to treat musculoskeletal diseases and injuries

▶ drugs used in the treatment of musculoskeletal disorders

Introduction

This chapter discusses injuries and disorders of the appendicular skeleton. Despite its seemingly dormant appearance, bone is a highly dynamic tissue that constantly adjusts to both internal and external influences. Bones serve several very important functions, including mineral storage, production of blood components, movement, support, balance, and protection of internal organs. Bones can actually modify their structure in response to weightbearing and external forces. The more bones are stressed, the more they respond by becoming stronger. Likewise, sedentary lifestyles promote a weak and porous bone structure.

Bones have a well-defined architecture that contributes to their structure and function. Review the various areas and components of bones, as shown in ■ **Figure 5-1**. Bones are surrounded by connective tissue called the periosteum that contains blood vessels, lymph vessels, and nerve fibers. Bones consist of two layers of tissue: cortical and cancellous. Cortical bone, which is the dense, compact, outer layer, makes up 80% of the skeletal bone mass. Cancellous bone, also called trabecular bone, makes up the inner layer and resembles a honeycomb. This spongy, mesh-like structure is designed to add strength to the bone while reducing the overall weight of the bone.

Physical Examination

The hands-on physical examination of bones, joints, and muscles is an integral part of an orthopedic evaluation. The examiner measures the degree of joint movement, referred to as range of motion (ROM), as shown in ■ **Figure 5-2**. **Passive range of motion (PROM)** is the degree of movement exhibited by a joint when the examiner moves the joint. **Active range of motion (AROM)** is the degree of movement exhibited by a joint when the patient attempts to move the joint without assistance. AROM may be assessed with and without **resistance**. Joints are also examined for swelling, stiffness, and tenderness. Instability is demonstrated by stressing the joint, which means passively moving the joint in a direction opposite its normal range of motion. Joints are also palpated for **crepitus** (a crackling sound caused by movement of air or gas) and **effusion**. Muscles are assessed for **motor strength**, symmetry, spasm, tenderness, and atrophy. Tests, signs, and maneuvers are applied to specific joints (see page 145) to assess the joint for injury,

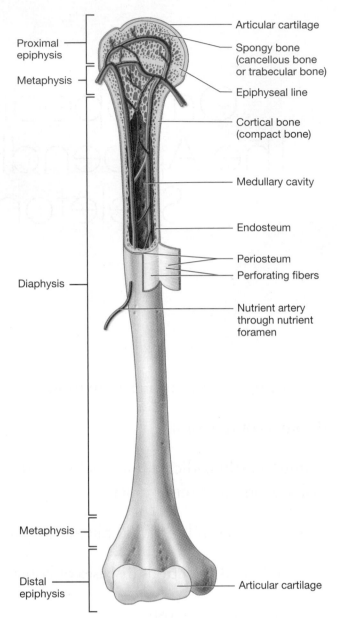

Proximal epiphysis
Metaphysis
Diaphysis
Metaphysis
Distal epiphysis

Articular cartilage
Spongy bone (cancellous bone or trabecular bone)
Epiphyseal line
Cortical bone (compact bone)
Medullary cavity
Endosteum
Periosteum
Perforating fibers
Nutrient artery through nutrient foramen
Articular cartilage

FIGURE 5-1 Architecture of bone.

instability, laxity, and other abnormalities. The examiner also observes the patient while walking and while getting up and down from the examination table.

> You may hear range of motion dictated as the acronym "rom". Passive range of motion is sometimes dictated as the acronym "prom".

> You may hear some dictators use the word crepitance, but there is no such term. The correct term is either crepitus (noun) or crepitant (adjective).

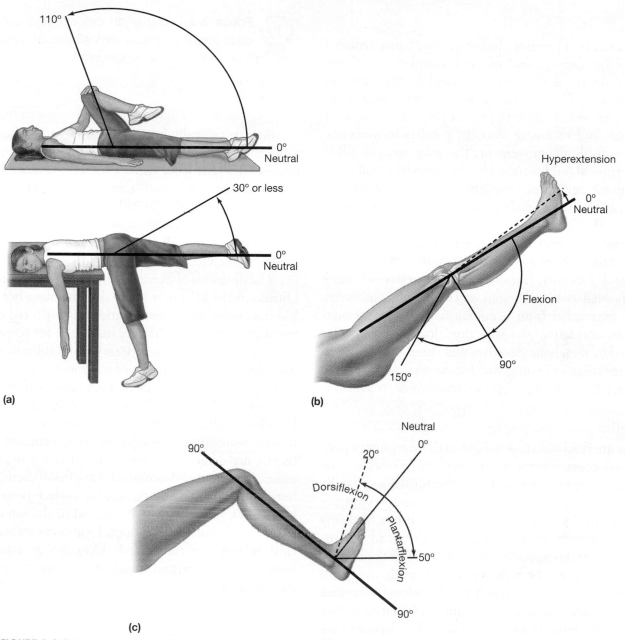

FIGURE 5-2 Range of motion for the (a) hip, (b) knee, and (c) ankle.

EXTREMITIES: Range of motion of the right hip to 90 degrees' flexion, 10 degrees' abduction, 20 degrees' adduction, 30 degrees' external rotation, 5 degrees short of neutral on internal rotation, with reproduction of his pain on internal rotation. The left hip has 90 degrees' flexion, 10 degrees' abduction, 10 degrees' adduction, 10 degrees' external rotation, 10 degrees short of neutral on internal rotation with reproduction of his pain on internal rotation. No leg-length discrepancy noted. Neurovascularly intact.

EXTREMITIES: The patient has marked valgus alignment about the right knee with range of motion from 0 to 25 degrees of flexion, 1+ pseudolaxity to varus and valgus stress. Neurovascularly intact. Well-healed arthroscopic portals.

 Be careful that you do not confuse the phrase "in flexion" with the word "inflection."

Disorders of Joints

Components of joints include cartilage, bursa, synovial membrane, capsule, and menisci. Cartilage is a dense connective tissue that can withstand flexing, tension, and pressure. The articulating surfaces of bones are covered by chondral tissue to protect the bone from wear and tear and to create smooth, painless movements. Also to facilitate movement, the joint space is filled with synovial fluid secreted by the synovial membrane. Hyaluronic acid causes the synovial fluid to be viscous. (1) The capsule is made of strong, fibrous tissue that encloses the joint. The capsule also helps stabilize the joint and prevents the joint from being pulled apart.

Disorders of the joints cause a significant amount of pain and disability. Joints incur degenerative changes from normal wear and tear as well as overuse syndromes. Joints may suffer from occupational and recreational injuries, accidents, and infection. Joints may also be affected by metabolic disorders that deposit crystals into the joint space or neurogenic diseases that decrease protective reflexes, proprioception, and muscle strength.

Bursitis

Bursae are fluid-filled cavities located near joints where friction occurs, such as where tendons or muscles pass over bony prominences. These fluid-filled sacs facilitate movement by reducing friction. **Bursitis** is inflammation of a bursa caused by overuse, injury, arthritis of the nearby joint, or infection of the nearby joint. Idiopathic and traumatic causes are the most common. Repeated trauma or recurrence of bursitis may lead to chronic bursitis, in which the bursal wall becomes thickened and the synovial lining proliferates. Adhesions, villus formations, tags, and chalky deposits may occur as a result of chronic inflammation. Typical sites of bursitis include the shoulder (subacromial or subdeltoid bursitis), olecranon (miner's or barfly's elbow), prepatellar (housemaid's knee), suprapatellar, retrocalcaneal, ischial (tailor's or weaver's bottom), greater trochanteric, pes anserine, and semimembranous gastrocnemius (**Baker cyst**).

> **Pause 5-1**   Why is an apostrophe used in disorders such as miner's elbow and housemaid's knee but not in eponyms?

Bursitis typically begins abruptly and causes focal tenderness and swelling directly over the bursae, as opposed to arthritis, which produces a more diffuse swelling. Chronic bursitis can last for several months and may recur. Persistent inflammation may affect the nearby joint by limiting range of motion. A ruptured Baker cyst causes calf pain and swelling that mimics thrombophlebitis.

The diagnosis of bursitis is typically made clinically. Ultrasound or MRI may be used to diagnose bursitis in less accessible areas that cannot be inspected or palpated (deep bursitis). Primary treatment for acute, nonseptic bursitis is rest, temporary immobilization, and high-dose NSAIDs. Range of motion exercises should be implemented as soon as pain allows. **Pendulum exercises** are helpful for bursitis involving the shoulder. Bursitis resulting from an underlying arthritis may require aspiration, especially for **tense effusion**. Antibiotics are given when septic arthritis is the primary cause. If oral antiinflammatories are insufficient, intrabursal injection of corticosteroids (triamcinolone) may be given. Chronic bursitis is treated in the same manner as acute bursitis, although long-term immobilization is not recommended. Exercise is especially important to maintain range of motion and prevent muscle atrophy.

> Her MRI scan of the right shoulder is positive for a moderate glenohumeral joint effusion and a subdeltoid bursitis and a downsloping lateral acromion as a potential source of rotator cuff impingement. There is also supraspinatus tendinitis.

> **(1)** Synovial fluid gets part of its name from the root word ova, meaning egg, because the fluid resembles the white of a chicken egg.
>
> **(2)** Purines and pyrimidines are the two classes of molecules that make up DNA and RNA.

Gout

Gout is a crystal-induced arthritis caused by **monosodium urate (MSU) crystals**. Urate is the final breakdown product of purine metabolism. (2) Gout usually affects a single joint (**monoarticular arthritis**), but when more than one joint is involved, the pattern is typically asymmetrical. Gout involving the first metatarsophalangeal (MTP) joint, called **podagra**, is the most common form of gout. The instep, ankle, knee, wrist, and elbow are also common sites. The onset of gout is acute with pain progressing to excruciating levels in a matter of hours. The joint swells and the skin over the joint becomes dusky red, warm, and tense. Fever is not uncommon.

Gout is caused by excess levels of urate (**hyperuricemia**) due to either overproduction or underexcretion of uric acid. (3) Decreased renal excretion is by far the most common cause of hyperuricemia. Many patients have a genetic predisposition to gout, but secondary causes include diuretics, low-dose aspirin therapy, cyclosporin, and niacin. Patients undergoing chemotherapy for leukemia, radiation therapy, or other treatments that cause rapid cell death may have increased uric acid levels because of the accelerated breakdown of nucleic acids.

Urate precipitates as needle-shaped MSU crystals. These crystals are deposited in cartilage, tendons, tendon sheaths, ligaments, and bursae of the smaller, cooler joints located distally (hands, feet, ears). **Tophi** (singular tophus) are crystal aggregates of MSU that form nodules in the joints and cutaneous tissue. Tophi can also be found in the kidneys. They appear as firm, yellow or white papules or nodules and commonly appear in the fingers, hands, feet, and around the olecranon and Achilles tendon. Tophi limit motion and cause deformities, resulting in **tophaceous gout**.

Gout is diagnosed by physical exam, serum urate levels (greater than 7.5 mg/dL), and analysis of synovial fluid. Polariscopic examination of joint aspirate shows needle-shaped, negatively birefringent urate crystals. X-ray images of the affected joint show punched out erosions with an **overhanging rim of cortical bone**, sometimes referred to as **rat bites** by the radiologist.

NSAIDs offer the best first-line treatment to reduce pain and swelling. Acute treatment may also use colchicine, which inhibits the deposition of urate in the joints. Long-term treatment may involve allopurinol, which blocks urate production. Urate excretion may be increased using **uricosuric drugs** such as probenecid. Tophaceous deposits may be reduced in size over time by reducing the serum urate level. Patients may complain of local desquamation (4) and pruritus during recovery.

Osteoarthritis

Osteoarthritis (OA), also called **degenerative joint disease (DJD)**, is the most common form of arthritis. OA often becomes symptomatic in individuals 40–50 years of age and affects most everyone to some degree by the age of 80. It is characterized by loss of joint cartilage and bone hypertrophy at the articular margins. A sedentary lifestyle and obesity may predispose individuals to DJD of the larger, weightbearing joints.

OA may be classified as primary or secondary. Primary generalized OA is a familial (5) arthritis that affects mostly middle-aged women and is seen in the small joints of the hands, namely the distal interphalangeal (DIP) joints, creating **Heberden nodes;** the proximal interphalangeal (PIP) joints, creating **Bouchard nodes;** the metacarpophalangeal (MCP) joints; and the carpometacarpal joints of the thumb. Larger joints affected by OA include the hips and knees. The cervical and thoracic spine may also be involved.

Secondary OA results from trauma, infection, joint abnormalities, or metabolic defects that affect the normal structure and function of the hyaline cartilage. Secondary OA may also be the result of overuse syndrome. Normally, hyaline cartilage protects the bony surface of joints from friction. Hyaline cartilage does not have a vascular supply, nerves, or lymphatic supply and consists mainly of water (95%), cartilage matrix, and chondrocytes. Weightbearing exercise causes compression of the cartilage, pumping fluid from the cartilage into the joint space. Decompression of the joint causes fluid and nutrients to reenter the cartilage. This mechanism of maintaining sufficient fluid in the joint spaces and hydration of the cartilage makes weightbearing exercise critical to the health of joints.

(3) A specific acid may be referred to in its acid form using the *-ic* suffix followed by the word acid (eg, uric acid) or as the salt of the acid using the *-ate* suffix (eg, urate). Other examples include citrate and citric acid, and lactate and lactic acid. It is incorrect to write the salt followed by the word acid (eg, *not* lactate acid).

(4) Desquamation is the shedding of skin.

(5) Familial means a disease affects more members of the same family than can be accounted for by chance. Familial is not necessarily the same as genetic or hereditary.

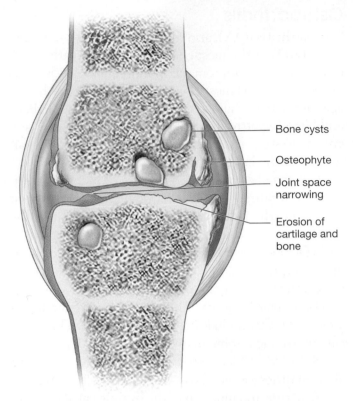

FIGURE 5-3 Joint changes associated with degenerative joint disease.

As OA progresses, subchondral bone stiffens and undergoes infarction. Cartilage breaks down and is gradually destroyed. Bone-on-bone contact develops in advanced disease. Without the protection of the cartilage, cysts (also called a **geode** when seen on x-ray), scar tissue, and **osteophytes** (bony outgrowths, spurs) form at the joint margins (■ **Figure 5-3**). The irritation causes an inflammatory response and the production of less viscous synovial fluid. Tendons and ligaments become stressed, leading to tendinitis and contractures.

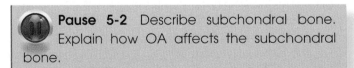

Pause 5-2 Describe subchondral bone. Explain how OA affects the subchondral bone.

Onset of symptoms is typically gradual. The first symptom is pain, often described as an ache, which may be worsened with weightbearing. Hip involvement may be felt in the inguinal area or greater trochanter or referred to the knee. Patients may complain of stiffness upon awakening that lasts 30 minutes or less and improves with movement. As the affected joint deteriorates, the joint enlarges and joint motion becomes restricted and crepitant. OA does not cause systemic symptoms.

Involvement of the knee joint causes the most disability among patients with OA. The ligaments of the knee become lax and the knee becomes unstable. The joint may feel **boggy** due to effusions. Some patients may develop a **varus deformity**.

X-rays are most useful for diagnosing OA. Imaging may show **narrowing of the joint space**, **sharpened articular margins**, osteophyte formation, cysts, increased density of the subchondral bone, **bony remodeling**, joint effusions, or **lipping of the marginal bone**. The degree of OA, as seen on plain radiographs, is reported as follows:

- grade 0: normal
- grade 1: possible joint space narrowing and subtle osteophytes
- grade 2: definite joint space narrowing, defined osteophytes and some sclerosis, especially in acetabular region
- grade 3: marked joint space narrowing, small osteophytes, some sclerosis and cyst formation and deformity of femoral head and acetabulum
- grade 4: gross loss of joint space with above features plus large osteophytes and increased deformity of the femoral head and acetabulum

Treatment goals include relieving pain, maintaining flexibility, and optimizing function. The mainstay of treatment for OA of the hips and knees is exercise and pain medications. Exercises that emphasize range of motion and muscle strength increase the capacity for tendons and muscles to absorb stress during joint motion. Daily stretching exercises prevent stiffness. Weight loss is also important for overweight patients.

Capsaicin cream, derived from cayenne pepper, applied topically may also relieve pain. Acetaminophen is effective early on. Tramadol (Ultram, Ultracet) may also be used. As the condition progresses, NSAIDs may be prescribed. Long-term treatment with NSAIDs is usually with COX-2 inhibitors because of the decreased gastrointestinal side effects associated with coxibs. Patients may also find relief with **glucosamine and chondroitin sulfate**, dietary supplements that are thought to help rebuild cartilage.

Treatments for refractory pain include intraarticular injections of corticosteroids such as triamcinolone or methylprednisolone acetate up to four times a year. Corticosteroids may also be given orally for acute episodes of OA associated with inflammation of the

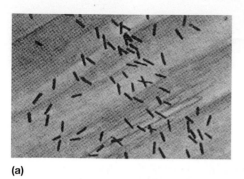
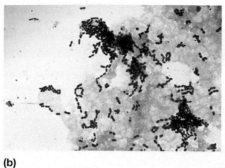
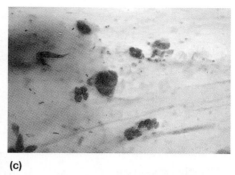

(a) (b) (c)

FIGURE 5-4 (a) E coli (gram-negative rods). *Source:* Courtesy of Centers for Disease Control and Prevention (CDC); (b) S pyogenes (gram-positive cocci) in the typical chain formation of streptococci. *Source:* Courtesy of Pearson Education; (c) N gonorrhoeae (gram-negative diplococci) that have been phagocytized by PMNs. *Source:* CDC/Joe Miller.

synovial membrane. Corticosteroids can only be used for short-term treatments due to the side effects of long-term steroid therapy. Patients may also benefit from serial (6) intraarticular injections of **hyaluronan**, a naturally occurring substance that acts as a lubricant and shock absorber. If an effusion of the knee is long-standing or recurs, a **medical synovectomy** (as opposed to a surgical synovectomy) can be performed by instilling a relatively large dose (30–50 mg) of triamcinolone hexacetonide followed by a strict regimen of rest. Laminectomy, osteotomy, and total knee and hip replacements are used only after medical management has failed and for patients with intractable pain and disability.

Septic Arthritis

Septic arthritis, also called infectious arthritis, is caused by bacterial, viral, or spirochetal infection of a joint. The infection occurs in the synovial or periarticular tissues. Untreated, septic arthritis can destroy joint structures in as little as two weeks. Septic arthritis caused by bacteria, by far the most common type of septic arthritis, is classified as either **gonococcal** or **nongonococcal arthritis**. Gonococcal arthritis primarily affects healthy, young adults, especially females of childbearing age, and nongonococcal arthritis is more common in patients with predisposing conditions such as rheumatoid arthritis, a previous history of joint infection, IV drug abuse, or a joint prosthesis.

Organisms may gain entry to the joint following joint trauma, surgery, or arthrocentesis. Infection may also result from hematogenous spread (through the blood stream) from a remote infection of soft tissue or from extension of an adjacent infection (eg, osteomyelitis or abscess). **Table 5-1** lists the most common organisms implicated in septic arthritis. Examples of bacteria are shown in ■ **Figure 5-4**. Gonococcal arthritis is associated with Neisseria gonorrhoeae and results when N gonorrhoeae spreads from infected mucosal surfaces (cervix, urethra, rectum, pharynx) via the bloodstream. Often, patients with gonococcal arthritis are co-infected with Chlamydia trachomatis.

Infection with nongonococcal organisms may be complicated by the organism's virulence factors such as adhesin produced by S aureus that allows bacteria to penetrate, infect, and remain within joint tissues. Endotoxins (produced by gram-negative organisms) and exotoxins (produced by gram-positive organisms), and antigen-antibody complexes (immune complexes) may further aggravate the joint and augment the inflammatory reaction.

Additional damage may be caused by the body's own defense mechanisms when white cells phagocytize the bacteria within the joint and then autolyse (break apart), releasing damaging lysosomal enzymes into the joint space. Chronic inflammation can result when the damaged cartilage becomes "antigenic" and the host launches an attack on itself, resulting in immune-mediated, **sterile synovitis**.

Symptoms include rapid onset of pain, swelling, heat, effusion, and restriction of both active and passive range of motion. Commonly affected joints include the hip, wrist, shoulder, and ankle. Infection in the hip causes pain that is referred to the groin. Infection caused by S aureus or P aeruginosa generally causes a more fulminant arthritis. Less virulent organisms, such as **coagulase-negative staphylococci** or Propionibacterium acnes, cause a less fulminant arthritis.

(6) Serial injections refer to several injections over a period of weeks or months.

Table 5-1 Bacteria Implicated in Septic Arthritis

Organism	Classification
**Neisseria gonorrheae (Figure 5-4)	gram-negative diplococci
Neisseria meningitidis	gram-negative diplococci
**Staphylococcus epidermidis	gram-positive cocci
**Staphylococcus aureus	gram-positive cocci
**Group B streptococci	gram-positive cocci
**Escherichia coli (Figure 5-4)	gram negative rod
**Pseudomonas aeruginosa	gram-negative rod
Enterobacter	gram-negative rod
Serratia marcescens	gram-negative rod
Salmonella	gram-negative rod
Streptococcus pyogenes (Figure 5-4)	gram-positive cocci
Streptococcus pneumoniae	gram-positive diplococci
Kingella kingae	gram-negative coccobacilli
Borrelia burgdorferi (Lyme disease)	gram-negative spirochete
Pasteurella multocida	gram-negative coccobacillus
Moraxella species	gram-negative diplococcus
Propionibacterium acnes	gram-positive rod
Peptostreptococcus magnus	anaerobic gram-positive cocci
Fusobacterium species	gram-negative spindle-shaped rod
Clostridium species	anaerobic gram-positive rod
Bacteroides species	anaerobic gram-negative rod

**most common causes

Gonococcal (GC) arthritis shows more systemic manifestations than nongonococcal disease. GC arthritis is marked by a distinctive dermatitis-polyarthritis-tenosynovitis syndrome with multiple skin lesions including petechiae, papules, pustules, hemorrhagic vesicles or bullae, necrotic lesions on mucosal surfaces and on the skin of the trunk, hands, or lower extremities. Arthralgias tend to be migratory (move from place to place), affecting the small joints of the hands, wrists, elbows, knees, and ankles. The axial skeletal joints are rarely affected. Recurrent disseminated gonococcal infection should prompt testing of a CH50 level for congenital deficiency of the complement components C7 and C8 (see Chapter 10 for more information on complement).

Synovial fluid examination provides the most definitive diagnosis. Fluid from an acutely infected joint usually shows a WBC greater than 20,000 consisting mostly of PMNs. (7) Gram stain may or may not be positive. Patients suspected of gonococcal arthritis should also have blood cultures and specimens taken from the urethra, endocervix, rectum, and pharynx. Specimens should be placed on **nonselective chocolate agar** or **Thayer-Martin agar**. Cultures for chlamydia should also be performed to rule out coinfection.

X-rays are not diagnostic in the early stages of septic arthritis, but after 10–14 days of infection, radiographs may reveal **joint-space narrowing**, erosions, or subchondral osteomyelitis. Gas within the joints suggests infection with anaerobic bacteria.

Treatment includes antibiotics and joint splinting (immobilization). Daily large-bore needle aspiration of pus, **tidal irrigation lavage**, **arthroscopic lavage**, or surgical debridement may be indicated. NSAIDs are helpful to reduce pain and inflammation. Sexual partners should also be treated when gonococcal arthritis is diagnosed.

Neurogenic Arthropathy

Neurogenic arthropathy, also referred to as **Charcot joint**, is characterized by joint destruction resulting from loss of pain perception or **proprioception**. (8) **Neuroarthropathy** is a secondary condition resulting from nerve damage due to diabetic neuropathy, spinal cord injury, pernicious anemia, peripheral nerve injury, and other disorders affecting the nerves. It is thought that impaired reflexes interfere with the joint's normal protective reflexes, allowing repeated minor episodes of trauma that produce periarticular fractures. Because the patient's perception of pain is reduced, the amount of articular damage does not typically correlate with the patient's complaints of pain. Damage becomes progressive as cartilage is destroyed, ligaments become lax, and muscle tone is decreased, resulting in joint dislocations.

In the early stages, physical exam shows an enlarged, boggy, often painless joint. A prominent, often hemorrhagic effusion and subluxation with joint instability may be noted. As the disease advances, the joint becomes deformed. Loose pieces of cartilage or bone may cause a coarse, grating sound.

X-rays show extensive cartilage erosion and osteophyte formation. In advanced disease, the joint becomes highly disorganized with multiple **loose bodies** within the joint space consisting of cartilaginous and osseous debris. Synovial effusion and joint subluxation may also be noted.

Treatment is directed toward the primary disease as well as immobilizing the joint with splints, boots, or calipers. Moderate to severe disease may be treated with

arthrodesis using internal fixation, compression, and/or bone graft. Hip and knee joints may be treated with total joint replacement, but loosening and dislocation of the prostheses are common. In extreme cases, amputation may be required.

Patellofemoral Syndrome

Patellofemoral syndrome (PS), also called **chondromalacia patella**, is the most common cause of knee pain in the primary care setting, particularly among adolescents and young adults. It involves softening and degeneration of the articular cartilage of the knee. PS is characterized by diffuse anterior knee pain around or under the patella that usually starts insidiously. Pain is aggravated by activities involving knee flexion, such as stair climbing or prolonged sitting (also referred to as a **theater sign** when there is pain with the first few steps after prolonged sitting). Most cases are caused by overloading of the patellofemoral joint related to overuse, lower extremity malalignments, poorly developed quadriceps muscles, or dysplastic changes about the patellofemoral articulation.

Physical exam reveals an abnormal **Q angle** (the angle made by the patellar and quadriceps tendons), **apprehension sign** (pain on compression of the patellofemoral joint), patellar maltracking, and a positive **patellar tilt test**. Axial views (**Merchant views**) may reveal subluxation, and lateral radiographs may reveal **patella alta** or **patella baja**. Chondromalacia patella is assessed using the Outerbridge scale, grades 1–4.

 Pause 5-3 Describe the terms patella alta and patella baja.

Treatment is primarily conservative and is aimed at strengthening the quadriceps and improving **patellar tracking** through physical therapy and a **home exercise program**. NSAIDs may be used for pain.

(7) Polymorphonuclear leukocytes (PMNs) are the most common form of white cells seen in a bacterial infection. They are usually referred to as "polys" and sometimes "PMNs." Rarely will you hear a dictator use the expanded term.

(8) Proprioception is the ability to sense the position and location of the body, especially the extremities.

- Joint disease may be caused by the degenerative effects of aging, overuse, metabolic disorders, neurogenic disorders, or infection.
- Bursitis is inflammation of a bursa caused by overuse, injury, arthritis of the nearby joint, or infection of the nearby joint.
- Gout is a crystal-induced arthritis caused by hyperuricemia, leading to accumulation of monosodium urate crystals in the joint. Arthrocentesis shows negatively birefringent urate crystals. Gout is treated with agents that block deposition of uric acid or increase excretion of uric acid.
- Osteoarthritis (OA), also called degenerative joint disease (DJD), begins with the destruction of cartilage and the formation of cysts, scar tissue, and osteophytes, leading to an inflammatory response, joint laxity, tendinitis, and muscle contractures.
- Septic arthritis is caused by bacterial, viral, or spirochetal infection of a joint and is classified as gonococcal or nongonococcal arthritis. Culture of synovial fluid provides the most definitive diagnosis.
- Neurogenic arthropathy is characterized by joint destruction resulting from loss of pain perception or proprioception.
- Patellofemoral syndrome is characterized by diffuse anterior knee pain caused by overloading of the patellofemoral joint related to overuse, lower extremity malalignments, poorly developed quadriceps muscles, or dysplastic changes about the patellofemoral articulation.

Orthopedic Injury

Orthopedic injuries include fractures, sprains, strains, tendinitis, and tendon ruptures. Injuries in healthy individuals typically result from sports, motor vehicle accidents, or recreational activities. Individuals with underlying bone or tendon disorders may suffer injury from daily activities or **falls from standing height**. Following an orthopedic injury, patients are instructed in weightbearing. The patient may be given one of the following instructions:

- **nonweightbearing:** no weight on extremity, or pressure
- **touch down** or **toe touch:** toe touch allowed for balance or to rest toe on ground
- **partial weightbearing:** patient may apply a percentage of their weight (25% to 50%) to the affected limb
- **weightbearing as tolerated:** apply weight to the affected limb as pain allows
- **full weightbearing:** no crutches needed

Fractures

Fractures may be classified as pathologic, accidental, or stress. **Pathologic fractures** result from mild or minimal force on a bone that is already weakened by a cyst, cancer, or osteoporosis. Accidental fractures occur from a single application of significant force. **Stress fractures** result from repetitive or overuse injuries to a bone.

In the presence of sufficient calcium and vitamin D, fractured edges that have been approximated and held in place with hardware, splints, or casts will heal within weeks to months. **Callus** forms at the fracture site to join the two fractured ends, and healing occurs in a process called **remodeling**. Callus formation can be seen on x-ray film and is indicative of healing. Complete remodeling eventually requires normal motion

Pause 5-4 Give two definitions for the term callus and compare the use of callus versus callous. Fill in the blanks with the correct term.

1. On physical examination, the patient is noted to have a periwound _____ at the right foot wound base.
2. X-ray of the fractured humerus shows adequate _____ formation and progression toward healing.
3. Examination of the foot shows a _____ area of the medial heel and big toe, indicating an improper gait.

and load-bearing stress. **Nonunion** describes a fracture that fails to heal within six months. **Delayed union** occurs when the bone has not completely healed within three to four months, although slow, progressive healing is occurring. **Malunion** describes a fracture that heals with the bone fragments misaligned.

The most serious complications of fractures include arterial damage (especially in fractures of the humerus and femur), compartment syndrome (see page 138), and bone infection (especially in open fractures). A complication of fractures of long bones is fat embolism caused by the release of fat from the bone marrow into the circulatory system, leading to **fat embolization syndrome** or pulmonary embolism. Disruption of the blood supply secondary to a fracture may cause aseptic necrosis of bone due to lack of nutrients. Fractures that extend into joints may damage cartilage and lead to scarring, osteoarthritis, and impaired joint function.

Fractures are diagnosed using x-ray imaging. When suspicion is high but an x-ray fails to reveal a definite fracture line, CT or MRI may be used. Several types of fractures are shown in ■ **Figure 5-5.**

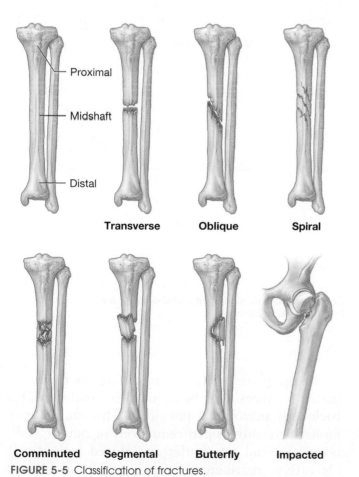

FIGURE 5-5 Classification of fractures.

The following terms are used to describe fractures:

- **open fracture**, also called a **compound fracture:** a fracture in which the bone punctures the skin, causing a visible wound

- **closed fracture**, also called a simple fracture: a fracture in which the bone does not puncture the skin

- **transverse:** a fracture perpendicular to the long axis of the bone

- **oblique:** a fracture angled across the bone

- **spiral:** a fracture resulting from a twisting motion that separates the bone in a circular pattern

- **comminuted:** a fracture that results in more than two bone fragments. A **comminuted segmental fracture** describes a bone with two separate breaks and a "floating" segment in the middle.

- **avulsion:** a fracture caused by a tendon dislodging or pulling away a bone fragment

- **impacted:** a fracture with fragments of bone forced into each other causing the bone to be shorter

- **torus** or **buckle:** a fracture occurring in children in which the bone cortex buckles

- **greenstick:** a fracture occurring in children in which the cortex is broken only on one side

- **epiphyseal:** a fracture involving the growth plate (physis) on the articular side of the plate (ie, the side closest to the joint). Epiphyseal fractures are classified using the **Salter-Harris classification** (designated I through VI and later modified to include VII through IX).

- **metaphysial:** a fracture within an area of bone composed of spongy cancellous bone

- **intraarticular:** a fracture occurring within a joint

- **nondisplaced:** a fracture that involves one or both cortices but does not cause the bones to lose their normal alignment. This fracture produces a **radiolucent line**, also known as a hairline fracture.

- **displaced:** a fracture causing the bone segments to be misaligned. Displacement is described in millimeters or as a percentage of bone width. Displaced fractures may be distracted or angulated (■ **Figure 5-6**).

- **distraction:** separation of bone in the longitudinal axis

- **angulation:** the angle of the distal fragment measured from the proximal fragment. Angulation may also be described as varus or valgus.

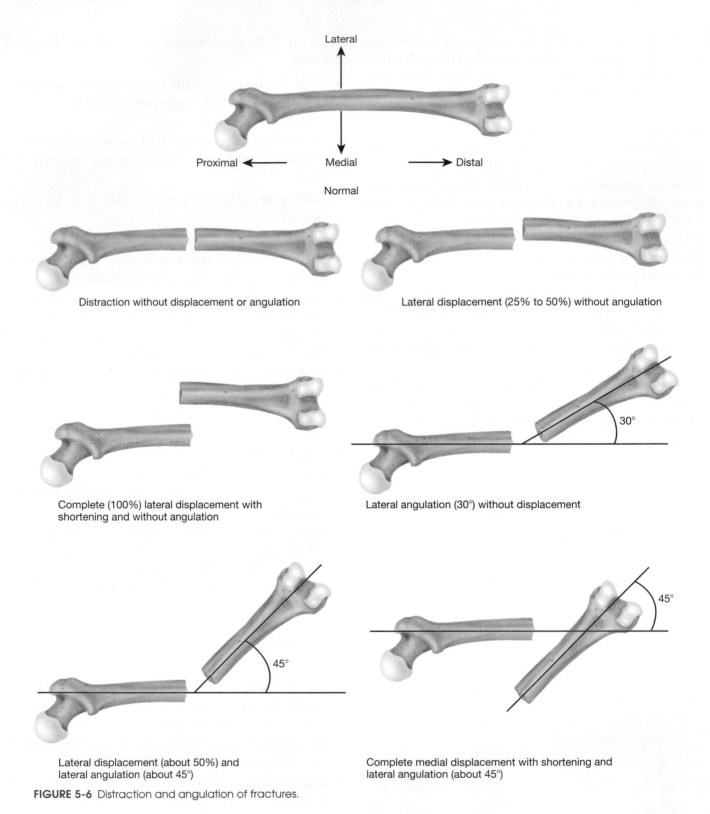

Lateral

Proximal ← Medial → Distal

Normal

Distraction without displacement or angulation

Lateral displacement (25% to 50%) without angulation

Complete (100%) lateral displacement with shortening and without angulation

Lateral angulation (30°) without displacement

Lateral displacement (about 50%) and lateral angulation (about 45°)

Complete medial displacement with shortening and lateral angulation (about 45°)

FIGURE 5-6 Distraction and angulation of fractures.

Open fractures must be treated operatively with **irrigation and debridement (I&D)** to decrease the risk of infection. Antibiotics and **tetanus prophylaxis** are given. Open fractures are often classified using the Gustilo and Anderson grading system using roman numerals I, II, III, IIIA, IIIB, and IIIC.

Before permanently immobilizing the bone, displaced fractures must be **reduced** (ie, realigned, put back into anatomical position). This may be performed surgically (**open reduction**) or nonsurgically using external manipulation (**closed reduction**). Operative treatment to repair and immobilize a fractured bone is referred to as **open reduction and internal fixation (ORIF)**. Internal fixation is carried out using hardware such as rods, plates, and/or screws. Examples of internal fixation devices include **reamed intramedullary nail**, **intramedullary rod**, plates, and screws.

When indicated, **external fixation** is used to maintain the bone in the proper alignment while remodeling occurs. External fixation involves the surgical insertion of bolts or wires directly into areas of uninjured bone on each side of the fracture. One end of the bolt is embedded in the bone and the other end extends beyond the surface of the limb to be attached to an **external fixator** (a metal supporting structure). A **monolateral fixator** uses a single rod to attach to the bolts. The **Ilizarov fixator** is circular and surrounds the limb. A significant complication of external fixation is **pin tract infection** (*not* pin track), where an infection develops around the bolt or pin.

> **Pause 5-5** Perform an image search using Google or other search engines to locate images of external fixation devices. Using copy and paste, add pictures of a monolateral fixator and Ilizarov fixator to your notes.

Stress Fractures

Stress fractures result when repeated stresses are applied to the bone faster than the bone can be repaired (remodeled). The bone gradually fatigues and eventually an actual break occurs. Stress fractures are most common in the lower extremities, with a higher rate of incidence in runners, military recruits, and athletes. Stress fractures may also be referred to as **march fractures** or fatigue fractures. Stress fractures may also occur with minimal trauma or stress in individuals with osteopenia, rheumatoid arthritis, or a metabolic bone disease.

Initially, patients may notice discomfort only during activity. On examination, patients acknowledge **point tenderness** over the stressed area of bone. Fractures may not be evident on plain radiographs. Bone scans are more sensitive and most useful when a femoral neck fracture is suspected. Stress fractures are graded 0–IV. Treatment involves activity reduction with either partial weightbearing or no weightbearing for six to eight weeks.

> **FINDINGS:** There is oblique, linear edema in the base of the left 4th metatarsal diaphysis, which raises concern for stress reaction/developing stress fracture. No full-thickness displaced fracture is seen. Otherwise, there is osteoarthritis of the midfoot and to a lesser degree the ankle. No other evidence to suggest fracture is seen by MRI. There is a large calcaneal spur.

Forearm Fractures

Forearm fractures involve the radius and ulna bones and oftentimes the wrist and the elbow, especially when the olecranon is involved. The most common cause is a fall on an outstretched arm. Forearm fractures fall into one of the following categories:

- **Monteggia fracture:** a forearm fracture with radial head dislocation
- **Galeazzi fracture:** a forearm fracture with distal radioulnar joint dislocation
- **both-bone forearm fracture:** a fracture involving both the ulna and radius
- **Colles fracture:** dorsally displaced or angulated fracture of the distal radius

> One of the more difficult orthopedic phrases to decipher is "both-bone fracture." Dictators often say this phrase very quickly, making it next to impossible to discriminate. Keep this phrase in mind when you are transcribing a report on a child involving the forearm.

Forearm fractures are evaluated with AP, lateral, and oblique views of the wrist, the entire forearm, and lateral views of the **ipsilateral** elbow. A **radiocapitellar view** should be obtained if radial head involvement is suspected. Radial head fractures may show a displaced anterior fat pad (**sail sign**).

> **Pause 5-6** A patient presents with right arm pain. A physician has ordered x-rays including AP, lateral, and oblique views of the wrist and lateral views of the ipsilateral elbow. Which elbow will be imaged?

Children under age 12 typically do not require anatomic reduction of forearm fractures. Injuries with minimal angulation and displacement may be treated with a sling or with a long-arm splint or cast with the elbow in 90 degrees of flexion. Surgical treatment of forearm fractures may involve percutaneous **Kirschner wire fixation (K-wire)** with **tension band wires**, external fixation, intramedullary nailing, or plate and screw fixation using 3.5 mm **dynamic compression plates**. Oblique fractures of the olecranon are repaired using **interfragmentary screw fixation** with tension band wire.

Femoral Shaft Fractures

Femoral shaft fractures occur in the diaphyseal region of the femoral bone, which is the largest bone in the body. The most common causes include blunt trauma from a motor vehicle collision, gunshot wounds, or falls from a significant height. Significant bleeding can occur with femoral fractures, so hemodynamic monitoring is important.

Diagnosis is made with x-rays using AP pelvis and internal rotation views of the ipsilateral femoral neck, and AP, lateral, and full-length views of the affected limb. Radiographically, fracture patterns are described as transverse, oblique, spiral, comminuted, segmented (three-part), or butterfly fragment (see Figure 5-5). A **CT scan with bone windows** may also be performed.

Treatment involves internal fixation using a reamed or unreamed intramedullary nail (■ **Figure 5-7**), a

blade plate, a **condylar screw-plate** device, or a **cephalomedullary (gamma type) nail**. Patients may require blood transfusions, so a type and cross (see page 425) may be ordered before surgery begins. Healing requires 12–16 weeks of protected weightbearing at 25% to 50% of the leg's normal load. Patients unable to undergo surgery or patients under age 11 may be treated with external fixation. Patients aged six months to eight years can be immobilized using a **spica cast**.

 Placement of an intramedullary nail is also referred to as IM nailing.

 Status post right hip fracture with IM nailing and weightbearing as tolerated.

 Pause 5-7 Why is "intermedullary nailing" incorrect?

Hip Fractures

Hip fractures (■ **Figure 5-8**) occur in the **intracapsular** (subcapital area, femoral neck) or the **extracapsular** area (trochanteric or subtrochanteric areas). In younger adults, a broken hip is typically caused by high-velocity trauma, but for adults over 50, pathologic fractures due to osteoporosis are the most common. Osteoporotic bone may have microfractures that become macrofractures due to repeated stress, or the osteoporotic bone may fracture acutely due to a fall from standing height. Fractures cause severe pain in the groin area that is exacerbated by **axial loading** (standing on the leg) and range of motion, especially internal rotation. The leg may be shortened.

Complications of hip fractures in the young include nonunion, malunion, and osteonecrosis (see page 141) of the femoral head. Morbidity is high in the elderly secondary to deep venous thrombosis and cardiopulmonary complications resulting from prolonged immobilization (ie, being bedridden).

Fractures of the hip are diagnosed on x-ray with AP pelvis and AP and lateral views of the hip and femur. Occasionally MRI or CT scan may be required to diagnose occult fractures. Extracapsular fractures are classified using the **Evans classification** (type I and type II),

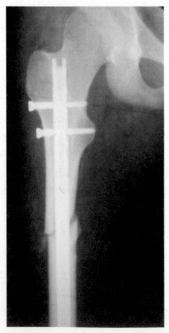

FIGURE 5-7 Intramedullary nailing of a femoral shaft fracture.
Source: Courtesy of Cheryl Wraa.

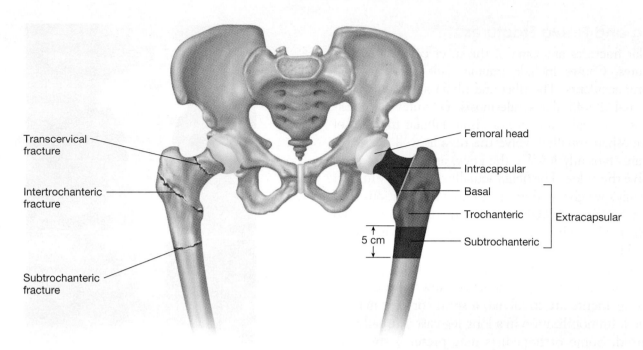

Transcervical fracture

Intertrochanteric fracture

Subtrochanteric fracture

Femoral head

Intracapsular

Basal

Trochanteric

Subtrochanteric

Extracapsular

5 cm

FIGURE 5-8 Intracapsular and extracapsular areas of the hip and types of hip fractures.

and intracapsular fractures are classified according to the **Garden classification** (stage I, II, III, and IV).

Intertrochanteric fractures are customarily treated by open reduction and internal fixation using a **dynamic hip compression screw** (■ Figure 5-9) or **nail plate** device. **Cerclage wires** may be used to reattach trochanteric fragments. Patients with femoral neck fractures may initially be placed in **Buck traction** with three to five pounds of weights. ORIF with early

ambulation is the treatment of choice for those who can tolerate surgery. Garden stage I and stage II fractures are repaired using **cannulated lag screws**. Partial or total hip replacement may be required, especially in the elderly.

A **patellar fracture**, commonly known as a broken kneecap, may result from a direct blow to the patella from a fall; a sudden, powerful quadriceps muscle contracture; or a motor vehicle collision. Patellar fractures are classified as vertical, transverse, **stellate**, or polar. These fractures are diagnosed on plain radiographs using AP, lateral, and **sunrise views**. Surgical treatment is indicated if there is a 3 mm separation of the fragments, greater than 2 mm **stepoff** of the articular surface, or an open fracture. Vertical fractures are repaired with 3.5 mm or 4.9 mm screws. Transverse fractures are repaired using a **tension-band technique** to resist the pull of the quadriceps muscle, which otherwise would displace the fracture. Stellate fractures require pins, screws, and wires and have the worst prognosis. Severely comminuted stellate fractures may be treated with **patellectomy**.

(a) Subcapital fracture repair

(b) Intertrochanteric fracture repair

FIGURE 5-9 Hip repair of (a) subcapital fracture using cannulated lag screws and (b) intertrochanteric fracture using dynamic hip compression screw.

Pause 5-8 Research the phrase "sunrise view." How did this radiographic view get its name?

Tibia and Fibula Fractures

Fibular fractures are some of the most commonly seen fractures. Causes include trauma, falls, missteps, and skating accidents. The tibia and fibula articulate at the **proximal tibiofibular syndesmosis**. Fractures are classified as proximal, midshaft, or distal. Fibular fractures of the midshaft usually involve the tibia as well. Proximal fractures typically involve the knee, and distal fractures involve the ankle. The fibula actually carries very little of the body's weight, so there are rarely complications with fibular fractures. A **Maisonneuve fracture** (pronounced *mā zho nuv*) involves the *proximal* fibula and a tear of the deltoid ligament of the *ankle*.

Diagnosis is by plain film using AP and lateral views of the shaft and knee, and **mortise views** of the ankle. If no ligaments are involved, a splint or cast may be applied. Immobilization in a long leg cast is usually not required. Some orthopedists may prefer a short leg walking cast or a **Cam Walker. (9)** Weightbearing is as tolerated. When fixation is needed, the fibula may be repaired using a **3.5 mm compression plate**.

Fractures of the tibia can involve the tibial plateau, tibial tubercle, tibial eminence, proximal tibia, tibial shaft, or tibial plafond. A fracture of the plafond is also called a pilon fracture. Tibial shaft fractures are the most common diaphyseal fracture. Tibial shaft fractures with more than 50% displacement or greater than 10% angulation are treated with an intramedullary nail, plates, screws, (■ Figure 5-10) or external fixator. The tibial shaft carries a significant amount of the body's weight and requires two to six months of nonweightbearing or protected weightbearing to heal.

> Patient shows a tibial tubercle fracture with tenderness over the anterior tibia. Patient cannot fully extend the knee and the patella is high-riding.

The distal tibia is also known as the "roof" or "plafond" over the talus, so fractures of the distal tibia are

(9) Cam Walker is written as two words in title case. Cam comes from the acronym CAM, meaning controlled ankle motion.

(10) A bivalved cast is split longitudinally down two sides to allow the cast to expand if the leg were to swell.

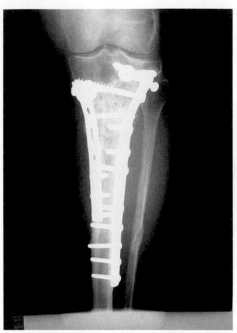

FIGURE 5-10 ORIF of the tibia using plates and screws.
Source: Courtesy of Cheryl Wraa.

called **plafond fractures**. A **tibial plateau fracture** involves the proximal weightbearing surface of the tibia (where the tibia articulates with the femoral condyles). These fractures are classified using the **Schatzker classification** and designated type I through type VI. Plateau fractures may be immobilized with a well-padded, long leg cast that is completely **bivalved. (10)**

> ASSESSMENT: Type II tibial plateau fracture in a young adult with good bone stock, treated with percutaneous elevation and cannulated cancellous screw fixation without bone grafting.

> ASSESSMENT: Type III tibial plateau fracture with central depression in an elderly person, treated surgically using percutaneous elevation, bone grafting, and cancellous screw fixation.

Ankle Fractures

Ankle fractures are common and usually involve both the bones and the ligaments. Fractures of the distal fibula and tibia are considered ankle fractures. The ankle consists of the malleolus of the tibia, the lateral

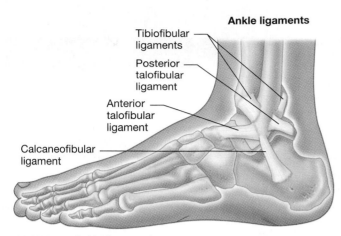

Ankle ligaments

Tibiofibular ligaments

Posterior talofibular ligament

Anterior talofibular ligament

Calcaneofibular ligament

FIGURE 5-11 Ankle ligaments.

malleolus of the fibula, the talus and calcaneus, as well as the navicular, cuboid, internal cuneiform, middle cuneiform, and external cuneiform bones. The ligaments include the deltoid ligament, the anterior and posterior talofibular ligaments, and the calcaneofibular ligament (■ **Figure 5-11**).

If fractures disrupt more than two of the structures stabilizing the ankle, the ankle becomes unstable. Disruption of the medial deltoid ligament also causes instability. Ankle fractures are classified using the **Weber system**. Weber A is a fracture below the ankle joint line; Weber B is a fracture at the joint line; and Weber C is a fracture above the joint line.

Stable fractures, which have a good prognosis, can be treated with a cast for six weeks. Ankle fractures are splinted using a **sugar-tong** method that employs a layer of padding, fiberglass or plaster, and an Ace bandage. An unstable ankle usually requires surgical repair. Widening of the joint, as seen on x-ray, is also an indication for surgical repair. A fibular fracture is plated through a lateral incision. Medial malleolar fractures are fixed with compression screws placed in a retrograde fashion. Open fractures or **comminuted pilon** fractures may require an external fixator and possibly an internal fixator as well. Early weightbearing and range of motion exercises are important to prevent stiffness.

Foot Fractures

Acute foot fractures of normal bones are usually caused by dropping heavy objects directly on the foot. They may also be caused by the stress of repetitive trauma. Fractures of the foot typically involve the metatarsal bones, most commonly the second and fifth metatarsals (MTPs). Single, point fractures are typically stable and treated with a short leg cast. A fracture of the proximal fifth MTP, called a **Jones fracture**, requires more aggressive treatment because the watershed blood supply to this area makes this type of fracture more susceptible to nonunion. **Table 5-2** outlines common fractures of the foot.

- Pathologic fractures result from minimal force on a bone that is already weakened by a cyst, cancer, or osteoporosis.

- Displaced fractures must be reduced (ie, realigned) using either open (surgical) or closed reduction.

- Stress fractures result when repeated stresses are applied to the bone faster than the bone can be remodeled.

- Forearm fractures involve either or both the radius and ulna bones.

- Femoral shaft fractures occur in the diaphyseal region of the femoral bone and are often repaired using intramedullary nails.

- Hip fractures occur in the intracapsular or the extracapsular area. Osteoporosis is the most common cause of hip fractures.

- Knee fractures are classified as vertical, transverse, stellate, or polar.

- Fibular fractures are some of the most commonly seen fractures and may be classified as proximal, midshaft, or distal. Fractures of the midshaft usually involve the tibia as well.

- Fractures of the tibia can involve the tibial plateau, tibial tubercle, tibial eminence, proximal tibia, tibial shaft, or tibial plafond.

- Ankle fractures are common and usually involve the distal fibula and the tibia as well as the ligaments.

- Fractures of the foot typically involve the metatarsal bones, most commonly the second and fifth metatarsals.

Table 5-2 Common Fractures of the Foot

Fracture Type	Location	Surgical Treatment	Medical Treatment
Lisfranc fracture-dislocation	second MTP	K-wires or 3.5 mm cortical screws or 4.0 to 4.5 mm cannulated screws	nonweightbearing short leg cast
chip or fleck fracture	cuneiform		short leg walking cast
Lisfranc dislocation	movement of the metatarsal bones away from the tarsal bones (disruption of the tarsometatarsal joints)	closed reduction with K-wires or 3.5 mm cortical screws or 4.0 to 4.5 mm cannulated screws	nonweightbearing short leg cast
dancer fracture	fracture of the fifth metatarsal bone base		
Jones fracture	fracture of the proximal fifth metatarsal bone diaphysis (shaft)	intramedullary malleolar screw	short leg cast
march fracture, marcher's foot (stress fracture)	fracture of a metatarsal bone		activity modification and protection in a cast or orthosis
pseudo-Jones	avulsion fracture proximal to the intermetatarsal articulation (fracture of the metatarsal tuberosity)		wooden-soled shoe only
toe fractures	proximal and distal phalanges	closed reduction when necessary	tape to adjacent toe (buddy taping or dynamic splinting)

 Pause 5-9 What is a watershed blood supply and how does this affect healing?

Dislocations

Dislocation is a complete separation of the bone ends that normally articulate to form a joint; subluxation is a partial separation. Dislocations most commonly occur in the shoulder, elbow, fingers, hip, knee, and ankle. Generally, dislocations cause pain, swelling, deformity and an inability to move the joint. Examinations involving dislocated joints should include a careful assessment of the associated neurovascular system because nerves may be impinged and vessels may be ruptured or torn. Treatment usually requires closed reduction, occasionally open reduction. Splints and slings are used to immobilize the joint for a short time while the ligaments heal. NSAIDs may be prescribed for swelling and pain. **Table 5-3** describes the most common dislocations.

Sprains, Strains, and Tears

A sprain is caused by a wrenching or twisting movement that stretches, tears, or ruptures ligaments and surrounding blood vessels. Patients often recall hearing a popping sound at the time of the injury. Swelling is immediate and pain can be moderate to severe. Ecchymosis is common. Sprains may be minimal (first-degree sprain), moderate to severe (second-degree sprain), or complete (third-degree sprain or tear). Third-degree sprains often cause joint instability because the ligaments are no longer holding the joint stable. A *strain* refers to the pulling or tearing of a muscle and/or its tendon. Third-degree strains prevent movement of the involved bone because the muscle responsible for movement is no longer attached.

Generally speaking, the most common treatment for sprains and strains is **rest, ice, compression, and elevation (RICE)** along with analgesics. Complete tears, also called **ruptures**, may require surgical repair. Physical therapy may be used in the acute or postacute stage to minimize swelling and effusion, normalize

Table 5-3 Common Dislocations

Area	Joint affected	Comments	Treatment
elbow	ulnohumeral joint		reduction with sustained, gentle traction after sedation and analgesia
	radial head subluxations (nursemaid's elbow)	occurs in toddlers	reduction without anesthesia or sedation
shoulder	glenohumeral		closed reduction with conscious sedation and traction-countertraction technique
	acromioclavicular and/or coracoclavicular	classified as grade I through IV	
finger	proximal interphalangeal (PIP) joint dislocations (dorsal or volar)	boutonnière deformity	closed reduction using digital-block anesthesia
knee	tibiofemoral joint	concomitant arterial injury with a spontaneously reduced knee dislocation and a large hemarthrosis	
	patellar joint	lateral dislocation	none; many spontaneously reduce
hip		may be complicated by avascular necrosis and sciatic nerve injury	reduction

pain-free range of motion, prevent muscular atrophy, maintain proprioception, and where appropriate, maintain cardiovascular fitness.

 The abbreviation RICE is pronounced as the acronym rīs.

Wrist Sprain

Wrist sprains typically occur from a fall on an outstretched hand. A wrist sprain involves partial stretching or disruption of the ligaments holding the radius and the carpal bones in alignment. Wrist sprains are graded I, II, and III, with grade I being no ligament damage, grade II being a partial tear, and grade III being a complete tear of the ligament. A wrist sprain should be differentiated from navicular or scaphoid fractures that are indicated by pain in the **snuffbox**. (11) A wrist sprain should also be differentiated from a scapholunate interosseous ligament tear or a **chip fracture** of the lunate or triquetrum bones. When fractures are suspected, AP, lateral and oblique (navicular) views of the hand are ordered. **Clenched fist views** or **coned**

views (ie, focused on a small area) may also be used to rule out injury to the scaphoid, lunate, or triquetrum bones. The wrist may be immobilized for comfort with activity as tolerated. A navicular fracture should be immobilized using a **thumb spica cast**.

Lower Extremity Sprains, Strains, and Tears

The hamstrings include the three long muscles in the posterior thigh (the long head of biceps, the semitendinosus, and the semimembranosus muscles) that originate at the ischial tuberosity and insert behind the knee. A pull or tear of one of the hamstrings is usually caused by quick starts with sudden hamstring contraction. Strains are classified as mild, moderate, or severe. A mild strain is characterized by muscle spasm but no tear. A moderate strain causes loss of function and possibly a hematoma. A severe strain is a full tear, often occurring at the origin or insertion. Some strains may

(11) The snuffbox, also called the anatomical snuffbox, is the small depression at the base of the thumb between the extensor and abductor tendons of the thumb.

be associated with ischial or fibular avulsion. Treatment in the acute phase is ice with an elastic wrap followed by a compressive wrap, rest, and crutches.

 Pause 5-10 Describe a fibular avulsion in layman's terms.

A sprain of the **anterior cruciate ligament (ACL)** is a very common knee injury and is typically caused by sudden decelerations such as stopping abruptly, pivoting, or landing after jumping. Physical examination may reveal a tense joint effusion with marked restriction in range of motion. **Lachman test** and the **anterior drawer sign** are positive. Evaluation involves MRI or arthroscopy to determine the extent of the tear. When torn, the collagen fibers appear as **mop ends**. Avulsion fractures may also occur at the ACL tibial insertion. The knee is placed in an immobilizer with weightbearing as tolerated. If knee instability persists, ACL reconstruction may be warranted.

Medial collateral ligament (MCL) injury is common, especially among teenagers and young adults. The injury is graded as I (microscopic strain), II (partial tear), or III (complete tear). X-rays may be ordered to rule out a concomitant fracture, but MRI is the diagnostic imaging of choice for ligamentous injury of the knee. The MCL typically heals with conservative treatment with a hinged brace. After healing, physical therapy should include quadriceps strengthening and range of motion exercises.

A meniscus is a crescent-shaped wedge of fibrocartilaginous tissue between two articulating bones that helps the bones conform to one another. The menisci of the knee are semilunar collagen wedges positioned between the femur and the tibia. The femoral condyles are round and the tibial plateau is relatively flat. The menisci are extensions of the tibia that allow the two bones to conform to each other. The menisci primarily provide load-bearing across the knee joint. Tears of the medial meniscus are the most common knee injuries. A tear results from a twisting action exerted on the knee joint while the foot is in a weightbearing position. A tearing or popping sensation is typically felt at the time of the injury. Patients may complain of clicking, catching, locking, pinching, or a sensation of giving way. Effusions associated with meniscal injuries are typically worse the day after the injury, and examination shows a **ballottable patella**. (12) Tenderness is localized to the **medial joint line**. Examination also shows a positive **McMurray test** and positive **Apley test**. An MRI will confirm a meniscal tear.

Tears are classified by their shape and direction: longitudinal tears (which may take the shape of a **bucket handle**); radial tears; oblique flap tears (described as a **parrot beak**); horizontal tears; and complex tears that involve more than one type of tear. Normal menisci have a homogeneous, low signal on MRI. Abnormal meniscal signals are classified using the following criteria:

- grade I—small area of increased signal within the meniscus
- grade II—linear area of increased signal that does not extend to an articulating surface
- grade III—abnormal increased signal that reaches the surface or edge of the meniscus

Grade I and II signals are common in older patients and are indicative of normal, degenerative processes. Grade III changes are considered meniscal tears.

(12) A ballotable patella describes a patella with inflammation and fluid accumulation in the suprapatellar space. Ballottement refers to an examination technique for detecting a floating object in the body.

(13) The red zone is the vascularized, peripheral area of the meniscus. The red-white zone is the transitional, central area of the meniscus, and the white zone is the central area with no vascularization.

 PREOPERATIVE DIAGNOSIS: Left knee medial meniscal tear with possible lateral meniscal tear.

POSTOPERATIVE DIAGNOSIS: Left knee medial meniscal tear with lateral meniscal tear and medial plica.

In most cases, treatment is conservative with elevation of the joint and application of a compression dressing and ice. Patients are instructed in limited weightbearing for several days. Complex tears are repaired arthroscopically. Tears in the avascular zone (**white zone**) (13) require a **partial meniscectomy** because the lack of blood supply prevents complete healing. Repairs involve smoothing and abrading the torn edges and bordering synovium to promote bleeding and healing. Likewise, **needle trephination** (poking holes) of the meniscal body may be performed to create vascular channels. Upon recovery, quadriceps-strengthening exercises are recommended.

> TECHNIQUE: MRI scans were performed through the right knee using 3.5 mm thick images acquired in the sagittal, axial, and frontal plane with T1 proton-density and T2-weighted pulse sequences with and without fat-suppression techniques.
>
> FINDINGS: A moderate joint effusion is noted. The patellofemoral joint is maintained. Fissuring of the patellar articular cartilage is noted, consistent with chondromalacia. The posterior horn of the medial meniscus shows a complex tear. Narrowing of the medial and lateral compartments of the knee joint is seen. Patellofemoral narrowing is also noted.

Inversion (varus) sprains of the ankle are the most common ankle sprains, especially among athletes and dancers. Ankle sprains involve the anterior talofibular ligament, the calcaneofibular ligament, or both. Swelling with ecchymosis on the lateral aspect of the ankle is immediate and weightbearing may be impossible. Ankle sprains are graded I through III. Grade I and II sprains are mild to moderate injuries with partial or complete tear of the ligaments. A grade III sprain involves a complete rupture of both ligaments. An ankle sprain is assessed using the anterior drawer sign.

Excessive anterior motion of the foot constitutes a positive test for a grade III sprain.

Ankle sprains are treated with rest, ice, compression, and elevation (RICE). A compression dressing is applied to control swelling and provide stability. An **Aircast ankle brace** may be used, as these provide more stability than an elastic support bandage. Crutches should be used to minimize weightbearing. Elevation reduces swelling and decreases pain.

Tendinopathy

Tendinopathy is an injury or disease process that affects a tendon. Specific forms of tendinopathy include tendinitis, tendinosis, and tenosynovitis. Tendinosis is a degenerative disease leading to scarring of the tendon. Tendinitis is inflammation of a tendon, and tenosynovitis is inflammation of the tendon and its surrounding sheath. Tenosynovitis occurs most commonly in the fingers, wrist, and ankle. Tendinitis and tenosynovitis are extremely common. Although the etiology is not always apparent, tendinitis is often the result of repetitive motion. Tendinopathy may result from repeated small tears or chronic degenerative changes. Calcium deposits may also form as a result of chronic inflammation. **Quinolone antibiotics** may also increase the risk of tendinitis or even tendon rupture. Rheumatoid arthritis may predispose the joint to tendinitis or tenosynovitis as well.

Movement of the involved tendon causes pain. Physical exam shows tenderness along the course of the affected tendon, and swelling may or may not be apparent. Treatment includes rest and splinting. If conservative treatment fails, the patient may require **surgical release** of the tendon or tendon sheath. **Table 5-4** outlines the most common forms of tendinitis affecting the upper extremities.

Table 5-4 Tendinitis of the Upper Extremities

Area affected	Tendon(s)	Comments
wrist (De Quervain syndrome)	abductor pollicis longus and extensor pollicis brevis	Pain occurs along the radial aspect of the wrist and with passive range of motion of the thumb. Finkelstein test is positive. Patient may require complete release of the abductor pollicis longus followed by splinting.
forearm and wrist	flexor carpi radialis or ulnaris, flexor digitorum	Pain occurs with resisted wrist flexion and ulnar deviation or on passive extension.
fingers (trigger finger)	digital flexor tendon volar flexor tendon	Snapping or popping feeling occurs during extension; the finger may lock in flexion, or "trigger," suddenly extending with a snap.

Lateral and Medial Epicondylitis

Tendinopathy of the elbow includes **lateral epicondylitis** (tennis elbow) and **medial epicondylitis** (golf elbow). These injuries involve minor tears in the tendons of the forearm's extensor and flexor muscles. Lateral epicondylitis typically affects the origin of the extensor carpi radialis brevis. Medial epicondylitis affects the flexor-pronator muscles (ie, pronator teres, flexor carpi radialis, palmaris longus, flexor carpi ulnaris, and flexor digitorum superficialis) at their origin on the anterior medial epicondyle. Grasping and squeezing items exacerbates the pain. Examination reveals pain at the site of the tendon insertion with point tenderness over the involved tendon. Treatment includes rest and NSAIDs for pain and swelling. A **counterforce brace** may improve symptoms during activities of daily living. For chronic cases, infiltration with triamcinolone and 1% lidocaine around the involved epicondyle may prove helpful. **Botulinum toxin injections** have been used for lateral epicondylitis. Botulinum toxin is a neurotoxin that decreases muscle contractions and spasms.

Rotator Cuff Disorders

The shoulder complex is comprised of several joints, including the sternoclavicular joint, acromioclavicular (AC) joint, glenohumeral (GH) joint, and scapulothoracic (ST) joint. Rotator cuff disorders (14) are the most common etiology of shoulder pain and may be caused by acute injury or chronic degenerative injuries to the musculotendinous structures of the shoulder. Inflammation is often due to impingement of the tendons between the humeral greater tuberosity and the lateral structures of the shoulder (acromion, coracoacromial ligament, coracoid process, and cricoclavicular ligament). Impingement can cause chronic bursitis or a complete tear of the rotator cuff (■ Figure 5-12). Degenerative tears and **full-thickness tears** are most common in the elderly.

Patients complain of shoulder pain, typically worse at night from sleeping on the affected shoulder, as well as catching, stiffness, weakness, instability, and pain in the upper deltoid that radiates down the arm. Pain is exacerbated by overhead activities. Onset of pain in the

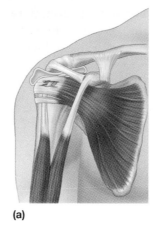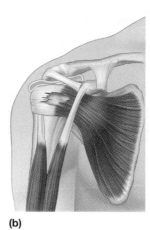

(a)   **(b)**

FIGURE 5-12 Partial and full-thickness tears of the rotator cuff.

elderly is often insidious due to the chronic, degenerative nature of the injury.

Physical examination reveals pain on active abduction and internal rotation with decreased motor strength. Reduced active and passive range of motion may indicate **adhesive capsulitis** (frozen shoulder). Appropriate x-ray views include AP, **supraspinatus outlet view**, and **axillary view**. Ultrasound may also be helpful, but MRI is the most definitive. An MRI can characterize the size and location of a rotator cuff tear. On MRI, a rotator cuff tear demonstrates a bright signal on T1-weighted images that increases on the T2-weighted images.

The vast majority of rotator cuff disorders respond to conservative management with NSAIDs, rest, and possibly corticosteroid injections. Physical therapy is recommended for range of motion, stretching, and strengthening, including **progressive resistive exercises (PREs)**, the use of **Thera-Bands**, and **plyometrics**. When indicated, surgical treatment involves direct suture of tendons along with **subacromial decompression** using an arthroscopic or open approach. The **Neer staging** system is used to classify shoulder impingement in stages I, II, and III.

> FINDINGS: No fracture, dislocation, or subluxation is seen. There is mild glenohumeral joint osteoarthritis with mild, asymmetric joint-space loss inferiorly. There is mild hypertrophic acromioclavicular degenerative joint disease that has a mild mass effect on the rotator cuff as well. There is a slight anterior downsloping of the anterior acromion.

(14) The rotator cuff consists of four muscles and their tendons that stabilize the shoulder: subscapularis, supraspinatus, infraspinatus, and teres minor.

Achilles Tendinitis

The Achilles tendon (also called the tendoachilles) is the largest and strongest tendon in the body. It is formed by the convergence of tendons from the soleus and gastrocnemius muscles and inserts at the posterior calcaneus. Achilles tendon injuries are quite common, especially in runners and other athletes. Repetitive forces from running without sufficient recovery time causes inflammation of the tissue between the tendon and its sheath, called the **paratenon**. Achilles injuries include **paratenonitis** (paratenon inflammation) with or without tendinosis. **(15)**

Physical examination reveals tenderness along the tendon from the musculotendinous junction to the calcaneal insertion (os calcis). Most pain is 3–5 cm proximal to the insertion on the calcaneus. Pain is elicited on dorsiflexion of the ankle.

Conservative treatment includes ice, rest, and orthotics. **Retrocalcaneal bursa injection** may also be given. Recalcitrant cases may be treated with a trial of cast immobilization with weightbearing. Surgery is reserved for patients that fail 6–12 months of conservative treatment. Physical therapy in the form of ultrasound therapy, **phonophoresis**, and **iontophoresis (16)** may improve healing. A heel wedge can be used to unload the tendon.

The Achilles tendon is also prone to rupture, typically 2–6 cm proximal to its insertion into the calcaneus (■ Figure 5-13). Patients experience a sudden snap in the back of the ankle with acute, severe pain and inability to walk on the affected ankle. Ruptures are typically caused by an abrupt, forceful change in direction when running, unexpected dorsiflexion of the foot, or violent dorsiflexion of the plantarflexed foot. Patients who have taken fluoroquinolone antibiotics or corticosteroids are at increased risk of rupture, even with minimal exertion. Chronic peritenonitis causes attrition of the tendon, making the tendon prone to rupture.

 Be sure you do not confuse peri*tenon*itis with peritonitis (inflammation of the peritoneum).

Physical examination shows swelling with a palpable gap along the Achilles tendon and decreased active plantarflexion strength. The patient will be unable to stand on their toes on the affected foot. **Thompson test** will be positive. A CT may be ordered to rule out avulsion of the calcaneus, and MRI will provide a definitive diagnosis when the differential

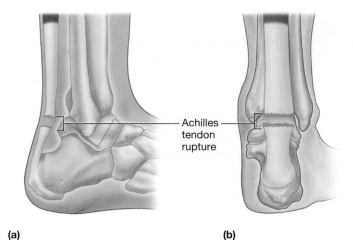

Achilles tendon rupture

(a)   **(b)**

FIGURE 5-13 Achilles tendon rupture.

diagnosis includes complete or incomplete rupture versus peritendinitis versus tendinosis.

Nonoperative treatment of ruptured Achilles tendon requires the foot to be in a short leg cast with the

> **FINDINGS:** There is diffuse, circumferential edema about the ankle and foot, including edema and fluid within the sinus tarsi. There is tendinosis and tenosynovitis of the medial and lateral flexor tendons of the ankle. No full-thickness or retracted tear of the posterior tibialis tendon is seen.
>
> There is also Achilles tendinosis. The deltoid ligament and fibular collateral ligament appear intact. The anterior and posterior talofibular ligaments as well as the anterior tibiofibular ligament appear intact. The posterior tibiofibular ligament is heterogeneous in appearance, with either a prominent blood vessel or, less likely, a serpiginous ganglion cyst associated at this level. The extensor tendons appear intact. There is heterogeneity of the plantar fascia, which can be seen with plantar fasciitis. There is a small ankle joint effusion. No full-thickness or retracted muscle tear is seen.

(15) Tendinosis is intrasubstance degeneration of the tendon.

(16) Phonophoresis is the use of ultrasound to improve the effect of topically applied medications. Iontophoresis uses a small electrical charge to improve the effect of topically applied medications.

- Dislocation is a complete separation of the bone ends that normally articulate to form a joint and most commonly occurs in the shoulder, elbow, finger, hip, knee, and ankle.
- A *sprain* is caused by a wrenching or twisting movement that stretches, tears, or ruptures ligaments and surrounding blood vessels.
- A *strain* refers to the pulling or tearing of a muscle and/or its tendon.
- A wrist sprain involves partial stretching or disruption of the ligaments holding the radius and the carpal bones in alignment.
- Sprains are graded I through III with grade III being a complete tear or rupture.
- Tendinopathy is an injury or disease process that affects a tendon and includes tendinitis, tendinosis, and tenosynovitis. Tenosynovitis occurs most commonly in the fingers, wrist, and ankle.
- Tendinopathy of the elbow includes lateral epicondylitis and medial epicondylitis and involves minor tears in the tendons of the forearm's extensor and flexor muscles.
- Rotator cuff disorders are the most common etiology of shoulder pain and may be caused by acute injury or chronic degenerative injuries to the musculotendinous structures of the shoulder.
- Achilles tendon injuries are quite common, especially in athletes, and include paratenonitis with or without tendinosis and complete rupture.
- Compartment syndrome, a possible complication of skeletal fractures, is caused by severe pressure increases within an enclosed space due to intercompartmental bleeding or swelling that compromise capillary flow.

foot in **maximal equinus** for four weeks followed by successive castings that gradually bring the foot back into the neutral position. Direct end-to-end anastomosis is recommended for acute ruptures.

Compartment Syndrome

Compartment syndrome (CS) is caused by severe pressure increases within an enclosed space that compromise capillary flow. Pressure may be increased within the muscle fascia due to a crush injury, bleeding from a fracture, or any trauma causing excessive swelling. Muscle tissue and nerves become ischemic with concomitant paresthesia. Untreated, CS quickly leads to muscle necrosis, nerve damage, and ultimately loss of the limb. If a large amount of muscle is affected, massive cell death releases large amounts of protein and intracellular constituents with subsequent tubular necrosis, hyperkalemia, and kidney failure. Compartment syndrome can occur in any limb following a major (or rarely minor) trauma, but it is most common in the shin and forearm.

The signs and symptoms of compartment syndrome are the five P's (pain, pallor, paresthesia, paralysis, and pulselessness). Any constrictive splints, casts, or dressings must be removed. Muscle necrosis is indicated by elevated serum **creatine phosphokinase (CPK)**. Treatment requires emergency fasciotomy to decompress the compartment. A longitudinal incision into the fascia is made to relieve pressure, and the wound is left open for several days followed by **delayed primary closure**.

Note the spelling of CPK; it is creatine (not creatinine) phosphokinase.

Common Disorders of the Feet and Hands

Plantar fasciitis is a common **enthesopathy (17)** of the foot. It is caused by strain on the plantar fascia at its insertion into the medial tubercle of the calcaneus as a result of excessive standing or improper footwear. Patients complain of pain on the bottom of the foot, especially upon the first steps out of bed. Physical exam shows pain with palpation over the plantar fascia's insertion on the medial heel. Treatment includes reduced standing and the use of arch supports and heel cushions. Arch supports bear more of the patient's weight and **unload the plantar enthesis**. NSAIDs may be used to reduce pain and inflammation.

(17) An enthesopathy is injury or inflammation at the site of insertion of muscle tendons and ligaments.

- Plantar fasciitis is a common enthesopathy caused by strain on the plantar fascia at its insertion into the medial tubercle of the calcaneus.

- Carpal tunnel syndrome is a neuropathy caused by compression of the median nerve that runs through the carpal tunnel. The pain is thought to be due to ischemia rather than physical damage of the nerve.

Carpal tunnel syndrome (CTS) is a neuropathy caused by compression of the median nerve that runs through the carpal tunnel, a spatially limited area that also encases nine long flexors of the wrist and fingers. Compression is caused by hypertrophy or edema of the flexor synovium. Risk factors include repetitive handwork such as assembly-line work, keyboarding, playing a musical instrument, or craftwork. Edema may be caused by increased fluid retention associated with pregnancy or the use of oral contraceptives. The tunnel is located at the base of the palm and is bounded by the carpal bones on three sides and anteriorly by the transverse carpal ligament. Compression of the nerve causes a decrease in **thenar muscle strength** and paresthesias in the median nerve distribution (the palmar surface of the first three and a half radial digits, especially the middle and index fingers). Patients complain of hand weakness or clumsiness with pain in the hand, wrist, or distal forearm. Patients are often awakened with pain or numbness in the hand. Pain is thought to be due to ischemia rather than physical damage of the nerve.

Be careful! It is very easy to confuse or mistype the terms medial and median.

Physical examination shows a positive **Tinel sign** (tapping the volar wrist over the median nerve with resultant paresthesia) and positive **Phalen sign** (hyperflexion of the wrist for 60 seconds with resultant paresthesia). CTS shows increased **2-point discrimination** (greater than 5–6 mm) in the tips of the fingers. Longstanding CTS may result in thenar muscle atrophy. **Electromyelography (EMG)** and **nerve conduction velocity (NCV)** studies may be performed to rule out proximal injury to the median nerve or to identify a peripheral neuropathy. Conservative treatment includes the use of a **cock-up wrist splint** to hold the wrist level and NSAIDs to reduce pain and inflammation. Diuretics and cortisone injections may also be useful. Surgical treatment in the form of a **carpal tunnel**

release (CTR) is indicated if EMG studies show increased **distal median nerve latency**. CTR involves an incision of the transverse carpal ligament through a longitudinal incision on the distal border of the transverse carpal tunnel ligament to the proximal wrist crease. Painful surgical scars may reduce the success of CTR. A few patients experience **flexion tendon bowstringing**.

Pause 5-11 Explain the phrase "distal median nerve latency" in layman's terms.

Disorders of the Bones

In addition to fractures and dislocations, bones may also become infected, necrotic, or weak due to metabolic changes or nutritional deficiencies.

Osteomyelitis

Osteomyelitis is a microbial infection of bone tissue. Causative agents may be bacteria, mycobacteria, or fungi. Organisms reach the bone by one of several routes: hematogenous, contiguous, or direct inoculation. Hematogenous spread is caused by seeding of the bone by bloodborne organisms that originate from a remote source. This condition is primarily seen in children. The highly vascular metaphysis of growing bones predisposes children to osteomyelitis, especially by staphylococcal bacteria.

Osteomyelitis may also be caused by contiguous spread from an overlying wound, decubitus ulcer, or an infected prosthetic joint. Direct inoculation of bone may occur with an open bone fracture, direct trauma, or contamination during surgery. Infections from direct inoculation, especially in cases of trauma, are often polymicrobial (ie, involving two or more organisms) and acute, displaying more localized symptoms. Depending on the infecting organism, the infection may cause a pyogenic or granulomatous reaction.

The most common causative agents include enteric gram-negative bacteria, Staphylococcus aureus, Pseudomonas aeruginosa, Serratia species, and Salmonella species. Candidal osteomyelitis (ie, infection with Candida species) most commonly occurs in debilitated or immunocompromised patients. Chronic infections persist or recur, regardless of their initial cause and in spite of aggressive treatment, and often create sequestra with multiple cavities that require curettage and occasionally bone grafting. Staphylococcus aureus is commonly implicated in chronic infections.

Peripheral vascular disease (vascular insufficiency) is often a predisposing factor for osteomyelitis because the decreased vascular flow results in impaired immune defenses. Patients with diabetes mellitus are also at higher risk of osteomyelitis.

> **Pause 5-12** Describe how diabetes mellitus puts patients at increased risk for osteomyelitis and possible amputation.

Patients present with pain, swelling, erythema, tenderness, fluctuance, and warmth over the affected area with decreased range of motion. Fever may or may not be present. The patient may mention recent weight loss and fatigue. Osteomyelitis affecting the vertebra may have an insidious onset and cause localized back pain and tenderness with **paravertebral muscle spasm**. Chronic osteomyelitis causes intermittent bone pain, tenderness, and **draining sinuses** that may recur over months or years.

> Fluctuation and fluctuance are synonymous. Fluctuants is not a word. The adjectival form is fluctuant.

Patients suspected of osteomyelitis undergo laboratory studies and diagnostic imaging tests. Blood tests include a CBC, blood cultures, ESR (erythrocyte sedimentation rate), and C-reactive protein. X-rays taken early in the infection show overlying soft-tissue edema. Between 14 and 21 days postinfection, **periosteal elevation** may be noted on x-ray followed by **cortical lucency** or **medullary lucency**. Bone destruction must be greater than 40% to 50% to cause detectable lucency on plain films. MRI, CT, and radioisotope bone scan using technetium 99m are also useful.

For optimal treatment, a biopsy with C&S should be performed to identify the causative agent and select the appropriate antibiotic therapy. Antibiotics are administered by IV for four to eight weeks. It may also be necessary to open the periosteum, drill the cortex, and débride any devascularized bone. Surgery may also be needed to drain concomitant paravertebral or epidural abscesses or to stabilize the spine to prevent injury.

Osteoporosis

Osteoporosis is a metabolic bone disease characterized by loss of bone density with subsequent breakdown in bone architecture and greatly increased risk of fracture. Osteoporosis increases the likelihood of fractures resulting from falls at standing height, especially in the wrist and hip. It is a significant cause of morbidity and mortality in the elderly, who are at increased risk of falls due to instability, weakness, or the side effects of medications. Hip fractures, while not primarily life-threatening, cause secondary mortality in the elderly population due to cardiopulmonary complications from being bedridden during recovery.

Normally bone formation and resorption are closely coupled. Slow but progressive bone loss results from an abnormal bone-remodeling cycle. Osteoblasts are responsible for laying down the organic matrix of bone that is subsequently mineralized. Mineralization with calcium, phosphorus, magnesium and other trace minerals strengthen the bone matrix. Osteoclasts, on the other hand, are responsible for resorbing bone. This destructive-creative dance is orchestrated by hormones (estrogen, calcitonin, and parathyroid hormone) and vitamin D and further affected by weightbearing exercise and good nutrition. Osteoporotic bone loss affects both cortical and cancellous bone, so the effects of osteoporosis typically appear in the appendicular skeleton first due to the predominance of cancellous tissue in long, tubular bones.

Although osteoporosis affects all bones, fractures of the wrist, thoracic and lumbar vertebrae, and proximal femur are the most common. Loss of bone mass in the vertebral bodies causes multiple compression fractures and loss of stature. In the thoracic spine, these compression fractures cause exaggerated cervical lordosis (**dowager's hump**). In the lumbar spine, osteoporosis is evidenced by progressive **flattening of the lordotic curve**. Abnormal stress of the spinal muscles and ligaments causes muscle spasm with chronic, dull, aching pain.

The majority of osteoporosis occurs in postmenopausal women due to declining estrogen. Postmenopausal osteoporosis may be classified as type I or type II. Type I shows an excess loss of cancellous bone with relative sparing of cortical bone, resulting in a predominance of wrist and vertebral fractures. Type II shows loss of both cortical and cancellous bone and an increased incidence of hip fractures. **Senile osteoporosis** occurs in individuals over 75 years of age and is primarily caused by poor calcium absorption. Other causes of osteoporosis include decreased calcium intake, malabsorption syndromes, low vitamin D levels, and secondary hyperparathyroidism.

Signs and symptoms of osteoporosis include pain with weightbearing, decreased stature, increased kyphosis, loss of lumbar lordosis, and chronic back pain. Examination reveals **paraspinal muscle spasm** with tenderness on palpation over the paraspinal area.

Bones begin to show **decreased radiodensity** after about 30% of the bone mass is lost. X-ray examination of vertebral bodies shows a striated appearance due to loss of trabecular bone. The cortices may be accentuated, creating a "picture-framing" appearance. Vertebral bodies with compression fractures show reduced vertebral body height and increased biconcavity.

The most useful diagnostic tool for osteoporosis is a **dual-energy x-ray absorptiometry (DEXA) scan**. This test measures bone density in the lumbar spine, hip, distal radius, and ulna. DEXA scans can be used to diagnose osteoporosis, assess risk of fracture, and monitor efficacy of treatment.

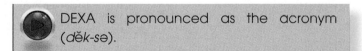

DEXA is pronounced as the acronym (dĕk-sə).

Treatment of osteoporosis includes **risk factor modification**, nutritional supplementation, and treatment with antiresorptive drugs. The goals of treatment are to maintain function, increase bone mass, reduce the risk of fracture, and decrease pain. To decrease risk factors, patients are advised to maintain proper body weight, increase weightbearing exercise, minimize caffeine and alcohol intake, and stop smoking. Strengthening exercises to increase stability and muscle coordination are also important to attenuate the risk of falls. Nutritional supplementation includes 1 to 1.5 g daily of calcium and 800–2000 units daily of vitamin D (prescription brand Drisdol). Antiresorptive medications such as the **bisphosphonates** are also given. Hip pads may be used to prevent hip fractures. **Vertebroplasty** or **kyphoplasty** may be used to relieve severe back pain. Vertebroplasty involves the injection of **methyl methacrylate** into the vertebral body. Kyphoplasty expands the vertebral body with a balloon.

Osteonecrosis

Osteonecrosis, also known as **avascular necrosis (AVN)**, is the death of cancellous bone tissue due to an interruption of the bone's blood supply and ensuing lack of oxygen. The lack of nutrients causes the bone to collapse, resulting in pain and loss of function. AVN typically affects the epiphysis of long bones, with the most common site of occurrence being the femoral head. Most often, both hips are involved. Other common sites include the scaphoid, mandible, talus, and humeral head. The process begins with an interruption of the blood supply, resulting in subchondral necrosis, subchondral fracture, and eventual collapse of the bone. New bone added atop the necrotic bone results in thick scar tissue (sclerosis) and abnormal bone remodeling, leading to even poorer vascularization. The articular surface becomes deformed, leading to osteoarthritis. In the later stages, the joint may be totally destroyed. Nonunion of fractures may occur due to lack of nutrients and substrates to repair the break. Secondary muscle atrophy results from lack of use.

The inciting event may be traumatic or atraumatic. The most common causes of traumatic osteonecrosis include femoral neck fractures, dislocation of the femoral head, displaced fractures of the scaphoid and talar neck, and four-part fractures of the humeral head. Bones with a single terminal blood supply and limited collateral blood supply are at higher risk of osteonecrosis. Atraumatic osteonecrosis is thought to be secondary to occlusion of the arterial wall or occlusion of the venous outflow vessels. Risk factors for osteonecrosis include trauma, corticosteroid use, ethanol use, sickle cell disease and other hemoglobinopathies, excessive radiation, and Gaucher disease. (18) Osteonecrosis is also associated with dysbarism, also known as caisson disease or the bends, in deep-sea divers. Patients with allogeneic organ transplants receiving lifelong immune suppressants are also at risk. **Table 5-5** lists the eponyms associated with osteonecrosis.

(18) Gaucher disease is pronounced gō-shā'.

Table 5-5 Eponyms Associated with Osteonecrosis

Eponym	Involved bone
Legg-Calve-Perthes	femoral head (in children)
Sever disease	calcaneus
Kohler disease	tarsal navicular
Freiberg infarction	second metatarsal head
Panner disease	capitellum
Kienböck disease	lunate

Patients typically present with pain of insidious onset as their primary complaint. The pain is exacerbated by weightbearing and is slowly progressive with a gradual loss of joint function.

An MRI and bone scan are used to diagnose osteonecrosis. Early in the disease process, MRI findings include decreased signal intensity (**water signal**) in the subchondral region on both T1- and T2-weighted images, suggesting edema of the surrounding tissue. In the middle stage of the disease, characterized by a reparative process, MRI shows a **low signal intensity** on T1-weighted scans and **high signal intensity** on T2-weighted scans.

Radionuclide bone scans are most helpful in the early stages of the disease. Early on, as the bone attempts to repair itself, osteoblastic activity and blood flow are increased, and these processes are highly visible on nuclear bone scans. The **doughnut sign**, which describes a central area of decreased nuclide uptake surrounded by a reactive zone of increased uptake, is pathognomonic for AVN. X-rays may be helpful in the later stages of the disease once bone deformities have occurred. A radiolucent line, called a **crescent sign**, can be seen on plain films. Osteonecrosis of the hip is divided into five stages: 0 through IV.

Even with early detection, it may be difficult to change the course of the disease. In the early stages, treatment involves limited weightbearing and pain control. Core decompression may be attempted by drilling a 4–10 mm tract through the area of necrosis. If the disease progresses, total joint replacement is performed on the hip, knee, and shoulder, and fusions are performed on the ankle and wrist.

X-RAYS: AP, pelvis, and frog-leg lateral of the left hip show avascular necrosis with early collapse of the femoral head.

FINDINGS: MRI study shows notable edema in the left femoral head, concerning for osteonecrosis. There is a linear component at the superior aspect of the femoral head, concerning for developing fracture. No significant flattening of the femoral head is currently seen. The edema extends into the femoral neck, but no definite cortical defect is seen in the femoral neck. There is osteoarthritis of the left hip with superior to central migration of the femoral head. There is no significant edema in the acetabulum, but mild sclerosis is noted. There is likely degenerative tearing of the labrum. No significant hip joint effusion. The visualized pubic symphysis appears intact. There is focal T2, high signal in the superior pubic ramus centrally on the left, which may be artifactual as there is no corresponding abnormality seen on the T1 exam. I would not totally exclude the possibility of a developing stress reaction, however. The muscles and soft tissues about the left hip are unremarkable for the technique.

Pause 5-13 Look up the term artifact/artifactual. How would you distinguish this term from artificial?

Deep Venous Thrombosis

Deep venous thrombosis (DVT) is a potentially life-threatening clot in the deep veins of the calf, thigh, or pelvis (■ Figure 5-14). The superficial femoral and popliteal veins in the thighs and the posterior tibial veins in the calves are most commonly affected. Thrombi are known to form following a fracture of the hip, pelvis, or leg. DVT may also occur following orthopedic procedures, illnesses causing prolonged immobility, congestive heart failure (CHF), myocardial infarction (MI), or stroke. Patients with cancer, obesity, and hypercoagulable states are also at increased risk of DVT. Estrogen use is associated with an increased incidence of thrombus formation in the deep veins.

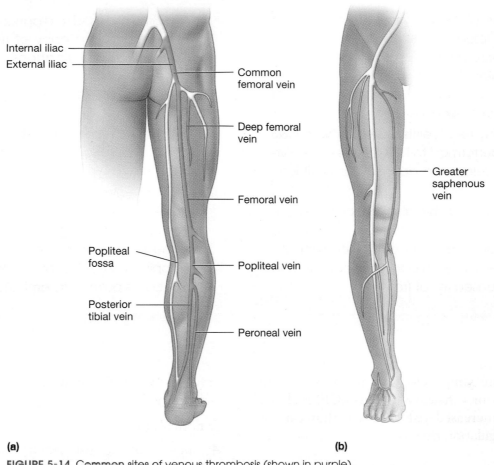

(a)   **(b)**

FIGURE 5-14 Common sites of venous thrombosis (shown in purple).

The clot typically forms in the valve cusps and consists of thrombin, fibrin, and RBCs but relatively few platelets. DVT becomes life-threatening if part of the thrombus breaks away and passes through the circulatory system to the lung (see also pulmonary embolus on page 253). Thrombi located below the popliteal fossa are not known to embolize, but half of all clots that form at or above the popliteal fossa will embolize. Clots typically propagate proximally. In addition to pulmonary embolus, complications of DVT include **chronic venous insufficiency** and **postphlebitic syndrome**.

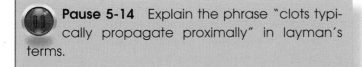

Pause 5-14 Explain the phrase "clots typically propagate proximally" in layman's terms.

Symptoms include pain and swelling of the leg and possibly phlebitis. Physical examination may show calf pain with increased pain with dorsiflexion of the foot while the knee is extended (**Homans sign**). Swelling of the dorsum of the foot and pitting edema may also be present. Leg circumference may be compared to the contralateral leg, with an increase of greater than 3 cm suspicious for DVT. Collateral superficial veins may also be seen. DVT can be diagnosed using venous ultrasound, **contrast venography**, or **impedance plethysmography**, which detects changes in electrical impedance between patent and obstructed veins. D-dimer may also be positive (see page 431).

Patients with known DVT are initially given injectable heparin (**unfractionated heparin** or **low-molecular-weight heparin**) followed by Coumadin (warfarin). Patients undergoing major orthopedic procedures are given prophylactic anticoagulants. Graduated compression devices such as **intermittent pneumatic compression (IPC)** sleeves, also called **sequential compression devices (SCDs)**, are used in the postoperative period to maintain blood flow in the lower extremities and to reduce venous stasis. This discourages clot formation by preventing the blood from pooling in the legs while lying in bed. Bedbound patients may also use compression devices, or they may be given **graduated compression stockings**, also called **TED hose**, that apply

- Osteomyelitis is a microbial infection of bone tissue caused by bacteria, mycobacteria, or fungi. Patients with peripheral vascular disease, peripheral paresthesias, and impaired wound healing are at increased risk of osteomyelitis.

- In cases of osteomyelitis, a biopsy with C&S should be performed to identify the causative agent and select the appropriate antibiotic therapy.

- Osteoporosis is a metabolic bone disease characterized by loss of bone density due to an abnormal bone-remodeling cycle with subsequent breakdown in bone architecture and greatly increased risk of fracture.

- DEXA scans are used to diagnose osteoporosis and monitor the efficacy of treatment with antiresorptive medications such as the bisphosphonates.

- Osteonecrosis, also known as avascular necrosis (AVN), is the death of cancellous bone tissue due to an interruption of the bone's blood supply. Osteonecrosis is associated with trauma and corticosteroid use.

- DVT is characterized by the formation of a clot in the deep veins of the lower extremities, causing pain and swelling. Patients undergoing orthopedic surgery are at increased risk of developing DVT. A life-threatening complication of DVT is pulmonary embolus.

progressively more compression running proximally to distally. An **inferior vena cava filter (IVCF)** is placed in patients at increased risk of DVT that cannot undergo anticoagulation therapy.

PLAN: Deep venous thrombosis prophylaxis with SCDs and TEDs.

Diagnostic and Therapeutic Procedures

The field of orthopedics relies heavily on diagnostic imaging studies and the physical examination, including hands-on tests, signs, and maneuvers. The laboratory plays a much smaller role in this medical specialty. The following sections summarize the most common signs, tests, and maneuvers used during the physical assessment as well as the basis of the imaging techniques employed by the orthopedist.

Muscle Strength Grading

Assessing muscle strength is an important part of an orthopedic examination. Normal strength is reported as 5/5 (dictated "five over five") based on a five-point scale. Decreases in strength are reported as 4/5 (four

over five), 3/5, etc. The following scale is used to report muscle strength:

5: normal strength

4: movement against gravity, weakness with resistance

3: marked weakness against resistance

2: some muscle or tendon movement when gravity is eliminated

1: only flicker of tendon movement

0: no movement

Signs, Tests, and Maneuvers

In the orthopedic setting, physical examinations are replete with signs, tests, and maneuvers to assess muscles, muscle groups, muscle strength, joints, tendons, sensation, and reflexes. The words "tests" and "signs" may be used interchangeably by the dictator (eg, McMurray test or McMurray sign). Technically, an orthopedic "test" is a procedure performed to elicit a "sign." Some signs are simply observations noted by the examiner as the patient moves about the room. Terminology in this area of orthopedics can be quite confusing and inconsistent, as eponyms vary by region and institution, and some tests are used in more than one anatomical area. **Table 5-6** lists some of the most common tests and signs used in an orthopedic physical examination.

Table 5-6 Common Orthopedic Tests and Signs

Area	Name	Comment
general	two-point discrimination	decreased sensation
	Semmes-Weinstein monofilament test	decreased sensation
knee	range of motion	normal range of motion: 3–5 degrees of hyperextension to 135 degrees of flexion
	blot test	knee effusion
	milk test and milk test II	knee effusion
	Q angle	patellar dislocation
	medial and lateral glide	medial and lateral restraints
	tilt test	lateral retinaculum
	apprehension test	patellar subluxation
	grind test	patellofemoral disease
	Lachman test	ACL injury
	anterior and posterior drawer test	ligamentous instability
	grasshopper patella patella alta patella baja	patellar position
	sag sign	PCL injury
	pivot-shift	ACL injury
	Steinman test	meniscal injury
	Apley test	ligamentous vs meniscal injuries
	McMurray	meniscal tears
	terminal J sign	patellar tracking
	varus and valgus stability	ligament stability
ankle	anterior drawer sign drawer sign	ligament injury
	Thompson test	Achilles tendon injury

Table 5-6 Common Orthopedic Tests and Signs (*Continued*)

Area	Name	Comment
hand and wrist	normal wrist range of motion	flexion: 70–80 degrees extension: 70–80 degrees radial deviation: up to approximately 20 degrees ulnar deviation: up to approximately 30 degrees supination: to 90 degrees pronation: 90 degrees
	Allen test	occlusion of radial or ulnar artery
	Tinel sign	carpal tunnel syndrome
	Phalen test	carpal tunnel syndrome
	Finkelstein test	De Quervain
hip	internal and external rotation	internal rotation 15–45 degrees external rotation 40–65 degrees abduction 35–70 degrees
	Trendelenburg sign	hip muscle weakness
	Trendelenburg test	abductor weakness
	Thomas test	hip joint flexion contracture
	Allis test	femoral neck fracture
shoulder	load and shift test	shoulder instability
	anterior apprehension sign apprehension test	shoulder subluxation or dislocation
	Fowler test	anterior shoulder instability
	Hawkins impingement test Neer impingement test	rotator cuff disorders
	drop-arm test	rotator cuff tear
	sulcus sign	shoulder instability

Imaging

Orthopedists make extensive use of imaging technology, including x-rays, MRI, and nuclear imaging techniques.

X-Rays

X-ray studies of the skeletal system can demonstrate bone density, pathologic changes (eg, necrosis, tumors, and infection), spurs, joint-space narrowing, synovial inflammation, nerve impingements, and soft-tissue changes. In the emergency setting, physicians may request a **wet reading**, which is an immediate report of the x-ray results. Most radiology departments have converted to digital technology and no longer use film as the imaging media, so this term is a throwback to a time when x-ray film was developed and read immediately (before the film had an opportunity to dry completely).

The orthopedist often orders specific views of a bone or joint based on their clinical suspicions. Standard x-ray views include anteroposterior (AP), lateral, and oblique. In addition, the following views may be ordered:

- any area: coned-down (note the word is coned, not cone)
- ankle: mortise
- knee: lateral and intercondylar notch views, tunnel, sunset, Merchant, Hughston (note unusual spelling of Hughston)
- shoulder: internal rotation, AP external rotation, axillary lateral, scapular Y view, supraspinatus outlet view
- hip: frog leg, crosstable lateral, push-pull
- wrist: AP with ulnar and radial deviation, carpal tunnel
- hand: clenched fist
- heel: plantar dorsal, axial

Plain films are often sufficient for diagnosing orthopedic pathology, but more complicated or occult fractures may require the two-dimensional, cross-section views provided by CT scans. CT combined with arthrography is also useful for assessing joint anatomy.

The most common **measurement** of bone density is the dual energy x-ray absorptiometry (DEXA) scan. This scan is used to both diagnose osteoporosis and to assess the risk of fracture. Sites measured include the lumbar spine, hip, distal radius, and ulna. DEXA results are reported as **T scores** and **Z scores**. A T score represents the number of standard deviations (the amount of difference) by which the person's bone density varies from a *young, healthy person of the same sex and race at peak density*. The Z score is the number of standard deviations by which the person's bone density varies from an *age-matched cohort.* (19) Osteopenia is defined as a T score of greater than 1, and osteoporosis is defined as a T score of greater than 2.5. This same technology can be used to assess vertebral deformities that may increase the risk of fracture. An assessment of the vertebra in the lower thoracic and lumbar spine is called a **vertebral fracture analysis**.

MRI

MRI technology is capable of producing highly detailed, two- and three-dimensional images of joints and surrounding tissue. MRI is best suited for studies of connective and soft tissues (ie, tissues with high hydrogen ion concentrations). In orthopedics, MRIs are used to

TECHNIQUE: Scans were performed through the lumbar spine, hip, and wrist with the Hologic Discovery C DEXA bone densitometer. Vertebral assessment was performed through the thoracic and lumbar spine in the AP and lateral projections.

FINDINGS

Lumbar Spine: Analysis of the vertebral bodies L1 through L4 demonstrates a composite bone mineral density of 0.955 g/cm^2, T score –0.8, Z score 1.1. Analysis of individual vertebral bodies demonstrates the lowest density at L3 at 0.934 g/cm^2, T score –1.4, Z score 0.7, corresponding to a WHO classification of osteopenia; at increased risk for fracture.

Left Hip: Analysis of the femoral neck demonstrates bone mineral density of 0.757 g/cm^2, T score –0.8, Z score 0.9, corresponding to a WHO classification of normal density.

Wrist: Analysis of the distal radius and ulna demonstrates bone mineral density of 0.613 g/cm^2, T score –1.2, Z score 0.6, corresponding to a WHO classification of osteopenia; at increased risk for fracture.

Note that when transcribing the densities of several contiguous vertebral bodies, the word "through" should be used, not a hyphen (eg, L1 through L4, not L1–L4).

assess muscles, tendons, ligaments, cartilage, menisci, masses, infection, avascular necrosis, and fractures that are not otherwise detected on x-ray. Adding the contrast agent gadolinium is useful in joint studies.

Magnetic resonance uses magnetic energy instead of radioactive energy to create images. It is most helpful in discriminating adjacent tissue densities. The patient is placed within a very strong, static magnetic field. In the excitation phase, a second magnetic field is applied at a right angle to the first, causing hydrogen ions (protons)

(19) A cohort is a group of people that share a common factor (eg, age or race). A cohort often describes a group of people from which statistical information is derived.

to change their orientation. As the second magnetic pulse is removed, the protons return to their original alignment, and in doing, so emit a detectable signal. The signal is directly proportional to the hydrogen ion concentration within the tissue. High signal density appears black and low signal density appears white on an MRI. Air or gas emits almost no signal. The time (denoted by the Greek letter tau) that it takes the protons to return to their original orientation is referred to as the **spin-lattice relaxation time** and is represented by T1. The very brief interval required for the protons to return to their previous state after the excitation phase is the **spin-spin relaxation time**, or T2. Excitation pulses and intervals can be manipulated to create T1-weighted images and T2-weighted images. **Table 5-7** lists terms commonly associated with MRI studies.

Table 5-7 Terms Associated with MRI Studies

Term	Description
T1-weighted image	Fluids with high water concentration (eg, urine and CSF) appear dark; blood, fat, and mucus appear bright.
T2-weighted image	Muscle and fat appear dark.
artifact	Images or features on an imaging study that are produced as part of the imaging process and not attributable to the patient's anatomy or pathology.
fat suppression	A technique that reduces the signal produced by hydrogen-containing lipids (mostly CH_2) compared to water-containing tissues; causes fat to appear black.
gating (gated)	A technique that synchronizes images with a phase of the cardiac or respiratory cycles; the synchronization may be prospective or retrospective.
functional magnetic resonance imaging (fMRI)	A technique that studies a biological function in addition to anatomy. For example, fMRI of the brain measures changes in blood flow and oxygen utilization.
short-T1 inversion-recovery (STIR)	A technique that suppresses the signal emitted by fat; helpful for elucidating fractures, especially occult hip fractures.
fluid-attenuated inversion-recovery (FLAIR)	A technique that suppresses the signal emitted by fluid; especially helpful for elucidating brain lesions.

In the context of an MRI technique, STIR and FLAIR are dictated as acronyms and are written in all uppercase.

Nuclear Medicine

A bone scan (also called bone scintigraphy) uses technetium 99 (Tc 99m) bound to the tracer **methylene diphosphonate (MDP)**. The radioisotope-tracer molecules are given by IV. The tracer binds preferentially to bone tissue, more so in areas of bone that are undergoing metabolic activity. Gamma cameras detect areas of radioisotope activity, creating images of the skeletal system. Areas of increased metabolic activity within the bone appear as **hot spots** on the images, indicating areas of fracture, infection, or tumor. Other nuclear bone studies include a **3-phase bone scan** (also called a **triphasic bone scan**) as well as studies that use the radioisotopes gallium 67 or indium 111. The amount of radioisotope administered is measured in **millicuries (mCi)**.

TECHNIQUE: The study was performed as a triphasic scan sequence following 25.0 mCi technetium 99m MDP administered intravenously. Flow and blood pool images of the feet were obtained. Delayed images were also acquired 2–4 hours later.

FINDINGS: The flow and blood pool images demonstrate hyperperfusion into the left lower extremity and hyperemia with uptake in the left second toe and first metatarsal. Delayed images demonstrate focal uptake identified in the distal phalanx of the left second toe and first metatarsal.

IMPRESSION
1. Hyperperfusion and hyperemia localizing to the left lower extremity with uptake identified in the distal phalanx of the left second toe and first metatarsal. The findings are consistent with osteomyelitis of the distal phalanx of the left second toe.
2. Increased uptake in the left first metatarsal. This is a nonspecific finding. This may represent osteomyelitis, degenerative changes, or fracture. Recommend clinical correlation.

When osteomyelitis is suspected, the scan may be performed by attaching Tc 99m to a monoclonal antibody specific for neutrophils. The antibodies attach to white cells that are concentrated in areas of infected bone.

A common phrase use by radiologists is **recommend clinical correlation**. This means the radiologist does not have enough information to make a decision about the significance of a finding and that the information should be interpreted in light of the patient's physical findings and complaints.

Laboratory Studies

Laboratory studies play a lesser role in orthopedics compared to some other medical specialties. Joint fluid analysis, enzymes, and metabolic byproducts are the main laboratory studies used by orthopedic surgeons.

Synovial Fluid Analysis

Synovial fluid obtained through arthrocentesis can be examined in the laboratory to determine the cause of joint pain and swelling. Results of the fluid analysis (**Table 5-8**) help differentiate inflammatory, noninflammatory, and infectious causes. An infected joint may have a white blood count (WBC) of 20,000 or higher with greater than 95% of the cells being PMNs.

Table 5-8 Normal and Abnormal Synovial Fluid Results

Test	Normal Results	Abnormal Results
clarity	clear	turbid, bloody
color	yellow	greenish, milky, red, or brown
viscosity	high	reduced, low
mucin clot	firm	friable
WBC	0–200/mcL	>200/mcL
polys (PMNs)	<25%	>25%
glucose difference (compared to serum)	0–10%	>10%
crystals	absent	present

Gram stain with aerobic and anaerobic cultures and antibiotic sensitivity (C&S) are performed when infection is suspected.

Crystal-induced arthritis is diagnosed by examining the fluid under a polariscopic microscope for the presence of **birefringent** or **negatively birefringent crystals**. The types of crystals found in synovial fluid include monosodium urate, **calcium pyrophosphate**, **calcium oxalate**, and **calcium phosphate**. Bloody joint fluid with white and red cell counts similar to peripheral blood may indicate **hemarthrosis** due to bleeding directly into the joint.

Viscosity is an important measure of synovial fluid's ability to lubricate and protect the joint. Low viscosity causes increased friction within the joint with resultant wear and degeneration. Viscosity is evaluated by visual examination and the mucin clot test.

Serum Studies

Serum studies related to orthopedics include enzymes, metabolic end products associated with muscle or bone destruction, and metabolic products that accumulate in the joints. **Table 5-9** outlines blood tests associated with orthopedic disorders.

Therapeutic Procedures

Orthopedists use a variety of procedures that range from simple, in-office procedures to extensive surgery. The following highlights the most common procedures performed for diagnostic and therapeutic purposes:

- arthrocentesis: the aspiration of synovial joint fluid for analysis.
- arthroscopy: visualization of internal structures of a joint by inserting fiberoptic devices (arthroscope) directly into the joint. Arthroscopic procedures can be diagnostic and therapeutic. Arthroscopic instruments can be used to remove synovium (synovectomy), remove **plica** (folds), repair tears, remove loose bodies, and shave cartilage.
- arthrodesis: the fusion of a joint by removing cartilage or placing bone graft materials (autografts, allografts, or synthetic graft materials). Arthrodeses may be categorized as compression, extraarticular, or intraarticular.

Arthroplasty

Arthroplasty refers to the surgical replacement of part (**hemiarthroplasty**) or all of a joint (**total joint arthroplasty**). The most common joints to undergo replacement are the hip, knee, and shoulder.

Table 5-9 Serum Blood Tests used in Orthopedics

Test Name	Description	Indication	Reference Range
alkaline phosphatase (alk phos)	found in various tissues, but 80% of serum alkaline phosphatase is derived from the liver and bone	osteoblastic bone disease, Paget disease, osteomalacia, hyperparathyroidism, osteogenic sarcoma, bone metastases	40–125 units/L
creatine kinase (CK)	CK consists of two subunits CK-B (brain type), CK-M (muscle type) which combine to form three specific isoenzymes: CK-MB, CK-BB and CK-MM	increased CK indicative of skeletal muscle damage (muscular dystrophy, trauma, rhabdomyolysis); increased levels of CK-MB is indicative of cardiac muscle damage	30–225 units/mL (CK-MB 0–5 ng/mL)
creatine phosphokinase (CPK)	synonym for creatine kinase (*not* creatinine)		
Ntx (N telopeptide)	increased with bone destruction such as osteoporosis	used to monitor antiresorptive therapy for osteoporosis; Ntx levels should decrease from baseline 3 months after initiating therapy	male: 21–66 nmol bone collagen equivalents/mmol creatinine female: 19–63 nmol bone collagen equivalents/mmol creatinine
uric acid	end product of purine metabolism	gout	2.5 to 7.8 mg/dL

Hemiarthroplasty of the hip involves replacement of the femoral head and neck. A **total hip replacement (THR)** involves the acetabulum as well as the femoral head and neck (■ **Figure 5-15**). Replacements may be described as **cemented** or **cementless**, referring to the use of a cement material to help set the joint into place.

The knee is divided into three sections: the medial, lateral, and patellofemoral compartments. Partial knee replacements involve replacing one or two compartments of the knee instead of all three. Replacement of a single compartment is a **unicompartmental** or **unicondylar knee replacement** (sometimes referred to as a "uni"). Replacing components of all three compartments is a **total knee arthroplasty (TKA)** (■ **Figure 5-16**).

Immobilization

Immobilization prevents movement of a joint or holds a bone in position during healing. Immobilization is accomplished using hardware, splints, casts, and braces.

Fixation devices used in orthopedics include:

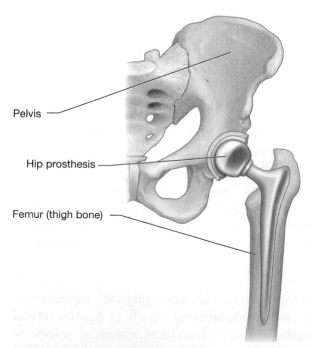

Pelvis

Hip prosthesis

Femur (thigh bone)

- K-wire (available in various diameters measured in thousandths of an inch, written 0.045, but often dictated as "four five K-wire"), cerclage wire
- nail plate
- condylar screw plate
- dynamic compression plate

FIGURE 5-15 Total hip replacement.

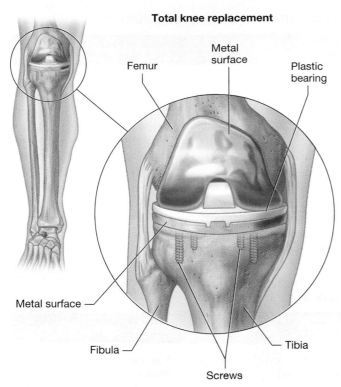

Total knee replacement

Femur

Metal surface

Plastic bearing

Metal surface

Fibula

Tibia

Screws

FIGURE 5-16 Total knee replacement.

- external fixator
- Ilizarov fixator
- monolateral fixator
- intramedullary rods
- reamed intramedullary nail
- cephalomedullary (gamma type) nail
- dynamic hip compression screw
- cortex or cortical screw
- cancellous bone screw
- interfragmentary screw
- Steinmann pin (eg, 3/32-inch Steinmann pin, dictated "three thirty two Steinmann")

Splints and casts (■ **Figure 5-17**) include:

- counterforce brace
- cock-up wrist splint
- Thomas splint: a traction splint used for hip and thigh fractures
- ulnar or radial gutter: a U-shaped splint (similar to the shape of a gutter) applied to either the ulnar or radial side of the forearm
- sugar tong splint: a common splint used for upper extremity fractures, often covered with a plaster cast

- wraparound: splints that can be wrapped around a limb but are easily removed for physical therapy or wound care
- spica (splint or cast): immobilizes an appendage by incorporating a part of the body proximal to that appendage. The most common are hip, thumb, and shoulder spicas.
- long arm cast: extends from palm and wrist to the axilla
- short arm cast: extends from wrist to elbow
- long leg cast: nonweightbearing cast, extends from upper thigh to toes
- long leg walking cast: extends from upper thigh to toes with rubber sole device called a walker
- short leg cast: extends just below knees to toes
- short leg walking cast: with rubber walker or reinforcement to accept cast shoe
- cast-boot: a strap-on boot that serves as a short leg cast

Dressings and Bandages

Orthopedics uses an array of dressings and bandages, most of which go by brand names with unusual spellings:

- Adaptic: nonadhesive mesh dressing
- Kerlix: broad, elastic gauze dressing
- Kling: narrow, elastic gauze dressing used for compression
- wet-to-dry: bandage soaked in saline and applied wet then allowed to dry
- Xeroform: fine mesh, nonadherent dressing impregnated with petrolatum
- Ace bandage: the brand name of a stretchable, elastic bandage used as a compression bandage
- Esmarch bandage: a tourniquet to exsanguinate a limb prior to and during surgery
- high Dye taping: a method of taping the ankle following an inversion injury (named for Dr. Ralph Dye)
- low Dye dressing: taping technique for plantar fasciitis

Pharmacology

The majority of medications used in the field of orthopedics are for treatment of pain and inflammation. Treatments for osteoporosis and gout, on the other hand, address the underlying disease.

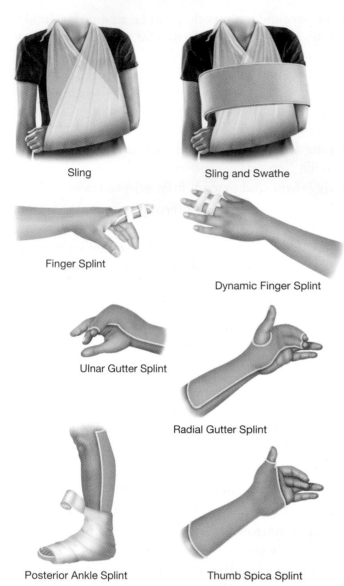

Sling

Sling and Swathe

Finger Splint

Dynamic Finger Splint

Ulnar Gutter Splint

Radial Gutter Splint

Posterior Ankle Splint

Thumb Spica Splint

FIGURE 5-17 Examples of splints and casts.

Corticosteroids

Corticosteroids have tremendous antiinflammatory action and are given both orally and by injection. Steroids may be injected directly into the affected joint (intraarticular injection). **Table 5-10** lists injectable corticosteroids used in orthopedics.

Hyaluronan

The synovial membrane of a joint secretes hyaluronic acid that helps to maintain the lubricating quality of the synovial fluid. Hyaluronan (**Table 5-11**), a derivative of hyaluronic acid, is injected into the joints of patients with OA to improve the viscosity and lubricating quality of the synovial fluid.

Table 5-10 Injectable Corticosteroids

Generic	Brand Name
hydrocortisone	Solu-Cortef
betamethasone	Celestone Celestone Soluspan
triamcinolone	Kenalog Aristospan
methylprednisolone	Depo-Medrol
dexamethasone	Decadron

Table 5-11 Hyaluronan

Generic	Brand Name
hyaluronic acid (hyaluronan, hyaluronate)	Euflexxa Hyalgan
	Orthovisc
	Supartz
	Synvisc

Muscle Relaxants

Muscle relaxants (**Table 5-12**) may be combined with analgesics and NSAIDs to treat strains and sprains and other musculoskeletal disorders that cause muscle spasm. Muscle relaxants do not actually relieve pain or inflammation, so they are typically prescribed along with other medications.

Table 5-12 Muscle Relaxants

Generic	Brand Name	Dose
carisoprodol and aspirin	Soma Compound	200/325 mg
cyclobenzaprine	Flexeril	5 mg, 10 mg
metaxalone	Skelaxin	800 mg
methocarbamol	Robaxin	500 mg, 750 mg
tizanidine	Zanaflex	2 mg, 4 mg, 6 mg

Pain Relievers

Pain relievers used in orthopedics include several classes of medication that relieve mild to severe pain as well as decrease pain by reducing inflammation. Classes include narcotic and nonnarcotic pain relievers and antiinflammatory medications including salicylates and nonsteroidal antiinflammatory drugs.

Nonnarcotic Pain Relievers

The most common nonnarcotic, nonaspirin analgesic is acetaminophen, known most commonly as Tylenol. Acetaminophen does not have antiinflammatory properties like NSAIDs. It is the drug of choice for OA in elderly patients because of its low side-effect profile. The chemical name for acetaminophen is n-acetyl-p-aminophenol, abbreviated **APAP** (dictated as the acronym, pronounced $\bar{a}$-$p\breve{a}p$). Many pain relievers are combined with acetaminophen for its synergistic effects, (**Table 5-13**) and when combined with other drugs, the abbreviation APAP is often used in the generic name. Brand names of drugs that are combined with acetaminophen often carry the suffix –*cet*.

Table 5-13 Nonnarcotic Pain Relievers with Acetaminophen

Generic	Brand Name	Dose
acetaminophen	Tylenol Extra Strength Tylenol	325 mg 500 mg
tramadol	Ultram Ultram ER	50 mg 100 mg, 200 mg, 300 mg
tramadol APAP	Ultracet	37.5/325 mg

Narcotics

Narcotics (**Table 5-14**) are used to treat moderate to severe pain. Narcotics bind to opiate receptors in the brain and block pain signals in the brain, not at the source of the pain. Narcotics also tend to give patients a sense of euphoria and many are highly sought after as **drugs of abuse**. Narcotic medications are potentially addictive and are classified as scheduled drugs, also called controlled substances. Many narcotics are combined with nonnarcotic drugs to decrease the amount of narcotic medication required and to address the pain at both the source and at the pain receptors in the brain.

Table 5-14 Narcotic Pain Relievers

Generic	Brand Name	Dose
hydrocodone APAP	Vicodin Vicodin ES Vicodin HP	5/500 mg 7.5/750 mg 10/660 mg
	Lorcet	10/650 mg
	Lortab	5/500 mg, 7.5/500, 7.5/500 mg, 10/500, 10/500 mg
	Norco	5/325 mg, 7.5/325 mg, 10/325 mg
hydrocodone ibuprofen	Vicoprofen	7.5/200 mg
hydromorphone	Dilaudid	2 mg, 4 mg, 8 mg
acetaminophen with codeine	Tylenol No. 3	300/30 mg
butalbital with APAP and caffeine	Fioricet Esgic	butalbital 50 mg, acetaminophen 325 mg, and caffeine 40 mg
oxycodone	OxyContin	10 mg, 15 mg, 20 mg, 30 mg, 40 mg, 60 mg, 80 mg, 160 mg

Nonsteroidal Antiinflammatory Drugs

The nonsteroidal antiinflammatory drugs (NSAIDs) are one of the most common classes of drugs used throughout medicine, but especially in the field of orthopedics. NSAIDs are used to treat mild to moderate pain, especially when pain is the result of inflammation such as bursitis, tendinitis, and arthritis. See also the discussion of NSAIDs on page 60. NSAIDs are structurally similarly to aspirin, and individuals allergic to aspirin should refrain from taking NSAIDs. Celebrex (celecoxib) is a member of a subgroup of NSAIDs that are selective COX-2 inhibitors (the coxibs) and are better tolerated by the GI tract. This medication is particularly helpful for arthritis because it has a safer profile for long-term use. Commonly used NSAIDs are listed in **Table 5-15**.

Drugs to Treat Gout

Drugs used in the treatment of gout (**Table 5-16**) either prevent the formation of uric acid or block the deposition of urate crystals in the joints. Urocit-K may be given to

Table 5-15 NSAIDs

Generic	Brand Name	Dose
indomethacin	Indocin	25 mg, 50 mg
meloxicam	Mobic	7.5 mg, 15 mg
piroxicam	Feldene	10 mg, 20 mg
naproxen	Naprosyn Anaprox Aleve	250 mg, 375 mg, 500 mg
ibuprofen	Advil Motrin	200 mg, 400 mg, 600 mg, 800 mg
celecoxib	Celebrex	50 mg, 100 mg, 200 mg, 400 mg
nabumetone	Relafen	500 mg, 750 mg
diclofenac	Cataflam	50 mg
	Voltaren Voltaren XR	75 mg 100 mg
etodolac	Lodine	200 mg, 300 mg, 400 mg, 500 mg, 600 mg

patients with gout to prevent the formation of uric acid stones in the urinary tract by increasing the urinary pH.

Table 5-16 Medications for Gout

Generic	Brand Name	Dose
colchicine	Colcrys	0.6 mg
allopurinol	Zyloprim	100 mg, 300 mg

Antiresorptive Drugs

Antiresorptive medications (**Table 5-17**) are used to prevent and reverse osteoporosis. Therapy for osteoporosis may include a bisphosphonate drug and/or hormone therapy. The bisphosphonates inhibit osteoclasts, therefore slowing the rate of bone resorption. Bisphosphonates are unusual in that they may be given orally on a daily, weekly, or monthly schedule or intravenously on a quarterly or yearly basis. When dictated, pay close attention to the dose and dose schedule to make sure they match. Also note the common suffix *adronate* used for bisphosphonates.

Table 5-17 Antiresorptive Medications

Generic	Brand Name	Dose
alendronate	Fosamax	5 mg, 10 mg, 35 mg, 40 mg, 70 mg (10 mg p.o. once a day or 70 mg p.o. once a week)
	Fosamax Plus D	70 mg alendronate with 2800 units cholecalciferol
ibandronate	Boniva	2.5 mg p.o. once a day or 150 mg once a month
pamidronate	Aredia	by injection only
risedronate	Actonel Actonel with calcium	35 mg per week risedronate 35 mg and calcium 1250 mg
zoledronate	Reclast	by injection only
	Zometa	by injection only

Estradiol inhibits the action of osteoclasts that break down bone. Menopause causes the rate of bone resorption to accelerate due to the decline in estradiol. Postmenopausal women may be prescribed conjugated estrogens (Premarin), estradiol (Estrace, Estraderm, Vivelle), or estropipate (Ogen, Ortho-Est).

Nutritional Supplements

Common nutritional supplements prescribed for bone health include vitamin D and calcium (**Table 5-18**). Calcium and vitamin D are both readily available over the counter (alone or in combination) or combined with prescription antiresorptive medications (eg, Actonel with Calcium and Fosamax Plus D).

Table 5-18 Nutritional Supplements for Bones

Generic	Brand Name	Dose
ergocalciferol (vitamin D_2 analog)	Drisdol	50,000 units
calcium and cholecalciferol (vitamin D)	Os-Cal 500+D	calcium 500 mg and vitamin D 400 units
tricalcium phosphate	Posture	calcium 600 mg and phosphorus 280 mg

Exercises

Using Context to Make Decisions

Use the sample report on page 156 to answer questions 1–9.

1. What word belongs in blank #1? _____
_____

2. What dictation error has occurred in the reported lab values? _____
_____

3. What transcription error occurred in the past medical history? _____
_____

4. What approach would you take to attempt to fill in blank #2? _____
_____

5. What drug name do you believe goes in blank #2?
_____

6. What is the most likely word that goes in blank #3?
_____

7. What transcription error has occurred beyond blank #2? _____

8. Which of the following would be a reasonable choice for blank #4?

   a. bone scan   **c.** ABI

   b. ultrasound   **d.** arthroscopy

9. Refer to sample report 5A on page 468 in Appendix B to answer this question: The patient presents for definitive management of avascular necrosis. Which of the following will be performed?

   a. The right hip joint will be fused.

   b. The right hip joint will be replaced.

   c. The right hip joint will be repaired.

   d. The right hip joint will be partially replaced.

10. Fill in the blanks with the correct term (effusion, diffusion, suffusion, affusion, perfusion, profusion, refusion).

    a. The patient was the front-seat passenger in a motor vehicle collision and hit her right knee on the dashboard. Examination shows tenderness and a palpable _____.

    b. The Esmarch bandage was removed and _____ occurred immediately.

    c. The left foot shows poor _____ due to severe peripheral vascular disease.

    d. Arthrocentesis showed a _____ of white cells but no blood.

11. Define the term *precipitate*. Write two sentences using this term as a noun and a verb. _____
_____

12. Explain why in*ter*fragmentary screws is the correct phrase as opposed to in*tra*fragmentary screws. ____
_____

Terms Checkup

Complete the multiple choice questions for Chapter 5 located at www.myhealthprofessionskit.com. To access the questions, select the discipline "Medical Transcription," then click on the title of this book, *Advanced Medical Transcription.*

Look It Up

Using the guidelines described on page xvii, complete a research project on Paget disease and osteomalacia.

Transcription Practice

1. Transcribe the key terms and phrases for Chapter 5.
2. Complete the proofing and transcription practice exercises for Chapter 5.

HISTORY OF PRESENT ILLNESS: This 75-year-old male is seen today for followup of a left second toe wound with history of associated osteomyelitis and arterial ____(1)____. At his last visit in June, 20XX, the toe wound on the left was actually healed following 2 courses of antibiotics for a methicillin-resistant S aureus. Also, his sedimentation rate had returned to normal at 160 and his CRP was down to 0.5. He has noticed that the left second toe wound has started draining again recently. He has been moderately active on it as well.

PAST MEDICAL HISTORY
1. Adult-onset diabetes.
2. Gout.
3. History of MRFA.
4. History of arterial insufficiency status post opening of peroneal and posterior tibial runoff.
5. History of osteomyelitis of the left second toe.

CURRENT MEDICATIONS
1. Metformin 500 mg b.i.d.
2. ____(2)____ -prim 100 mg.

PHYSICAL EXAMINATION: On vascular examination, I could palpate a weak popliteal pulse on the left but no pedal pulses. The left second toe had a distal wound, full thickness, with some scabbing and undermining.

IMPRESSION: Recurrent opening of the left second toe wound with history of ____(3)____ and arterial sufficiency.

PLAN: Repeat imaging studies of the left foot with CT and ____(4)____.

PEARSON
myhealthprofessionskit™

To access the transcription practice exercises for this chapter, go to www.myhealthprofessionskit.com. Select the discipline "Medical Transcription," then click on the title of this book, *Advanced Medical Transcription*.

Orthopedics: The Spine

6

Preview Terms
Before studying this chapter, make sure you understand the following terms. Definitions can be found in the glossary.

axial skeleton
foramen,
    pl. foramina
myelopathy
paraspinal muscles
process
radiculopathy

Learning Objectives

After completing this chapter, you should be able to comprehend and correctly transcribe terminology related to:

▶ orthopedic disorders of the back and neck

▶ signs and maneuvers used to diagnose disorders of the spine

▶ laboratory and imaging tests used to diagnose and monitor disorders of the spine

▶ therapeutic procedures used to treat disorders of the spine

▶ drugs used in the treatment of neuropathic pain

Introduction

Neck and back pain are among the most common reasons for physician visits. Most spine pain is mechanical in origin as opposed to infectious or malignant. Vocational spine injuries as well as degenerative changes that accompany aging cause a significant amount of pain and disability. Derangement of any part of the spine may lead to muscle strain, ligament sprain, or muscle spasm. Oftentimes, several symptoms are present, and the pain may be exacerbated by fatigue, stress, and physical deconditioning.

Anatomy of the Spine

Understanding the anatomy of the spine is important to correctly transcribing reports involving the vertebrae, nerves, and muscles of the neck and back. Study ■ **Figure 6-1** carefully to become familiar with the intricate parts of vertebral anatomy.

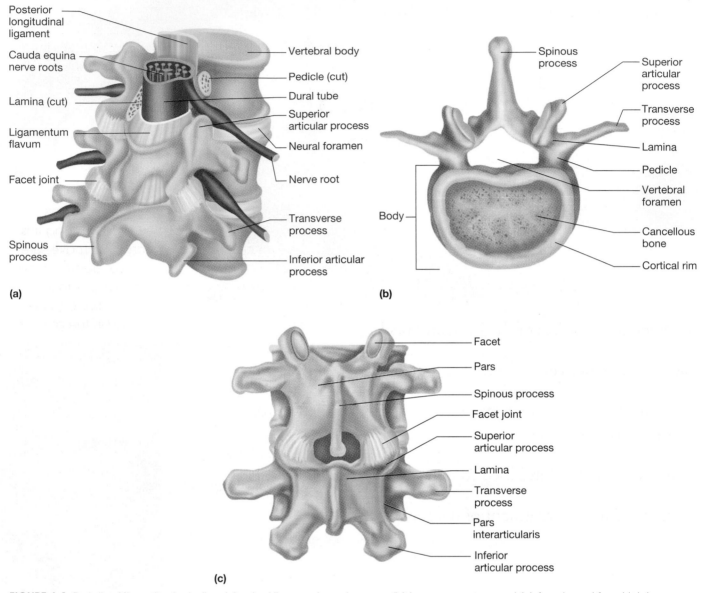

FIGURE 6-1 Details of the spine including (a) spinal ligaments and nerves, (b) bony processes, and (c) facets and facet joints.

The spine consists of a column of 24 vertebral bodies. Although cervical, thoracic, and lumbar vertebrae vary in their size and shape, they all have a single spinous process as well as bilateral transverse, superior, and inferior bony processes that form an opening called the **vertebral foramina**. The cervical vertebrae are easily distinguished from thoracic and lumbar vertebra by the bilateral foramina in the transverse processes that allow passage of the vertebral arteries. Vertebral bodies are located on the anterior side of the spine and form the anterior wall of the vertebral foramina. The **lamina** (a plate-like structure) of each vertebra forms the posterior wall of the vertebral foramina and serves as a base for the processes. The vertebral bodies give the spine structure and substance, and the bony processes give the spine flexibility and stability.

The **ligamenta flava** (literally the yellow ligaments), located on the posterior wall of the vertebral foramina, connect the lamina of adjacent vertebrae. The **anterior longitudinal ligament** runs along the anterior side of the vertebral bodies. The spinal canal, created by the vertical and horizontal alignment of the vertebral foramina, runs the length of the spine, surrounding and protecting the spinal cord. Extending posteriorly from each lamina is a spinous process. On either side of the spinous process are the **superior and inferior articular processes** that connect to the vertebral bodies through the **pedicles** and terminate in **facets**, somewhat flat areas that articulate with the adjacent vertebra. The thoracic vertebrae also have **costal facets** where the ribs articulate with the spine. The pars are segments of bone that connect the articular processes to the lamina. The **pars interarticularis** is the segment of bone between the superior and inferior articular processes of the lumbar vertebrae.

Each vertebral body is separated by an **intervertebral disk**. The two facet joints at the same level along with the intervertebral disk function as a three-joint complex. Each vertebral unit is referred to as a level. Each level is numbered, starting at the number one for each region of the spine (cervical, lumbar, thoracic, or sacral). Disks are referenced by the adjacent vertebral bodies positioned above and below (eg, C1-C2, T3-T4, L5-S1). The bony and ligamentous structures of the spine contribute to many back pain syndromes by pressing on the spinal cord or nerve roots. (1)

> A hyphen is only used when referencing a single disk, not a range of disks. Listen carefully for the word "through," indicating several levels. For example, "The spine was fused at levels C2 through C4" (*not* C2-C4).

The spinal cord is protected by the **dura mater**, also called the **thecal sac**. The spinal cord runs the length of the cervical and thoracic spine and terminates at about the first lumbar disk to become the **cauda equina**, which is a bundle of nerve roots contained within the arachnoid space of the lumbar spinal column. Cauda equina means "horse tail," and this bundle of nerves derives its name from its appearance. Nerve fibers originating in the spinal cord exit in pairs through the right and left **neural foramina** of the lumbar spine at various levels, causing the bundle to taper like a horse's tail.

> Be very careful that you do not accidentally transcribe fecal sac instead of thecal sac. The two words sound very similar and without paying close attention, it is easy to transcribe the phrase incorrectly.

> The correct phrase is neural foramen or neural foramina, not the combined forms neuroforamen or neuroforamina, although many dictators will pronounce it in the combined form. The adjectival term neuroforaminal *does* take the combined form.

The intervertebral disks (2) are made of a tough, fibrous **annulus** (ring) (3) surrounding a gel-like center, called the **nucleus pulposus** (literally the inner pulp). The annular ring gives the disk shape, and the nucleus pulposus acts as a cushion between the vertebral bodies and gives the disk its shock-absorbing qualities.

Orthopedic Disorders of the Back and Neck

The vast majority of pain syndromes involving the back and neck are caused by structural changes of the vertebrae and disks, leading to disruption or compression of nerves with subsequent muscle spasm. A careful history, physical examination, and imaging studies are typically required to accurately diagnose chronic pain related to the spine and paraspinal muscles. The etiology of the pain may fall into four general categories: arthropathy, muscular spasm, radiculopathy, or myelopathy.

Disruption of the spine's anatomy causes reflexive spasms of the paraspinal muscles that can be extremely painful. **Radicular pain** is caused by compression or irritation of a nerve root as it exits the spinal cord. Radicular pain causes symptoms that radiate distally along the distribution of that nerve with impairment in strength, sensation, and reflexes. When a nerve emanating from the lumbar region is involved, the radiculopathy is commonly referred to as **sciatica**.

> The point where the nerve exits the spinal cord is the "root" (hence the term "radicular"). Although a radiculopathy infers pain along the route (path) of the nerve, the phrase "nerve route" is incorrect.

Pain or impairment caused by involvement of the spinal cord itself is referred to as myelopathy. Myelopathy causes impairment of strength, sensation, and

(1) Vertebral disks may be written with the letter repeated for each vertebral body in the level (C1-C2) or only written one time per level (C1-2).

(2) Disk (spelled with a /k/) is the preferred spelling for all anatomical disks with the exception of the optic disc (spelled with a /c/).

(3) Annulus has two acceptable spellings: anulus and annulus.

reflexes served by the nerves extending from the affected spinal cord level and all levels below, referred to as **segmental neurologic deficits**. Involvement of the cauda equina may cause **bowel or bladder dysfunction**, loss of perianal sensation, erectile dysfunction, urinary retention, and loss of rectal tone and sphincter reflexes.

Several types of disk disease are shown in ■ **Figure 6-2**. The most common causes of back pain include:

- degenerative disk disease
- disk herniation
- spondylolisthesis
- spinal stenosis
- compression fracture
- osteoarthritis of the facet joints

A thorough interrogation of the patient's history is important to determine the nociceptive **(4)** source. Questions should include the quality of the pain, onset, duration, severity, and location. The clinician should also note accompanying symptoms such as stiffness, numbness, paresthesias, weakness, urinary retention, and incontinence. Pain-modifying factors are also important, such as rest, activity, changes in position, weightbearing, time of day, and relationship to sleep.

Cervical Subluxation

Cervical subluxation may occur at the **atlantoaxial joint**, which is the joint formed by the **atlas** (C1) and the **axis** (C2). This particular joint is a synovial joint so it may be affected by rheumatoid arthritis. Atlanto-axial instability is also associated with Down syndrome and is caused by laxity of the transverse ligament that holds the **dens (5)** against the **anterior arch**. Subluxation with stenosis at C1-C2 may result from major trauma and can be life threatening. Atlantoaxial subluxation is often asymptomatic but may cause vague neck pain, occipital headache, or occasionally cervical spinal cord compression. Conservative treatment includes cervical immobilization with a **cervical collar**. Surgery may be required to stabilize the spine.

---

(4) Nociceptive means causing pain.

(5) The dens, also called the odontoid process, is a tooth-like structure that projects upward from the axis. The atlas rotates around the dens.

Examples of Disk Problems

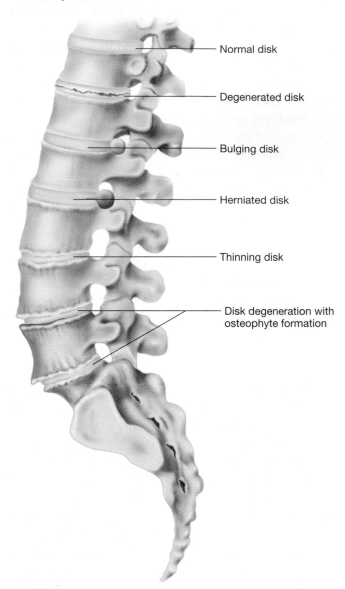

- Normal disk
- Degenerated disk
- Bulging disk
- Herniated disk
- Thinning disk
- Disk degeneration with osteophyte formation

FIGURE 6-2 Examples of disk disease.

Degenerative Disk Disease

Degenerative disk disease (DDD) is primarily a disease of aging, mostly affecting those of middle age. DDD can occur anywhere along the spine but it most commonly occurs in the lumbar spine. The exact etiology of DDD is not entirely clear, but many believe it begins with microscopic tears of the tough, fibrous annulus. These small tears gradually give way to bulges or frank herniation. The disks may also become desiccated with loss of the nucleus pulposus. **Internal disk degeneration (IDD)** describes annular fissuring of the disk without external bulges or herniation. The disks themselves contain nerve endings capable of generating pain. **Diskogenic pain** from DDD may be due to changes in the disk itself or by compression of nerve roots caused by displacement of the nucleus pulposus or malalignment of vertebral structures. As the quantity of nucleus pulposus declines (due to resorption or **desiccation**), the space between the vertebral bodies narrows (**disk space narrowing**). In advanced disease, diskogenic pain results from **endplate destruction**, (6) disk fibrosis, and osteophyte formation.

Physical examination of the paraspinal muscles and spine stabilizers often elicits tenderness and tightness due to reactive muscle spasm. Muscle atrophy in one leg may be evident in the midthigh or midcalf, as demonstrated by comparing the circumference of each leg. Hips, knees, and ankles should be examined for range of motion, crepitus, and effusions. Specific maneuvers, such as **pelvic rocking**, sustained hip flexion, or the **straight leg raise test** will elicit pain when disks are involved and give further clues as to the etiology and location (spinal level) involved. The examiner should assess the patient in flexion, extension, **lateral bending** (also called **sidebending**), and rotation for pain and limited range of motion. Plain films of the spine show degenerative changes in the disk spaces. **Flexion and extension views** help to assess stability.

DDD is first treated conservatively with single or combination therapies including activity modification, muscle relaxants, physical therapy, chiropractic, osteopathic manipulation, NSAIDs, or spinal injections of corticosteroids. Patients with neck pain may be treated with intermittent immobilization using a soft, cervical collar. Most patients recover within six months but often have recurrence. Surgery may be recommended if two to three months of conservative treatment fails. Indications for surgery include limitations in **activities of daily living (ADLs)**, weakness or numbness in the arms or legs, or difficulty walking or standing. Surgical procedures used in the treatment of DDD are described on page 176.

> The patient's MRI was reviewed. It shows a moderate size posterior central disk herniation at L5-S1, mildly impinging the thecal sac and the S1 nerve root sheaths bilaterally. She also has evidence of disk desiccation with a darkened disk at this level. There is also moderate foraminal stenosis laterally.

Herniated Nucleus Pulposus

Herniated nucleus pulposus (HNP), sometimes erroneously referred to as a slipped disk, may be caused by degenerative disk disease or by acute trauma that places sudden, excessive pressure on a disk, such as heavy lifting, a fall from a significant height, or a motor vehicle collision. Herniations may be classified as **protruding** or **bulging**, in which case the annulus is intact; **extruded**, characterized by an actual break in the annulus; or sequestered, in which case a fragment of the disk detaches and becomes trapped within the spinal canal. In most cases, the displaced disk material compresses the spinal cord, the cauda equina, or the nerve root as it exits the spinal cord and passes through the neural foramina. **Central herniation** refers to an HNP that impinges on the spinal canal. A **lateral herniation** is located lateral to the pedicles and may compress the nerve root. A damaged disk may also cause a chemical radiculitis in which the nucleus pulposus releases substances that irritate the root even though there is no direct contact with the root. HNP is more common in the middle-aged patient; after age 50, the nucleus pulposus begins to dry out and the disk becomes smaller, so it is less likely to bulge or herniate. Osteoarthritic changes and spinal stenosis are more common among the elderly.

> The abbreviation HNP sounds very much like H&P when dictated. Be sure to listen in context to distinguish these two abbreviations.

HNP of the cervical spine causes neck pain, occipital pain, arm pain, shoulder-girdle pain, and symptoms in the upper extremities including weakness, paresthesias, hypesthesia, and decreased reflexes. The **Spurling test** re-creates the radicular symptoms. Symptoms of cervical myelopathy may include gait deterioration with falls, impaired manual dexterity (eg, difficulty buttoning a shirt), and generalized weakness, as well as bowel and bladder dysfunction. Examination shows a positive **Babinski reflex** in the lower extremities and a positive **Hoffmann reflex** in the upper extremities.

(6) Vertebral endplates are cartilaginous plates that attach the disks to the vertebral bodies and supply nutrients to the annulus and nucleus pulposus.

> Reflexes were 2+ biceps, 2+ brachioradialis, 2+ triceps, 2+ patellar, and 2+ Achilles. Babinski's were downgoing bilaterally. Sensory exam was intact to light touch and pinprick, proprioception and vibration in all 4 extremities.

> TECHNIQUE: Scans were performed through the cervical spine. A series of T1- and T2-weighted scans along with T2 inversion-recovery weighted scan sequences were acquired pre-contrast, sagittally, axially, and coronally.
>
> FINDINGS: Scans through the cervical spine performed following contrast demonstrate mild scoliosis. The cerebellar tonsils are normal in position. Cisterna magna is normally formed. Cervical vertebral body heights are preserved. Disk heights are narrowed at C3-4, C4-5, and C5-6. At C2-3, the disk margins are intact. Canal and foramina appear patent. Facets are normal. At C3-4, a broad-based annular disk bulge is seen, resulting in mild contour deformity of the ventral surface of the sac. No evidence of cord compression. No evidence for nerve root sleeve entrapment. At C4-5, a mild annular bulge is seen. No evidence of disk herniation. The bulge is seen centrally, contouring the ventral surface of the sac. No evidence for cord effacement. At C5-6, there is right paracentral disk herniation. Medial right foraminal disk herniation is noted, resulting in foraminal encroachment on the right side at C6-7 and C7-T1. Disk margins are intact.

HNP of the lumbar spine occurs most commonly at L4-5. Central herniation in the lumbar region typically compresses the nerve root as it exits the foramen located below the herniated disk. A herniated disk of the lumbar spine with nerve root irritation causes low back pain with pain radiating down the buttocks and

(7) Saddle anesthesia is decreased sensation of the perineal region, such as loss of the ability to feel toilet paper touching the skin.

below the knee. Patients complain of bilateral leg weakness and **saddle anesthesia**. (7) Bowel or bladder incontinence or impotence is indicative of **cauda equina syndrome**. The straight leg test and the **crossed straight leg test** are positive when there is nerve root irritation at L4-5 or L5-S1.

> Bowel incontinence may also be dictated as fecal incontinence. Be careful that you do not transcribe thecal incontinence.

A thorough physical examination is especially helpful in the diagnosis of lumbar HNP. Assessment should include all dermatomes and the motor strength of all muscle groups. Patients are asked to rate their pain **on a scale of 1–10** with 1 being no pain and a 10 being the worst pain. Patients may also indicate their level of pain using a **Visual Analog Scale (VAS)**. Patients should be observed while walking for the presence of gait disturbances or **foot drop**. Patients should also undergo a rectal exam that includes assessment of rectal tone, perianal sensation, and the **anal wink**. Positive straight leg raise test and positive crossed straight leg raise test are common.

Specific symptoms may give the clinician clues as to the vertebral level of the affected disk. Herniation at L3-4 causes anterior tibialis weakness, decreased knee jerk, and medial knee sensory changes. Herniation at L4-5 causes altered sensation over the lateral aspect of the calf and first dorsal web space and weakness in the extensor hallucis longus. Symptoms of herniation at L5-S1 include decreased ankle jerk, decreased plantarflexion strength, and diminished sensation in the lateral aspect of the foot. Symptoms of cauda equina include saddle anesthesia and changes in bowel and bladder function. Cauda equina syndrome requires **nerve decompression** on an emergent basis.

A **CT myelogram** is the test of choice to assess the degree of compression and to determine whether the compression is caused by bony or soft tissues. A **diskogram** may be performed to diagnose diskogenic pain. As with DDD, most patients will respond to conservative treatment and will heal within six months. Treatment includes education as well as NSAIDs and muscle relaxants. Patients with symptoms of myelopathy or those who fail conservative treatment may be treated surgically with **anterior cervical diskectomy (ACD)** or **ACD with fusion (ACDF)**. Surgical treatment for

- Cervical subluxation occurs at the atlantoaxial joint (C1-2). It may result from osteoarthritis, congenital abnormalities, or from trauma. Most patients are asymptomatic or complain of vague pain, but sudden, traumatic injury at this joint can cause paralysis or death.

- Degenerative disk disease affects almost everyone to a degree by middle age. Over time, the disk annulus becomes damaged and/or the disk desiccates. Subsequent bulges, herniations, and loss of disk height cause a shift in spinal elements, resulting in muscle spasm and pain. If conservative treatment fails, steroid injections and eventually diskectomy may be performed.

- Herniated nucleus pulposus is characterized by extrusion of disk material through the disk annulus, resulting from degenerative disk disease or by sudden, acute trauma. Radiculopathy and myelopathy result from compression of nearby nerves. CT myelogram is the test of choice to assess nerve compression. Diskectomy may be performed after failure of conservative therapy.

the lumbar spine includes a **microdiskectomy (8)** with a posterior approach. A hemilaminotomy is performed to remove the disk fragment that is impinging on the nerves. If fusion is required, a **transforaminal lumbar interbody fusion (TLIF)** may be performed.

PHYSICAL EXAMINATION: The patient has numbness, burning, and stabbing down the right arm and right leg. She does have some hyperreflexia in the lower third of her extremities. She does have normal sensation bilaterally. The cervical motion is about 30% of normal with worse pain with flexion and sidebending to the right. Her lumbar motions are about 30% of normal, with worse pain with flexion. Straight leg raise is 90 degrees on the left but only 30 degrees on the right.

IMAGING: Her MRI shows that she has a herniated disk, right paracentral at C4-5 as well as C5-6 with cord compression at both of these levels. The lumbar MRI shows significant herniated disks at L4-5 and L5-S1. These are both very large herniations.

RECOMMENDATIONS: I would recommend 2-level ACDF and decompression of the spinal cord at C4-5 and C5-6. We discussed the risks and benefits, and she is going to consider these recommendations.

Her MRI shows that she has a herniated disk at L2-3 with massive facet hypertrophy and complete destruction of the spinal canal at this level. I would recommend that she have a decompression with diskectomy and TLIF.

Spondylolisthesis

Spondylolisthesis is an **anteroposterior subluxation** of two vertebral bodies relative to each other. In other words, a vertebral body slides forward relative to the disk below it. A vertebra may slide out of position due to a congenital defect in the pars interarticularis, age-related degeneration of the disk, facet joint incompetence, or stretching of the posterior ligamentous-bony restraints. Spondylolisthesis occurs in the lumbar spine, especially at L5-S1. Spondylolisthesis may be classified as **spondylolytic** (also called isthmic), degenerative, traumatic, pathologic, or iatrogenic (due to a defect following spine surgery). Spondylolisthesis caused by major trauma can cause spinal cord compression with neurologic deficits. Spondylolisthesis is graded 1–4 to indicate the degree of vertebral subluxation as viewed in the sagittal plane (■ **Figure 6-3**).

(8) Microdiskectomy uses a surgical microscope and microsurgical techniques.

Grades of Spondylolisthesis

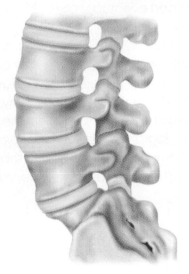

Normal spine

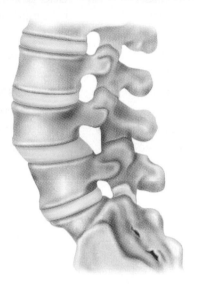

Grade 1
< 25% slippage

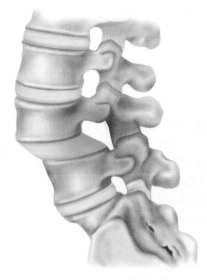

Grade 2
25% to 50% slippage

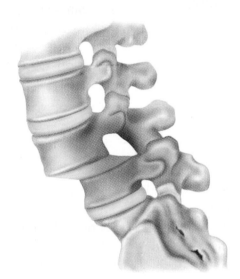

Grade 3
50% to 75% slippage

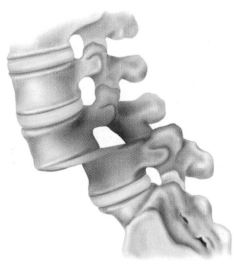

Grade 4
> 75% slippage

FIGURE 6-3 Spondylolisthesis

PHYSICAL EXAMINATION: Her cervical motion is about 20% of normal in flexion, extension, lateral rotation, and sidebending, with most pain on flexion. Positive Tinel in the upper extremities bilaterally, as well as some numbness in the C5-6 distribution, more on the left.

IMAGING: X-rays of the cervical spine show that she has a grade 1 spondylolisthesis at C3-4 and C4-5.

Spondylolysis, which is the degeneration or deficient development of a portion of a vertebra, is the most common cause of spondylolisthesis. A congenital defect, most commonly found in the pars interarticularis, causes the vertebra to be vulnerable to fractures. Adolescents and young adults active in sports are most prone to this form of spondylolisthesis. A bilateral break in this region, also referred to as the **neural arch**, cleaves the vertebra into two pieces. The section of the vertebra posterior to the break remains fixed and the remainder of the vertebra slides anteriorly relative to the spine below (anterolisthesis).

Degenerative spondylolisthesis occurs in older adults, often due to instability of the ligaments or disks, allowing movement of the vertebra and subsequent stress on the pars interarticularis, the thinner area of the vertebra. Osteoarthritic changes in the facet joints can also lead to spondylolisthesis. Eburnation and erosive changes of these joints lead to malalignment of the articular surfaces and decreased stability. The slip most commonly occurs at L4-5 and less commonly at L3-4. Radicular symptoms may result from **lateral recess stenosis** (9) caused by **facet hypertrophy** or **ligamentous hypertrophy** and/or disk herniation.

> **Pause 6-1** Explain this sentence in layman's terms: "Eburnation and erosive changes of these joints lead to malalignment of the articular surfaces and decreased stability."

Retrolisthesis, which is slippage in the posterior direction, may also occur in some individuals with degenerative disorders of the spine. Mild to moderate subluxation (less than 50%) may be asymptomatic, especially in young persons, but will predispose the patient to spinal stenosis later in life.

Patients with symptomatic spondylolisthesis may present with back or leg pain (radiculopathy), abnormal gait, neurogenic claudication, or hyperlordotic posture. Younger patients may report a recent history of sports-related trauma. Physical examination should include a rectal exam and straight leg raise test. Examination may reveal limited lumbar flexion with significant hamstring tightness and an inability to flex hips with the knees fully extended. High-grade slips will cause a palpable stepoff.

Imaging studies are important to the diagnosis and staging of spondylolisthesis. Oblique, plain-film views show the characteristic **Scottie dog** shape (■ Figure 6-4). A break in the pars interarticularis makes it look as if the dog is wearing a collar. **Spot lateral views** show the presence and degree of spondylolisthesis and are typically used for staging. Flexion and extension views assess stability. CT myelography is used to assess the degree of neural compression. MRI is also used to assess the degree of neural compression and also indicates the extent of disk desiccation. Traumatic spondylolisthesis may cause **jumped facets** or fractures of the articular processes and/or lamina. **Diskography** or selective spinal blocks can determine if the pain is from the disk or a defect of the pars.

Most cases of spondylolisthesis can be managed conservatively. Operative treatment is indicated when symptoms are incapacitating or if radiculopathy, neurogenic

> **(9)** The lateral recess is the space within the spinal canal adjacent to the exit zone of the nerve roots.

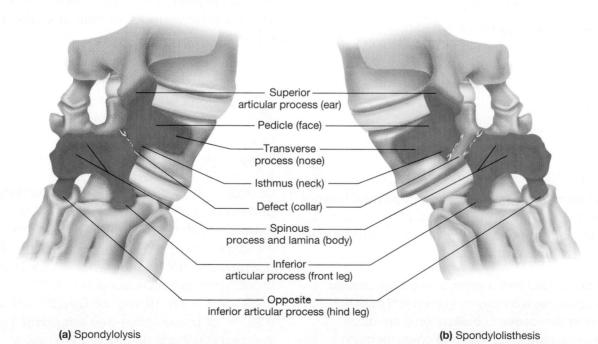

Superior articular process (ear)
Pedicle (face)
Transverse process (nose)
Isthmus (neck)
Defect (collar)
Spinous process and lamina (body)
Inferior articular process (front leg)
Opposite inferior articular process (hind leg)

(a) Spondylolysis

(b) Spondylolisthesis

FIGURE 6-4 An x-ray in the oblique projection shows (a) spondylolysis leading to (b) spondylolisthesis with the typical appearance of a Scottie dog with a collar.

claudication, or postural or gait abnormalities develop. The goal of operative treatment is to stabilize the joint, decompress nerves, and restore sagittal alignment.

Spondylosis

Spondylosis is a general term reserved for acquired, age-related degenerative changes of the spine (ie, diskopathy or facet arthropathy). **Lumbar spondylosis** describes bony overgrowths (osteophytes, **bridging osteophytes**), predominantly those at the anterior lateral, and less commonly, posterior aspects of the superior and inferior margins of vertebral bodies (see Figure 6-2). **Cervical spondylosis**, also called **degenerative arthritis**, is a collective term describing degenerative changes that occur in the apophysial joints (10) and intervertebral disk joints with or without neurologic signs.

> This 59-year-old woman presented with a spastic gait and weakness in her upper extremities. A T2-weighted sagittal MRI shows cord compression from cervical spondylosis with cervical spondylotic myelopathy. Signal changes were noted in the cord at C4-5, with ventral osteophytosis, buckling of the ligamentum flavum at C3-4, and prominent loss of disk height between C2 and C5.

> **Pause 6-2** The terms spondylosis, spondylolysis, spondylolisthesis can be difficult to distinguish. Write out the definitions of these three terms and devise your own method for remembering the difference between them.

Facet Arthropathy

The facet joints, also called the **zygapophyseal joints** (or **Z joints**), are the joints in the posterior aspect of the spine formed by the superior articulating

> **(10)** An apophysial joint is formed by a bony process. An apophysis is a bony outgrowth that does not have its own center of ossification (from *apoa* meaning separated from and *physis* meaning growth (growth plate).

processes of one vertebra and the inferior articulating processes of the vertebra above it. These particular spinal joints are synovial joints (ie, have hyaline cartilage and capsules), and as such, are susceptible to degenerative and inflammatory arthropathies as well as hypertrophy. The facets are innervated by the **medial branch nerve**, which senses pain in the facet joint capsule (■ **Figure 6-5**). The medial branch nerves do not control sensation in the back, arms or legs, so they can be blocked or ablated without detrimental consequences to motor strength or sensation.

Unfortunately, there are no physical examination maneuvers, imaging tests, or noninvasive tests that will definitively diagnose **facet joint arthropathy**. When facet joint pain is suspected and other sources of pain have been ruled out, fluoroscopic-guided **medial branch blocks** (steroid injections) are performed to both diagnose and temporarily treat the source of the pain. If pain subsides after steroid injection, the pain can then be attributed to the facet joint. A single medial branch innervates two facet joints, so adjacent vertebral levels must be treated.

A second treatment modality, called **radiofrequency ablation (RFA)** or **radiofrequency rhizotomy**, destroys the nerve, thereby eliminating any sensory input from the painful joint. This procedure uses energy generated by radio waves to heat the medial branch nerve until it no longer transmits pain signals. The nerve may regenerate over the course of 9–18 months with subsequent return of the pain. If so, the treatment can be repeated.

> OPERATION: Radiofrequency neurotomies of the right L3-4, L4-5, and L5-S1 medial branch nerves using a Stryker RF generator via fluoroscopic guidance using a C-arm fluoroscope.
>
> DETAILS: Using the Fisher N-50 radiofrequency generator, sensory and motor tests were performed at 2 Hz and 50 Hz, demonstrating no pain radiating down the lower extremity. Subsequently, the right L3-4, L4-5, and L5-S1 medial branch nerves were lesioned at 80 °C for 60 seconds and then 10 mg of Depo-Medrol and 0.25 mL of preservative-free lidocaine 1% were injected into each medial branch nerve.

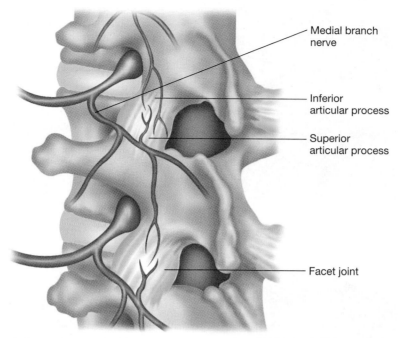

FIGURE 6-5 Medial branch nerves innervate the facet joint capsule and may be blocked using steroid injections to reduce pain from facet joint arthropathy.

Stenosis

Spinal stenosis refers to narrowing of the spinal canal (vertebral foramina) or neural foramina (**intervertebral foramina**) due to spondylosis and/or degenerative disk disease. Stenosis typically occurs in the cervical and lumbar spine and rarely in the thoracic area. Stenosis occurs when bony structures, disks, ligaments, cysts, or masses compress a nerve root laterally or press on the spinal cord or cauda equina centrally. Stenosis may be classified as **central canal stenosis** or lateral recess stenosis. Symptoms may result from nerve root compression or compression of nutrient arterioles that supply the nerve roots.

Primary stenosis refers to congenital malformations and developmental flaws. Primary stenosis presents in younger patients and is often easier to diagnose since younger patients have fewer comorbid conditions. **Secondary stenosis**, also called acquired stenosis, may be iatrogenic, or it may be caused by trauma or degenerative changes.

Osteophytes, the most common bony structures to cause stenosis, form in response to physiologic stress on the bone surface and are a part of the degenerative effects of aging. The formation of osteophytes, called **osteophytosis**, occurs at the superior and inferior margins of the vertebral body. Osteophytes that form on the posterior surface cause lateral recess stenosis, impinging on the nerve roots of the caudad vertebra.

Pause 6-3 Explain the meaning of "caudad vertebra" as it is used in the following sentence, "Osteophytes that form on the posterior surface cause lateral recess stenosis, impinging on the nerve roots of the caudad vertebra."

Osteoarthritic changes, including synovial cysts and **hypertrophy of the facet joints**, also lead to stenosis. Degenerative spondylolisthesis can further compromise the canal. Compression fractures that lead to instability and structural changes can cause spinal stenosis. Metastatic tumors that impinge on the nerve roots or spinal cord also cause stenosis.

A congenitally narrow canal is more prone to diskogenic causes of stenosis such as bulging of the disk annulus, a herniated disk, or desiccated disks. Large disk herniations can compress the **dural sac** and compromise its nerves, particularly at the more cephalad lumbar levels where the dural sac contains more nerves. Hypertrophy of the posterior longitudinal ligament or the ligamenta flava (see Figure 6-1) may also encroach on the nerve pathways. The ligamenta flava tends to ossify as a person ages, leading to hypertrophy. When disk height is reduced, the spinal column shortens and the ossified ligament buckles inward, compressing the

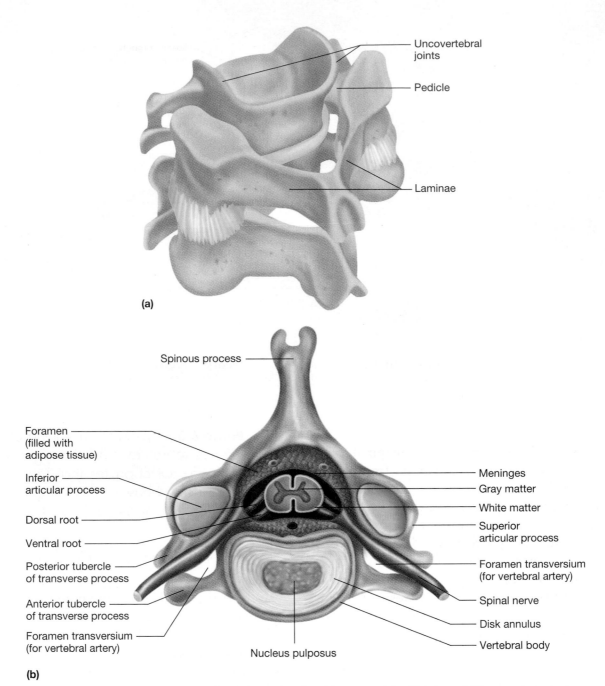

(a)

(b)

FIGURE 6-6 Two views of the cervical vertebrae showing (a) uncovertebral joints and (b) normal cervical vertebral anatomy.

spinal sac and nerve roots. In the cervical spine, **unco-vertebral joint hypertrophy** (11) (■ **Figure 6-6**) may also be a causative factor.

Patients with cervical stenosis usually present with cervical radiculopathy, with or without myelopathy. Patients complain of radiating arm pain with numbness and paresthesias. Muscle weakness may also be evident. Stenosis involving the spinal cord can cause clumsiness and difficulty walking due to spasticity and impaired proprioception. Examination may reveal **long-tract signs** such as hyperreflexia and clonus.

(11) Uncovertebral joints are the synovial joints between adjacent lateral lips of the cervical vertebral bodies of C3 through C7, also called Luschka joints.

 The correct phrase is long-tract signs, not long-track signs.

Patients with lumbar stenosis present with a constellation of complaints including low back pain, sciatica, and **neurogenic claudication** (pain with walking that is relieved with sitting or with back flexion). Severe stenosis produces cauda equina syndrome characterized by bilateral leg weakness, loss of bowel control due to sphincter dysfunction, and urinary retention due to atonic bladder. MRI and CT myelogram are the studies of choice for spinal stenosis. Flexion-extension views on plain film will show spinal instability. A **Torg ratio** is a measure of the degree of stenosis and is calculated as the diameter of cervical canal to the width of cervical body.

> **Pause 6-4** Neurogenic claudication can be distinguished from true claudication by examining the pedal pulses. What is the expected finding on examination of the pulses in neurogenic claudication compared to true claudication? What other physical signs may be seen with claudication that might not be present with neurogenic claudication?

Nonsurgical treatments include physical therapy, antiinflammatory drugs, and **epidural steroid injections (ESI)**, including **caudal ESI**, **interlaminar ESI**, and **transforaminal ESI**. Gabapentin and tricyclic antidepressants (TCAs) are also prescribed to lessen neurogenic pain. Acute pain relief can come from 24–48 hours of bed rest in a recumbent position with the head of the bed elevated about 30 degrees (**semi-Fowler position**). Patients may also be advised to lose weight to reduce lumbar lordosis.

Surgical treatment involves decompression of the involved nerves by performing **laminectomy** (■ Figure 6-7) and/or **foraminotomy** at several levels. Diskectomy with limited laminotomy is used to treat disk herniations. A microdiskectomy (removing the disk using microscopic instruments) may be performed if the herniation is localized. (12) Cervical stenosis may be treated surgically with either an anterior or a posterior approach. A posterior approach is used to treat multiple levels or to decompress nerves due to a **hypertrophied ligamentum flavum**. Cervical laminoplasty may also be performed, which is often preferred for unilateral decompressions because it preserves the contralateral facet joint. Disruption of bilateral cervical facet joints may result in **swan-neck deformity**. Cervical diskectomies are often accompanied by cervical fusions using allograft or autograft material. A **fusion with instrumentation** such as an **anterior cervical plate** is indicated when more than one level is involved.

(12) A microdiskectomy is a form of minimally invasive spine surgery. A small incision is made in the back to allow the insertion of dilators that create an operating port large enough to insert a microscope and specially designed instruments.

Lumbar Laminectomy

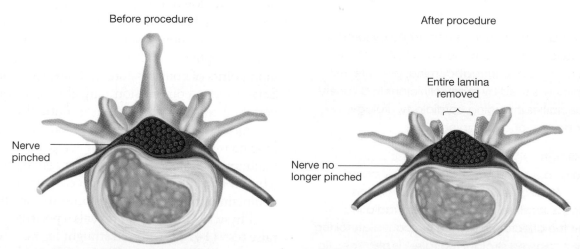

Before procedure

Nerve pinched

After procedure

Entire lamina removed

Nerve no longer pinched

FIGURE 6-7 A laminectomy procedure removes the lamina (including the spinous process) to relieve pressure on the spinal cord.

- Spondylolisthesis is an anteroposterior subluxation of two vertebral bodies caused by a congenital defect in the pars interarticularis or degeneration in the disk, facet joints, or ligaments.
- Spondylolysis is the degeneration or deficient development of a portion of a vertebra, causing vertebrae to become malaligned. It is the most common cause of spondylolisthesis. Spondylolysis is seen as a Scotty dog with a collar on oblique views of plain film.
- Spondylosis is a general term for acquired, age-related degenerative changes of the spine.

- Facet arthropathy is osteoarthritic disease of the synovial facet joints. Medial branch nerve blocks are used to both diagnose and treat facet arthropathy. A rhizotomy may be performed on the medial branch nerves if pain persists.
- Spinal stenosis is narrowing of the spinal canal or neural foramina. Primary stenosis is congenital, and secondary stenosis is acquired through degenerative changes, trauma, or surgery. Degenerative changes causing secondary stenosis include osteophyte formation and hypertrophy of the posterior longitudinal ligament and/or the ligamenta flava.

Pause 6-5 Explain this sentence in layman's terms: Cervical laminoplasty may also be performed, which is often preferred for unilateral decompressions, because it preserves the contralateral facet joint.

The patient's MRI shows a left herniated disk at C6-7, but this study was done in 20XX. She also had plain films in our office today, which show significant degenerative disk disease with anterior and posterior osteophytes and disk-space collapse at C5-6 and C6-7 as well as congenital spinal stenosis with a Torg ratio of less than 80%.

On MRI, lateral and axial views demonstrate right L4 lateral recess stenosis secondary to combination of far-lateral disk protrusion and zygapophyseal joint hypertrophy.

Sciatica

Sciatica is pain that radiates along the sciatic nerve, which runs from the lumbar spine through the buttocks and down the posterior aspect of the thigh, terminating below the knee. Typical causes include nerve compression due to intervertebral disk herniation, osteophytes, and spinal stenosis. The most common points of compression are L3-4, L4-5, and L5-S1. Sciatic nerve compression may also occur outside the vertebral column in the pelvis or buttocks.

(13) The Valsalva maneuver is performed by forcing exhalation against a closed glottis. It increases intrathoracic and intraabdominal pressure. This technique is used by many clinicians in a variety of specialties including cardiology, urology, orthopedics, and otolaryngology.

(14) The straight leg raise test may cause pain that radiates down the leg when the leg is raised above 60 degrees and sometimes less. This finding is sensitive for sciatica. Pain radiating down the affected leg when the contralateral leg is lifted (crossed straight leg raise) is also specific for sciatica.

Patients complain of burning, lancinating, or stabbing pain with or without low back pain. The **Valsalva maneuver** (13) or coughing may aggravate the pain when a herniated disk is involved. Patients may also complain of numbness or weakness in the affected leg.

Physical examination reveals a positive straight leg raise test. (14) The crossed straight leg raise test is even more specific for sciatica. MRI or CT may be performed to determine the exact location of the compression and to determine if more than one level is affected. Conservative treatment includes a brief period of bed rest (24–48 hours) in the semi-Fowler position. NSAIDs and acetaminophen are commonly prescribed. Patients may also be prescribed medications for **neuropathic pain** such as gabapentin and tricyclic antidepressants. **Diathermy (15)** may help reduce muscle spasm and pain after the acute stage. Surgical treatment, such as microdiskectomy, is used when six weeks or more of conservative treatment fails.

Sacroiliac Joint Dysfunction

The sacrum is made of five fused bones, forming a triangular-shaped bone at the end of the spine (■ Figure 6-8). The sacroiliac (SI) joints (■ Figure 6-9) are formed by the junction of the sacrum with the right and left iliac bones, joining the spine and the pelvis. The SI joints are somewhat C-shaped, diarthrodial joints (ie, synovial joints) that contain numerous ridges and depressions that allow the bones to interlock, although a slight amount of motion is allowed across these joints. The SI joints bear a large amount of weight while in the standing position, and like other weightbearing joints, are subject to degenerative arthritis.

The sacrum and iliac bones are held together by a collection of strong ligaments tying the sacrum and ilia to the piriformis, biceps femoris, gluteus maximus and minimus, and erector spinae, latissimus dorsi, thoracolumbar fascia, and iliacus muscles. This creates a broad spectrum of pain patterns associated with the SI joints. **SI joint dysfunction** is common in pregnancy due to relaxation and stretching of the ligaments, an effect of hormones associated with pregnancy as well as the change in lumbar lordosis.

There is no definitive pain pattern that points to SI joint dysfunction, but often patients present with a dull ache or sharp, stabbing pain in the area of the **posterior superior iliac spine (PSIS)**, buttocks, back of the thigh, or even the upper back. The patient may be able to point specifically to the **sacral sulcus** (the dimple in the PSIS) and reproduce the pain in that one spot (**Fortin finger sign**).

Conservative treatment consists of physical therapy modalities such as ultrasonography, phonophoresis, deep and superficial heat, and cold packs. Deep

(15) Diathermy is the treatment of pain using locally applied heat.

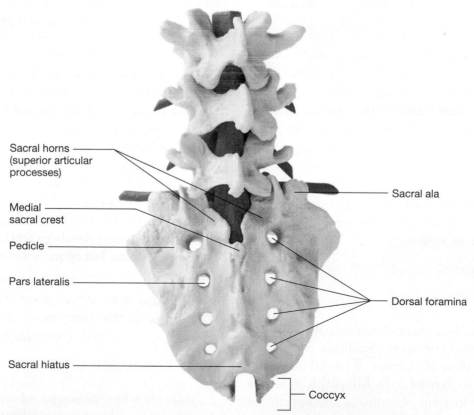

Sacral horns (superior articular processes)

Medial sacral crest

Pedicle

Pars lateralis

Sacral hiatus

Sacral ala

Dorsal foramina

Coccyx

FIGURE 6-8 The sacrum with important landmarks noted. *Source:* Patricia Hofmeester/Shutterstock.com

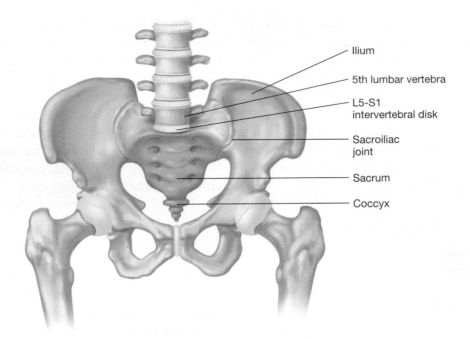

FIGURE 6-9 The lumbar spine, sacrum, and iliac bones. Note the C-shaped sacroiliac joints.

tissue massage, **myofascial release**, and stretching are also helpful. NSAIDs and muscle relaxants are used to treat the inflammation and muscle spasm. Steroid injections of the SI joint may be given if conservative treatment fails.

> The right gluteus maximus was preanesthetized with 10 mL of lidocaine 1% over the inferior pole of the right sacroiliac joint. Using AP and oblique views of the fluoroscope, a 20-gauge, 4½-inch Quincke needle was inserted into the inferior pole of the right sacroiliac joint. Next, 1 mL of Omnipaque 150 contrast was injected, showing an excellent arthrogram and good needle placement. Subsequently, 2 mL of preservative-free lidocaine 1% and 30 mg of Depo-Medrol were injected.

Scoliosis

Scoliosis is a complex, three-dimensional deformity of the spine's normal curvature. Scoliosis is typically defined as greater than 10 degrees of lateral deviation of the spine from its central axis. **Idiopathic scoliosis** is the most common form of scoliosis and appears in adolescence. Scoliosis may be associated with spondylolysis and spondylolisthesis.

Scoliosis can usually be diagnosed on physical exam. With the patient standing, shoulder, rib, and hip symmetry are examined. The patient is also examined posteriorly while bending forward (**Adams forward-bending test**). When bending forward, scoliosis in the thoracic spine causes the ribs to rotate and produce a rib hump. The difference in the rib heights (the **rib slope**) can be measured using a **scoliometer**. The scapula on the same side becomes more prominent. The most common curve is a right thoracic curve, which causes the right shoulder to rotate forward and the medial border of the right scapula to protrude posteriorly.

In the lumbar region, the pelvis becomes more prominent, producing a high-riding hip opposite the rib hump. Leg lengths will be uneven. Examination should also include assessment of hamstrings for tightness, lower extremity reflexes, and screening tests for ataxia and proprioception (**Romberg test**). Examination may also reveal **café au lait spots** or neurofibromas.

> **Pause 6-6** What are café au lait spots? How is this term pronounced? How are these spots associated with scoliosis?

Scoliosis is best appreciatetd on a plain film of the entire spine in the AP view. Spine films show the iliac crests and allow determination of the **Risser** stage (0 through V), which is the amount of ossification of the iliac growth cartilage. Risser 0 indicates an immature skeleton and Risser V indicates a fully mature skeleton.

Treatment of scoliosis depends on the degree of curvature. Patients who present with minimal curvature are treated with **watchful waiting** and periodic radiographs to monitor curve progression. Patients who are still growing may be braced using a **Milwaukee brace** or a **thoracolumbosacral orthosis (TLSO)**. Surgery is indicated for curvatures that exceed 45 degrees. Surgical correction of scoliosis involves vertebral fusion with instrumentation in the form of contoured rods, wires, and screws. The instrumentation helps maintain the fusion until the bone grafts mature. Types of instrumentation systems used to surgically correct scoliosis include:

- Cotrel-Dubousset (CD) instrumentation
- Luque-To
- TSRH (Texas Scottish Rite Hospital)
- Isola

Compression Fractures

Compression fractures of the spine are caused by severe trauma or by minimal or no trauma in pathologically weakened bone. Most fractures occur in the thoracic and lumbar spine. Traumatic fractures are often due to motor vehicle collisions that cause flexion and flexion-and-distraction fractures. Falls from a significant height can cause **burst fractures**. Osteoporosis is the underlying cause of most pathological fractures. Metastatic disease can also weaken bone, leading to fracture. Primary carcinoma from the lung, prostate, breast, and kidney are all known to spread to the spine, and in some cases, back pain due to a compression fracture is the first symptom to cause the patient to seek medical care. Multiple myeloma and lymphoma cause primary bone lesions that may lead to compression fractures.

Fractures caused by osteoporosis may be initially asymptomatic with an insidious onset of pain. Midline back pain with **point tenderness** is the hallmark symptom. The fracture often causes collapse of the vertebral body, leading to severe pain, deformity, nerve compression, and loss of stature. The most common type of fracture is an **anterior wedge fracture** (■ Figure 6-10), which causes the anterior portion of the vertebral body to collapse, altering normal load-bearing on both the fractured vertebra and the surrounding vertebrae and increasing thoracic kyphosis. Patients attempt to compensate for the pain and deformity by changing their posture with secondary pain in the hips, sacroiliac joints, and spinal joints. **Hip flexor contractures** due to **iliopsoas shortening** may also occur.

As with hip fractures, morbidity and mortality in elderly patients with compression fractures are

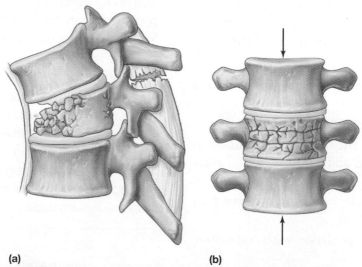

(a)   **(b)**

FIGURE 6-10 Two types of vertebral fractures: (a) anterior wedge compression fracture with disruption of the ligament caused by a flexion injury and (b) compression fracture of a vertebral body caused by axial loading forces.

- Sciatica refers to nerve pain that radiates from the low back down to the legs. Neuropathy may be caused by disk herniation, osteophytes, or spinal stenosis. Diskectomy may be required if conservative therapy fails.
- Sacroiliac joint dysfunction is caused by osteoarthritis of the synovial joints that join the sacrum to the iliac bones. Patients often have a positive Fortin finger sign. Treatment includes physical therapy and SI joint injections.
- Scoliosis is a complex, three-dimensional deformity of the spine, most commonly appearing during adolescence. Treatment may include bracing with TLSO, or in extreme cases, spinal fusion with placement of contoured rods, wires, and screws to straighten the spine.
- Compression fractures of the vertebral bodies are often the result of osteoporosis but may also be caused by metastatic disease or severe trauma. Fractures cause the vertebral body to collapse, leading to deformity and pain. Morbidity and mortality are associated with prolonged immobilization. Treatment includes vertebroplasty.

typically due to secondary medical conditions such as pneumonia, deep vein thrombosis, pulmonary embolism, skin breakdown, and gastric ulceration associated with prolonged bed rest. Protracted inactivity also worsens osteoporosis. Treatment may include a TLSO brace and inpatient rehabilitation. Fractures due to osteoporosis may be treated with vertebroplasty or kyphoplasty.

Diagnostic Studies

Physical examination and imaging studies play the most significant role in the diagnosis and treatment of spinal disease.

Tests, Signs, and Maneuvers

Common orthopedic tests, signs, and maneuvers performed during the physical examination of the spine include:

- Babinski: positive for myelopathy affecting the lower extremities
- café au lait spots: may be present in scoliosis
- fabere sign: acronym for the maneuvers included in the Patrick test (**f**lexion, **ab**duction, **e**xternal **r**otation, **e**xtension)
- femoral nerve stretch test: positive for nerve root irritation at L3-L4
- Gaenslen (gānz'-lən): positive with sacroiliac disease
- Lhermitte (lār'-mēt): positive for cervical cord injury or unstable cervical spine
- Patrick test: positive for sacroiliac joint disorders

- skin crease: indicative of spondylolisthesis
- Spurling test: indicative of nerve root compression in the cervical spine
- straight leg raise, also called Lasègue (lah-sāg'): positive for sciatica

The acronym fabere is easily confused with Faber, an eponym associated with anemia. This acronym is written in all lowercase.

On physical examination, he only has about 20% of normal lateral rotation. He has no forward flexion. He has about 20% of normal extension and positive Spurling sign on the left. His neurologic exam shows that he has a positive Tinel over the left wrist. He also has some sensory changes in the left C6-7 distribution. He has increased reflexes in the lower extremities compared to the upper as well as 2-beat clonus bilaterally, but negative Babinski signs. He also has some sensory changes in the left L5-S1 distribution, and straight leg raise is positive at about 70 degrees. His lumbar motion is restricted to 30% of normal, with most pain on flexion.

Pause 6-7 What is a 2-beat clonus?

Imaging

Imaging techniques play a central role in the diagnosis of spinal disease. X-rays, MRI, and myelography are the mainstays of diagnostic imaging techniques for spinal pathology.

X-Ray Views

X-rays of the spine are typically taken in the AP, lateral, and oblique views. An **open-mouth view** is used to detect **odontoid fractures**. The odontoid process (dens) is a vertical projection of C2 that is attached to the skull base by way of ligaments. This particular bone may be fractured in forceful flexion movements as might occur in a motor vehicle collision.

> TECHNIQUE: Multidetector, multislice CT was performed with multiplanar reformatting in sagittal, coronal, and axial reconstructions with very thin 0.7 mm axial sections.
>
> FINDINGS: Vertebral heights are well maintained. Minimal anterolisthesis at L4-5. Severe disk space narrowing at L5-S1. Mild foraminal narrowing at L3-4, moderate at L4-5, and severe at L5-S1 secondary to facet hypertrophy. Mild canal stenosis at L5-S1. Mild disk bulges at L3-4 and L4-5.

Myelography

Myelography is an imaging technique for visualizing the spinal structures. Using a needle, contrast material is injected into the subarachnoid space of the spinal cord. Real-time images using fluoroscopy are taken that allow examination of the spinal cord, nerve roots, blood vessels, and meninges to document spacial abnormalities and nerve compressions. A CT myelogram combines injection of contrast material with computed tomography to better define the spinal anatomy. CT myelography can detect disk herniations, nerve root compression, spinal cord compression, and degenerative changes of the spine. CT myelography is most useful in planning surgical procedures of the spine.

> Axial cervical CT myelogram demonstrates marked hypertrophy of the right facet joints, resulting in tight restriction of the neuroforaminal recess and lateral neural foramen.

MRI

MRI studies are particularly useful for diagnosing spinal disease, especially disk herniations and other soft-tissue related disorders of the spine.

> A T2-weighted sagittal MRI shows multilevel disk herniation and spondylosis causing bilateral neuroforaminal stenosis and moderate central canal stenosis. There is no myelomalacia.

> An ovoid ventral epidural defect is present just inferior to the L5-S1 disk, resulting in mass effect on the right S1 nerve root and causing ventral flattening of the thecal sac. This abnormality demonstrates intermediate signal intensity on the T1-weighted image and becomes mildly hyperintense on T2-weighted sequences.

> Short recovery time T1-weighted spin-echo sagittal MRI scan demonstrates marked spinal stenosis of the cervical canal at C1-2 resulting from formation of a pannus surrounding the dens in a patient with rheumatoid arthritis. Long recovery time T2-weighted fast spin-echo sagittal MRI scan shows the effect of the pannus on the anterior canal.

Therapeutic Procedures

There is an array of procedures used to treat back pain. First-line therapy begins with physical therapy, patient education, and NSAIDs. Steroid injections into the affected area of the spine are quite common and are used if more conservative modalities fail. As a last resort, surgical procedures may be performed.

Spinal Injections

The spinal nerves are protected by the dura and the sleeve-like space around the dura called the epidural space. Nerves exit the spinal cord and pass through the epidural space. Epidural steroid injections are both diagnostic and therapeutic; relief of the patient's pain confirms the source of the pain. Using **fluoroscopic localization** to ensure exact placement of the needle and flow of the injectate, an anesthetic is injected to immediately numb the nerve and then corticosteroids are injected to relieve the inflammatory component of the radicular pain. Maximum relief typically occurs two to three days following the injection after the inflammation has had time to subside. Injections typically use Omnipaque (a nonionic contrast media) to localize the needle followed by instillation of preservative-free lidocaine 1% to deaden the nerve and then a corticosteroid such as preservative-free Depo-Medrol or Celestone to reduce inflammation. Injections may be given in a series of three treatments over the course of several months.

 Pause 6-8 Compare the terms instillation and installation.

Epidural steroid injections (ESI) and are often abbreviated **CESI** (cervical), **TESI** (thoracic), and **LESI** (lumbar) and dictated as initials, not acronyms. Epidural injections at any level of the spine can be performed using an interlaminar or transforaminal approach. Lumbar injections may also take a caudal approach. Interlaminar injections deliver medication to the posterior epidural space by passing the needle through the ligamentum flavum. This approach may use a **loss-of-resistance** technique to sense the needle placement within the epidural space. A transforaminal epidural steroid injection involves injection of an anesthetic and corticosteroid mixture through the neural foramen to treat the nerve roots.

A caudal epidural steroid injection is a procedure for injecting anesthetic and a corticosteroid through the **sacral hiatus**. Medication spreads in the cephalad direction to treat the L5-S1 joint and the lower lumbar levels.

> PROCEDURE: Transforaminal epidural steroid injection of the right L4 and L5 nerve roots under fluoroscopic guidance using a C-arm fluoroscope.
>
> DESCRIPTION: ... A 22-gauge, 3½-inch Quincke needle was directed in a gun-barrel fashion toward the tip of the pars. Then 0.5 mL of Omnipaque 150 contrast was slowly injected and delineated the nerve root and epidural space but did not spread to the vascular plexus. Subsequently, 0.5 mL of preservative-free lidocaine and 6 mg of preservative-free Celestone were injected.

Medial branch blocks are steroid injections directed at the medial branch nerves to treat facet arthropathy. Medical branch blocks may be performed in the cervical, lumbar, or lumbosacral areas.

> PROCEDURE: Left C2-3, C3-4, and C4-5 medial branch nerve blocks under fluoroscopic guidance using an OEC 9800 Super C-arm fluoroscope.
>
> DESCRIPTION: ... A 23-gauge, 2½-inch Quincke needle was directed toward the left C2-3, C3-4, and C4-5 articular pillars at the direct center where the medial branch nerves are located. Then 0.25 mL of Omnipaque 150 contrast was injected at each site to confirm needle placement. Subsequently, 3 mg of preservative-free Celestone and 0.25 mL of preservative-free lidocaine 1% were injected.

Spinal Surgery

Invasive spinal surgery is usually considered a treatment of last resort. After conservative and minimally invasive modalities have been exhausted and the patient has neurologic symptoms or symptoms that interfere significantly with activities of daily living, surgery may be performed.

Spinal Fusion

Spinal fusion is a type of arthrodesis that affixes two spinal levels, preventing movement between the two, and therefore preventing nerve compression. Fusions are performed after removing a disk, vertebral body, lamina, or bilateral facets. To fuse two vertebral bodies, the intervertebral disk is removed and a 1 to 2-inch piece of bone, called a **strut graft**, is put in its place. The strut maintains the position of the vertebral bodies and provides a substrate for new bone to build upon until eventually the two bones are stitched together as a single unit. Bone grafts may consist of the patient's own bone (an autograft) or **cadaveric bone** (allograft or **allogeneic bone**). A third option is the use of **bone morphogenetic protein (BMP)** that stimulates bone growth (osteoinduction). An autograft consists of morsels of bone taken from the patient's iliac crest, or the graft may be local bone obtained from the concurrent decompression (ie, bone retrieved from the laminectomy, corpectomy, or facetectomy).

To increase the success of the fusion, anterior or posterior **interbody cages** (■ **Figure 6-11**) may be used. These cages are packed with bone-graft material and placed on their side in the interbody space. The mesh-like structure of the cage allows the graft material to expand through the walls of the cage to completely fuse the two bones. The cage itself is rigid so it maintains the disk-space height. Cages may be made of carbon fiber, **PEEK** (polyethylethylketone), or titanium (eg, brand name **BAK cage**). PEEK cages are radiolucent whereas titanium cages are radiopaque.

> Review of his CT scan of the lumbar spine shows he has had a previous 4-level fusion. L4-5 and L5-S1 are fused with BAK cages. At L2-3, there is an interbody PEEK cage that is not fused, and L4-5 looks like it had a posterior fusion that is not fused. He has a dynamic fixation at L2-3 and L3-4.
>
> My recommendation would be to revise the upper 2 levels to remove the loose screws and do an interbody fusion at L3-4 and then a redo posterolateral fusion with redo instrumentation at L2, L3, and L4.

A vertebral fusion can take up to a year to complete, so hardware may be used to hold the vertebral components in position until the bones completely fuse. This hardware, also referred to as instrumentation, includes **pedicle screws**, rods, anterior or posterior cervical plates, cervical wiring, and facet screws (eg, Magerl screw). The fused vertebrae and hardware may be referred to as a **construct**. In most cases, the hardware remains in place indefinitely, but occasionally the hardware itself causes pain or becomes loose and must be removed.

> His x-ray shows good position of his construct, but there is a little bit of windshield-wiper effect around the screws, which indicates some mild loosening.

Posterior Lumbar Interbody Fusion

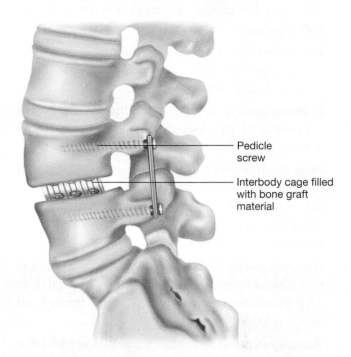

Pedicle screw

Interbody cage filled with bone graft material

FIGURE 6-11 An interbody cage is used to maintain the disk space and also provide structure for the bone graft material while it engrafts. Screws are placed in the pedicles with a plate to provide stability.

Decompression Procedures

The following list describes various surgical procedures used to relieve compression of a nerve caused by disk herniation, stenosis, or malalignment of a spinal component. The procedures described below may be performed on a single vertebral level or multiple levels.

Corpectomy (literally removal of a body): a surgical procedure that removes a vertebral body and the adjacent intervertebral disks. This procedure is typically performed for patients with a spinal fracture, tumor, or infection that is compressing a nerve. After removing the vertebra, the spine must be stabilized with a bone graft and instrumentation. This procedure in particular carries the risk of spinal cord damage leading to quadriplegia. To help prevent this, spinal cord function can be monitored intraoperatively using **somatosensory evoked potentials (SEPs)**.

Facetectomy: a surgical procedure to remove part of the facet joint. This procedure is used to decompress nerves or to gain access to the disk space when approaching the spine from the posterior aspect. Bilateral facetectomy requires concurrent instrumentation for spinal stability.

Foraminotomy: a surgical procedure to enlarge the neural foramen to treat unilateral nerve compression.

Laminoplasty: a surgical procedure with a posterior approach that repositions the lamina to increase the size of the vertebral foramen.

Laminotomy: a surgical procedure that removes a portion of the lamina to decompress spinal nerves.

Hemilaminectomy and laminectomy: a surgical procedure that removes part or all of the lamina to decompress a spinal nerve (see Figure 6-7). Laminectomies may also be performed to gain access to the intervertebral disk.

Anterior cervical diskectomy (ACD): a surgical procedure to remove a cervical intervertebral disk. This procedure approaches the spine through an incision made in the front of the neck.

Anterior cervical diskectomy and fusion (ACDF): a surgical procedure to remove a cervical intervertebral disk followed by placement of graft material to fuse two or more spinal levels (■ Figure 6-12). Instrumentation, such as a cervical plate or rods and screws, may also be used to immobilize the joint

until the fusion is complete. Because the incision is made in the front of the neck, an anterior surgical approach to the cervical spine carries the risk of vascular injury of the carotid and vertebral arteries, injury to the **recurrent laryngeal nerve** with vocal cord paralysis, and dysphagia from esophageal damage.

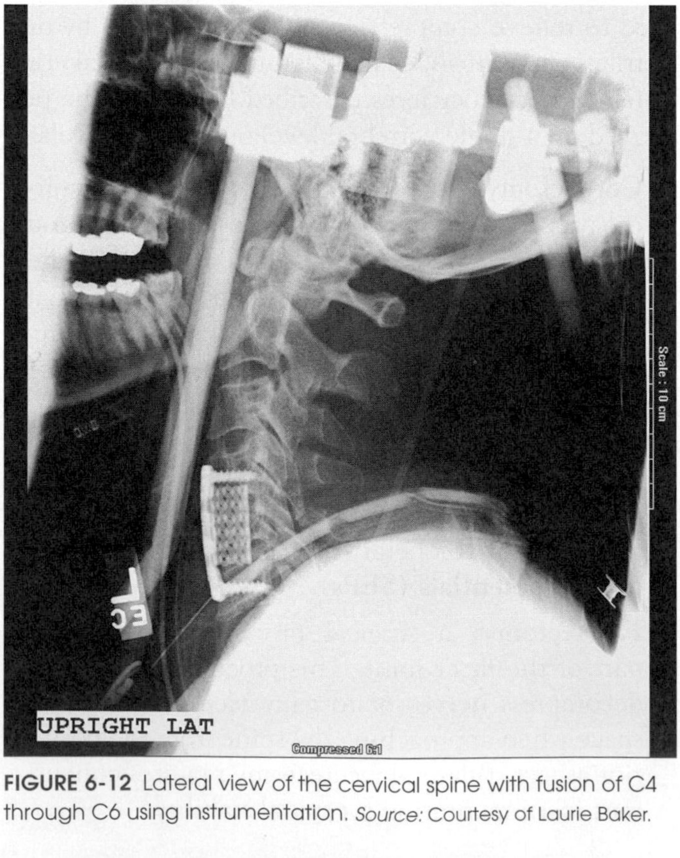

> The abbreviation ACDF is almost always dictated as opposed to the expanded phrase, but this abbreviation is fraught with problems. Three out of four of the letters in this abbreviation are difficult to distinguish (/a/ versus /h/, /d/ versus /z/ or /p/, /f/ versus /s/). As with all abbreviations, evaluate carefully and make sure the expanded term fits the current context.

Anterior lumbar interbody fusion (ALIF): a surgical procedure to remove a lumbar intervertebral disk. The surgery approaches the spine through the abdomen using a retroperitoneal or transperitoneal approach. Once the spine is reached, the anterior longitudinal ligament is raised and disk material is removed piecemeal using curettes and **pituitary rongeurs.** The endplates are removed and graft material is placed in the intervertebral space. Instrumentation may be applied to stabilize the construct. The anterior approach leaves the back muscles and nerves undisturbed, but carries the risk of ileus as well as bleeding from accidental nicking of major abdominal vessels.

Transforaminal lumbar interbody fusion (TLIF): a surgical procedure that approaches the lumbar spine from the posterior aspect. This procedure goes through the neural foramen to access and remove the disk material. A fusion is performed using one or two interbody cages.

Posterior lumbar interbody fusion (PLIF): a surgical procedure to remove a lumbar intervertebral disk and fuse the vertebral bodies. This procedure approaches the vertebra using a posterior approach with a midline incision directly over the disk. A posterior approach to the disk requires the removal of part or all of the lamina. After removal of the disk, a bone graft is placed to promote fusion of the vertebral bodies. Fusion may be aided by

UPRIGHT LAT

Compressed 6:1

FIGURE 6-12 Lateral view of the cervical spine with fusion of C4 through C6 using instrumentation. *Source:* Courtesy of Laurie Baker.

an interbody cage. Instrumentation may be used to immobilize the joint until complete fusion has occurred.

> TLIF and PLIF are often dictated as *P-līf* and *T-līf*. The P and T are extremely difficult to distinguish. Listen carefully for contextual clues or flag the abbreviation for clarification by the dictator.

Extreme lateral interbody fusion (XLIF): a minimally invasive procedure that approaches the disk space from the patient's side. The patient is placed in the lateral decubitus position during this procedure and a working port (a long tube with a retractor) is inserted through the patient's side, past the psoas muscle (transpsoas) until the port abuts the lateral side of the disk. The disk is removed and an interbody cage is placed. A lateral plate with screws may be placed to add stability to the fusion. This approach is less invasive and requires less recovery time because no back muscles are cut and a laminectomy or facetectomy is not required to access the disk space (as is required from a posterior approach). XLIF can be performed on lumbar levels L4 and above.

Axial lumbar interbody fusion (Axial LIF): a minimally invasive procedure that accesses the L5-S1 disk by passing a working port under the sacrum (entering just lateral to the coccyx) and through the S1 vertebral body. The L5-S1 disk material is removed and a stabilizing screw is placed through S1 and into the L5 vertebral body.

Intervertebral disk arthroplasty, also called **artificial disk replacement (ADR)** or **total disk replacement (TDR):** a surgical procedure that replaces degenerative intervertebral disks with artificial disks. This procedure does not require fusion or instrumentation.

Intradiscal electrothermal therapy (IDET), also referred to as **intradiscal electrothermal annuloplasty (IDEA):** a minimally invasive procedure to treat diskogenic pain that uses radiofrequency energy (heat) to seal (ie, repair) fissures in the disk annulus and perhaps deaden nerves (nociceptors) within the disk to reduce pain.

Vertebroplasty

Vertebroplasty is a minimally invasive procedure to inject orthopedic cement into a fractured vertebra to increase strength and the ability to withstand physiologic loads while the patient is erect. Using fluoroscopy to guide placement of an 11- to 13-gauge bone biopsy needle, a trocar is introduced into the fractured vertebra through the pedicle (**transpedicular approach**). **Polymethylmethacrylate (PMMA)** is injected directly into the vertebra, often on both the right and left sides of the vertebral body. The methylmethacrylate polymer is initially a thick paste but quickly hardens. An antibiotic, such as tobramycin, may be added to the paste to decrease the chance of infection. Barium or tantalum may also be added to make the cement radiopaque. The procedure can be performed under local or general anesthesia.

Kyphoplasty is a form of vertebroplasty that uses an inflated balloon to expand the vertebral body before injecting the cement polymer. The fractured vertebra is first drilled out to make a hollow space for the balloon, called a **bone tamp** (brand name KyphX). The balloon is inflated to tamp down (compact) the trabecular bone fragments and elevate the collapsed endplate. The balloon is deflated and removed before injecting the polymer. Kyphoplasty carries less risk of cement extrusion into the spinal canal compared to vertebroplasty because the polymer is placed inside a cavity. In addition, a larger amount of polymer can be placed in the vertebra, making the vertebral body stronger, restoring the original vertebral height, and lessening spinal deformity. Proper **load bearing** is also restored to adjacent vertebrae, lessening the chance of subsequent fractures on either side of the repaired vertebra. Kyphoplasty is not appropriate for burst fractures because the integrity of the posterior vertebral cortex may be disrupted, allowing cement to leak into the spinal canal.

Pharmacology

In addition to the medications covered in Chapter 5, two other classes of drugs, tricyclic antidepressants and anticonvulsants, are commonly used to treat back and neck pain, especially chronic pain.

Neuropathic Analgesics

Several medications originally prescribed for epilepsy have also been found to be helpful in alleviating neuropathic pain. The most common neuropathic drug prescribed to treat neuralgia and peripheral neuropathy is gabapentin (brand name Neurontin). Gabapentin was originally prescribed for epilepsy but it, along with other anticonvulsants (**Table 6-1**), is commonly prescribed for chronic neurological pain.

Table 6-1 Neuropathic Analgesics

Generic	Brand Name	Dose
gabapentin	Neurontin	100 mg, 300 mg, 400 mg, 600 mg, 800 mg
carbamazepine	Tegretol Tegretol XR	100 mg 100 mg, 200 mg, 400 mg
pregabalin	Lyrica	25 mg, 50 mg, 75 mg, 100 mg, 150 mg, 200 mg, 225 mg, 300 mg

Tricyclic Antidepressants

A specific class of antidepressants, referred to as the tricyclic antidepressants (TCAs), have pain-relieving properties in addition to their psychiatric indications. These medications (**Table 6-2**) are especially helpful to patients suffering from chronic pain because protracted periods of pain are known to induce clinical depression.

Table 6-2 Tricyclic Antidepressants

Generic	Brand Name	Dose
amitriptyline		10 mg, 25 mg, 50 mg, 75 mg, 100 mg, 150 mg
desipramine	Norpramin	10 mg, 25 mg, 50 mg, 75 mg, 100 mg, 150 mg
imipramine	Tofranil	10 mg, 25 mg, 50 mg
nortriptyline	Pamelor	10 mg, 25 mg, 50 mg, 75 mg

Exercises

Using Context to Make Decisions

Use sample report A on page 182 to answer questions 1–7.

1. Would blank #1 be "severely limited" or "within normal limits"? _____

_____

2. All cranial nerves tested normal. How would you fill in blank #2 _____

_____

3. Gaenslen and Patrick signs relate to which diagnosis?

_____

4. How likely is it that diagnosis #4 would be sciatica?

_____

5. Is diagnosis #3 transcribed correctly? If not, how would you correct it? _____

_____

6. What word is transcribed incorrectly in the Plan? _____

7. Which side of the back will be injected 2 weeks following the first injection? _____

_____

Use sample report B on page 183 to answer questions 8–10.

8. What word was transcribed incorrectly in Finding #1? _____

9. What word was transcribed incorrectly in Conclusion #2? _____

10. The radiologist dictated this patient's age as 33, but the date of birth calculates the age to be 73. Which is more likely to be correct? _____

_____

11. Explain why "intraarticular injections" is the correct phrase and not "interarticular injections."

_____

12. What word best completes the following statement?

_____

The MRI shows involvement of the cauda equina, although the patient does not complain of _____ or bladder dysfunction.

13. What medication would complete the following dictation? _____

_____

ASSESSMENT: Failed back surgery syndrome status post ALIF at L3-L4 and L4-L5. Will renew her prescription for _____ 300 mg t.i.d. to titrate up to 600 mg t.i.d. (total 1800 mg per day) over the next week.

14. Which area of the spine is described in the following MRI? _____

There is evidence of ACDF with plate and screws seen anteriorly. The cord is normal in size and signal intensity. Cerebellar tonsils are normal in position. Medulla is normal. Mild degenerative change is seen in the atlantoaxial joint. Odontoid appears intact.

15. In the following excerpt, why is L4 and L5 written with "and" instead of hyphenated (L4-L5)? _____

_____

OPERATION: Transforaminal epidural steroid injection of the right L4 and L5 nerve roots under fluoroscopic guidance using a C-arm fluoroscope.

Terms Checkup

Complete the multiple choice questions for Chapter 6 located at www.myhealthprofessionskit.com. To access the questions, select the discipline "Medical Transcription," then click on the title of this book, *Advanced Medical Transcription.*

Look It Up

Using the guidelines described on page xvii, complete a research project on failed back surgery syndrome.

Transcription Practice

1. Transcribe the key terms and phrases for Chapter 6.
2. Complete the proofing and transcription practice exercises for Chapter 6.

Sample Report A

PHYSICAL EXAMINATION

BACK: There is no pathologic kyphoscoliosis, scars, or masses. Lumbar range of motion is _____(1)_____ in all planes. Flexion is 20 degrees. Extension and right and left lateral flexion are 10 degrees. There is tenderness over both SI joints. Gaenslen sign and Patrick sign are strongly positive on the right only. Straight leg raise is negative bilaterally.

NEUROLOGICAL: Cranial nerves _____(2)_____ are intact. There is sensory loss at the left L4 dermatome. Deep tendon reflexes are 2+ Achilles and patellar symmetrically. She has an antalgic, short-stride, heel-toe gait with both knees flexed at 30 degrees during midstance, and her trunk is hunched over forward. She can do the toe walk and the heel walk.

DIAGNOSES

1. Bilateral lumbar _____(3)_____ syndrome.
2. Right _____(4)_____ joint dysfunction.
3. L5, S1 disk herniation.
4. _____.

PLAN

We will schedule her for right L3 through S1 medial branch nerve blocks to decrease the back pain and to increase her lumbar range of motion. In 2 weeks we will schedule her for the same injections on the contralateral side. If she gets good relief from the medial branch nerve blocks we can then advance to radiofrequency neuropathies of the medial branch nerves that innervate the lower lumbar facet joints. This will provide her with at least half a year of significant pain relief. Will also inject her right sacroiliac joint to decrease the lower back and buttock pain.

Sample Report B

FINDINGS
1. Two views of the lumbar spine demonstrate multilevel degenerative disk disease with endplate cupping, which may be secondary to the disk disease and/or the patient's osteoporosis. No high-grade compression fracture, deformity, or spondylolysis identified. There may be very slight left lateral listhesis of L2 in relation to L3, secondary or concurrent with disk disease.
2. Facet arthropathy in lower lumbar levels.
3. Pelvis and bilateral hips appear grossly intact.
4. The sacrum appears intact.

CONCLUSION
1. Degenerative disk disease, scoliosis, and osteoporosis of the spine.
2. Endplate cupping deformity, particularly at the T12-L1 and L1-2 levels, likely reflects the patient's degenerative disk disease and/or osteoporosis. Known high-grade compression fracture deformity identified.
3. Mild, left lateral listhesis of L2 in relation to L3.
4. Sacroiliac joints are sclerotic, suggesting sacroiliitis.

7

Urology and Nephrology

Learning Objectives

After completing this chapter, you should be able to comprehend and correctly transcribe terminology related to:

▶ renal failure, chronic kidney disease, and glomerular disease

▶ infection of the upper and lower urinary tract

▶ voiding dysfunction

▶ urinary calculi

▶ urinary obstruction

▶ prostatic disease

▶ laboratory and imaging tests used to diagnose and monitor diseases of the urinary tract

▶ therapeutic procedures used to treat diseases of the urinary tract

▶ drugs used to treat disorders of the urinary tract and to maintain electrolyte and fluid homeostasis

Introduction

The kidneys play a critical role in fluid and electrolyte homeostasis, and disorders of the kidneys can have profound effects on the entire body. The kidneys receive 21% of cardiac output (about 1200 mL/min), indicative of the tremendous amount of work they must accomplish. The kidneys play a key role in:

- maintaining electrolyte balance, critical for nerve and muscle function
- regulating acid-base balance, critical for respiration
- maintaining the hematocrit through the production of erythropoietin
- regulating blood pressure through the release of renin
- activating vitamin D and regulating serum calcium and phosphate
- regulating osmolality of the extracellular fluid
- eliminating metabolic waste

Anatomy and Physiology

Understanding the architecture of the kidney is extremely helpful in understanding disorders of the kidney. Review ■ Figure 7-1, carefully noting the anatomy of the kidney.

The capillaries that make up the glomerulus have a unique vessel-wall structure that is integral to the filtering function of the glomerulus. Glomerular capillaries have a fenestrated endothelium, a basement membrane, and an epithelium consisting of podocytes. Together, these three layers selectively filter the blood, allowing water, electrolytes, glucose, amino acids, creatinine, urea, as well as other waste products to pass through to the capsular space while retaining platelets, red and white cells, and protein molecules (■ Figure 7-2). Cells are prevented from passing due to their size. Proteins are retained within the capillary space by both their size and their electrical charge. The basement membrane of the glomerular capillaries has a net negative charge that repels the negatively charged protein molecules, preventing them from passing through to the capsular side of the capillary wall. The majority of plasma calcium

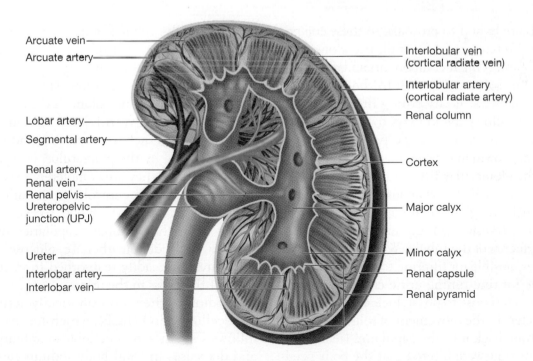

Renal artery → Segmental arteries → Lobar arteries → Interlobar arteries → Arcuate arteries → Interlobular arteries → Afferent arterioles → Glomerulus → Efferent arterioles → Peritubular capillaries → Interlobular veins → Arcuate veins → Interlobar veins → Lobar veins → Renal vein

FIGURE 7-1 Renal anatomy including renal circulation.

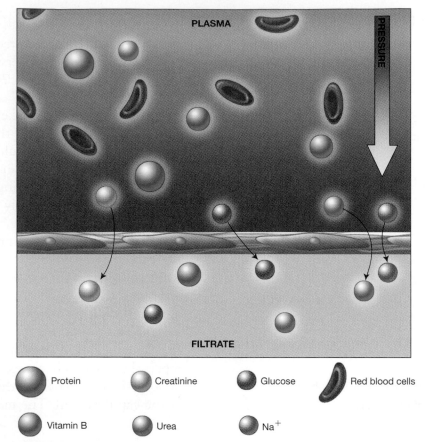

PLASMA

PRESSURE

FILTRATE

| | Protein | | Creatinine | | Glucose | | Red blood cells |

| | Vitamin B | | Urea | | Na$^+$ |

FIGURE 7-2 Depiction of glomerular filtration and selectivity of membrane.

and fatty acids are bound to proteins, so these components are not filtered either. Overall, the glomerulus retains proteins and cellular components and allows the majority of other solutes to pass into the glomerular filtrate. This somewhat undiscerning first step of the filtration process allows the kidneys to excrete a high percentage of toxins with a single pass through the glomerulus. The Bowman capsule has a capsular space that collects the **glomerular filtrate**.

The kidney normally filters about 180 liters of fluid each day through the glomerular capillaries. The glomerular filtrate is transformed into urine as is traverses the various segments of the tubule. While the glomerulus is largely responsible for filtering toxins, the tubules are responsible for fine-tuning urine composition and concentration in response to physiologic needs. Tubular reabsorption refers to the movement of solutes from the glomerular filtrate back into the capillaries (ie, retrieving components that were filtered that the body needs to retain). Tubular secretion refers to the elimination of unneeded components by moving items from the tubular circulation into the tubular lumen (■ **Figure 7-3**). Reabsorbed items are returned to the general circulation and secreted items are removed through the urine.

Within the tubules, glucose and amino acids are reabsorbed into the peritubular capillaries, and adjustments are made to the concentrations of sodium (Na$^+$), potassium (K$^+$), hydrogen ions (H$^+$), and bicarbonate (HCO$_3^-$). Normal urine volume is 0.6 to 2 L/d, but most people produce between 1.0 and 1.5 L/d.

Metabolites such as creatinine and urea are completely filtered by the glomerulus, and since they are not reabsorbed, they are completely excreted. Tubular secretion is used to control the amount of potassium and hydrogen ions in the blood, so excess potassium is secreted from the peritubular capillaries into the tubule. Sodium, chloride, bicarbonate, glucose, amino acids, and water are readily reabsorbed from the tubules to prevent their loss in the urine.

Sodium is the most osmotically active ion in the extracellular fluid (ECF), which means water always follows sodium across cellular membranes. Increases and decreases in total-body sodium cause concomitant increases or decreases in total-body water. The kidneys contribute to total-body fluid volume by excreting more or less sodium in response to dietary intake and other physiologic conditions. Increased sodium excretion (**natriuresis**) causes increased water

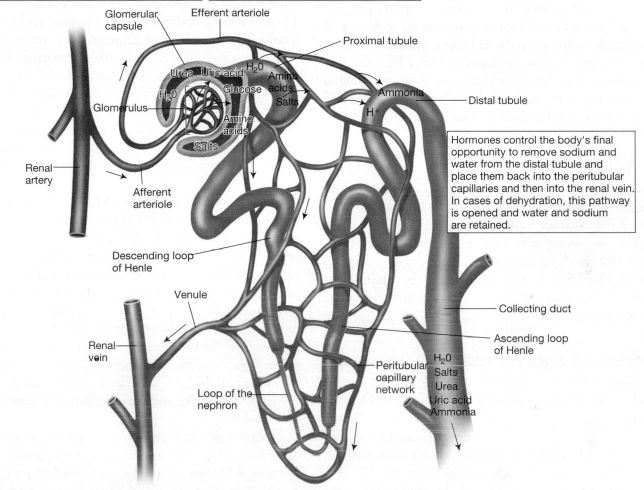

Glomerular Filtration

Blood from the renal artery is filtered in the glomerulus. The filtered product which contains water, salts, nutrients, and waste products is called the glomerular filtrate.

Tubular Reabsorption

Nutrients and salts are actively reabsorbed and transported to the peritubular capillary network and some water is passively reabsorbed into the peritubular capillaries.

Tubular Secretion

Some substances are actively secreted from the peritubular capillaries into the distal tubule for removal from the body.

Hormones control the body's final opportunity to remove sodium and water from the distal tubule and place them back into the peritubular capillaries and then into the renal vein. In cases of dehydration, this pathway is opened and water and sodium are retained.

FIGURE 7-3 Filtration, reabsorption, and secretion within the nephron.

excretion (**diuresis**). It is imperative that the body maintain plasma sodium concentrations within a normal range of 136–145 mEq/L, so sodium may be excreted in the urine or shifted to extracellular spaces in order to maintain the correct plasma sodium concentration. Therefore, plasma sodium levels are not indicative of total body sodium and do not reflect dietary levels of sodium.

The **glomerular filtration rate (GFR)** is a measure of the volume of fluid that passes through the glomerulus per unit of time. The GFR is an important indicator of kidney function. To respond to physiologic needs, the body adjusts the GFR and the rate of reabsorption within the tubules by adjusting the resistance (ie, the hydrostatic pressure) in the afferent and efferent arterioles. Resistance is increased by constricting the vessels and decreased by dilating the vessels (compare this to the rate of water flowing through a large-diameter tube compared to a small-diameter tube—the smaller diameter decreases the rate of flow). Increased resistance in the peritubular capillaries causes blood to flow more slowly through the tubules, resulting in more time for reabsorption to occur. For example, when systemic blood pressure falls, pressure sensors within each nephron trigger the release of renin, causing the efferent arterioles to constrict, thereby raising the arterial resistance and pressure. This causes movement of filtrate through the tubules to slow down, allowing more sodium and water to be reabsorbed. Urine volume decreases, total-body fluid volume increases, and the systemic blood pressure rises.

Acute Renal Failure

Renal failure is traditionally categorized as acute or chronic. **Acute renal failure (ARF)**, also called **acute renal injury**, is a life-threatening disorder caused by injury to both kidneys that results in rapidly progressive deterioration of kidney function in a matter of hours or days. Injury to the kidneys is typically secondary to trauma, illness, or surgery, or may be caused by an intrinsic disorder of the kidney itself. Impaired renal function is manifested by an inability to maintain fluid homeostasis (fluid and electrolyte balance) with widespread systemic consequences.

There are many causes for ARF, and the causes are divided into three major categories: prerenal, intrinsic (also called intrarenal), and postrenal. The categories refer to the location of the initiating event. Prerenal causes are systemic disorders that originate on the incoming side of the kidney's circulation. Postrenal are those causes that occur on the outgoing side of the kidneys (ie, in the ureters, bladder, or urethra). Intrinsic ARF is caused by direct insult to the nephrons.

Prerenal Renal Failure

Prerenal ARF is the most common and is due to inadequate **renal perfusion**. Filtration within the kidneys is dependent upon blood pressure to "push" the blood through the glomerulus. When the pressure of the blood coming into the kidneys is decreased, the kidney's ability to adequately filter the blood is greatly diminished. In addition, markedly decreased perfusion reduces oxygen available to the cells and the kidney tissue suffers necrosis. The vast majority of energy expenditure within the kidney occurs in the tubular epithelium, so the tubules are the most likely structures to suffer irreversible damage from hypoxemia.

Hypoperfusion may be the result of cardiac disease with decreased cardiac output (eg, myocardial infarction, valvular damage). A decrease in systemic blood pressure may also be caused by shock (systemic vasodilation), dehydration, or the shift of fluids from the intravascular space to the extravascular space. **Renal artery stenosis** caused by atherosclerosis, embolism, or thrombosis can also lead to ARF. If the underlying condition is addressed quickly, prerenal ARF is often reversible. Nephrons cannot regenerate, so the damage is not reversible if tubular necrosis occurs.

Intrinsic Renal Failure

Intrinsic renal failure is marked by parenchymatous damage to the kidney. Damage can begin in the glomerular capillaries, any of the small renal vessels, renal tubular epithelium, or in the renal interstitium. There is some overlap between prerenal and intrinsic renal failure, as prerenal causes can evolve to intrinsic damage if not corrected within a matter of hours. Structural and functional damage may be caused by cytotoxic insults. Inflammatory states caused by pyelonephritis or autoimmune disorders such as systemic lupus erythematosus are also implicated. Kidney disease that begins as a glomerular disorder (discussed in the following section) can also lead to intrinsic disease.

Acute tubular necrosis (ATN) is the most common form of intrinsic renal failure and accounts for the majority of hospital admissions due to acute renal failure. The function of the renal tubules and the renal capillaries are interdependent and damage to one typically leads to damage to the other, kicking off a vicious cycle of injury that is difficult to stop. The hallmark of ATN is **isosthenuria**, which is the inability to adjust the concentration of urine in response to physiologic conditions. Urine osmolality is an indicator of the tubules' ability to concentrate urine; values below 50 mOsm/kg indicate impaired concentration ability.

Exogenous and endogenous nephrotoxins can also cause ATN. The most common exogenous toxins to cause ATN are aminoglycoside antibiotics (gentamicin, streptomycin, and tobramycin) and radiographic contrast media. Renal failure can begin after 5–10 days of exposure to an aminoglycoside. Measurement of **peak and trough levels** of gentamicin is important for attaining therapeutic levels while minimizing toxicity. A "**gent trough**" (gentamicin trough) is the blood concentration of gentamicin immediately preceding a dose (presumably the point of lowest blood concentration). The "**gent peak**" is the blood level taken 30 minutes following administration of gentamicin, presumably the point of highest blood concentration.

Other nephrotoxic drugs include NSAIDs, ACE inhibitors, ARBs, cyclosporin, acyclovir, indinavir, methotrexate, and amphotericin B. These drugs have a direct cytotoxic effect on tubular epithelial cells. The risk of toxicity increases in patients with comorbidities. Ethylene glycol, the main ingredient in antifreeze, is also nephrotoxic.

Hypoxia causes the epithelial cells of the tubules to slough off, plugging the tubules with dead cells. The tubules may also become occluded with casts (1) composed of heme pigments (from hemoglobin and myoglobin) when renal concentrations rise due to widespread hemolysis or severe muscle damage. Crystal formation from megadoses of vitamin C or uric acid deposits from hyperuricemia can also occlude the tubules. These tubular occlusions evolve to a secondary postrenal failure.

Postrenal Failure

Postrenal causes of kidney failure include obstruction of the ureters, bladder, or urethra. Obstruction may be caused by **benign prostatic hypertrophy (BPH)**, prostate cancer, **neurogenic bladder**, stone disease, or a clot within the urinary collecting system. Strictures, tumors, and phimosis may also obstruct flow of urine through the urethra. Regardless of the location of the obstruction, urine backs up into the renal medulla, causing intraluminal fluid pressures to be exerted in the opposite direction of the normal flow and decreasing the GFR. Tubular filtering mechanisms that depend on pressure gradients and concentration gradients fail in these circumstances. Postrenal failure overlaps with intrinsic renal failure when crystals or proteins obstruct the tubules. A unilateral obstruction is typically compensated by the contralateral kidney, but bilateral obstruction quickly progresses to renal failure.

The first noticeable signs of renal failure may be weight gain from water retention and peripheral edema. Since ARF is oftentimes secondary to other medical conditions, symptoms of the primary illness may show themselves first. As uremia increases, the patient experiences headache, anorexia, nausea, vomiting, weakness, myoclonic jerks, seizures, confusion, asterixis, and hyperreflexia. Coma may ensue. The patient's breath may smell of ammonia. Electrolyte imbalances lead to **anasarca** (total-body edema). The renal tubules lose their ability to excrete hydrogen ions, producing a **high anion gap acidosis**. The respiratory system tries to compensate for the acidosis with **Kussmaul respirations** (deep, sighing respirations). The renal tubules also fail to regulate potassium, and the resultant hyperkalemia causes muscle weakness and potentially cardiac failure.

Diagnosis and Treatment

Laboratory studies of blood and urine are used to diagnose and monitor the course of acute renal failure. The metabolite creatinine is produced by muscle tissue throughout the body at a constant level. Because the only route of excretion for creatinine is through the kidneys, serum creatinine levels and the urine-to-plasma ratio of creatinine are important markers of renal function. A progressive, daily rise in serum creatinine is diagnostic of acute renal failure. Other laboratory studies used in the management of ARF include:

- specific gravity
- glomerular filtration rate (GFR)
- fractional excretion of sodium (FENa) (U/P Na ÷ U/P creatinine)
- urine osmolality
- urine-to-plasma osmolality
- urine sodium
- BUN-to-creatinine ratio
- plasma HCO_3^- (bicarbonate)
- serum phosphorus
- serum potassium
- renal failure index (Urine Na ÷ U/P creatinine ratio)

Ultrasound and ultrasound with Doppler may be useful in the diagnosis of acute renal failure. These studies are used instead of CT and MRI because contrast materials used in these imaging modalities are contraindicated in the setting of renal failure.

Unfortunately, management of acute renal failure is difficult and it carries a high mortality rate. The primary illness leading to acute renal failure must be addressed and reversed if possible. Nephrotoxic medications (eg, contrast materials, nephrotoxic antibiotics, heavy metal preparations, chemotherapeutic agents, NSAIDs) as well as medications that are cleared through renal excretion must be withdrawn or used with extreme caution.

Treatment of acute renal failure focuses on achieving volume homeostasis and correcting electrolyte imbalances. The problems encountered in acute renal failure are similar to those with chronic kidney failure, only the timeframe is protracted. Specific treatment strategies are similar and are explained in detail below under treatment

(1) Casts consist of a matrix of protein and may contain formed elements such as RBCs, WBCs, or tubular epithelial cells. Casts take on the shape and width of the tubules and are usually associated with a pathological process.

for chronic kidney disease. In the acute setting, treatment includes infusion of fluids with meticulous monitoring of **intake and output (I's & O's)** to prevent fluid overload. **Continuous renal replacement therapy** (ie, dialysis) may be required when fluid overload cannot be controlled or in the setting of **multiple organ dysfunction syndrome (MODS)**. Infection is the most common cause of death.

Patients at risk of nephrotoxicity from radiocontrast materials may be treated prophylactically with IV fluids and N-acetylcysteine (NAC) administered the day before and the day after imaging studies that use contrast materials.

Chronic Kidney Disease

Whereas acute renal failure develops over hours or days, **chronic kidney disease (CKD)** is marked by progressive deterioration of renal function over months to years. One in nine adults in the United States is affected by chronic kidney disease, which results from many types of renal insults and disorders, both genetic and acquired. The most common cause in the United States is diabetic nephropathy followed by **hypertensive nephroangiosclerosis**. The disease may be asymptomatic for years because of the slowly progressive nature of the disease plus the fact that the kidneys have tremendous capacity. Symptoms begin to appear when approximately two-thirds of glomerular filtration capacity is lost. Patients may have **renal insufficiency** that leads to end-stage disease. **End-stage renal disease (ESRD)** is defined as the loss of seven-eighths of the kidneys' filtration capacity, represented by a glomerular filtration rate of 10–15 mL/min or less.

In the early stages of the disease, the ability to concentrate urine is lost. As the disease progresses, the kidney loses the ability to adjust concentration and the urine osmolality becomes fixed at about 300 mOsm/kg, approximately the same osmolality as plasma. In advanced disease, the kidney can no longer regulate phosphate, acid (hydrogen ions), potassium, or phosphorus. Chronic kidney disease may be staged as follows:

stage 1: normal GFR (greater than 90 mL/min/ 1.73 m^2) with either persistent albuminuria or known structural or hereditary renal disease

stage 2: mild decrease in GFR (60–89 mL/min/ 1.73 m^2)

stage 3: moderate decrease in GFR (30–59 mL/ min/1.73 m^2)

stage 4: severe decrease in GFR (15–29 mL/ min/1.73 m^2)

stage 5: renal failure (GFR less than 15 mL/ min/1.73 m^2)

Risk factors for developing chronic kidney disease include:

- being African-American
- genetic predisposition
- polycystic kidney disease
- diabetes mellitus
- hypertension
- potassium deficiency
- urinary tract obstruction
- chronic glomerular disease
- chronic infection

The first and most common complaint of renal insufficiency is fatigue. Patients also complain of weakness, malaise, pruritus, and muscle cramps in the calves, especially at night. Anorexia with nausea and vomiting are common, as is a metallic taste in the mouth (**dysgeusia**). Neurological symptoms include irritability, difficulty concentrating, insomnia, memory defects, restless legs, and twitching. The patient often appears chronically ill with a yellowish color to the skin. A **uremic fetor** (fishy odor of the breath) may be noted and **uremic frost** (crystalized urea from sweat) may be seen on the skin.

The broad range of symptoms is indicative of the widespread systemic changes that occur when fluid homeostasis is lost. Chronic kidney disease eventually involves all body systems and is associated with significant morbidity and mortality. Manifestations of chronic kidney disease include:

Volume overload: the kidney loses the ability to control sodium concentration and excrete water, resulting in fluid retention and volume overload (hypervolemia).

Hypertension: elevated blood pressure resulting from hypervolemia is present in nearly all patients with advanced CKD. It may also be caused by activation of the renin-angiotensin-aldosterone system.

Hyperkalemia: increased serum potassium develops when the GFR falls to 10–20 mL/min. Changes in potassium levels from both endogenous (eg, hemolysis or trauma) or exogenous (diet, medications that decrease potassium secretion) sources are not well compensated and quickly lead to hyperkalemia. Potassium-sparing diuretics, ACE inhibitors, beta-blockers, NSAIDs, cyclosporine, tacrolimus, and ARBs can exacerbate hyperkalemia.

Metabolic acidosis: early on, the tubules lose the ability to excrete excess hydrogen ions (H^+), producing a mild acidosis (pH 7.30 to 7.35). Advancing disease leads to severe acidosis (pH less than 7.3). The blood pH must be maintained within a very tight range, so the acidosis is buffered by pulling calcium carbonate and calcium phosphate from the bone stores. Over time, the leaching of minerals from the bone leads to **renal osteodystrophy.**

Pericarditis: the lining of the heart becomes inflamed (pericarditis), presumably due to irritation of toxins that are not adequately removed from the blood. Symptoms include fever and pleuritic chest pain. Examination reveals pulsus paradoxus (2) and a pericardial friction rub.

Congestive heart failure: patients with ESRD have a high cardiac output due to fluid overload and chronic anemia. The additional cardiac workload causes **left ventricular hypertrophy.**

Anemia: ESRD causes severe anemia due to decreased production of red cells and decreased red cell survival. Erythropoietin production falls relative to the loss of functional renal mass, and the resultant decreased stimulation causes the bone marrow to produce fewer red blood cells. Decreased production may also result from deficiencies of iron, folate, and vitamin B_{12}.

Bleeding: platelet counts are only mildly decreased, but coagulopathy results from dysfunctional platelets. Platelets show decreased adhesiveness and aggregation resulting in a prolonged bleeding time. Patients typically have petechiae and purpura.

Disrupted mineral metabolism: impaired phosphorus excretion leads to **hyperphosphatemia** and a decrease in plasma **ionized calcium** due to calcium ions binding to phosphate molecules. The reduction in ionized calcium stimulates the parathyroid gland to secrete parathyroid hormone (PTH). High PTH levels stimulate osteoclasts and increase bone resorption, resulting in **osteitis**

fibrosa cystica. Bone lesions are most prominent in the phalanges and lateral ends of the clavicles.

Neuropathy: more than half of patients on dialysis suffer **sensorimotor polyneuropathy**, usually in a stocking-and-glove distribution. Deep tendon reflexes are also decreased, and patients complain of distal pain.

Encephalopathy: when the GFR falls below 10–15 mL/min, **renal encephalopathy** ensues. The encephalopathy is thought to be related to toxic levels of PTH, so control of hyperphosphatemia is important.

Diagnosis and Treatment

A diagnosis of renal insufficiency is made based mainly on serum and urine chemistries. Occasionally, ultrasound studies and renal biopsy are helpful. A stable but abnormal serum creatinine on successive days is most consistent with chronic kidney disease (compared to a rapidly climbing creatinine level that occurs in acute renal failure). Laboratory studies are notable for abnormal serum electrolytes, BUN, creatinine, phosphate, and calcium. Although creatinine is not a major contributor to the symptoms of kidney disease, it is a marker for other substances, many of which have yet to be identified, that do cause symptoms. A urinalysis is also integral to the diagnosis, including a microscopic study of the urinary sediment (typically referred to as a **UA with micro**). The sediment may reveal **broad, waxy casts** indicative of dilated, hypertrophic nephrons. Ultrasound studies typically reveal small, **echogenic kidneys.**

Pause 7-1 Which of the laboratory results in the sample dictation below are not within normal limits? Do they support a diagnosis of renal insufficiency? Why or why not?

Glucose 97, BUN 51, creatinine 3.4, potassium 4.7, sodium 146, chloride 104, CO_2 22.

---

(2) Pulsus paradoxus describes a situation when the pulse becomes weaker with inspiration and stronger with expiration. Normally, the situation is reversed.

Treatment focuses on managing or reversing any underlying disorders that may have led to chronic kidney disease. Once the disease has gotten underway, it is very difficult to stop the progression. The goal is to control fluid, electrolyte and mineral imbalances, slow progression to ESRD, and delay dialysis. Strict dietary compliance is needed and a multitude of carefully monitored therapeutic agents is required. Symptoms are treated as follows:

- Metabolic acidosis is treated with alkaline compounds such as sodium bicarbonate, calcium bicarbonate, and sodium citrate.

- Hypervolemia is controlled using **loop diuretics**. Furosemide (Lasix) is effective but must be given at high doses (80–240 mg p.o. b.i.d.). ACE inhibitors are also used to help control hypervolemia because they promote natriuresis.

- Hypertension is typically due to volume overload, so control of salt intake and water retention are the most important strategies for reducing blood pressure. Diuretics and controlled dietary intake of salt help reduce hypertension.

- Hyperkalemia is treated with dietary restriction of potassium. When potassium approaches life-threatening levels of greater than 7, **sodium polystyrene sulfonate (PSP)**, brand name Kayexalate, is used to bind potassium in the GI tract.

- Anemia can be treated with administration of erythropoietin in the form of epoetin alfa (EPO) or darbepoetin alfa along with IV ferrous fumarate, folate, and B_{12} supplementation. The goal is to maintain a hemoglobin level of 11–12 g/dL.

- The prolonged bleeding time is treated only if surgery is needed. Prior to surgery, desmopressin acetate (DDAVP) or **conjugated estrogens** are given to improve platelet function.

- Hyperphosphatemia is treated with dietary restriction of phosphorus and administration of calcium carbonate. The goal is to prevent elevated PTH with subsequent leaching of calcium from bone stores. A phosphate binder called sevelamer (brand name Renagel) may also be used. Vitamin D supplements are also given to promote dietary calcium absorption.

Dialysis is initiated when the GFR drops below 15 mL/min or when hyperkalemia and heart failure become imminently life-threatening. Life expectancy on dialysis is often less than five years. Renal transplantation has a high success rate and increases life expectancy considerably. Living-related donors or unrelated donors matched with **HLA typing** (see page 313) are the most successful. **Cadaveric donors** (deceased donors) are commonly used but have a higher rate of transplant rejection compared to matched, living donors.

Glomerular Disease

Kidney diseases classified as glomerular are those that begin with damage to the major components of the glomerulus. As individual glomeruli fail, the kidney compensates for the decreased function by increasing arterial pressure in the remaining glomeruli. Chronically increased arterial pressures within the nephrons cause arteriosclerosis and further loss of function, thus beginning a vicious cycle of decreasing function. As more nephrons are lost, the concentrating ability of the kidney is lost because the increased arterial pressure forces fluids through the tubules at a faster rate, allowing less time for water molecules to be reabsorbed. The problem can be compared to working a manufacturing line where you have to grab specific items off a conveyer belt. The faster the belt, the more difficult it becomes to selectively grab the items passing by.

Glomerular syndromes are caused by damage to the major components of the glomerulus: the epithelium, **glomerular basement membrane (GBM)**, capillary endothelium, or mesangium. Glomerular disorders are loosely classified as either **nephritic** or **nephrotic**. Nephritic disorders are inflammatory reactions that manifest as hematuria. Nephrotic syndromes are marked by proteinuria.

 Listen carefully to distinguish the terms nephritic and nephrotic.

Nephritic Syndromes

Glomerulonephritis (GN) is an inflammatory reaction within the glomeruli. It may be acute or chronic and is typically immune-mediated. **Postinfectious glomerulonephritis**, often referred to as **acute glomerulonephritis**, is caused by an immune reaction

Table 7-1 Autoimmune Disorders Associated with Glomerulonephritis

Disorder	Description	Serology Tests
IgA nephropathy (Berger disease)	IgA antibodies deposited in the glomerular mesangium	IgA, serum complement
ANCA-associated GN	autoimmune reaction directed against capillaries	antineutrophil cytoplasmic antibodies (p-ANCA and c-ANCA)
anti-GBM nephritis, also known as Good-pasture syndrome	autoimmune reaction directed against the glomerular basement membrane	anti-GBM

following an infection such as impetigo or bacterial pharyngitis caused by **group A beta-hemolytic streptococci.** The infection itself does not spread to the kidney, rather the body's reaction to the infection leads to kidney damage. Anywhere from one to three weeks following the acute infection, antigen-antibody complexes form and precipitate in the glomerulus. The antigen-antibody complexes cause a local inflammatory reaction. The integrity of the glomerular membrane is damaged, allowing albumin and RBCs, which normally do not pass through the glomerulus, to escape into the glomerular filtrate and appear in the urine. Most people recover fully from postinfectious glomerulonephritis but a few will progress to chronic kidney disease.

Noninfectious glomerulonephritis also begins with the precipitation of antigen-antibody complexes within the glomerulus that have been instigated by an autoimmune reaction. Autoimmune disorders causing glomerulonephritis are listed in **Table 7-1.** Inflammation follows the accumulation of immune complexes, and the ongoing inflammation causes normal glomerular tissue to be replaced with fibrous, sclerotic tissue with subsequent loss of functioning nephrons. When the disease progresses over days to weeks, it is referred to as **rapidly progressive glomerulonephritis (RPG).**

Patients may present with hematuria, edema, and oliguria. The edema may first appear in regions of low tissue pressure such as the periorbital or scrotal areas. The urine may be described as cola-colored due to the presence of red blood cells. Laboratory examination reveals dysmorphic RBCs and **RBC casts** in the urinary sediment. Proteinuria and elevated serum creatinine are also present, and serum complement levels are low (see page 314). Serology tests may be performed to determine if the disease is caused by an autoimmune disorder (**Table 7-1**). Renal biopsy may be required for a definitive diagnosis. The disease may be described as **crescentic glomerulonephritis** if 50% or more of the glomeruli have an abnormal crescent shape seen on tissue biopsy.

Treatment focuses on reducing fluid overload and hypertension, as the increased pressure within the glomeruli furthers the damage. Antihypertensives such as ARBs and ACE inhibitors are used to reduce systemic blood pressure as well as intrarenal pressure. Sodium restriction and diuretics help to control hypervolemia. Progress is monitored with GFR and creatinine clearance studies.

Nephrotic Syndromes

Nephrotic syndrome is defined by heavy proteinuria with urinary excretion of greater than 3 g of protein per day accompanied by hypoalbuminemia, hyperlipidemia, and edema. The underlying cause is increased permeability of the glomerular membrane, allowing protein to pass into the glomerular filtrate. The large amount of albumin that is allowed to "spill" into the urine causes hypoalbuminemia. Serum albumin is a primary contributor to the intravascular colloid osmotic pressure (3) that retains water in the intravascular spaces. Loss of albumin causes water to flow out of the vasculature and into the interstitial spaces (edema).

(3) Colloid osmotic pressure is the effect of dissolved particles pulling water across a semipermeable membrane.

Nephrotic disorders may be classified as primary disease or secondary renal disorders caused by systemic diseases. Primary renal disorders include:

- minimal change disease (4)
- membranous nephropathy
- focal segmental glomerular sclerosis

Examples of systemic diseases that lead to (secondary) renal disorders include:

- amyloidosis
- systemic lupus erythematosus
- preeclampsia
- diabetic nephropathy

Diabetic nephropathy is the most common cause of end-stage renal disease in the United States. Diabetes mellitus (types 1 and 2) causes changes in the capillaries of the kidneys, just as the disease causes vascular changes throughout the body. For this reason, many patients with diabetic retinopathy also have nephrotic syndrome. Diabetics should be screened routinely for microalbuminuria for the early detection of diabetic nephropathy.

The tremendous loss of protein characteristic of nephrotic syndrome causes an array of complications. **Table 7-2** lists the proteins lost and the ensuing consequences.

Edema is the hallmark of nephrotic syndrome. Patients may also complain of anorexia, malaise, and dyspnea (from fluid retention). The high protein concentration makes the urine "frothy." Examination may reveal parallel white lines in the fingernail beds called **Muehrcke lines (mŭr'kə)**.

Diagnosis is confirmed on laboratory studies that show a urine protein-to-creatinine ratio of greater than 3, proteinuria of greater than 3 g in a 24-hour period (normal protein excretion is less than 150 mg/d), hypoalbuminemia (less than 3 g/dL), and total protein less than 6 g/dL. A **spot urine** (ie, a random sample) is also tested for proteinuria. Urine

Table 7-2 Proteins Lost Due to Nephrotic Syndrome

Protein	Consequence
erythropoietin	decreased red cell production
transferrin	decreased iron
hormone-binding proteins	hypothyroidism and other endocrine disorders
apoproteins	hyperlipidemia due to disrupted lipid metabolism
albumin	edema
antithrombin and plasminogen	thrombosis and pulmonary embolism
vitamin-D binding protein	hypovitaminosis D, hypocalcemia, and subsequent bone disease
immunoglobulins	predisposition to infection

sediment may be positive for RBCs and casts (**hyaline**, **granular**, **fatty**, or **waxy**). **Lipiduria** may be evident as oval fat bodies (lipid accumulations within tubular cells seen in the urine) or as fatty globules in the urine itself. Urinary cholesterol forms crystals that appear in a **Maltese cross** pattern under polarized microscopy. Positive **Sudan staining** indicates the presence of triglycerides.

ACE inhibitors and ARBs are given to slow the rate of progression to end-stage renal disease. Salt restriction helps to minimize edema. Fluid overload is also treated with thiazide and loop diuretics. Dyslipidemia is also treated aggressively with antilipemic medications. Patients with coagulopathies are treated with anticoagulants to prevent or reverse **renal vein thrombosis** or deep vein thrombosis.

---

(4) Minimal change disease is marked by a change in the electrical charge of the glomerular basement membrane. This change in the membrane allows proteins to pass through the basement membrane and appear in the urine.

Pause 7-2 Summarize key differences between nephrotic syndrome and nephritic syndrome. What are some clues that you may be able to draw from the context of a report to help you distinguish these two terms when dictated?

- Renal failure may be categorized as acute or chronic. Acute renal failure is rapidly progressive, occurring over hours to days. Chronic kidney failure progresses slowly over a number of years.
- Prerenal kidney failure is due to inadequate renal perfusion leading to necrosis.
- Acute tubular necrosis is the most common form of intrinsic renal failure and is often caused by nephrotoxins.
- Postrenal causes of renal failure include obstructive disorders such as BPH, neurogenic bladder, and stone disease.
- Acute renal failure has widespread systemic ramifications including edema, respiratory disturbances, and a high mortality rate.
- Chronic kidney disease is marked by years of renal insufficiency that leads to ESRD. The most common cause of CKD is diabetic nephropathy.
- Symptoms of CKD include hypertension, hyperkalemia, metabolic acidosis, heart disease, anemia, mineral imbalances, bleeding, neuropathy, and encephalopathy.
- Treatment of CKD focuses on correcting electrolyte, mineral, and hormone imbalances, slowing the progression of the disease, and delaying dialysis.
- Glomerular diseases of the kidney are marked by primary damage to the glomerular apparatus, which leads to damage to the remainder of the nephron.
- Nephritic disorders are marked by inflammatory reactions within the glomerulus caused by postinfectious or autoimmune antigen-antibody complexes precipitating in the glomerulus, triggering a local inflammatory reaction.
- Nephrotic syndromes are marked by edema, proteinuria, and accompanying hypoalbuminemia caused by increased permeability of the glomerular membrane. The most common cause of nephrotic syndrome is diabetes mellitus.

Urinary Tract Infections

Urinary tract infections (UTIs) include infection of the urethra, prostate, bladder, or kidneys. Normally, the urinary tract is sterile, but it may become contaminated by colonic and fecal bacteria (normal flora of the bowel). Contamination from bacteria is kept in check by urination, which flushes bacteria from the bladder and urethra. Other protective defenses include the acidic pH of the urine, high osmolality of urine, ureterovesical and urethral sphincters, and mucosal barriers. The vast majority of infections occur when bacteria ascend the urethra, infect the bladder, and then further ascend through the ureters to the kidneys. Hematogenous spread causes only about 5% of UTIs. Severe UTIs can also lead to bacteremia and systemic infection.

The most frequent causative agents are commensal (5) gram-negative bacteria, with greater than 75% of **community-acquired UTIs** (6) attributable to a single agent, E coli. Other enteric gram-negative rods and gram-positive enterococci play a larger role in **hospital-acquired infections**. Most acute, uncomplicated cases of UTI are caused by a single agent, but chronic UTIs often involve more than one organism. Microbial agents commonly implicated in UTIs are listed in **Table 7-3**.

Pause 7-3 What is hematogenous spread?

(5) Commensal describes an organism that derives benefit from another organism (the host) but does not harm the host organism.

(6) A community-acquired UTI simply means it was contracted outside the hospital or long-term care setting.

Table 7-3 Microorganisms Commonly Associated with UTIs

Organism	Description
Escherichia coli	gram-negative enteric rod
Klebsiella species	gram-negative enteric rod
Proteus species	gram-negative enteric rod
Enterobacter species	gram-negative enteric rod
Serratia species	gram-negative enteric rod
Staphylococcus saprophyticus	gram-positive cocci
Enterococcus faecalis	gram-positive cocci
Staphylococcus aureus	gram-positive cocci

Anatomical abnormalities may predispose individuals to urinary tract infections. In children, incompetent **ureterovesical valves** with **vesicoureteral reflux (VUR)** increase the risk of UTIs. Diabetes increases the risk of infection due to a higher incidence of neurogenic bladder and also due to the higher urinary glucose concentrations that promote bacterial growth.

In general, women are more prone to urinary tract infections because of the anatomically short urethra and the close proximity of the urethral meatus to the vaginal introitus and anus. Males are at much less risk of contracting UTIs, and in the absence of sexual behavioral risk factors, a single infection in a male may prompt further investigation for underlying causes such as cancer.

Lower Urinary Tract Infections

UTIs can be divided into two categories: lower tract infections and upper tract infections. The lower tract includes the urethra, prostate, and bladder. The upper tract includes the ureters and the kidneys. Localization of the infection is not always possible and only really necessary in more complicated cases of UTI.

The diagnosis is confirmed by a **clean-catch voided urine** culture that shows a single organism at a concentration greater than 10^5 **colony forming units (CFU)/mL** of urine. A *catheterized* urine specimen is considered positive if it shows a single organism at a concentration of 100 CFU/mL. A CBC will typically show **leukocytosis with a left shift**. Urinalysis is positive for pyuria, bacteriuria, hematuria, WBCs, or **WBC casts**. A positive nitrite by **urine dipstick** is also indicative of UTI.

The **leukocyte esterase** test is positive when WBCs are present in the urine at greater than 10 WBCs/mcL.

 Urinalysis tests for nitrites (spelled with an /i/), not nitrates (spelled with an /a/).

 Pause 7-4 Why would catheterized urine have a smaller threshold for a positive diagnosis of UTI?

 Urine culture is positive for quinolone-resistant Escherichia coli, greater than 50,000 CFU/mL.

Urethritis

Urethritis is inflammation of the urethra. The inflammation may be caused by bacteria, protozoa, viruses, or fungi. Common agents include **Chlamydia trachomatis**, **Neisseria gonorrhoeae**, **Trichomonas vaginalis**, and **herpes simplex virus (HSV)**. Urethritis occurs when organisms infect the female urethra or the periurethral glands in the **bulbous** or **pendulous urethra** of the male. **Nongonococcal urethritis (NGU)** is one of the most commonly seen sexually transmitted diseases in men. The main symptom of urethritis is dysuria. The diagnosis of urethritis may be confirmed by a clean-catch voided urine culture that shows a single bacterial species in colony counts from 10^2 to 10^4 CFU/mL (lower counts than the threshold for diagnosing cystitis).

Cystitis

Acute cystitis is an infection of the bladder mucosa and is very common in females. Cystitis in men is rare and usually implies a pathologic process. Because intercourse increases the risk of cystitis in females, it is sometimes referred to as **honeymoon cystitis**. Symptoms include irritative voiding, hematuria, low-grade fever, and suprapubic discomfort. Irritation is manifested by frequency and urgency, obstruction, a sensation of incomplete bladder emptying, a need to void again shortly after urinating, or nocturia. Pneumaturia may occur if the infection results from a **vesicoenteric** or **vesicovaginal fistula** or from **emphysematous cystitis**.

Physical examination may reveal suprapubic tenderness, but otherwise the exam is rather benign. A **midstream clean-catch urine** is collected for dipstick

- Urinary tract infections are among the most common urinary disorders. Infection may be in the urethra, prostate, bladder, or kidneys.
- The majority of acute, uncomplicated UTIs are caused by E coli ascending the urethra and infecting the bladder, ureters, or kidneys.
- Diagnosis is suspected by a positive dipstick test for nitrite and leukocyte esterase; diagnosis is confirmed by a clean-catch urine culture showing greater than 10^5 CFU/mL.
- Urethritis in males is usually caused by sexually transmitted organisms including chlamydia, gonorrhea, trichomonas, and herpes.
- Cystitis is common in women but rare in men.
- Pyelonephritis often results from ascension of bacteria from the lower urinary tract, especially in women.

analysis and possibly for culture. UA shows pyuria, turbidity, bacteriuria, hematuria, white cells, and possibly white cell casts. Treatment of uncomplicated cystitis includes antibiotics, phenazopyridine (an analgesic), and increased fluid intake. Women who suffer recurrent cystitis (three or more infections per year) are given prophylactic antibiotics to take either nightly or immediately following coitus. Drinking cranberry juice daily has been found to reduce pyuria and bacteriuria. Antibiotics used to treat cystitis include trimethoprim-sulfamethoxazole (TMP-SMZ), nitrofurantoin, and cephalexin.

ASSESSMENT AND PLAN: Urinary tract infection, positive for E coli susceptible to Cipro. She is now on IV Cipro. This has been a recurring problem after her bladder suspension. We will go ahead and place her on low-dose prophylaxis after she finishes her Cipro therapy.

Upper Urinary Tract infections

Acute pyelonephritis, a very common renal disorder, is a suppurative (pus-forming) bacterial infection of the kidney parenchyma and renal pelvis. Pyelonephritis is far more common in women than men, mainly due to the higher prevalence of lower urinary tract infections that ascend upward through the urinary tract to the kidneys. Pyelonephritis is also a significant cause of community-acquired bacteremia in women.

Risk factors for infection include neurogenic bladder, urinary obstruction, sexual activity, pregnancy, and diabetes. **Instrumentation** of the urinary tract (eg, catheterization, cystoscopy, urologic surgery) also increases the risk of pyelonephritis.

Patients present with symptoms very similar to lower urinary tract infection, including chills, fever, tachycardia, flank pain, nausea, vomiting, and irritative voiding symptoms. Patients may note a fishy or ammonia-like smell to their urine. Physical examination may reveal a palpably enlarged kidney with tenderness on percussion of the **costovertebral angle (CVA)**. Urine culture will be positive with greater than 100,000 CFU/mL.

Less severe infections are treated with a quinolone antibiotic or nitrofurantoin orally. Patients with a severe infection or complications should be treated with IV antibiotic combinations such as ampicillin and gentamicin, SMX-TMP plus fluoroquinolone, or ceftriaxone. Parenteral therapy should be continued until **defervescence** or other signs of clinical improvement occur. A **nephrostomy** may be placed for drainage if ureteral obstruction is present.

Voiding Dysfunction

The act of voiding is a deceptively complex physiologic process involving both the somatic and autonomic nervous systems. The detrusor is a layer of smooth muscle within the urinary bladder that is arranged in spiral, longitudinal, and circular bundles. Contraction of the **detrusor muscles** expels urine from the bladder into the urethra. **Rugae**, or folds, within the bladder flatten out as the bladder stretches to accommodate more urine. The flattening of the folds allows the bladder to enlarge without significantly increasing the internal pressure within the bladder. Normally, the urinary bladder holds 300–500 mL. The first urge to avoid normally occurs with bladder volumes of 150–300 mL. A threshold volume, which varies from one person to another, triggers awareness of the need to void. **Voiding dysfunction** includes functional incontinence, urinary incontinence, mixed incontinence, and overactive bladder. Mixed incontinence is a combination of urge and stress incontinence or urge with functional incontinence.

The physical examination and patient history are very important in the assessment and correct diagnosis of urinary incontinence. Patients may be asked to keep a **voiding diary** (7) for several days. A full assessment should include neurologic, pelvic, and rectal examinations. The neurologic assessment should include mental status, gait, upper and lower extremity function, and signs of peripheral or autonomic neuropathy. The spine should be examined for spondylosis and stenosis.

The urethral sphincter and the anal sphincter share the same sacral roots, so testing perineal (8) sensation, **volitional anal sphincter contraction**, the **anal wink reflex**, and the **bulbocavernosus reflex** will provide clues as to the neural status of the urethral sphincter. The pelvic exam should include the vaginal mucosa, the anterior and posterior vaginal walls, and a **bimanual exam**. A cotton swab test (**Q-Tip test**) may be performed to assess urethral mobility.

 Pause 7-5 Explain the "volitional anal sphincter contraction" in layman's terms.

She reports multiple urologic concerns including a mixture of obstructive and irritative voiding symptoms, a reported history of recent acute renal failure, frequent urinary tract infections, mixed incontinence, and "cysts" on her bladder.

Functional Incontinence

Functional incontinence is not due to any faulty urinary tract mechanisms or interrupted neural pathways, rather the patient suffers cognitive, psychological, or physical impairments that interfere with voiding. The patient may not be cognizant of the need to urinate, not know where the toilet is located, or be unable to ambulate to a toilet.

(7) A voiding diary includes a record of fluid intake, time of each void, accidents, and episodes of leakage.

(8) Listen carefully for perineal, peritoneal, and peroneal.

Urinary Incontinence

Urinary incontinence can be divided into three categories: urge, stress, and overflow incontinence. **Urge incontinence (UI)** is the uncontrolled leakage of urine following a sudden, irrepressible urge to void. It is the result of **uninhibited contractions** of the detrusor muscle. Detrusor hyperactivity may be idiopathic or result from cerebrovascular accidents, cervical stenosis, or bladder inflammation (cystitis, stones, or neoplasms). Atrophic vaginitis, common after menopause, is evident by thinning of the urethra with subsequent irritation and leakage of urine. The use of diuretics can exacerbate UI, especially in individuals with physical impairments that impede their ability to reach a bathroom quickly.

 Pause 7-6 Explain "uninhibited contractions" in layman's terms.

A form of urge incontinence is **overactive bladder syndrome (OAB)** characterized by urgency, frequency, and nocturia. When an overactive bladder is not associated with urine loss, it is referred to as **overactive bladder dry**. Another variant of UI is **detrusor hyperactivity with impaired contractility (DHIC)**. This syndrome is also marked by irritative bladder symptoms as well as a weak flow rate, urinary retention, bladder **trabeculation**, and a **postvoid residual volume** greater than 50 mL. DHIC can mimic prostatism in men or stress urinary incontinence in women.

Treatment for urge incontinence is generally pharmaceutical. The goal of therapy is to improve the symptoms of frequency, nocturia, and urgency. Treatment options include anticholinergics (eg, tolterodine, brand name Detrol, and solifenacin, brand name VESIcare), antispasmodic agents (hyoscyamine and oxybutynin, brand name Ditropan), and TCAs (imipramine). Patients may also be treated with electrical stimulation of the nerves using a device marketed under the name InterStim.

Stress incontinence (SI) is leakage of urine due to sudden, increased intraabdominal pressure that occurs with bending, laughing, sneezing, coughing, climbing stairs, and other activities that increase pressure within the abdominal cavity. The amount of urine leaked is small to moderate. SI results from weakened pelvic floor muscles or weakened endopelvic fascia following multiple vaginal deliveries, or from **atrophic urethritis** caused by hypoestrogenism. The weakened supporting structures cause the **urethrovesical junction** to descend, the bladder neck to shorten, and the urethra to become **hypermobile**. These anatomical shifts cause the pressure in the urethra to fall below that of the bladder. The decreased muscle tone causes urine loss at lower abdominal-pressure thresholds. Less commonly, SI may be due to impaired intrinsic sphincter function (called **intrinsic sphincter deficiency**) following pelvic surgery.

On cystoscopy, the physician may see a **lead pipe urethra**, which describes a urethra that remains open at the sphincter. In males, prostatectomy is a common cause of damage to the sphincter, posterior urethra, or bladder neck. SI causes a positive **cough test** (leakage of urine when coughing) in either the lithotomy or standing position.

Medical treatment for SI in postmenopausal females may include topical estrogen cream to reverse atrophic changes in the urethra and vagina. Alpha-agonists such as midodrine (ProAmatine) or pseudoephedrine (Sudafed) may improve symptoms of mild stress incontinence. Imipramine, a tricyclic antidepressant, has been shown to have modest efficacy.

Conservative (nonsurgical) treatments for SI include collagen injections, **pessaries** or occlusive devices, pelvic floor conditioning (**Kegel exercises**), and bladder training. Behavioral therapy and biofeedback may also be helpful, especially when combined with other therapies. Kegel exercises have been shown to increase the strength of the levator ani group of muscles and tighten the connective tissues supporting the urethra.

Surgical treatment of SI focuses on stabilization of the bladder by placing it back into its appropriate anatomic location and lengthening of the urethra. A common procedure is a **bladder sling suspension** with a transvaginal or suprapubic approach (**colpocystourethropexy**) to raise the bladder neck and better align the bladder and urethra. A sling is a band of material placed directly under the bladder neck or midurethra that acts as a physical support to prevent bladder and urethral descent.

Overflow incontinence (OI) results from an overly full bladder that continually leaks small amounts of urine. Patients may complain of weak urinary stream, dribbling, hesitancy, frequency, nocturia, and constant leakage. Patients may mention that their bladder never feels empty. They may also complain of difficulty voiding, even when the urge is felt. The primary contributing factor is urinary retention. Overflow incontinence may be caused by impaired detrusor function that prevents the bladder from completely emptying. Neurological problems affecting the detrusor muscle include spinal cord injuries, spinal stenosis, and radiculopathy, as well as peripheral or autonomic neuropathies. Overflow incontinence is associated with diabetes mellitus and neurological disorders such as Alzheimer disease, Parkinson disease, and multiple sclerosis. A neurogenic bladder, caused by damage to the sacral nerves, may also cause OI due to a loss of the sensation to urinate.

Bladder outlet obstruction may also cause the bladder to remain too full, thereby overcoming urethral resistance, allowing dribbling or seepage. Obstruction may be caused by tumors, stones, **pelvic organ prolapse**, or an enlarged prostate. Benign prostatic hypertrophy is often associated with overflow incontinence. One form of bladder outlet obstruction is caused by **detrusor sphincter dyssynergia (DSD)**. In this disorder, the sphincter contracts at the same time as the detrusor muscle. The sphincter "clamps down" instead of opening to release the urine, effectively resulting in an obstruction. Dyssynergia is marked by severe bladder trabeculation, diverticula, a **Christmas-tree shape** to the bladder, hydronephrosis, and ultimately renal failure.

> Since she has been continuing to complain of increased urinary frequency and urgency and slowing of her urinary stream, a urodynamic study was performed in our office. This indicated the presence of a diminished bladder capacity with a prolonged, slow urinary stream. Due to the significant slowing of her urinary stream, cystoscopy was performed, which indicated some mild urethral stenosis. Urethral dilation was then performed gently with sounds up to a #20-French.

The history and physical examination are key to determining the etiology of OI. Diagnostic tests may include cystometry, uroflow, **voiding cystourethrogram (VCUG)**, and sphincter electromyography (EMG). Treatment for neurogenic bladder and overflow incontinence is limited. Available treatments focus on alleviating the urinary retention. Patients may be taught bladder evacuation techniques such as the **Credé method**, Valsalva maneuver, or **intermittent catheterization**. Credé method involves applying manual pressure over the lower abdomen. Valsalva is performed by forcing exhalation against a closed glottis. The most efficacious treatment for urinary retention is intermittent catheterization, also called **intermittent self-catheterization**. Using a catheter, patients empty their bladder every three to eight hours to keep urine volume low. Indwelling catheters may also be

- Voiding dysfunction includes urinary incontinence, functional incontinence, mixed incontinence, and overactive bladder.
- An assessment for voiding dysfunction should include a complete history and a thorough physical examination including a neurological examination.
- The three types of incontinence include urge, stress, and overflow.
- Urge incontinence is the uncontrolled leakage of urine following a sudden urge to void. Urine is released due to uninhibited contractions of the detrusor muscle caused by neurological disorders, infection, neoplasm, or the effects of aging.
- Overactive bladder is a form of urge incontinence and is characterized by urgency, frequency, and nocturia. Treatment includes the use of anticholinergics, antispasmodics, and TCAs.
- Stress incontinence is the leakage of urine due to sudden increased intraabdominal pressure. Common causes of SI include weakened pelvic muscles, atrophic urethritis, and prostatectomy. SI may be treated medically or with bladder slings.
- Overflow incontinence results from an overly full bladder that continually leaks small amounts of urine. The primary cause of OI is impaired detrusor function due to neurological disorders. OI may also be caused by bladder outlet obstruction resulting from tumors, stones, pelvic organ prolapse, or an enlarged prostate.
- Diagnosis of voiding dysfunction is aided by uroflow studies, cystometry, VCUG, and EMG.

used if the patient or a caregiver is unable to perform intermittent catheterization, but indwelling catheters are prone to infection. Treatment may be augmented with anticholinergic medications such as oxybutynin.

Some patients may require urethral stents to maintain the urethral opening. Men may opt for laser ablation of sphincter tissue or a sphincterotomy. Removing the sphincter will cause permanent incontinence and require the use of a condom catheter and leg bag. If conservative measures fail and the kidneys are at risk of damage, urinary diversion or cystectomy may be needed.

A urinary flow study was performed that indicates a moderate voided volume with a slow, prolonged urinary flow but a small amount of residual urine, based on an ultrasound study.

Urinary Calculi

Nephrolithiasis refers to a condition in which calculi (stones) form in the kidney. **Ureterolithiasis** refers to the presence or formation of stones in the ureters. Renal stones almost always begin in the kidney but may enlarge as they pass through or become lodged in the ureters. The pain produced by ureterolithiasis is referred to as **renal colic**. Morbidity and mortality increase when stones cause obstruction accompanied by upper urinary tract infection. In these situations, the patient is at risk of **pyelonephritis**, **pyonephrosis**, and **urosepsis**, requiring emergent treatment to remove the obstruction and treat the infection.

Urinary stones are aggregates of crystals and organic matrix. Over 80% of stones consist of calcium oxalate or calcium phosphate and result from **hypercalciuria** (defined as urine calcium greater than 275 mg/d in men and greater than 250 mg/d in women). Approximately 10% of stones are composed of uric acid and the remainder is either **cystine** or **struvite** (magnesium ammonium phosphate.) A calculus forms when substances in the urine come out of solution (precipitate) due to supersaturation. Given the proper pH, particles precipitate and aggregate, forming a small stone that grows in size. Foreign bodies as well as all types of crystals can act as a **nidus**, on which calcium, uric acid, cystine, and magnesium can build.

Listen carefully for oxalate (ox-**al**′āt), which sounds very much like oscillate and oxylate.

Also, note the correct spelling of cystine in this context (*not* cysteine).

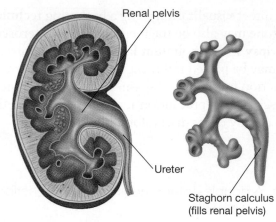

FIGURE 7-4 A staghorn calculus.

The patient is in today for a followup of his ureteral calculus. He had a 100% calcium oxalate monohydrate stone. He is not interested at this time in a metabolic stone evaluation. Therefore, I would like to see him back in 1 year with a KUB. The stent was removed at today's office visit.

Although stones may develop anywhere within the urinary tract, the majority of stones begin in the renal pelvis or calyces of the kidney. A **staghorn calculus** is a stone that lodges in the renal pelvis and enlarges until it completely fills the pelvis of the affected kidney (■ **Figure 7-4**). Stones may remain within the kidney or pass into the ureters. Stones can cause damage by pressing on tissues, causing pressure necrosis, or by abrading tissues as the jagged edges pass through the ureters. Stones may become lodged in the ureters, especially in the **ureteropelvic junction (UPJ)**, in the distal ureter where it crosses over the iliac vessels, or at the **ureterovesical junction (UVJ)**. Stones typically must be greater than 5 mm in diameter to become lodged. Stones that obstruct the flow of urine cause **hydroureter** and possibly **hydronephrosis**.

Predisposing factors for stone formation include infection, oliguria, dehydration, increased calcium or uric acid excretion, decreased secretion of citrate (**hypocitruria**) or magnesium, or any condition that results in urinary stasis. Inherited metabolic defects are a major causative factor in stone disease. Diet modifications in the form of restricted sodium intake and reduced protein intake along with increased fluids play an important role in the prevention of stones in these individuals.

Hereditary metabolic disorders that disrupt calcium homeostasis can also cause stones. One such metabolic disorder is marked by normal serum calcium with hypercalciuria. Hypocitruria, another metabolic disorder, also promotes calcium stone formation because citrate normally binds calcium, preventing it from crystalizing and aggregating into stones.

Uric acid stones develop in the presence of increased urine pH (less than 5.5) or with **hyperuricosuria** (urinary uric acid greater than 1500 mg/d). Uric acid stones are often a combination of calcium and uric acid, as the uric acid crystals provide a nidus for calcium to bind. Cystine calculi result from a rare hereditary disorder that causes cystinuria. Struvite stones form in the presence of urinary tract infections caused by urea-splitting bacteria such as Proteus and Klebsiella species. These particular stones are infectious and must be removed.

Nonobstructing stones, even large ones, are usually asymptomatic. The first symptom may be hematuria or a gravel-like substance in the urine. Patients may also present with symptoms of a UTI. Symptoms of bladder irritation are common when the stone is lodged in the **intramural ureter**. (9)

Patients with **obstructive ureterolithiasis** typically present to the emergency department with sudden-onset renal colic. The pain is usually excruciating and accompanied by nausea and vomiting. The pain may travel from the CVA to the flank, downward to the suprapubic area and the external genitalia. Patients typically pace or shift constantly in response to the pain, compared to patients with acute abdomen who prefer to lie still.

The diagnostic test of choice for suspected stone disease is a **spiral (helical) CT scan** without contrast. Calcium stones are radiopaque and show up nicely on x-ray studies. Uric acid stones are not radiopaque but are typically mixed with calcium, so they appear radiopaque. A **KUB study** (x-ray of the <u>k</u>idneys, <u>u</u>reters, and <u>b</u>ladder) can assist with followup and further treatment. A plain radiograph or a **scout reconstruction** of the CT scan (10) can help visualize the size, shape, and position of the stone.

(9) The intramural ureter is the distal portion of the ureter that runs obliquely along the bladder wall.

(10) A scout reconstruction is a CT image formatted to look like a plain radiograph.

In the absence of complicating factors such as hydronephrosis or infection, initial treatment for **ure-terocolic** focuses on pain control while allowing the stone to pass spontaneously. In the emergency department, patients are given narcotics such as codeine, oxycodone, or hydrocodone combined with acetaminophen (see page 153), and NSAIDs for pain relief. Antiemetics are given to relieve nausea and vomiting. Patients unable to tolerate oral intake are given IV morphine, fentanyl (Sublimaze), or ketorolac (Toradol), and ondansetron (Zofran) for nausea.

Once pain control has been achieved, treatment of the stone depends on the stone's size and composition. Calcium stones cannot be dissolved with oral medications or diet modifications. Stones comprised of pure cystine or uric acid (with minimal calcium contamination) are amenable to medical therapy using **alkalinizing agents** such as potassium citrate (Urocit K) that maintain the urine pH between 6.5 and 7. Patients with pure uric acid stones and documented hyperuricemia are treated with allopurinol to decrease uric acid excretion (see also page 154). D-penicillamine (Cuprimine) is used in the treatment of cystinuria.

Stones measuring 3 mm or less are most likely to pass spontaneously. Stones that measure 4–10 mm in diameter will often pass within two to six weeks with the aid of **medical expulsive therapy (MET)** consisting of the calcium channel blocker nifedipine (see page 304) and terazosin (Hytrin) or tamsulosin (Flomax), both alpha blockers. MET helps relax ureteral smooth muscle and lower urinary tract muscles, facilitating passage of the stone. Once the stone passes through the ureter into the bladder, it can be passed through the urethra with minimal discomfort.

Larger stones and those that do not respond to medical therapy may be treated with endoscopy or lithotripsy. If both obstruction and infection are present, decompression on an emergent basis is required. A symptomatic calculus measuring 1 cm or less may be treated with **extracorporeal shockwave lithotripsy (ESWL)**, which shatters the stone into fragments small enough to expel. ESWL combined with MET is highly effective.

Distal stones may require removal endoscopically. A ureteroscope is inserted into the urethra and through the bladder to the distal ureter. The stone is removed under direct visualization using a **basketing technique**. The stone may also be fragmented using **ureteroscopic lithotripsy** with a **holmium laser**. A **double-J ureteral stent** may be placed following ureteroscopy to prevent obstruction from ureteral spasm and edema. Physicians may eschew this precaution in some patients, as these stents usually cause discomfort.

 A double-J stent should *not* be transcribed as "JJ stent."

Proximal and midureteral stones (those located above the inferior margin of the SI joint) may be treated with lithotripsy or a ureteroscope inserted in an antegrade direction through the kidney. If ureteroscopy or lithotripsy fails, a **percutaneous nephrostomy tube** may be inserted directly into the kidney. **Sandwich therapy**, which is a combination of ESWL and **percutaneous nephrostolithotomy**, may be used for complicated stone cases or staghorn stones.

Individuals who form their first stone before the age of 50 (typically in their 20s or 30s) or those patients with a family history of stone disease are likely to have recurrence. In these patients, dietary modifications and medical management are recommended to help prevent recurrence. Analysis of the stone composition and metabolic tests are necessary to plan a preventive course of action. Patients are given a urine strainer to recover stones or fragments to be analyzed.

Laboratory evaluation for metabolic factors includes serum electrolytes, creatinine, calcium, uric acid, parathyroid hormone, and phosphorus. A 24-hour urine specimen is collected and analyzed for pH, calcium, oxalate, uric acid, sodium, phosphorus, citrate, magnesium, creatinine, and total volume. A second 24-hour urine may be collected following a calcium- and sodium-restricted diet.

The most common findings on 24-hour urine studies include hypercalciuria, hyperoxaluria, hyperuricosuria, hypocitraturia, and low urinary volume. Hyperuricosuria may indicate **gouty diathesis**. (11) Magnesium and citrate normally bind calcium and increase excretion of calcium; consequently, hypomagnesuria and hypocitraturia promote the formation of calcium-based stones. Potassium citrate is prescribed to increase urine citrate.

(11) Gouty diathesis is increased stone production associated with high serum uric acid.

- Renal stones, which are aggregates of crystals and organic matrix, typically form in the kidney but may be found anywhere within the urinary tract.
- The majority of renal stones consists of calcium in the form of calcium oxalate or calcium phosphate resulting from hypercalciuria.
- Hereditary disorders that lead to hypercalciuria, hypocitraturia, or cystinuria cause renal stone formation.

- Complications of renal stone disease include hydroureter and hydronephrosis.
- Diagnosis of acute renal colic is by spiral CT scan.
- Treatment may include lithotripsy, nephrolithotomy, or medical treatment to dissolve the stone.
- Stone analysis and metabolic evaluation are used to determine prophylactic treatment.

Her 24-hour urine revealed an elevated oxalate level and low-normal citrate level. I have recommended that she begin potassium citrate therapy.

Stones consisting of predominately calcium cannot be dissolved, but medications are available for long-term chemoprophylaxis. In addition to dietary changes (low sodium, increased potassium, reduced animal protein, and augmentation of fluid intake), medical management of hypercalciuria might include thiazide diuretics, intestinal-calcium binders, or phosphate supplementation. Parathyroid disorders that increase urinary calcium should be addressed when applicable.

The urinary pH is also an important parameter to evaluate, as acid pH (below 5.5) is conducive to uric acid and cystine stones. A pH greater than 7.2 is suggestive of a struvite stone caused by a urinary tract infection.

Urinary Obstruction

Obstruction within the urinary tract is a common renal disorder encountered in both primary care and in the emergency setting. There are many causes of urinary obstruction with a wide range of outcomes. Hindrance of normal urine flow is referred to as **obstructive uropathy**. When obstruction leads to renal dysfunction, it is termed **obstructive nephropathy**. The obstruction can occur anywhere along the urinary tract, from the intrarenal collecting system to the urethral meatus. Obstruction typically leads to hydronephrosis (also called **pelvocaliectasis**) or hydroureter. Hydronephrosis is a dilation of the renal pelvis and calyces; hydroureter is characterized by dilation of the ureter. The

ureters can actually dilate until they become tortuous. When both the ureters and the renal pelvis show signs of dilation, it is termed **hydroureteronephrosis**. Hydronephrosis or hydroureter may also be caused by functional obstruction, which is not an actual physical blockage (eg, a stone or stricture) but any cause that prevents the normal progression of urine through the urinary tract (eg, neurogenic bladder or vesicoureteral reflux).

In children, the most common causes of obstructive uropathy are anatomic abnormalities such as strictures at the ureterovesical junction (UVJ) or ureteropelvic junction (UPJ). In young adults, stones are a major causative factor, and in older adults benign prostatic hypertrophy (BPH) and tumors play a major role.

The abbreviations UVJ and UPJ are extremely difficult to distinguish because V and P sound similar. Use context, not sound, to determine the correct abbreviation.

Causes of hydronephrosis and hydroureter may be classified as intrinsic, extrinsic, or functional. Examples of intrinsic causes include strictures or obstructions, papillary necrosis, ureteral folds, clots, tumors, stones, ureterocele, or urethral atresia. Functional causes include infection, reflux, and neurogenic bladder. Examples of extrinsic causes include BPH, prostate cancer, retroperitoneal masses, abdominal or pelvic masses, aortic aneurysm, pregnancy, and uterine prolapse.

Patients with an acute obstruction typically present with severe pain associated with nausea and vomiting. Chronic causes for obstruction are often slowly progressive and insidious and do not cause the severe pain characteristic of acute obstruction.

On examination, the hydronephrotic kidney may be palpable, and **CVA tenderness** is noted. Lower extremity edema may be noted. A palpably distended bladder may also be noted if the obstruction is in the lower urinary tract. Imaging studies are performed to determine the exact location and cause of the obstruction. **Intravenous pyelogram (IVP)**, KUB, CT, ultrasound, or nuclear medicine studies may be performed.

Chronic urethral strictures and partial obstructions lead to bladder diverticula. Severe, prolonged obstruction leads to loss of renal function that may not be recovered. The presence of infection adds to the urgency, as sepsis may quickly ensue. Treatment may include **retrograde ureteral stent placement**, placement of percutaneous nephrostomy tube, procedures to remove or dissolve stones, and in some cases laparoscopy or laparotomy.

> ▶ This is a 17-year-old with a history of left renal and ureteral calculi, hydroureteronephrosis, and infections, status post cystoscopy with double-J stents and ultimate stone passage with removal.

> ▶ A cystoscopy was performed that showed a tight bladder-neck contracture. The patient was counseled appropriately and was offered transurethral bladder neck incision in order to relieve bladder-neck obstruction and symptoms. No medications are going to be of benefit at this point.

> ▶ On the left, there is evidence of a grade 2 hydronephrosis. There is also dilatation of the entire length of the left ureter down to the vesicoureteral junction, indicative of left hydroureter. By history, the patient is known to have a lesion involving the bladder. Therefore, there is the possibility of a mucosal lesion encroaching on the left vesicoureteral junction producing left hydronephrosis and left hydroureter.

Prostatic Disease

The prostate gland is a donut-shaped gland about the size of a walnut located below the urinary bladder anterior to the rectum (■ **Figure 7-5**). The prostate gland

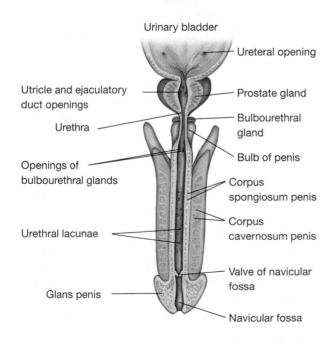

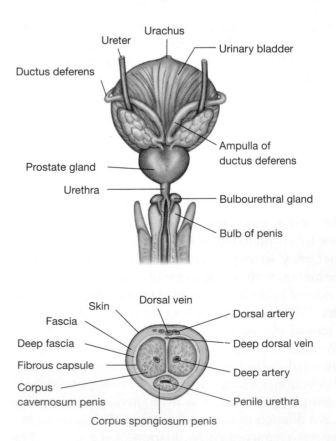

FIGURE 7-5 Anatomy of the prostate gland and penis.

surrounds the prostatic urethra. The prostate's role is to secrete prostatic fluid into the semen to increase the pH and help sperm survive in the acidity of the female vagina.

Benign Prostatic Hypertrophy

Benign prostatic hypertrophy (BPH) is the most common benign tumor in men. The hypertrophy is thought to be mediated by the hormone dihydrotestosterone (DHT). The increased size of the prostate causes obstruction, which may be either mechanical or dynamic. Mechanical obstruction is caused by the prostate pressing on the urethra and bladder outlet. Dynamic obstruction is caused by the effects of increased muscle tone within the prostate tissue in response to autonomic stimulation. Bladder outlet obstruction causes increased work on the detrusor muscles, leading to muscle hypertrophy, hyperplasia, and collagen deposition within the bladder walls. These changes are seen as trabeculations on cystoscopy.

Symptoms of BPH include obstructive and irritative voiding. Patients may complain of hesitancy, decreased force and caliber of stream, a sensation of incomplete bladder emptying, **double voiding** (urinating twice within two hours), straining to urinate, or postvoid dribbling. Sequelae of untreated BPH include recurrent UTIs, gross hematuria, bladder stones, and renal insufficiency.

Patients are assessed using a **seven-question** symptom index with a symptom score ranging from 0–35. The index was developed by the American Urological Association (AUA) and may be referred to as the **AUA score**. Scores between 10 and 20 correlate to moderate symptoms and a score greater than 20 indicates severe symptoms. Physical examination, including a digital rectal exam (DRE), typically shows an enlarged, smooth, firm, elastic prostate. Induration is more indicative of prostate cancer. A normal prostate ranges in size from 20 to 40 g.

Treatment recommendations are based on the patient's AUA score. Low scores may be treated with watchful waiting. Symptoms caused by smooth-muscle contraction are treated with alpha-blocker therapy (eg, Cardura, Flomax, and Hytrin). Hypertrophy may be reduced with the long-term use of **5-alpha-reductase inhibitors** (eg, finasteride) that block DHT production. Procedures to treat prostatic hypertrophy are listed on page 223.

Prostatitis

Prostatitis, also referred to as **prostatodynia**, is inflammation of the prostate gland. The most common cause is bacterial prostatitis, which may be acute or chronic. Bacteria implicated are the typical urinary tract pathogens (Klebsiella, Proteus, E coli, and chlamydia). Symptoms typically include irritative voiding (frequency, urgency, nocturia, double voiding). Pain may be experienced in the perineum, top of the penis, lower back, or testes. Acute prostatitis may produce flu-like symptoms. Digital rectal exam may reveal an **exquisitely tender** prostate that feels swollen, boggy, or indurated.

Often patients are treated empirically with antibiotics. If therapy fails, laboratory studies may be performed. **Prostate specific antigen (PSA)** test is typically drawn to assess the degree of prostate inflammation. Urinalysis and culture may be performed on two separate urine samples. The first sample is a midstream urine collection. The second collection follows digital prostate massage. UA may be positive for pyuria, bacteriuria, and hematuria.

If cultures are negative, the diagnosis is **abacterial prostatodynia (nonbacterial prostatitis)**. The etiology for abacterial prostatodynia is not known. To better reflect the lack of understanding of this disease, it has been reclassified as **inflammatory chronic pelvic pain syndrome (CPPS)**. These patients show increased leukocytes in expressed prostate secretions but the culture is negative. Even though the cultures are negative, a trial of antibiotics is given with the assumption that the causative agent is a fastidious organism that is difficult to culture such as Ureaplasma, mycoplasma, or chlamydia.

> Be careful that you correctly transcribe "abacterial infection" and not "a bacterial infection." These terms sound the same but are opposite in meaning.

Antibiotics used to treat bacterial prostatitis include ampicillin, aminoglycosides, trimethoprim-sulfamethoxazole, carbenicillin, erythromycin, cephalexin, or fluoroquinolones. Treatment may be required for 6–12 weeks. Obstructive prostatitis with urinary retention requires a **percutaneous suprapubic tube** for drainage, as catheterization is contraindicated in the setting of a swollen, infected prostate.

- Obstruction of the urinary tract causes obstructive uropathy or obstructive nephropathy and may lead to hydroureter, hydronephrosis, or hydroureteronephrosis.
- Causes of obstruction include physical barriers such as stones, strictures, tumors, and BPH as well as functional obstruction caused by a neurogenic bladder or vesicoureteral reflux.
- Treatment should address the primary cause of the obstruction and may also include a ureteral stent or nephrostomy tube. Prolonged obstruction causes permanent loss of renal function.
- BPH, the most common benign tumor in men, causes obstructive and irritative voiding symptoms. The AUA score is used to assess symptoms of BPH.
- Treatment of BPH may include medical management to shrink the prostate or to decrease the intensity of smooth-muscle contractions within the prostate. If medical management fails, minimally invasive procedures are available to reduce the size of the prostate or to remove the prostate.
- Prostatitis is inflammation of the prostate gland, usually caused by infection. Patients with a slightly elevated PSA value are usually treated empirically with antibiotics. Recurrent prostatitis requires long-term antibiotic therapy lasting 6–12 weeks.

Diagnostic Studies

Urology and nephrology make tremendous use of diagnostic imaging, diagnostic procedures, and laboratory tests in the evaluation and treatment of urological disorders.

X-rays

Imaging studies based on x-ray technology have a large role in the diagnosis and treatment of urological disorders, especially urinary tract masses or disorders involving calcium-based stones. Plain radiographs as well as imaging utilizing computed tomography and contrast media play important roles in the diagnosis of urinary tract disorders.

Kidneys, Ureters, Bladder

An x-ray of the kidneys, ureters, and bladder (KUB) is an anteroposterior flat-plate x-ray using plain film to evaluate the urinary tract for stones or masses. It may also be used to locate a double-J stent. When a KUB precedes another diagnostic study, it is typically referred to as a **scout film**. When reading a KUB film, the radiologist may comment on the presence of **phleboliths**, calcified lymph nodes, an **appendicolith**, granuloma, or other calcified masses. Plain film images combined with CT images provide the best diagnostic information for the treatment of stone disease.

Pause 7-7 What are phleboliths and appendicoliths?

FINDINGS: The KUB demonstrates what appears to be a small triangular calculus in the midpole calyx, 6 mm, left kidney. The right kidney is unremarkable. In the pelvis, phleboliths are seen. Bilateral hip replacements are noted. Degenerative disk changes are seen throughout the lumbar spine and in the SI joints.

CONCLUSION: No definite right renal or ureteral calculi seen, although there is suspicion for a triangular, 6 mm calculus in the midpole of the left kidney.

Intravenous Pyelogram

An intravenous pyelogram (IVP), also referred to as **excretory urography (EXU)**, uses intravenous radiopaque contrast media to produce a series of x-ray images of the entire urinary tract. A scout film is taken immediately before the administration of contrast. A bolus of intravenous contrast material (eg, Optiray) is given and x-ray images are taken at intervals (1, 5, 10, and 15 minutes or until contrast is seen filling both ureters). The contrast media can first be seen as a "blush" in the cortical area of the kidneys. A few minutes later, the contrast outlines the calices and the renal pelvis. At the next interval, contrast is seen within the ureters and eventually the bladder. Blockages within the kidney or ureter will extend the time required to complete the test. After the contrast reaches the bladder, the patient is asked to void and a postvoid image is taken.

An IVP is useful for identifying hydronephrosis and hydroureter. It can also show nonopaque stones as a filling defect. The progression of the contrast media is indicative of the functional status of the kidney as well. The patient must have intact renal function with a creatinine less than 2.0 in order to undergo an IVP because patients with impaired renal function are at risk of renal failure after administration of IV contrast material. Due to the risk of allergic reaction and renal failure following administration of IV contrast media, the IVP has largely been replaced by **noncontrast CT scans**.

Retrograde Pyelogram

A **retrograde pyelogram** is the ideal test for determining the anatomy of the urinary system, especially for presurgical planning. A retrograde pyelogram is performed under general anesthesia. A ureteral catheter is inserted through the urethral meatus (as opposed to intravenously) and contrast media is injected into the ureters up to the UPJ. Radiographic images are obtained (■ Figure 7-6). This test visualizes the ureters, UPJ, renal pelvis, and calices. The test aids in the

---

> ▶ TECHNIQUE: Scout KUB followed by standard-protocol IVP after the administration of 100 mL of Ultravist intravenously.
>
> SCOUT KUB: There is either a 17 mm stone or at least 2 side-by-side stones in the left renal pelvis region. No definite right nephrolithiasis is seen. No definite urolithiasis is seen. Mild degenerative changes of the spine, sacroiliac joints, and hips. Soft tissues are unremarkable.
>
> The 1-minute view demonstrates symmetric uptake of contrast from the kidneys. On the 3- and 5-minute views, there is more notable opacification of the left ureter. There is no definite obstruction of the right ureter, although mild pelvocaliectasis is noted on the right. The right ureter is segmentally visualized without definite stone or stricture demonstrated. The left ureter was seen in its entirety without evidence of stone or stricture. The urinary bladder is within normal limits. There is no significant postvoid residual. On the 10-minute and postvoid examinations, there is a punctate, calcific density, which at first projects over the left femoral head and then to the left of the sacrum. This is likely not in the ureter.
>
> IMPRESSION
> 1. Left nephrolithiasis with one or multiple side-by-side stones in the left renal pelvis. However, no significant hydronephrosis, urolithiasis, or obstruction is seen.
> 2. Mild pelvocaliectasis on the right with an otherwise unremarkable exam of the right kidney and ureter.
> 3. No significant postvoid residual.

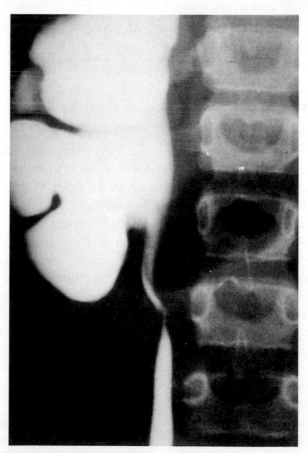

FIGURE 7-6 Retrograde pyelogram showing a constriction in the ureter. *Source:* Courtesy of Philip E. Gleason, MD.

evaluation and diagnosis of structural disorders such as stones, filling defects, ureteral kinks, ureteral strictures, vesicoureteral reflux, fistulas, diverticula, and urinary tract tumors. This procedure is also used to determine the required length and width of an indwelling double-J stent prior to placement. Patients with known reactions or contraindications for the use of intravenous contrast agents may be evaluated with a retrograde pyelogram because the contrast media does not enter the blood stream or pass through the nephrons.

Voiding Cystourethrogram (VCUG)

A voiding cystourethrogram (VCUG) is a radiographic study of the lower urinary tract. A catheter is inserted through the urethra and the bladder is filled with contrast media. X-rays are taken of the bladder and urethra during filling and also while the patient voids. The test is useful in diagnosing bladder outlet obstruction, sphincter abnormalities, ureterocele, bladder wall abnormalities, and vesicoureteral reflux.

> I reviewed the VCUG and there is no urinary reflux. The bladder has a normal capacity and normal shape. There is no postvoid residual. No urinary reflux. The entire exam is normal.

CT

Noncontrast helical CT has become the test of choice in the evaluation of renal colic. Helical CT takes multiple, incremental images of the entire urinary system and can be performed without IV contrast. A helical CT is the most sensitive and specific test for localizing urinary stones, including radiolucent stones that are not visible on KUB. It can also distinguish between stones and blood clots. CT scans are also useful for detecting ureteral dilation, renal enlargement (**nephromegaly**), hydronephrosis, and inflammatory changes seen as **perinephric stranding** or **streaking in the perinephric fatty tissue**. The abdominopelvic images include the kidneys, renal blood vessels, ureters, and bladder as well as other abdominal and pelvic structures. **CT urography** combines a CT study with an IVP.

Phleboliths are commonly seen and must be distinguished from ureteral stones. Oftentimes, stones create a local inflammatory reaction with edema. This creates a **rim sign** (also described as a halo or ring) around the stone on CT images and is a distinguishing factor. Uric

acid stones as well as stones consisting of cystine, matrix, and **xanthine** appear as bright white spots and are easily distinguished from calcific stones and the surrounding tissue.

> A CT scan of the abdomen and pelvis was performed for complaint of left renal colic along with gross hematuria. This indicates a large obstructing distal left ureteral calculus with hydroureteronephrosis proximal to the stone. In addition, there are stones in both the right and left lower poles of both kidneys. Due to the symptomatic nature and large size of the distal left ureteral stone, this will be treated with a transurethral ureteroscopic laser lithotripsy and placement of a double-J ureteral stent.

> **Pause 7-8** Draw a simple diagram of the kidneys and ureters and mark the location of the stones and hydroureter as described in the sample dictation above.

Ultrasound

Ultrasound imaging is very useful in the evaluation and management of urinary tract disorders. Renal ultrasound is performed through the abdomen or back, and bladder ultrasound is performed through the lower abdominal wall. Ultrasound studies are helpful in assessing the size and location of the kidneys, the presence of hydronephrosis, hydroureter, cysts, obstructions, and as a screening test for medical renal disease (eg, glomerulonephritis).

Renal cysts are the most common masses detected on renal ultrasound, and the vast majority of cysts are benign. Most patients over the age of 55 will show some renal cyst formation. A **multicystic kidney** contains multiple simple cysts that increase in numbers as the patient ages. A fluid-filled cyst appears **anechoic** while cysts containing solid material or debris appear more **echogenic**. Cysts may be classified as simple or complex. Simple cysts are collections of serous fluid and do not require treatment. Simple cysts may contain blood (hemorrhagic cysts) or be infected. Hemorrhagic and infected cysts are highly echogenic. Complex cysts may be described as unilocular (ie, have a single chamber) or septated, also called multilocular (ie, have multiple chambers). Although ultrasound cannot definitively determine if a cyst is benign or malignant, the **Bosniak classification** system, based on ultrasound characteristics, gives diagnostic guidance.

> Multiple bilateral renal cysts. Large complex cyst in the inferior pole of the right kidney measuring 8.7 x 5.5 x 4.9 cm. This is likely a Bosniak IIF lesion. Recommend further characterization with MRI to exclude neoplastic soft tissue component.

Illnesses such as glomerulonephritis, diabetes, hypertension, and autoimmune diseases cause the kidneys to appear more hyperechoic and oftentimes smaller than normal. Edematous areas of the kidneys appear hypoechoic. Swelling or hemorrhage within the kidney may be detected by **effacement of the corticomedullary boundaries**. Pyelonephritis caused by gas-producing bacteria may be detected by the presence of gas, referred to as **emphysematous pyelonephritis**.

Bladder ultrasound can detect bladder wall abnormalities, bladder stones, tumors, or diverticula. Fistulas can also be visualized. Ultrasound is also used to determine postvoid residual volumes. Ultrasound studies are typically performed with a full bladder. Water is hypoechoic, so distortions of the bladder wall (eg, diverticula) or intraluminal masses appear echogenic against the black outline of the water/urine. The addition of Doppler technology to an ultrasound study can evaluate renal blood flow, especially thromboembolic disease.

> FINDINGS: Right kidney measures 13.3 cm. Left kidney measures 12.8 cm. Normal cortical echogenicity and thickness bilaterally. No hydronephrosis. Exophytic upper pole cyst on the right measures 3.6 x 3.0 cm. Additional upper pole cyst on the right measures 1.4 x 1.1 cm. These are simple in appearance. Parapelvic cyst in the mid left kidney measures 8 x 8 mm. Varices in the inferior pole on the right, described on prior MRI, are not seen on the current study.

Nuclear Medicine Scans

Both functional and anatomical information can be gained through nuclear medicine scans, also called **scintigraphy**. A radionuclide is injected and images are obtained at timed intervals using a gamma camera. Progression of the radionuclide through the urinary system is helpful in the evaluation of **renovascular disorders**, tubular function, vesicoureteral reflux, or renal obstruction. Several different radionuclide pharmaceuticals are used, two of which use technetium 99m:

- ^{99m}Tc-mercaptoacetyltriglycine (^{99m}Tc-MAG3)
- ^{99m}Tc-diethylenetriamine pentaacetic acid (^{99m}Tc-DTPA)
- ^{131}I–hippurate

> **Pause 7-9** Review the guidelines in the *Book of Style* for transcribing radioisotopes. List the two different ways isotopes may be written.

Cortical scintigraphy is a nuclear imaging study of the renal parenchyma. It is used to diagnose pyelonephritis, scarring, and solid renal masses. It can also be used to determine relative renal function (comparing the function of left and right kidneys), **renal ectopia**, infarction, and thrombosis. Renal scintigraphy is used to evaluate renal blood flow as well as renal function. The venographic phase of a renal scan is useful for diagnosing renal vein thrombosis. The obstructed kidney will be photopenic, indicating no perfusion of the radionuclide through the kidney.

Nuclear imaging studies may be combined with furosemide (**diuretic renography**) to enhance the functional information gathered. After administration of ^{99m}Tc-MAG3, furosemide is given. Normally, a **washout** is observed as the kidney rapidly excretes the radionuclide. The time required to excrete half the radionuclide from the renal pelvis is the T½. Retention of the radionuclide following furosemide indicates obstruction. Vesicoureteral reflux (VUR) is indicated if tracer activity within the collecting system decreases and then increases again.

Pause 7-10 Explain why the tracer activity decreases and then increases when VUR is present.

TECHNIQUE: The patient received an IV injection of 10.3 mCi of ^{99m}Tc-MAG3, and 30-minute dynamic-acquisition scans were obtained.

FINDINGS: The renal perfusion images demonstrate diminished flow to both kidneys. The functional image shows diminished cortical uptake of radiotracer by the left kidney. A photopenic defect in the medial aspect of the left kidney subsequently fills with activity over time, consistent with a dilated collecting system. Images of the right kidney demonstrate good cortical uptake with prompt appearance of activity in the right collecting system.

IMPRESSION
1. Mildly impaired flow and function of the left kidney.
2. Mildly impaired flow with good function of the right kidney.

Endoscopy

Direct visualization of the urinary tract using endoscopes is a common and highly utilized diagnostic and therapeutic modality. **Urethroscopy**, cystoscopy, and **cystourethroscopy** use a cystoscope inserted through the urethral meatus to examine the entire length of the urethra, bladder **urothelium**, **trigone**, and ureteral orifices. (12) Indications for cystoscopy include hematuria, recurrent UTI, voiding disorders

(12) The urothelium is the epithelial lining of the urinary tract. The trigone is the triangular space at the base of the bladder formed by the two ureteral orifices and the bladder outlet.

as well as diagnosis and surveillance of bladder cancer. The cystoscope can also be used to obtain urothelial biopsies or to remove lesions and foreign bodies. Urethral strictures can be treated and double-J stents can be placed.

Using the obturator, the #17-French Olympus cystoscope was passed into the bladder. The obturator was removed and replaced with a 70-degree lens. A thorough evaluation of the bladder mucosa revealed no abnormalities. Both ureteral orifices were in their normal position and configuration, exuding clear urine. There were no stones. There were no calculi, tumors, or irregularities of the bladder mucosa. A 30-degree lens was then placed to allow visualization of the urethra, which was intact and normal.

CYSTOSCOPY: Flexible cystoscope was passed without difficulty. Urethra is normal. Bladder is entered, and flexible cystoscope used to systematically visualize the entire bladder mucosa. No evidence of mucosal lesions or tumors. Both ureteral orifices seen to efflux clear urine. Scope is retroflexed on the bladder neck and it is normal. However, the external and internal sphincters are wide open, allowing for total incontinence. He has a large-capacity, compliant bladder without any bladder contractions during the cystoscopy.

Ureteroscopy is an endoscopic procedure for examining the ureters and evaluating filling defects previously identified on radiologic studies. Indigo carmine dye, which turns the urine blue, may be administered intravenously or directly into the ureters to help detect leaks or reflux. A ureteral brush biopsy may also be performed. The intrarenal collecting system can be examined with the use of a **flexible ureteropyeloscopy**.

> **FINDINGS:** Using a cystoscope, the urinary bladder was examined and found to be intact with no evidence of suture or puncture injury. A #5-French whistle-tip catheter was inserted into bilateral ureters and passed without difficulty. Indigo carmine was noted to drain from bilateral ureteral orifices. The patient tolerated the procedure well.

Nephroscopy, which is the direct visualization of the kidney, is performed through a percutaneous tract using a nephroscope. This procedure can be used to extract renal stones, as a **second-look procedure** to remove residual renal calculi, or to diagnose upper urinary tract pathology.

Urodynamic Studies

A **urodynamic study (UDS)** includes a series of tests to investigate the lower urinary tract. A UDS assesses the bladder, urethra, and sphincter to determine the cause and appropriate treatment of urinary incontinence, irritative voiding symptoms, incomplete voiding, and recurrent urinary tract infections. Components of a UDS may include uroflow, cystometry, leak point pressure, electromyography, and videourodynamics.

Uroflow is a noninvasive procedure for evaluating bladder outlet obstruction or abnormal voiding patterns. The procedure measures the peak flow of urine in milliliters per second. Decreased flow may be indicative of urethral obstruction, a weak detrusor, or a combination of both.

Cystometry evaluates the anatomic and functional status of the bladder. A cystometer measures the contractile force (ie, the pressure) within the bladder during filling and voiding, effectively measuring **detrusor activity**, sensation, capacity, and compliance. The graph generated from the cystometric analysis is called a **cystometrogram (CMG)**, which plots the volume of urine voided against intravesical pressure.

Simple cystometry only detects abnormal detrusor compliance. A **multichannel** (or **subtracted) cystometrogram (CMG)** simultaneously measures intraabdominal and detrusor pressures by placing a catheter in the urethra and a probe in the rectum or vagina. Pressures are measured while filling the bladder and again while voiding. Subtracting the pressure readings taken from the bladder and the abdomen allows involuntary detrusor contractions to be distinguished from intraabdominal pressure. A CMG combined with uroflow, referred to as a **pressure flow study**, can distinguish bladder outlet obstruction from detrusor dysfunction.

> **FINDINGS:** On initial uroflow, he voided 74 mL and had 630 mL of postvoid residual urine with a peak flow of 3.1. Then the test was stopped and he voided another 25 mL. The cystometrogram was carried out. He has a normally compliant bladder with a capacity of approximately 200 when he had the first sensation and 491 was his capacity. He has detrusor contraction measuring peak pressure of 64 cm H_2O with near-zero flow with quieting of his external sphincter.
>
> **ASSESSMENT:** High-pressure bladder and low-flow, high-grade outlet obstruction.

Measurement of the **abdominal leak point pressure (ALPP)** is used to evaluate stress urinary incontinence and can be taken as part of a multichannel urodynamic study. The ALPP test measures the amount of abdominal pressure required to overcome the intrinsic sphincter pressure, resulting in leakage of urine. The test is performed with the bladder approximately half full. The patient is asked to cough and to perform the Valsalva maneuver, successively increasing the amount of abdominal pressure exerted on the bladder with each cough or maneuver. The pressure at which leakage occurs is the ALPP. Patients with normal continence should not leak any urine.

Electromyography (EMG) studies may be added to a urodynamic study to evaluate for discoordinated voiding. Needle electrodes are placed on the external sphincter. Failure of the urethra to relax during bladder contraction is indicative of detrusor sphincter dyssynergia.

Videourodynamic studies combine the radiographic findings of a voiding cystourethrogram (VCUG) with multichannel urodynamics. A urodynamic catheter (eg, a Cook dual-lumen, pigtailed catheter), a rectal tube, and EMG electrodes are placed. Room-temperature contrast is used to fill the bladder to produce fluoroscopic images. With the aid of fluoroscopy, urodynamic studies are performed, including uroflow studies, a static cystogram (to detect cystoceles), VCUG, ALPP, and EMG.

Joaquin came in for videourodynamic study to evaluate for neurogenic bladder. This was performed under sterile conditions. A #6-French double-lumen catheter was placed in the urethra. The rectal catheter was inserted. The contrast was infused at the flow rate of 5 mL. The bladder was slowly filled, and under fluoroscopy the bladder appeared to be smooth and spherical in shape. There was no trabeculation.

The detrusor pressure remained fairly stable, below 40 cm H_2O. During the procedure, Joaquin was moving constantly; therefore, there are a lot of artifacts. However, I did not notice uninhibited contractions.

The bladder was filled to almost 100 mL. This is well over his anatomical capacity at this age. Joaquin began to leak at about 94 mL. He is not able to generate very effective bladder contractions. I also noticed urine leaking with straining; therefore, this indicates Valsalva voiding. At the end of voiding, Joaquin still had about 30 mL of postvoid residual. I also noticed mild, right-sided, grade 1 reflux after the voiding phase.

Pause 7-11 Explain "uninhibited contractions" as the phrase is used in the above sample dictation.

Laboratory Studies

Laboratory studies of blood and urine play a dominant role in the diagnosis, treatment, and management of urological disorders. Urine collections may be random,

(13) Laboratory tests may be classified as qualitative or quantitative. Qualitative tests typically give a "positive/negative" or "present/absent" result, while quantitative tests give an actual value, volume, or measurable quantity. Screening tests are often qualitative, while confirmatory tests are typically quantitative.

which means they are collected at any time during the day, or they may be first-morning collections. First-morning urine is typically more concentrated and contains a higher percentage of solutes than a random specimen. Some laboratory studies require a 24-hour urine collection in which all urine voided within a 24-hour time frame is collected into a single container. Blood collections, likewise, may be random or may coincide with the collection of a random urine sample or at the beginning or end of a 24-hour urine collection. Correlating blood and urine levels of certain constituents can give important diagnostic information in the diagnosis of kidney disorders, since the kidneys are responsible for clearing substances from the blood. Theoretically, as concentrations of a given substance (that is known to be excreted by the kidneys) decreases in the blood, urine levels of the same substance should increase.

Urine may be obtained through a catheter or by voiding. A clean-catch urine sample is preferred for most urine studies. This method requires external cleansing of the urethral opening with a nonfoamy disinfectant soap to reduce contamination from normal flora of the external genitalia. A midstream urine sample refers to the capture of urine several seconds after the beginning of flow, after approximately 5 mL has been expelled. The next 5–10 mL is collected into a sterile container. A midstream catch reduces contamination from bacteria normally found in the urethra. Urine may also be collected following prostatic massage in order to capture prostatic secretions.

Urinalysis

Urinalysis with microscopic examination of the sediment (UA with micro) is the most common urine test performed. A urinalysis includes a visual examination of the urine for color (eg, straw, yellow, dark yellow, brown) and turbidity (eg, cloudy, hazy, clear), measurement of the specific gravity, and a dipstick test using a reagent strip. The dipstick is a small, thin strip with 10 different test pads impregnated with test reagents (■ **Figure 7-7**). Each pad reacts with the urine and changes color to indicate a positive or negative reaction. Components of a urine dipstick analysis are described in **Table 7-4**. The dipstick test gives qualitative, quantitative, and semiquantitative results. Qualitative values are reported in terms such as trace, small, moderate, or large, or 1+, 2+, etc. Semiquantitative values are reported as the lowest value in a range (eg, see comment under glucose in Table 7-4). (13)

Table 7-4 Components of a Dipstick Urinalysis

Component	Reference Range	Comments
specific gravity	1.002 to 1.030	
urine pH (■ Figure 7-8)	5.0 to 8.0	Alkaline urine in a patient with suspected UTI suggests infection with Proteus, Klebsiella, or Pseudomonas; acidic urine in patients with urolithiasis suggests uric acid or cystine stones.
protein	negative	Dipstick detects albumin concentrations as low 30 mg/dL. Urine protein concentrations are reported as 30, 100, 300, or 2000 mg/dL.
urobilinogen	trace	Increased levels are indicative of liver disease.
bilirubin	negative	Increased levels are indicative of liver disease. Positive result may be confirmed with Ictotest.
glucose	negative	Increased levels seen in diabetes mellitus and diabetes insipidus. Glucose is reported as 100, 250, 500, 1000, or >1000 mg/dL.
ketones	negative	Levels elevate with diabetic ketoacidosis, increased protein, and decreased carbohydrate catabolism. Color reactions are categorized as trace, small, moderate, and large, corresponding to ketone concentrations of 5, 15, 40–80 and 80–160 mg/dL of urine, respectively.
nitrites	negative	Nitrites suggest infection with gram-negative bacteria that reduce normally occurring nitrates to nitrite. Results are reported as positive or negative.
leukocyte esterase	negative	Esterase indicates presence of PMNs that contain leukocyte esterase. Positive results are reported semiquantitatively as trace, 1+, 2+, or 3+ or (alternatively) small, moderate, or large.
blood	negative	Test reagents react with the heme component of blood; a positive test indicates presence of hemoglobin or myoglobin but cannot distinguish between intact RBCs and free heme molecules; reported as small, moderate, or large.

The **specific gravity** is an important component of the urinalysis. It is a relative measure of the amount of dissolved solids in the urine and is indicative of the kidneys' ability to concentrate urine. The specific gravity of pure water is 1.000. All urine contains some solutes, so the specific gravity of urine will always be greater than 1.000. A low specific gravity of 1.016 indicates dilute urine, and a high specific gravity of 1.030 represents highly concentrated urine. Normally, the kidneys should be able to produce urine with a range of specific gravity values in response to physiologic needs. Abnormal specific gravity values are often indicative of renal tubular disease. **Hyposthenuria** refers to a persistently low urine specific gravity of less than 1.007. Patients with late-stage renal tubular disease can only produce isosthenuric urine with a fixed specific gravity of 1.010. Specific gravity

values above 1.035 are physiologically impossible and may be due to contamination with contrast media such as Renografin or Hypaque. Dipstick test strips typically contain a test pad for determining specific gravity, but values may also be determined using a refractometer.

Most often, the specific gravity value is dictated without the decimal. For example, 1.020 would be dictated "ten twenty." Always transcribe the value with the decimal, even when not dictated. Always transcribe all three decimals following the decimal point, even if the last decimal is zero.

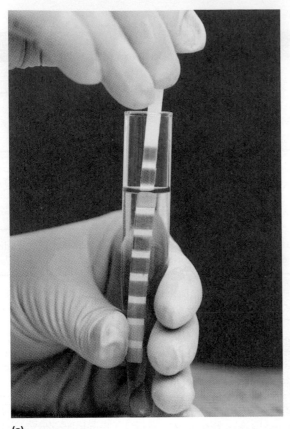

(a)

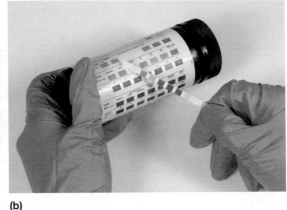

(b)

FIGURE 7-7 Urine dipstick test is performed by (a) dipping the reagent strip into a urine sample. *Source:* ©zilli/ iStockphoto.com. (b) comparing the color changes of each of the reagent squares on the dipstick. *Source:* David Gold/iStockphoto.com.

A microscopic examination of urine reports the presence of formed elements such as cells, casts, and crystals. If all dipstick urinalysis parameters are normal, the microscopic examination may not be necessary. Physicians may order a **UA with reflex to micro, (14)** meaning the microscopic exam is only performed if the dipstick results indicate a need for further examination.

To perform the microscopic examination, a 10 mL aliquot **(15)** of urine is centrifuged, forcing any formed elements or particulate matter to the bottom of the test tube. Then 9 mL of the supernatant is decanted **(16)**, leaving a 10-fold concentration of urine sediment (■ **Figure 7-9**). A small drop of the concentrated

(14) When used in reference to a laboratory test, the term reflex means a positive test result should automatically trigger an order for a followup test. Given a normal test result, the reflex test is not performed.

(15) An aliquot (*al'-i-kwot*) is a portion (sampling) taken from the whole.

(16) The supernatant is the clear liquid that results from removing particulate matter from a fluid, either by gravity (natural settling) or by gravitational force (centrifuging). Decant means to carefully pour off the supernatant so as not to disturb the particulate matter in the bottom of the test tube.

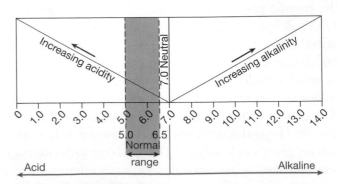

FIGURE 7-8 Urine pH scale.

Table 7-5 Formed Elements Reported on a Microscopic Evaluation of Urine.

Formed Element	Reference Range	Comments
leukocytes	0–5 WBC per high-power field	>5 WBC per high-power field is positive for pyuria; suggests infection or injury to the urinary tract.
erythrocytes	0–5 RBC per high-power field (may be higher in females)	>5 RBC per high-power field is positive for hematuria and warrants further investigation.
epithelial cells	small numbers normally present	Large numbers of squamous epithelial cells indicate contamination; many large clumps are suspicious for neoplasm.
bacteria and yeast	none	Small numbers of bacteria or yeast seen in each high-power field has a high correlation with bacterial infection.
casts	none (rare epithelial, hyaline or granular cast may be considered normal)	Examined under low power; types of casts include broad, waxy, hyaline, RBC, WBC, and granular.
crystals	none	Uric acid, oxalate, and phosphate crystals may be seen in normal individuals and in stone formers. Cystine crystals indicate cystinuria and are always pathologic. Other crystals of clinical significance include leucine and tyrosine.

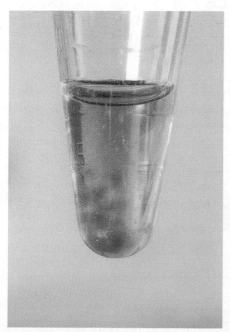

FIGURE 7-9 The urine sediment that remains in the test tube after decanting the supernatant is examined under a microscope. *Source:* Michal Heron/Pearson Education.

urine is placed on a microscope slide and examined for formed elements (**Table 7-5**). A **high-power field** is magnified 40 times (40X) and a **low-power field** is magnified 10 times (10X). The number of each formed element is reported as the average number of elements seen in one field of the microscope. When there are too many elements to reasonably count, the number is reported as **too numerous to count (TNTC)**.

> Formed elements are dictated as the number of elements seen per microscopic field. White cells may be dictated as "five to ten WBCs per high-power field," which is transcribed as "5–10 WBC per high-power field." Casts are reported as the number seen per low-power field. For example, "The UA with micro showed 1–2 broad, waxy casts per low-power field."

Formed elements (eg, white cells, red cells, casts) in the urinary sediment may also be reported using semiquantitative descriptions:

- occasional   0–3
- few   3–6
- moderate   6–12
- many   12 or more
- TNTC   Too numerous to count

Creatinine

Serum creatinine is the most widely used indicator of renal function. Creatinine is a byproduct of muscle metabolism, and its production rate is proportional to muscle mass. Individuals with greater-than-average muscle mass typically have higher creatinine levels while smaller individuals and those with muscle wasting or amputations have lower baseline levels. Women generally have lower creatinine levels than men, and the elderly also have decreased baseline creatinine levels. The creatinine clearance value is used to calculate the glomerular filtration rate (GFR) for several reasons: the level of creatinine production is fairly constant for any given individual, its only route of excretion is the kidneys, and it is not reabsorbed or secreted by the tubules. Reference values for creatinine and GFR are shown in **Table 7-6**.

Decreased glomerular filtration results in less creatinine filtered and a concomitant rise in blood levels. To determine the creatinine clearance, urine is collected for 24 hours. A blood sample is drawn to coincide with the urine collection. A 24-hour urine collection accounts for the diurnal variation in the excretion of creatinine and therefore gives results that are more accurate. Creatinine clearance is calculated using the following formula:

$$\left[\frac{urine\ creatinine \times urine\ volume}{serum\ creatinine \times min.\ of\ duration} \right] = \frac{mL}{min}$$

The glomerular filtration rate is determined by calculating the creatinine clearance and then adjusting for the patient's height and weight. Laboratories typically are not given the patient's height and weight, so this calculation cannot be reported by the lab. Instead, laboratories report the GFR using an average value to represent the body surface area (BSA), so the result reported by the lab is written in milliliters per minute divided by a constant value for the BSA (1.73 m²). Values below 60 mL/min/1.73 m² indicate slight impairment. Values in the 30- to 40-range suggest moderate renal impairment, and values of 28 or below represent severe renal impairment.

An estimate of the GFR can be calculated using the serum creatinine value and the **MDRD equation**, named for the Modification of Diet in Renal Disease (MDRD) Study. This equation does not require the collection of a 24-hour urine sample.

 Using the MDRD, with an age of 73, his estimated GFR is only 17 mL/min. His 24-hour urine creatinine and protein are pending. Given his history of hepatitis C, he is at risk for chronic membranoproliferative glomerulonephritis related to the hepatitis C infection.

Pause 7-12   Why are GFR values above 60 not clinically significant?

Blood Urea Nitrogen

Blood urea nitrogen (BUN) is the major end product of protein catabolism and is produced in the liver. Urea is freely filtered through the glomeruli but it is

Table 7-6 Creatinine and GFR Reference Values

Test Name	Reference Range	Comment
serum creatinine	0.6 to 1.3 mg/dL (males) 0.4 to 1.1 mg/dL (females)	
urine creatinine	0.8 to 2.0 g/24 hours (male) 0.6 to 1.8 g/24 hours (female)	
glomerular filtration rate	60–180 mL/min/1.73 m²	Only values below 60 are reported; values above 60 are reported as "above 60 mL/min/1.73 m."

also reabsorbed to a certain extent in the distal tubules. Because it is also reabsorbed, it is not as accurate as creatinine for determining glomerular filtration. Other variables such as nutrition status, liver function, and hydration status can affect the BUN value, so this metabolite alone is not a good indicator of renal function. But taken together, the BUN and creatinine values can be informative (**Table 7-7**). The BUN-to-creatinine ratio is normally 10. Increases or decreases in the ratio may indicate that the abnormal BUN values are due to renal impairment, liver impairment, hemolysis, or other causes. The BUN does, however, correlate well to uremic symptoms and can be used to determine the timing of dialysis and the adequacy of a dialysis treatment.

> Most dictators will dictate blood urea nitrogen as the abbreviation b-u-n, but occasionally you will hear it pronounced as the acronym "bun."

Table 7-7 BUN

Test Name	Reference Range
BUN	5–20 mg/dL
BUN-to-creatinine ratio	10

Note: Ratios have no parameters since the upper value (numerator) and the lower value (denominator) in the fraction use the same units, which are canceled out in the calculation.

$$\frac{20 \, mg/dL}{2 \, mg/dL} = 10$$

Ionized Calcium

Monitoring ionized calcium (also called free calcium) is important in managing the critically ill patient. Extreme hypocalcemia or hypercalcemia can cause cardiac arrest. Calcium exists in the plasma in three different forms. Half is ionized, meaning it is not attached to any other molecule and it carries an electrical charge (in the case of calcium, the charge is positive). The remainder of calcium in the plasma is bound to protein molecules such as albumin or to anions (negatively charged molecules) such a bicarbonate, citrate, or phosphate. Only ionized calcium is biologically active; bound calcium can be decoupled from its binder to serve as an immediate resource when more ionized calcium is needed (**Table 7-8**).

Table 7-8 Plasma Calcium

Test Name	Reference Range	Comments
total plasma calcium (Ca)	8.8 to 10.2 mg/dL	
ionized calcium (Ca$^+$)	4.5 to 5.3 mg/dL	Critical values are <3.5 mg/dL and >6.4 mg/dL.

Sodium

Sodium is the most abundant cation (positively charged electrolyte) in the extracellular fluid and is the most osmotically active electrolyte as well. The kidney plays a central role in the feedback mechanisms that control the body's total sodium and water. The body attempts to maintain a tight range of plasma sodium concentration at about 136–145 mEq/L. There are dire consequences when sodium reaches critical values of less than 120 mEq/L or greater than 155 mEq/L. Hyponatremia, defined as a serum sodium level of less than 125 mEq/L, is the most common electrolyte imbalance among hospitalized patients.

When hyponatremia is present, concomitant measurement of urine sodium helps determine the site of sodium loss. Elevated sodium in the urine (greater than 20 mEq/L) is indicative of renal loss. Hyponatruria indicates an extrarenal loss of sodium, which can occur with prolonged diarrhea and vomiting or third spacing of fluids.

> There is no such term as **hyper**natruria. It is possible to have *too little* sodium excreted in the urine but there is no *normal* upper level of sodium excretion that defines **hyper**natruria.

Urine sodium levels (**Table 7-9**) may be measured to determine the cause of hyponatremia or to assess the function of the renal tubules. Urine sodium may be reported as sodium measured in millimoles per liter (mmol/L) or as the relative amount of sodium excreted compared to creatinine, called the **fractional excretion of sodium (FENa)**. In addition to sodium excretion, the **fractional excretion of urea (FEUrea)** may also be used to assess kidney function. FEUrea is more accurate when diuretics are used because urea excretion is not affected by diuretic medications whereas sodium is heavily influenced by diuretics. Note that calculations of fractional excretions are reported as either decimals or percents.

Table 7-9 Plasma and Urine Sodium

Test Name	Reference Range	Comments
plasma sodium	136–145 mEq/L	critical values: <120 and >155
urine sodium (random sample)	15–301 mEq/L or 15–301 mmol/L	<20 mmol/L (prerenal) >30 mmol/L (intrinsic) >40 mmol/L (late postrenal)
fractional excretion of sodium (FENa)	0.01 to 0.02 (or 1% to 2%)	<1% (prerenal) >2% to 3% (intrinsic) >3 (late postrenal)
fractional excretion of urea (FEUrea)	0.35 to 0.5 (or 35% to 50%)	<35% (prerenal) >50% (ATN)

The conversion factor for sodium, potassium, and chloride used to convert milliequivalent measurements to millimole measurements is 1, so for these three electrolytes, milliequivalent values are the same as millimole values.

Osmolality

Osmolality is a measure of the total number of dissolved particles in a liquid. Serum osmolality is maintained by a feedback system involving the hypothalamus, pituitary gland, and the kidneys. Sodium, chloride, glucose, and urea are major contributors to serum osmolality, and both serum and urine osmolality are important indicators of renal function (**Table 7-10**).

Table 7-10 Urine and Serum Osmolality

Test Name	Reference Range
osmolality, urine	50–1200 mOsm/kg H_2O
osmolality, serum	275–301 mOsm/kg H_2O

Urine osmolality is closely tied to hydration status. Urine osmolality decreases with excessive fluid intake (more dilute urine) and rises with dehydration (concentrated urine). Urine osmolality is significantly decreased in patients with acute tubular necrosis because the kidneys are no longer able to concentrate urine.

Osmolality is reported in osmoles per kilogram of water (Osm/kg H_2O). An osmole is a unit of measure to express the osmolar activity of a given solute. It indicates the amount of osmotic pressure exerted by the fluid due to the concentration of dissolved solids. Remember, osmotic pressure is the force that causes water to flow through a semipermeable membrane (in the direction of the solute). The laboratory reports physiologic values in milliosmoles (mOsm), which is one thousandth of an osmole.

Parathyroid Hormone

Parathyroid hormone, secreted by the parathyroid gland, is an important regulator of calcium metabolism. In the context of nephrology, parathyroid hormone (**Table 7-11**) is used to monitor patients with disruptions in calcium and phosphorus metabolism due to kidney disease. Hypocalcemia and hyperphosphatemia cause secondary hyperparathyroidism, resulting in increased levels of PTH. Increased PTH draws calcium from the bone stores, leading to renal osteodystrophy. PTH is reported in **picograms per milliliter**. A picogram is a trillionth of a gram (1×10^{-12}).

Table 7-11 Parathyroid Hormone

Test Name	Reference Range
parathyroid hormone (PTH)	50–330 pg/mL

Prostate Specific Antigen

Prostate specific antigen (PSA) is a glycoprotein produced in the prostate gland (**Table 7-12**). Normally, only a small amount reaches the general circulation, but a significant derangement in the cellular architecture of the prostate gland can cause more to leak into the peripheral blood. Elevated levels of PSA in the blood are highly specific for prostate inflammation and steadily increasing levels are highly suspicious for prostate cancer. A single, high PSA reading that returns to normal after antibiotic therapy is typical of prostatitis.

Table 7-12 Prostate Specific Antigen

Test Name	Reference Range
prostate specific antigen (PSA)	0–4 ng/mL

Serial PSA readings may be taken to determine the **PSA velocity**, which is the rate of increase in the PSA value over time. When PSA values are still low, a consistent increase in serial PSA readings (ie, an increasing PSA velocity) is highly suspicious for prostate cancer. Patients with a high suspicion for cancer may undergo a **sextant prostate biopsy** (a biopsy of six different sites within the prostate). Once a cancer diagnosis is established, PSA values are used to monitor for metastatic disease or recurrence. After complete prostatectomy, serum PSA values should be less than 0.05. PSA is reported in **nanograms per milliliter**. A nanogram is one billionth of a gram (1×10^{-9}).

Urine Culture

Although many urinary tract infections are easily diagnosed based on symptoms and urinalysis, persistent or recurrent UTIs and pyelonephritis require culture and sensitivity tests to select the most appropriate antibiotic therapy. If the patient is able to void, a midstream clean-catch specimen is used; otherwise, a sample is obtained through a catheter.

To perform a urine culture, 1 mL of urine is plated (spread evenly across the surface of a culture plate) and incubated for 24 hours. The lab reports the results of a urine culture based on the number of colony forming units. A bacterial "colony" is a distinct area of growth as seen on a bacterial culture plate. A CFU represents

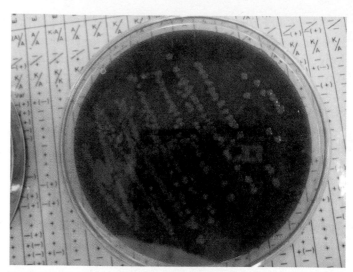

FIGURE 7-10 Colonies of E coli appear as tiny, distinct mounds on the surface of the culture plate with each colony representing a single bacterium at the time the culture was plated.

a single bacterium that has multiplied repeatedly to create a single colony (**Figure 7-10**).

After culturing the causative agent, a sensitivity test is performed. A sample of bacteria is taken from the culture plate and tested against an array of antibiotics to determine which antibiotic will provide the most effective therapy.

Therapeutic Procedures

Therapeutic procedures used in urology and nephrology are often both diagnostic and therapeutic.

Stenting

A **ureteral stent** is a hollow, plastic tube used to keep the ureteral lumen patent, especially following urological procedures or to aid in the passing of stones. Stents are also used to prevent **urinomas** (collections of urine outside the urinary collecting system) or stricture formation following urological surgery. The most commonly used urological stent is the double-J stent. The stent begins in the renal pelvis, passes the length of the ureter, and ends inside the bladder. Each end of the stent coils into a J shape to keep the stent from slipping out of the kidney pelvis or the bladder. Stents come in a range of lengths from 20–30 cm and a range of flexibility. Stents also come in three different diameters, measured on the French scale (6-, 7-, and 8.5-French). Retrograde pyelogram films are often performed before placing the stent to help select the correct stent size.

Although the stents have coils on either end to hinder movement, they can still migrate or become dislodged. They may also become blocked, kinked, or infected. Since stents are radiopaque, a KUB or abdominal flat plate is useful for assessing stent placement. Stents may cause bladder irritation, spasm, and reflux, which can be treated with pain medications, anticholinergics such as oxybutynin or tolterodine, and analgesics such as Pyridium.

Percutaneous Endourology

Percutaneous endourology refers to diagnostic and therapeutic procedures that use endoscopic instruments inserted through the skin directly into the renal collecting system. A guidewire is first passed percutaneously into the renal pelvis and dilators are inserted over the guidewire to create a tract for inserting endoscopic instruments for **nephrostomy tubes**.

When drainage of an obstructed kidney is warranted, a **percutaneous nephrostomy** may be performed with placement of a nephrostomy tube. Commonly used nephrostomy tubes include the **Malecot** (tulip-shaped) and the **pigtail (locking-loop or Cope-loop) catheters**. These tubes are preferred when active infection is present, as retrograde placement of a double-J stent may exacerbate an infection by promoting the ascension of bacteria into the kidney. Percutaneous placement of a catheter can be performed under local anesthesia using ultrasound to localize the renal pelvis, so this procedure is preferred for patients that are too hemodynamically unstable to tolerate general anesthesia. This technique is also preferred for pregnant patients because it does not expose the patient or the fetus to radiation. Using a **Seldinger technique**, a tube ranging in size from 8- to 12-French can be placed.

> **Pause 7-13** Using a Google image search, locate a picture of a Malecot and pigtail stent used for percutaneous nephrostomy.

To remove stones or masses, endoscopic instruments can be inserted through the percutaneous tract for **direct visualization** of the renal collecting system. **Percutaneous nephrolithotomy** is performed to remove kidney stones, especially when there is a large **stone burden**. **Percutaneous nephrolithotripsy (PCNL)**, used to break up large stones such as staghorn calculi, is performed through the endoscope using ultrasound

applied directly to the stone (■ **Figure 7-11**). Percutaneous routes are preferred for removing infectious stones because they can be promptly evacuated, lessening the chance of spreading the infection.

Lithotripsy

Lithotripsy refers to any of several methods for breaking up stones within the urinary system. The method used to remove stones depends on the stone's composition, size, and location. Treatment methods may be extracorporeal (directed from outside the body) or intracorporeal (occurring within the body). Intracorporeal approaches use either rigid or flexible endoscopes or percutaneous ports to reach the stone.

Extracorporeal shockwave lithotripsy is a commonly used modality for pulverizing stones. ESWL uses an external energy source applied to the skin to create acoustic shockwaves focused on the stone to break the stone into fragments. ESWL may be performed with the patient submerged in a tank of water that helps dissipate the energy of the shockwaves. Late-model lithotripters incorporate a water-filled drum or silicone cushion applied directly to the patient's skin at the point where shockwaves are focused, eliminating the need to submerge the patient and decreasing anesthesia requirements. Ultrasound or fluoroscopy is used to localize the stone during treatment. The fragments created by the shockwaves are typically small enough to pass on their own. ESWL may be used for calculi smaller than 1 cm in diameter that are located in the renal pelvis, proximal, or midureter. Stones in the lower pole of the kidney may break apart using ESWL, but they are more difficult to pass because they are in a dependent portion of the kidney and the stone fragments are too heavy to drain into the renal pelvis. Patients with a history of cardiac arrhythmias may be treated with **gated lithotripsy** that only fires shockwaves during the R-wave portion of the cardiac cycle. ESWL is associated with hematuria that is typically mild and transient. Perinephric, subcapsular, and intrarenal hematomas can occur, causing severe pain, ileus, or shock.

> Note the spelling of gated lithotripsy (not gaited).

Bladder stones and distal ureteral stones may be removed under direct vision using an endoscope and a **basket-extraction technique** (also called basketing). In this procedure, endoscopes are inserted using a

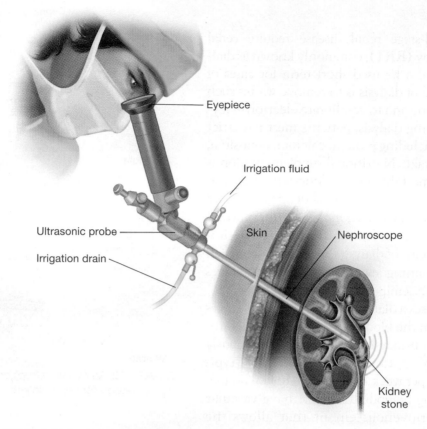

Eyepiece

Irrigation fluid

Ultrasonic probe

Skin

Nephroscope

Irrigation drain

Kidney stone

FIGURE 7-11 Percutaneous nephrolithotripsy.

retrograde approach. **Endoscopic lithotripsy** (also called **intracorporeal lithotripsy**) may be required to break up large stones before removing with basketing. This technique uses endoscopes to localize and directly visualize the stone while simultaneously breaking up the stone using the direct application of energy. Endoscopic **lithotrites** use ultrasonic, electrohydraulic, mechanical, or laser energy to fragment the stone into smaller pieces for easier removal. Baskets or graspers are passed through one of the endoscopic ports to retrieve the fragments. A commonly used endoscopic laser is the **holmium:YAG (yttrium-aluminum-garnet)**.

Stones in the renal pelvis or proximal ureters may require percutaneous nephrolithotripsy that enters the renal pelvis through the skin and uses a rigid or semirigid endoscope. The rigid endoscope allows the application of ultrasonic energy directly to large stones in the renal pelvis. Rigid endoscopy with ultrasonography is also the preferred method for treating infectious calculi. The hollow core of the rigid scope allows for simultaneous fragmentation and evacuation (suction) of infectious stone fragments to prevent the spread of infection.

In some cases, a combination therapy may be used. **Stone pushback** refers to the endoscopic manipulation

of a stone before applying ESWL. Stones in the proximal ureter may need to be pushed backward into the renal pelvis to optimize shockwave therapy. Stents may also be placed within the ureter before treatment of large ureteral stones to decrease the chance of **steinstrasse** (German for "stone street"). Steinstrasse is seen as multiple, small stone fragments lined up like cobblestones in the ureter following ESWL.

A CT scan of the abdomen and pelvis was performed. This indicates a large obstructing distal left ureteral calculus with hydroureteronephrosis proximal to the stone. In addition, there are stones in both the right and left lower poles of both kidneys. Due to the symptomatic nature and large size of the distal left ureteral stone, this will be treated with a transurethral ureteroscopic laser lithotripsy and placement of a double-J ureteral stent. The stones in the lower poles of the right and left kidneys will be treated subsequently with ESWL procedures.

Dialysis

Patients with end-stage renal disease require **renal replacement therapy (RRT)**, commonly known as dialysis. Dialysis may also be used short-term for cases of poisoning. The goal of dialysis is to remove wastes such as urea and creatinine and to equilibrate electrolyte levels. While undergoing dialysis, patients must pay strict attention to diet, including protein, calcium, potassium, and phosphorus intake. Nutritional supplementation is also required. The mortality rate for long-term dialysis is high, with a five-year survival rate of about 33%. Several dialysis techniques are available, including **intermittent hemodialysis**, **continuous hemofiltration**, and **peritoneal dialysis**. All forms of dialysis use a dialysate, which is a solution containing electrolytes that exchanges components across a semipermeable membrane.

Hemodialysis uses a dialyzing machine that removes waste products from the blood and equilibrates electrolyte levels. Filtration may be performed continuously (continuous hemofiltration) or intermittently (typically three sessions per week lasting three to five hours). Patients undergoing hemodialysis must have **vascular access** to an arteriovenous circuit that allows the removal of blood to be filtered and the return of blood that has been dialyzed. Long-term hemodialysis is performed through an **arteriovenous fistula (AV fistula)**, **arteriovenous graft (AV graft)**, or **arteriovenous shunt** placed in the forearm (■ Figure 7-12). The AV graft is the most common type of access. This approach uses a **Gore-Tex** tube that is implanted into the forearm and anastomosed to an artery at one end and a vein at the other. An AV fistula may also be created. This approach opens an artery and a vein in close proximity and creates an anastomosis. The fistula must **mature** for several weeks or months before it can be used for dialysis. On physical examination, a patent fistula will have a **bruit** on auscultation and a **thrill** on palpation over the fistula. A common complication of AV fistulas is **vascular steal syndrome** caused by the diversion of arterial blood. The extremity becomes pale, cool, and painful. When dialysis must be started emergently, central venous access is used, typically through the internal jugular vein, until a permanent graft has been placed and allowed to mature.

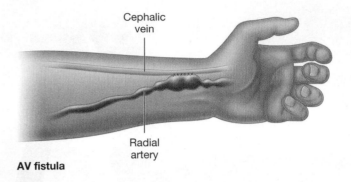

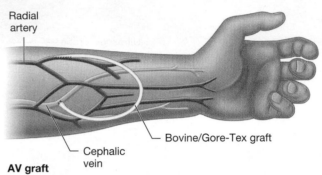

FIGURE 7-12 An AV fistula (top) or an AV graft can be used as venous access for hemodialysis.

 Patient is status post left arm AV graft placement 4 weeks ago. The swelling in the left arm has markedly improved. There is a palpable thrill and positive bruit over the graft.

Peritoneal dialysis uses the peritoneum as a natural semipermeable membrane through which water and solutes can equilibrate. Waste products diffuse across the capillary membranes and then across the peritoneal membrane into the dialysate. Water and solutes equilibrate across this membrane by osmosis, diffusion, and active transport of molecules. Peritoneal dialysis does not require vascular access; two separate abdominal catheters are used to infuse dialyzing fluid into the abdominal cavity and to drain the dialysate containing wastes. Catheters are made of soft silicone rubber or porous polyurethane with polyester fabric cuffs that allow tissue ingrowth around the **catheter exit site**. The cuffs create a watertight seal that also protects from infection along the **catheter tract** or at the catheter exit site.

Peritoneal dialysis can be performed at home while the patient goes about normal activity, although it does require motivation and participation on the part of the patient to infuse dialysate and drain the accumulated fluid several times a day. **Continuous ambulatory**

Note the correct spelling of steal (not steel) in the phrase vascular steal syndrome.

peritoneal dialysis (CAPD) requires the infusion of 2–3 L of dialysate four to five times a day and again at night. Using gravity, the solution is drained every four hours. **Continuous cyclic peritoneal dialysis (CCPD)** uses a long daytime interval (called a **long dwell**) and three to six nighttime exchanges performed by an automated cycler. The most significant complications of peritoneal dialysis include infection at the catheter exit site or peritonitis. Symptoms of peritonitis include abdominal pain, cloudy peritoneal fluid, fever, nausea, and tenderness to palpation.

Prostate Procedures

An enlarged prostate causes a variety of urologic symptoms, ranging from bothersome to life-threatening. There is a variety of minimally invasive and surgical procedures used to reduce the size of the prostate or to completely remove the prostate. Most procedures use a transurethral approach that inserts surgical instruments (cutting devices, heating devices, etc) through the pendulous urethra until contact is made with the prostate. Minimally invasive techniques include:

- **transurethral microwave thermotherapy (TUMT)**, which uses a microwave antenna positioned within the prostate to heat and destroy hyperplastic prostate tissue.

- **transurethral laser-induced prostatectomy (TULIP)**, which uses **neodymium:yttrium-aluminum-garnet (Nd:YAG)** and holmium:YAG to vaporize prostate tissue.

- **photovaporization of the prostate (PVP)**, which uses high-power potassium-titanyl-phosphate (KTP) laser (also called a green-light laser) to vaporize prostate tissue.

- **transurethral needle ablation of the prostate (TUNA)**, which uses radiofrequency needles passed through the urethra to heat the prostate tissue to 110° C at 456 kHz. Heat-induced coagulation causes necrosis of the prostatic tissue.

- **high-intensity focused ultrasound (HIFU)**, which uses a transrectal probe to focus high-intensity ultrasound at the prostate gland to create thermal lesions.

Surgical procedures for treatment of an enlarged or diseased prostate include:

- **transurethral resection of the prostate (TURP)**, which uses electrosurgical techniques such as monopolar and bipolar probes to remove the prostate.

- **transurethral incision of the prostate (TUIP)** uses electrosurgical techniques to make incisions in the prostate to relax the prostatic tissue, decreasing resistance to urine flow. Prostatic tissue is not removed in this procedure.

- **open simple prostatectomy** uses a suprapubic or retropubic approach to completely remove the prostate. It is required when the prostate gland is greater than 75 g.

> Most of the prostate procedures above are dictated as acronyms including TULIP (like the flower), HIFU (*hī-fū*), TURP, and TUNA (like the fish). Even TUMT is often pronounced as an acronym.

Bladder Slings

Bladder slings are used to treat incontinence due to intrinsic sphincter deficiency and/or urethral hypermobility. These procedures place a hammock-like physical support under the proximal or midurethra to prevent urethral descent. Two common surgical approaches include the retropubic bladder-neck suspension and the transvaginal sling. **Pubovaginal slings** may be anchored to the **fascia lata** or the **rectus fascia**.

A minimally invasive procedure for treating stress incontinence involves placement of **tension-free vaginal tape (TVT)** using a strip of material similar to the mesh used to repair hernias. Using a transvaginal approach, the TVT is wrapped around the urethra and passed upward toward the pubic bone (but the ends are not anchored to the bone). Scar tissue forms around the tape to hold it in place.

Injection Therapy

Injection therapy for stress incontinence caused by intrinsic sphincter deficiency artificially inflates the submucosal tissues of the bladder neck and urethra. Products used for injection therapy include Contigen (bovine collagen), autologous fat taken from the abdomen, carbon beads (Durasphere), calcium hydroxylapatite (Coaptite), Teflon paste, and polydimethylsiloxane (Macroplastique). Injectables are placed in the periurethral space, especially around the bladder neck. These **urethral bulking** procedures are simple to perform, can be performed in the office or in an outpatient surgical setting (except suprapubic antegrade approaches that require an operating room), and are associated with minimal risk. Injectable therapy is not a permanent cure, but the procedure can be repeated as needed.

Pharmacology

Urology and nephrology make tremendous use of pharmaceutical preparations for managing infection, stone disease, and the complications of renal insufficiency and renal failure.

Antibiotics

Antibiotics play a significant role in the management of urinary disorders because the urinary tract is quite prone to infection. Several classes of antibiotics (**Table 7-13**) are used to treat urinary tract infections including aminoglycosides, quinolones, sulfonamides, and cephalosporins.

Urinary Analgesics

Urinary analgesics exert a local pain relieving effect on the mucous membranes of the urinary tract. They are commonly prescribed for UTI or interstitial cystitis (**Table 7-14**).

Table 7-14 Urinary Analgesics

Generic	Brand Name	Dose
phenazopyridine	Pyridium AZO-Standard	100 mg, 200 mg 95 mg
dimethyl sulfoxide (DMSO)	Rimso-50	instilled directly in the bladder
pentosan	Elmiron	100 mg

Diuretics

Diuretics are divided into several subclasses including loop diuretics, thiazide diuretics, potassium-sparing diuretics, and osmotic diuretics. All diuretics, except for the osmotic diuretic mannitol, act on the loop of Henle and/or the convoluted tubule.

Loop Diuretics

Loop diuretics (**Table 7-15**) are used to treat fluid retention (edema). Loop diuretics act at the proximal convoluted tubule, the distal convoluted tubule, and

Table 7-13 Antibiotics for Urinary Tract Infections

Generic	Brand Name	Antibiotic Class	Dose
ampicillin		penicillin	250 mg, 500 mg
gentamicin		aminoglycoside	
ciprofloxacin	Cipro Cipro XR	quinolone	250 mg, 500 mg, 750 mg 500 mg, 1000 mg 500 mg, 1000 mg
trimethoprim-sulfamethoxazole (TMP-SMZ)*	Bactrim Septra	sulfonamide	sulfamethoxazole 400 mg and trimethoprim 80 mg
	Bactrim DS Septra DS		sulfamethoxazole 800 mg and trimethoprim 160 mg
cephalexin	Keflex	first generation cephalosporin	250 mg, 500 mg
nitrofurantoin	Macrodantin		25 mg, 50 mg, 100 mg
	Macrobid		100 mg
ceftriaxone	Rocephin	third-generation cephalosporin	500 mg, 1 g

*You may also see sulfamethoxazole abbreviated SMX and trimethoprim abbreviated TMP. The combination drug may be written with sulfamethoxazole listed first or trimethoprim first.

the loop of Henle. This class of diuretic blocks the reabsorption of sodium and potassium. Since water follows sodium across semipermeable membranes, more water is excreted in the urine, reducing total body water. Loop diuretics increase secretion of potassium, so a potassium supplement is often prescribed along with the diuretic to prevent hypokalemia (see page 49). Note the common suffix –ide used in the names of the loop diuretics.

Table 7-15 Loop Diuretics

Generic	Brand Name	Dose
furosemide	Lasix	20 mg, 40 mg, 80 mg
bumetanide	Bumex	1 mg
torsemide	Demadex	5 mg, 10 mg, 20 mg, 100 mg

Thiazide Diuretics

Thiazide diuretics (**Table 7-16**) act on the loop of Henle and the distal convoluted tubule to block the reabsorption of sodium and potassium. This class includes **hydrochlorothiazide (HCTZ)**, the most commonly used diuretic. Hydrochlorothiazide is combined with a great number of other medications used in the treatment of heart disease and renal insufficiency. Patients with hypercalciuria may also be treated with thiazide diuretics to lower urine calcium excretion and prevent calcium oxalate stone formation.

Table 7-16 Thiazide Diuretics

Generic	Brand Name	Dose
chlorthalidone	Hygroton	15 mg, 25 mg, 50 mg, 100 mg
hydrochlorothiazide (HCTZ)	Microzide	12.5 mg, 25 mg, 50 mg
metolazone	Zaroxolyn	2.5 mg, 5 mg, 10 mg

Potassium-Sparing Diuretics

Diuretics may be described as **potassium sparing**, meaning they do not increase the excretion of potassium. Potassium-sparing diuretics (**Table 7-17**) cause water and sodium to be excreted, but their mode of action spares potassium. The advantage of this medication is that it does not require a concomitant dose of potassium to prevent hypokalemia.

Table 7-17 Potassium-Sparing Diuretics

Generic	Brand Name	Dose
amiloride	Midamor	5 mg
spironolactone	Aldactone	25 mg, 50 mg, 100 mg
triamterene	Dyrenium	50 mg, 100 mg

Osmotic Diuretics

The osmotic diuretic mannitol (**Table 7-18**) acts in the glomerulus. It is the only diuretic that does not act somewhere along the loop of Henle or the other sections of the tubule. The drug increases the osmolality of the glomerular filtrate, thereby holding water in the tubules instead of allowing the water to be reabsorbed.

Table 7-18 Osmotic Diuretics

Generic	Brand Name
mannitol	Osmitrol

Nutritional Factors

Patients with CKD require close monitoring of nutritional factors as well as control of calcium, especially patients who develop secondary hyperparathyroidism. The following are commonly used supplements and medications to control vitamin and mineral levels (**Table 7-19**).

Table 7-19 Nutritional Factors for CKD

Generic	Brand Name	Description
B complex	Nephro-Vite Nephrocaps Rena-Vite	B vitamins
sevelamer	Renagel	phosphate binder
calcium acetate	PhosLo	phosphate binder
calcitriol (1,25 dihydroxychole-calciferol)	Rocaltrol	vitamin D analog for treatment of hypocalcemia
doxercalciferol	Hectorol	vitamin D analog; treatment of secondary hyperparathyroidism
paricalcitol	Zemplar	vitamin D analog; treatment of secondary hyperparathyroidism
cinacalcet	Sensipar	calcimimetic; treatment of secondary hyperparathyroidism

Alpha-Adrenergic Blockers

Alpha-1-adrenergic blockers (**Table 7-20**) are used to treat benign prostatic hypertrophy. This class of medication relaxes striated and smooth muscle thereby inhibiting contractions of the prostate and allowing urine to flow more freely.

Table 7-20 Alpha-Adrenergic Blockers

Generic	Brand Name	Dose
doxazosin mesylate	Cardura Cardura XL	1 mg, 2 mg, 4 mg, 8 mg 4 mg, 8 mg
tamsulosin hydrochloride	Flomax	0.4 mg
terazosin hydrochloride	Hytrin	1 mg, 2 mg, 5 mg, 10 mg
prazosin	Minipress	1 mg, 2 mg, 5 mg

Alpha-Reductase Inhibitors

The hormone dihydrotestosterone (DHT) promotes tissue growth of the prostate. The class of drugs known as 5-alpha-reductase inhibitors (**Table 7-21**) inhibits the conversion of testosterone to DHT and thereby decreases the size of the prostate gland. Medications in this class have a common suffix –asteride.

Table 7-21 Alpha-Reductase Inhibitors

Generic	Brand Name	Dose
finasteride	Proscar	5 mg
dutasteride	Avodart	0.5 mg

Antispasmodics

Antispasmodics (**Table 7-22**) are used to relax smooth muscle and inhibit involuntary detrusor muscle contractions for the treatment of overactive bladder and urge incontinence. Antispasmodics are anticholinergic medications that block choline receptors. The first generation medications (eg, oxybutynin) used to treat overactive bladder and urinary incontinence are nonselective cholinergic antagonists. These medications cause side effects such as dry mouth, constipation, blurred vision, and drowsiness. A subclass of anticholinergics are the antimuscarinics (eg, tolterodine, solifenacin,

Table 7-22 Antispasmodics

Generic	Brand Name	Dose
tolterodine	Detrol Detrol LA	1 mg, 2 mg 2 mg, 4 mg
oxybutynin	Gelnique (topical gel)	topical gel
	Oxytrol (transdermal)	transdermal
	Ditropan Ditropan XL	5 mg 5 mg, 10 mg, 15 mg
darifenacin	Enablex	7.5 mg, 15 mg
solifenacin	Vesicare	5 mg, 10 mg

darifenacin), which are more selective for smooth muscle of the bladder and therefore have fewer side effects.

Erythropoietins

Anemia associated with CKD is due to decreased red cell production. The kidney is responsible for secreting erythropoietins that act on the bone marrow to promote red cell production. Loss of kidney mass or kidney function decreases production of erythropoietins, leading to anemia. Treatment is with erythropoiesis-stimulating agents (ESAs), also called colony stimulating factors (**Table 7-23**).

Table 7-23 Colony Stimulating Factors

Generic	Brand Name
darbepoetin alfa	Aranesp
epoetin alfa	Epogen Procrit

Exercises

Using Context to Make Decisions

1. Based on the laboratory results in the sample excerpt, which of the following could be true about the patient?

   LABS: Sodium 139, potassium 4.1, chloride 100, bicarbonate 29, BUN 31, creatinine 1.2, glucose 95, albumin 4.2, calcium 8.6, phosphate 3.1, ALT 63, AST 34, alkaline phosphatase 69, total bilirubin 0.3, white blood cell count 9.5, hematocrit 35.7, MCV 109, platelets 331. UA was negative for leukocytes and nitrites.

   a. Results indicate a low suspicion for UTI.

   b. Results are highly suspicious for liver disease.

   c. Results are indicative of acute kidney failure.

   d. Results indicate a need for further evaluation of the parathyroid gland.

Use the sample report on page 230 to answer questions 2–11.

2. What word is missing in blank #2?_____
   _____

3. Which of the following would correct the sentence containing blank #1?

   a. He had a Foley catheter placed, and a Murphy drip was started.

   b. He had a leeway Foley catheter placed, and a Murphy drip was started.

   c. He had a Shumway Foley catheter placed, and a Murphy drip was started.

   d. He had a 3-way Foley catheter placed, and a Murphy drip was started.

4. What word is missing in blank #4?_____
   _____

5. Which item number listed under the Past Medical History has a transcription error? What information in the report supports your answer? _____
   _____

6. What is the significance of the physical exam finding, "no costovertebral angle tenderness"?

   a. The patient probably does not have spinal stenosis.

   b. The patient probably does not have pyelonephritis.

   c. The patient probably does not have rib pain.

   d. The patient probably does not have cystolithiasis.

7. What is the correct way to write the specific gravity result?

   a. ten oh three   c. 1003

   b. 10.03   d. 1.003

8. What test name has been transcribed incorrectly in the Laboratory Data section? What is the correct term?_____
   _____

9. Under the Laboratory Data heading, what does "large leukocytes" mean?

   a. A large number of white cells are noted on the microscopic exam.

   b. White cells seen on the microscopic exam are larger than normal.

   c. The dipstick test indicates a large number of white cells are present in the urine.

   d. The white cells are larger than the red cells.

10. What word should be transcribed in blank #3?__
    _____

11. Which of the following terms would be appropriate for blank #5?

    a. infer   c. confer

    b. defer   d. refer

12. Which of the following would complete this sentence? The stone was located in the distal ureter at the _____.

    a. UVJ
    b. UPJ
    c. urethrovesical junction
    d. TMJ

13. Which of the following would complete this sentence? She is noted to have bladder diverticula and a stricture just below the _____.

    a. urethrovesical junction
    b. ureterovesical junction
    c. prostatovesical junction
    d. ureteropelvic junction

14. Compare the terms invaginate and evaginate. Which of the two terms completes the following excerpt? _____

    Chronic urethral strictures or partial obstruction lead to bladder diverticula, which begin as outpouchings of mucosa that _____ between detrusor muscle bundles. These outpouchings progress to herniation of the bladder mucosa to form diverticula.

15. In the following context, what is a nidus?_____

    _____

    Foreign bodies as well as all types of crystals can act as a nidus on which calcium, uric acid, cystine, and magnesium can build.

Terms Checkup

Complete the multiple-choice questions for Chapter 7 located at www.myhealthprofessionskit.com. To access the questions, select the discipline "Medical Transcription," then click on the title of this book, *Advanced Medical Transcription*.

Look It Up

Using the guidelines described on page xvii, complete a research project on interstitial cystitis and ureteral reflux.

Transcription Practice

1. Transcribe the key terms and phrases for Chapter 7.
2. Complete the proofing and transcription practice exercises for Chapter 7.

INDICATIONS: Gross hematuria.

HISTORY OF PRESENT ILLNESS: The patient is a 73-year-old male with a known history of metastatic prostate cancer, currently on a regimen of palliative chemotherapy with Taxotere and prednisone. His last cycle was on July 10, 20XX. He has been followed previously by Dr. Smith for bilateral ureteral obstruction secondary to locally advanced disease, managed with bilateral ureteral stents. He was sent to the hospital yesterday by Dr. Jones with increasing hematuria with blood clots. He did complain of some increased weakness and fatigue. Urinalysis was consistent with an infection. Serum sodium was 120. He had a _____(1)_____ Foley catheter placed, and a Murphy drip was started. In spite of this, he has had ongoing hematuria with passage of clots. He was initially placed on Levaquin for his presumptive urinary tract infection. Urine culture shows multidrug-resistant Escherichia coli. Infectious disease consult was requested.

PAST MEDICAL HISTORY
1. Widely metastatic prostate cancer.
2. Atrial fibrillation.
3. Hypertension.
4. Bilateral ureteral obstruction.
5. Chronic hypernatremia.
6. Deep venous thrombosis.
7. Hypertension.
8. Gastroesophageal reflux disease.

PAST SURGICAL HISTORY
1. Cystoscopy and bilateral stent placement.
2. Bilateral _____(2)_____ for prostate cancer.

ALLERGIES: Alprazolam.

PHYSICAL EXAMINATION
VITAL SIGNS: The patient is 5 feet 10 inches and weighs 160 pounds. Blood pressure is 110/78, temperature 99.1, pulse 105, saturation 97% on room air.
GENERAL: This is a well-developed male who is resting comfortably in bed. He is alert and oriented x3. Pleasant and cooperative during our interview. He is in no distress at the time of my interview.
HEENT: Normocephalic and atraumatic. Pupils are equal, round, and reactive to light bilaterally. The extraocular motions are intact. The oropharynx is clear.
NECK: Supple. No lymphadenopathy.
CHEST: Breathing unlabored.
ABDOMEN: Soft, nontender, nondistended. No palpable mass. No hepatosplenomegaly. No suprapubic distention or tenderness. No costovertebral angle tenderness. No inguinal adenopathy.

GENITOURINARY: Uncircumcised phallus. Foreskin is readily retractable. He has a Foley catheter in place draining clear urine at this time with mild to moderate bladder irrigation.
EXTREMITIES: The patient is noted to have bilateral lower extremity edema. No clubbing or cyanosis.

LABORATORY DATA: Sodium 132, potassium 5.1, chloride 106, CO_2 20, BUN 11, creatinine 1.1, WBC 8.56, hemoglobin 10.7, and platelets 373. Urinalysis shows a pH of 5.0, specific gravity ten oh three, nitrate positive, large leukocytes, small blood. Culture shows a multidrug-resistant E coli.

RADIOLOGY: Renal ultrasound was ordered and is currently pending.

IMPRESSION

1. Widely metastatic prostate cancer, status post bilateral orchiectomy, on palliative chemotherapy.
2. Bilateral ureteral ___(3)___, managed with indwelling stents.
3. Gross ___(4)___, on Murphy drip.
4. Multidrug-resistant Escherichia coli urinary tract infection.

PLAN

1. Would continue the patient's Murphy drip for the time being. I suspect his hematuria was exacerbated by his cystitis. It seems to be clearing at this point, and hopefully we can get him off his drip and remove his Foley catheter in the next few days. Will ___(5)___ selection of appropriate antibiotic to infectious disease.
2. Will certainly follow up on his renal ultrasound. I would be surprised if he had occluded his stents this soon after stent placement, although that is a possibility.

Pulmonology

8

Preview Terms

Before studying this chapter, make sure you understand the following terms. Definitions can be found in the glossary.

atelectasis
CO
CO_2
cor pulmonale
cyanosis
dyspnea
hemoptysis
hypercapnia
hypoventilation
hypoxemia
hypoxia
O
perfusion
ventilation

Learning Objectives

After completing this chapter, you should be able to comprehend and correctly transcribe terminology related to:

▶ disorders causing airway obstruction

▶ pleural disease

▶ lower respiratory infection

▶ disorders of pulmonary circulation

▶ respiratory failure

▶ laboratory and imaging tests used to diagnose and monitor pulmonary disease

▶ drugs used to treat respiratory disease and infection

Introduction

The goal of respiration is to provide oxygen to the tissues and to remove CO_2, the byproduct of metabolism. In addition to respiration, the lungs also play a critical role in maintaining arterial pH by controlling the concentration of carbon dioxide. The functional components of respiration include ventilation (the inflow and outflow of air), diffusion (movement of O_2 and CO_2 across the alveolar membrane), transport of O_2 and CO_2 to and from the tissues, and regulation of blood gasses and pH.

Anatomy and Physiology

Air passes from the trachea to the two main right and left bronchi, which split off from the trachea at the **carina**. The main bronchi branch into the lobar (secondary) bronchi that successively branch into **segmental** and **subsegmental bronchioles**, with up to 25 generations of branches that finally terminate at clusters of tiny alveoli measuring a mere 200–300 microns in diameter (■ **Figure 8-1**). The trachea is supported by annular cartilaginous fibers that prevent airway collapse. The bronchi are supported by cartilaginous plates with smooth muscle in between.

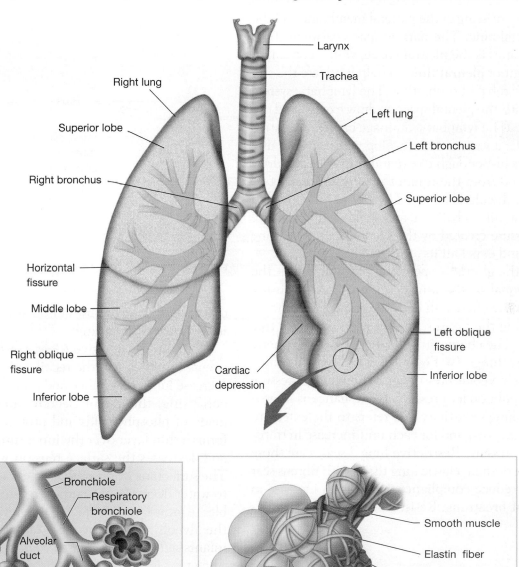

FIGURE 8-1 Anatomy of lung, alveolar sacs and alveoli with capillaries.

The plates of cartilage gradually diminish so that the terminal bronchioles have no fibrous supports. These bronchioles are about 1.5 mm in diameter with walls consisting almost entirely of smooth muscle fibers. These terminal bronchioles are held open by the same elastic forces that keep the alveoli open. These tiny airways are prone to obstruction due to constriction of smooth muscle, especially due to the action of histamine released from **mast cells (1)** within the alveoli.

The lungs' only point of attachment is the mediastinum; they are otherwise suspended within the thoracic cavity. The lungs are surrounded by a double membrane consisting of the parietal membrane and the visceral membrane. The narrow space between these two membranes is the **pleural space**, which contains a small amount of **pleural fluid** to help lubricate the surfaces as they rub past each other. The lymphatic system connects with the pleural space to draw excess fluid out of the space. The lymphatic drainage causes a negative pressure (like a vacuum) to develop within the pleural space that is just enough to expand the lungs and draw them outward from the hilum to maintain their position within the chest cavity. The normal lung has an elastic quality like a balloon, and without the negative pleural pressure created by the pleural space, the lung will recoil and expel all its air through the trachea.

When the glottis is open, the pressure within the alveoli is equal to the atmospheric pressure. During inspiration, the chest wall expands and the diaphragm drops, causing the pressure within the respiratory tree to decrease. The change in pressure draws atmospheric air into the lungs (■ Figure 8-2). The difference between the alveolar pressure and the pleural pressure is the transpulmonary pressure. **Compliance** is a measure of the lung's elasticity and refers to the extent to which the lungs expand for each unit increase in transpulmonary pressure. Restrictive lung diseases are those that replace normal, elastic lung tissue with fibrous scar tissues and reduce compliance, causing an increase in the **work of breathing**. Resistance within the airways

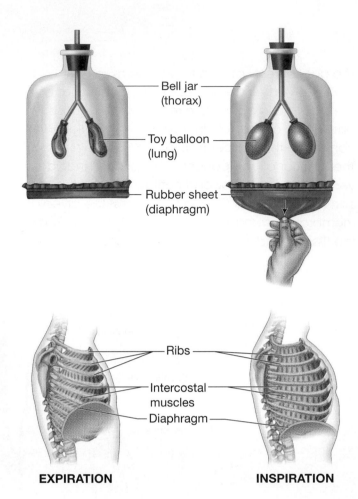

FIGURE 8-2 Mechanism of breathing.

due to narrowing or obstruction also causes an increase in the work of breathing.

Expiration is passive (does not require work) and occurs simply due to the recoil action of the lungs. To increase lung compliance and prevent the alveoli from collapsing, the alveoli secrete **surfactant**, which is made of phospholipids and proteins. The surfactant forms a thin layer over the inner surfaces of the alveoli and decreases the surface tension within the alveoli. The surfactant works in the same way that adding soap to water decreases the surface tension and allows bubbles to grow larger. Reducing the surface tension within the alveoli reduces the work of breathing. Premature infants suffer from increased work of breathing because surfactant is not produced within the alveoli until the last few weeks of gestation.

The pulmonary artery carries deoxygenated blood from the left ventricle. The pulmonary artery extends only 5 cm from the apex of the left ventricle and then divides into the right and left branches that lead to each respective lung. The walls of the pulmonary artery

(1) Mast cells are a type of immune cell (similar to basophils) that are found within the tissues. Mast cells release histamine and chemotactic substances that initiate immune responses. Be careful that you do not transcribe "mass cells" or "mass of cells."

are thin and the diameter larger than most arteries. These features give the pulmonary artery a large degree of compliance, allowing the lungs to accept a dramatically increased coronary output during physical exertion with only a modest increase in vascular pressure. Systolic pulmonary arterial pressure averages about 25 mmHg, with diastolic pressure being approximately 8 mmHg and mean pressure of 15 mmHg. Blood also flows to the lungs through several bronchial arteries that carry oxygenated blood to service the lung parenchyma. Lymphatic vessels surround the alveoli to help remove particulate matter, support the action of the immune system in protecting the lungs from infection, and also to absorb protein molecules that leak from the lung capillaries, thereby preventing edema.

Exchange of oxygen and carbon dioxide is accomplished by simple diffusion across the alveolar-capillary membrane. Gas molecules are in constant motion due to kinetic energy. (2) The constant movement causes the molecules to collide with one another in a random fashion, effectively bouncing the molecules back and forth across the alveolar-capillary membrane. Although the molecules move in both directions across the membrane, the net movement is always from highest concentration to lowest concentration. When red blood cells come in contact with an alveolus, the concentration of oxygen is highest in the alveolus, so the net movement of oxygen molecules is from the alveolus into the red blood cell (■ Figure 8-3). Likewise, deoxygenated blood arriving at the alveoli has a higher concentration of CO_2 than atmospheric air on the alveolar side of the membrane, so the net movement of CO_2 is from the capillaries to the alveoli.

The collision of gas molecules against a surface is known as gas pressure, which is directly proportional to the number of gas molecules hitting the surface. Measuring the pressure of a gas is a way of expressing the amount or concentration of a gas. The total pressure exerted against a surface by a mixture of gases is the sum of the individual pressures. The pressure exerted by each individual gas is known as the **partial pressure** of that gas.

Both atmospheric air and the capillary blood passing through the alveoli contain a mixture of gases (oxygen, carbon dioxide, nitrogen), so physiologic concentrations of gases are expressed as partial pressures. The partial pressure of a gas is designated with a /P/, so the partial pressure of oxygen is written PO_2, and the partial pressure of carbon dioxide is written PCO_2. When reporting the partial pressure of gases contained in arterial blood, as in the arterial blood gas study, the abbreviations include the lowercase /a/ and are written PaO_2 and $PaCO_2$ and expressed in millimeters of mercury (mmHg). A normal PaO_2 is 80–100 mmHg and $PaCO_2$ is 35–45 mmHg. Gas pressures, especially those used during surgical procedures, may also be expressed in **atmospheres** (atm); one atmosphere equals 760 mmHg.

Respiration is most efficient when the amount of oxygen within the alveolar sacs (ventilation) is matched to the amount of blood reaching the alveolar membrane (perfusion), expressed as the **ventilation-perfusion ratio (V/Q ratio)**. Even under normal circumstances, the V/Q ratio is not 1:1 because not all lobes of the lungs are ventilated equally. In addition, 2% to 4% of cardiac output flows through the bronchial vessels and is not oxygenated, contributing to a normal V/Q ratio of less than 1.

A **V/Q mismatch** occurs when there is either disruption of blood flow or poor ventilation (■ **Figure 8-4**). Intrapulmonary shunts occur when areas of the lung have adequate perfusion in the setting of nonfunctioning alveoli (due to airspace filling or collapse). Blood passes through these alveoli without picking up oxygen (wasted ventilation), resulting in a reduced V/Q ratio. **Shunt** is characterized by the persistence of hypoxemia despite 100% oxygen inhalation.

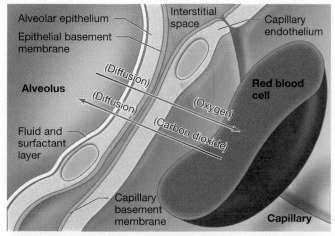

FIGURE 8-3 Oxygen and carbon dioxide move across the alveolar-capillary membrane in the direction of highest to lowest concentration.

> **(2)** Gas molecules are in constant motion, and kinetic energy is the energy a molecule possesses due to its motion.

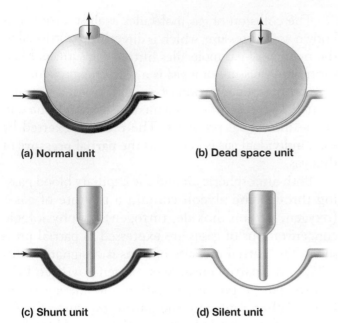

FIGURE 8-4 Ventilation-perfusion relationships: (a) normal unit, (b) dead space, (c) shunt unit, and (d) silent unit.

A high V/Q ratio indicates a problem with perfusion. If the capillaries are underperfused, from either damage to the capillary bed, blockage, or decreased cardiac output, the normally functioning alveoli contain oxygen that is never taken up by the red cells. Alveoli may be intact and receiving oxygen (ie, adequate ventilation), but the alveolar capillaries are obstructed or hypoperfused. These areas are referred to as dead space. When there is a large amount of dead space, the work of ventilation is wasted effort because the blood never achieves a sufficient oxygen concentration. The bronchi and the bronchioles do not participate in gas exchange, so there is always a given amount of anatomic dead space within the airways.

The efficient exchange of oxygen and carbon dioxide is heavily dependent upon the arterial pH. Drastic changes in pH, outside the tightly controlled range of 7.2 to 7.4, have profound effects on respiration. Because of this, the lungs not only participate in gas exchange but also in acid-base balance. The kidneys also play a role in maintaining blood pH by excreting or reabsorbing hydrogen ions, but the kidneys require several days to fully adapt. The lungs are capable of affecting the pH much faster by increasing or decreasing the ventilation rate. An increase in CO_2 decreases the pH because CO_2 combines with water to create carbonic acid, thereby decreasing the pH. An example of the lungs attempting to correct pH can be seen with metabolic acidosis. To compensate for acidosis, the respiratory rate is increased substantially (**hyperventilation**) in an attempt to "blow off" more CO_2, thus raising the pH (ie, making the blood less acidic).

Physical Examination

The physical examination of a patient with respiratory complaints and suspected respiratory disease is a critical component of the diagnostic process. Examination includes inspection, palpation, percussion, and auscultation of the chest as well as observation of breathing patterns, use of **accessory muscles of respiration**, and extrapulmonary signs of disease.

Normal lung sounds noted over the periphery of the lungs are called **vesicular breath sounds. Adventitious breath sounds** (abnormal breath sounds) include wheezes, rhonchi, fine or coarse crackles, stridor (high-pitched crowing), and pleural friction rub. Percussion helps identify solid areas due to masses and areas filled with air or fluid. **Dullness to percussion** signifies areas of **consolidation** (alveoli filled with fluid) or pleural effusion, and **hyperresonant** areas suggest emphysema or **pneumothorax** (areas filled with air). Reference points for describing the location of sounds include the trachea, nipple line, sternum, **anterior axillary line, midaxillary line, midclavicular line** as well as the ribs and intercostal spaces (■ Figure 8-5).

Observation is an important part of the physical assessment of a patient with suspected or known respiratory disease. The diaphragm is the primary muscle used for respiration. The use of **accessory muscles**, including the intercostal muscles, sternocleidomastoid muscles, scalene, and trapezius muscles, indicates high work of breathing and is a sign of significant pulmonary impairment. **Nasal flaring** also indicates increased work. The normal rate of breathing is 12–14 breaths per minute, with the normal ratio of time spent in inspiration compared to expiration being 2:3. Tachypnea describes an increased rate of breathing (greater than 20 breaths per minute) that is typically accompanied by decreased volume of inspired and exhaled air (decreased **tidal volume**). Chest **excursion** is the increase in the chest's girth during inhalation and may be reduced in patients with pulmonary injury or disease.

Pursed-lip breathing, characterized by exhaling through the lips held slightly apart, extends the exhalation phase and may be exhibited by patients with obstructive airway diseases. **Kussmaul breathing**, which describes rapid, large-volume breathing, indicates intense stimulation of the respiratory center and is seen in metabolic acidosis. **Cheyne-Stokes respiration,**

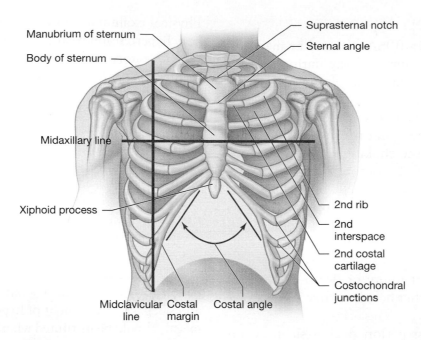

Manubrium of sternum

Body of sternum

Suprasternal notch

Sternal angle

Midaxillary line

Xiphoid process

2nd rib

2nd interspace

2nd costal cartilage

Costochondral junctions

Midclavicular line   **Costal margin**   **Costal angle**

FIGURE 8-5 Reference points used in the physical examination of the lungs.

which is a rhythmic waxing and waning of both rate and tidal volumes with regular periods of apnea, is seen in patients with end-stage left ventricular failure, persons with neurologic disease, or in healthy individuals at high altitude.

Extrapulmonary signs of disease include digital clubbing, marked by structural changes at the base of the nails, softening of the nail bed, and a convex and enlarged distal phalanx. Cyanosis, **elevated central venous pressure**, and lower extremity edema may also be noted in patients with respiratory disease.

Hemoglobin in arterial blood is normally 97% to 100% saturated with oxygen (referred to as the **O₂ saturation**), and venous blood is approximately 75% saturated. A simple test of oxygen saturation is **pulse oximetry**. The oximeter is typically placed on the fingertip or the bottom of an infant's foot. The infrared light emitted by the oximeter is reflected by the oxygenated hemoglobin molecule, and the amount of reflection is indicative of the degree of saturation of hemoglobin.

Vital signs: Blood pressure 98/64, pulse of 108, respirations 34, O₂ saturation 97% on nonrebreather mask with 15 L/min of oxygen.

Airway Obstruction

Airway obstruction is a major cause of respiratory disability. Obstruction may be caused by aspiration of a foreign body, compression by extrinsic masses, or an intrinsic pulmonary mass. Obstruction may also be caused by a decrease in the internal caliber of the airway due to mucus, swelling of the bronchial walls, collapse of the airways, or constriction of the smooth muscles of the airways. Airway obstruction may be described as reversible, partially reversible, or nonreversible.

A typical dictated phrase is "Oh-two sats are 98% on room air," which would be transcribed as "Oxygen saturation is 98% on room air." This means the patient is breathing room air (ie, not receiving oxygen therapy) and is maintaining normal oxygen saturation levels.

Remember, mucous is an adjective and mucus is the noun. These terms are easily confused because they are pronounced the same way but are actually different parts of speech. Use "mucus" when the word stands alone but "mucous" when the word precedes another noun (eg, mucous membrane, mucous gland).

Obstructive Sleep Apnea

Obstructive sleep apnea (OSA), caused by mechanical obstruction of the upper airway during sleep, is characterized by paroxysms of inspiratory effort and periods of breathing cessation lasting ten seconds or more, leading to poor gas exchange. Patients with OSA exhibit restlessness and snoring during sleep, and roommates may note choking, gasping, or snorting. Patients complain of morning headache, excessive daytime sleepiness, cognitive difficulties, and memory impairment due to a lack of restorative sleep. Repeated, intermittent hypoxemia throughout the night often leads to cardiac dysrhythmias, systemic hypertension, and pulmonary hypertension. Patients are at increased risk of injury or death from motor vehicle crashes and other accidents due to excessive daytime **somnolence**.

Upper airway obstruction during sleep occurs when the pharyngeal muscle tone is reduced, allowing the pharynx to collapse during inspiration. Risk factors for developing OSA include obesity and anatomical variants such as a narrowed upper airway (**micrognathia**); a **pendulous uvula;** a crowded oropharynx caused by a short or retracted mandible; a prominent tongue base (**macroglossia**); tonsillar hypertrophy; thick, lateral pharyngeal walls or lateral parapharyngeal fat pads; **bull neck** (short, thick neck); a neck circumference greater than 43 cm, or craniofacial anomalies. Obstruction of the sinuses due to a deviated nasal septum or sinus infection may also contribute to OSA. Use of alcohol or **hypnotics** (sleep aids) are known to exacerbate OSA. Many patients with OSA have concomitant hypertension, heart failure, diabetes, GERD, acromegaly, a history of stroke, and/or hypothyroidism.

Diagnosis of OSA is based on the patient's history, physical examination, and results of polysomnography, including daytime symptoms of fatigue and **hypersomnolence**, nighttime symptoms, and observation of five or more episodes of hypopnea and/or apnea per hour.

Physical examination may reveal systemic or pulmonary hypertension with cor pulmonale.

Laboratory studies may show erythrocytosis due to compensation of long-standing oxygen deprivation. Observations during polysomnography include apneic periods of up to 60 seconds and low oxygen saturation. Cardiac abnormalities include sinus bradycardia, sinus arrest, atrioventricular block, tachydysrhythmia, paroxysmal supraventricular tachycardia, atrial fibrillation, and ventricular tachycardia. Results of polysomnography are expressed as the **apnea-hypopnea index (AHI)**, which is the total number of episodes of apnea and hypopnea occurring during sleep divided by the hours of sleep time. An AHI greater than 5 is indicative of sleep apnea.

Treatment begins with control of modifiable risk factors including weight loss and avoidance of alcohol and sleep aids. Treatment of hypothyroidism and acromegaly should be instituted where appropriate. Patients typically struggle to lose the 10% to 15% of body weight necessary to improve OSA, and often patients require bariatric surgery to aid in weight loss.

Some patients may benefit from **nighttime appliances** that prevent the mandible from retruding, but the most successful and specific treatment for obstructive sleep apnea is **nasal continuous positive airway pressure (nasal CPAP)** or **bilevel positive airway pressure (BiPAP)**. These devices prevent the collapse of the airway by continuously applying positive air pressure into the pharynx using air pressures ranging from 3–15 cm H_2O. (3) Although the treatment is extremely effective, patient compliance is usually poor.

 The abbreviation CPAP is dictated "see-pap" and BiPAP is dictated "bye-pap."

Surgical treatment of OSA may include an **uvulopalatopharyngoplasty (UPPP)**. This procedure enlarges the upper airway by resecting pharyngeal soft tissue including submucosal tissue from the tonsillar pillars to the **arytenoepiglottic folds**, resection of the adenoids, and removal of approximately 15 mm of the free edge of the soft palate and uvula.

(3) Ventilation pressures are sometimes expressed in centimeters of water (cm H_2O) instead of partial pressures. The concept is similar to pressures expressed in millimeters of mercury in that it represents the amount of air that will displace a given height in a column of water or mercury as measured by a manometer.

 UPPP may also be dictated as UP3 ("you pee three").

Asthma

Asthma is a chronic inflammatory disorder that causes intermittent, *reversible* airway obstruction. It is characterized by diffuse airway inflammation, hyperresponsive airways, and limitation of airflow due to bronchoconstriction, swelling, airway remodeling, and plugs of mucus. The immune system plays a major role in the pathophysiology of asthma. Mast cells, eosinophils, T lymphocytes, macrophages, and neutrophils release histamine, cytokines, and leukotrienes that perpetuate inflammatory reactions. These inflammatory cells infiltrate the airway epithelium and smooth muscle, causing remodeling of the airways that can be seen as desquamation, fibrosis, collagen deposition, and smooth muscle hypertrophy. Smooth muscle hypertrophy narrows the airway lumen and increases reactivity to stimulants such as allergens, infectious agents, and pollutants. Increased mucus also plugs the airways, further restricting the flow of air. **Atopy (4)** is a common predisposing factor to the development of asthma. **Exercise-induced asthma (EIA)**, also called **exercise-induced bronchospasm (EIB)**, is a variation of asthma that is triggered by physical activity.

Most patients have intermittent episodes of asthma that are marked by respiratory distress with increased respiratory rate, tachypnea, diaphoresis, and use of accessory muscles of respiration. Patients may be noted to have chest tightness, coughing, wheezing, and reduced exercise tolerance. The expiratory phase of respiration is prolonged with an inspiratory-to-expiratory ratio of at least 1:3. Symptoms of severe exacerbations may include pulsus paradoxus (a fall of systolic BP greater than 10 mmHg during inspiration), altered consciousness, cyanosis, and respiratory failure. Patients with mild symptoms are asymptomatic between episodes. Triggers include environmental allergens (eg, pollens, dust mites) chemical irritants (eg, smoke, pollution), ozone, respiratory infection, sinusitis, rhinitis, aspirin, GERD, tartrazine dyes, and exercise. Some patients have catamenial asthma, which occurs at predictable times during the menstrual cycle. Extrapulmonary symptoms include **atopic dermatitis** and eczema. Complications of asthma include exhaustion, dehydration, airway infection, cor pulmonale, tussive syncope, and respiratory failure.

Asthma severity may be categorized as intermittent, mild persistent, moderate persistent, or severe persistent. **Status asthmaticus** describes severe, intense, prolonged bronchospasm that is refractory to treatment. Asthma control may be described using the phrases well controlled, not well controlled, or very poorly controlled.

Diagnosis is based on a thorough physical examination as well as **pulmonary function tests (PFTs)** that measure airflow rates, lung volumes, and the ability of the lung to transfer gas across the alveolar-capillary membrane. The primary pulmonary function tests used in the evaluation of asthma include:

- **forced expiratory volume in one second (FEV$_1$)**, which is the volume of air forcefully expired during the first second after taking a full breath
- **forced vital capacity (FVC)**, which is the total volume of air expired with maximal force
- **flow-volume loops (FVL)**, which are simultaneous spirometric recordings of airflow and volume during forced maximal expiration and inspiration

Patients with airflow obstruction show a reduced FEV$_1$ and an **FEV$_1$-FVC ratio** of less than 75% (see pulmonary function testing on page 261). An improvement of at least 12% in FEV$_1$ and 200 mL in FVC after administration of a bronchodilator confirms the diagnosis of reversible airway disease. A decrease in these parameters after provocation with a bronchoconstrictor (**bronchoprovocation testing**) such as **methacholine** further supports the diagnosis of airway hyperreactivity and asthma. Flow-volume loops should also be performed to rule out **vocal cord dysfunction**, which can mimic asthma.

Listen carefully for the abbreviations FEV and FVC. The /f/ often sounds like an /s/ and /v/ is easily confused with /b/.

Reactive airway disease (RAD) is sometimes incorrectly used as an alternative name for asthma, but technically, symptoms of reactive airway disease do not meet the criteria established by American Thoracic Society for diagnosing asthma, and the terms should not be used interchangeably.

(4) Atopy is a genetically determined predisposition toward an allergic response and plays a central role in asthma, atopic dermatitis, and hayfever. Be careful that you do not confuse atopy and atopic with ectopy, ectopic, or myopic.

Patients with a severe exacerbation should be monitored with pulse oximetry as well as **peak expiratory flow (PEF)** or FEV$_1$ measurements. **Arterial blood gas analysis (ABGs)** may be drawn to evaluate patients in marked respiratory distress or impending respiratory failure.

> **Pause 8-1** What does "reversible airway disease" mean? Why is asthma considered a "reversible" airway disease?

Treatment for asthma includes fast-acting agents for quick relief of asthmatic attacks and long-acting medications for ongoing asthma control. Quick-relief medications, also called **rescue medications**, promptly reverse acute airflow obstruction by relaxing the bronchial smooth muscles. These same medications are also used to prevent an attack of exercise-induced bronchospasm. Medications used for long-term control (referred to as maintenance, controller, or preventative medications) are taken daily, independent of symptoms, in order to attenuate airway inflammation.

Classes of medications used in the long-term maintenance and acute treatment of asthma include:

- **long-acting beta 2-agonists (LABA)** for maintenance of bronchodilation
- **short-acting beta 2-agonists (SABA)** for bronchodilation in an acute exacerbation
- anticholinergics to reverse vagally mediated bronchospasm (ie, not allergy-induced reactions)
- inhaled corticosteroids (ICS)
- **mast cell stabilizers** that modulate mast cell response and eosinophil recruitment (5)
- phosphodiesterase inhibitors for mild bronchodilation
- leukotriene modifiers to dampen the immune response
- monoclonal antibodies (eg, Xolair) to reduce allergic responses mediated by IgE antibodies

> **(5)** Immune cells are known to release chemicals that cause other immune cells to come toward the site of injury or inflammation. The chemoattraction of immune cells to a site of injury or infection is referred to as "recruitment."

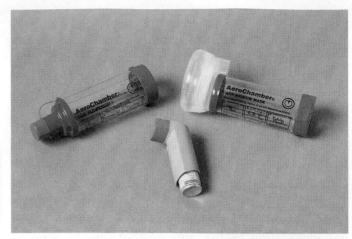

FIGURE 8-6 A variety of metered-dose inhalers. *Source:* Michal Heron/Pearson Education.

> **Pause 8-2** Using layman's terms, describe the action of "mast cell stabilizing drugs that modulate mast cell response and eosinophil recruitment" and how these drugs contribute to the treatment of asthma.

Many of the inhaled medications are packaged in **metered-dose inhalers (MDI)** that deliver a prescribed dose of aerosolized medicine (■ Figure 8-6). Patients are encouraged to monitor the efficacy of their prescribed treatment regimen with daily **peak-flow monitoring** using peak expiratory flow meters (■ Figure 8-7).

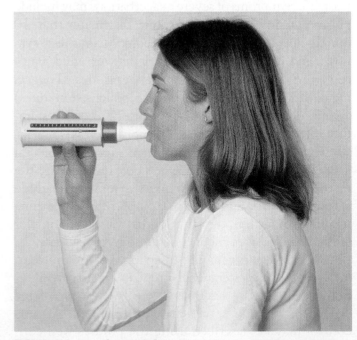

FIGURE 8-7 Use of a peak-flow meter. *Source:* © Dorling Kindersley.

These handheld meters give the patient and the clinician objective measurements of treatment efficacy. Patients suffering an acute attack are instructed to self-administer two to four puffs of an inhaled, short-acting beta 2-agonist such as albuterol (Ventolin) and to measure PEF.

In the emergency department setting, inhaled bronchodilators in the form of beta 2-agonists and anticholinergics are given using an **MDI with a spacer**. When indicated, larger doses can be given using a **nebulizer** instead of an MDI. Patients unable to inhale medications may be given bronchodilators subcutaneously. Ipratropium (Atrovent) helps decrease tonicity of the airways and may be given along with albuterol. Children are typically treated with terbutaline or subcutaneous epinephrine instead of beta 2-agonists. Systemic corticosteroids are administered to speed recovery.

Chronic Obstructive Pulmonary Disease

Chronic obstructive pulmonary disease (COPD) is a significant cause of morbidity and is among the top five causes of mortality in the US. COPD is a progressive disease characterized by obstruction of airflow and loss of elastic recoil caused by long-standing inflammation. The disease process has features of both emphysema and chronic bronchitis with involvement of the large and small airways as well as the lung parenchyma.

Chronic bronchitis is defined as excessive secretion of bronchial mucus accompanied by a productive cough for three months or more in two consecutive years. Chronic bronchitis causes a narrowing of the lumen of the airways and an increase in airway resistance. Changes in the airway are mediated by inflammatory responses that lead to pathological changes in the bronchial architecture. Mucous gland enlargement is seen on histological studies along with ciliary abnormalities, smooth muscle hyperplasia, and bronchial wall thickening. Obstruction results from hypersecretion of mucus, mucosal edema, bronchospasm, and peribronchial fibrosis.

Emphysema is defined as a permanent enlargement of airspaces distal to the terminal bronchioles with loss of elastic recoil, lung hyperinflation, destruction of alveolar septa, and subsequent formation of **bullae** (airspaces of 1 cm or more in diameter). Emphysematous changes are thought to be mediated by increased numbers of activated polymorphonuclear leukocytes and macrophages that release elastases, which break down alveolar walls (septae) and destroy the pulmonary capillary beds. Cell necrosis is accelerated due to the increased activity of free radicals found in cigarette smoke as well as those released by inflammatory cells. Destruction of the alveoli prevents adequate oxygenation of blood even in the presence of sufficient oxygen intake (ie, adequate ventilation) due to damage or loss of the alveolar-capillary membrane. Even though there is actually more air contained within the emphysematous lung, the loss of alveoli decreases the surface area available for exchanging gas across the alveolar-capillary membrane.

The leading risk factor for COPD is a history of cigarette smoking, especially 40 or more pack-years. In patients with a genetic predisposition, inhalation of cigarette-related toxins provokes an inflammatory response that leads to pathological changes. Less than 1% of cases of emphysema occurs in nonsmokers and is caused by the genetic disorder **alpha-1-antitrypsin (ATT) deficiency**. This enzyme is produced by the liver and inhibits the action of neutrophil elastase in the lungs, protecting the lungs from overproduction of elastase by the neutrophils. In this patient population, emphysema is typically diagnosed around the age of 50 for nonsmokers and age 40 for smokers.

COPD is a slowly progressive disease, and patients may be asymptomatic for years. A productive cough is often the first symptom. Beginning with dyspnea on exertion, breathlessness advances to dyspnea with mild exertion and then with activities of daily living. The increased work of breathing raises calorie requirements and leads to weight loss. Patients may complain of morning headache due to nocturnal hypercapnia or hypoxemia. Patients typically display one of two symptom patterns referred to as **pink puffers** (resulting from emphysematous changes) and **blue bloaters** (resulting from changes of chronic bronchitis). Late-stage COPD is complicated by cardiac arrhythmias, recurrent pneumonia, pulmonary hypertension, and cor pulmonale. Cause of death is often respiratory failure.

Diagnosis of COPD involves a thorough history and physical examination along with imaging studies and pulmonary function tests. Physical examination reveals an increased respiratory rate with increased work of breathing, increased expiratory phase of breathing, and lung hyperinflation manifested as a **barrel chest** (increased AP diameter of the thorax as shown in ■ **Figure 8-8**). Patients are often noted to

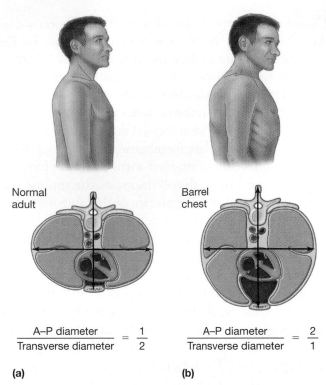

Normal adult

Barrel chest

$$\frac{\text{A–P diameter}}{\text{Transverse diameter}} = \frac{1}{2}$$

$$\frac{\text{A–P diameter}}{\text{Transverse diameter}} = \frac{2}{1}$$

(a)   (b)

FIGURE 8-8 Patients with COPD may develop a barrel chest.

display pursed-lip breathing and paradoxical indrawing of the lower intercostal spaces, known as the **Hoover sign**. Auscultation and percussion of the chest may reveal wheezing, decreased breath sounds, hyperresonance on percussion, and coarse crackles. Patients with advanced disease may have cor pulmonale evidenced by peripheral edema, elevated **jugular venous pressure (JVP), splitting of the first and second heart sounds (split S1 and S2)**, and murmur due to tricuspid valve insufficiency.

> The phrase jugular venous pressure does *not* take the combined form jugulovenous (there is no such term).

CBC shows erythrocytosis as the body tries to compensate for decreased oxygen by increasing the number of circulating red cells. Patients with COPD often have positive sputum cultures showing Streptococcus pneumoniae, Haemophilus influenzae, or Moraxella catarrhalis.

X-ray images of chronic bronchitis may demonstrate **bibasilar increase in peribronchial and perivascular markings** due to bronchial-wall thickening. Radiographic images of patients with emphysema show pathognomonic bullae, seen as radiolucent areas surrounded by arcuate, **hairline shadows**. Hyperinflation of the lungs is manifested as an increased AP diameter, **flattening of the diaphragm, rapid tapering of hilar vessels**, and increased retrosternal airspace. High-resolution CT scanning (HRCT) is also helpful in the diagnosis of emphysema. Bullae, which may not be visible on plain films, are easily seen on CT.

Pulmonary function tests play a key role in the diagnosis and staging of COPD (see also page 261 for more information on PFTs). Key components of pulmonary function studies used in the diagnosis of COPD include FEV_1, FVC, and FVL. Reductions of FEV_1, FVC, and the ratio of FEV_1-FVC (also called the **FEV_1%**) are the hallmark of airflow limitation. In healthy lungs, 70% to 75% of all the air exhaled after maximum inhalation (FVC) is exhaled within the first second (FEV_1). Patients with COPD have an FEV_1% of less than 70%. **Table 8-1** outlines key findings in patients with COPD.

> **Pause 8-3** Perform a Google Image search using the keywords x-ray and COPD. Study the x-ray images and describe the difference between normal lungs and lungs with chronic obstructive disease.

> A recent CT scan showed bullous emphysema, more prominent in the upper-lobe distribution. The patient had pulmonary function tests, and these surprisingly showed only a mild obstructive airway defect with an FEV_1 of 90% of predicted and an FEV_1-FVC ratio of 69%, and a midexpiratory flow rate of 50% of expected. His DL_{CO} was 72% of expected, which is also very surprising in view of the extent of his emphysematous change on CT scan.

Treatment of COPD involves oxygen therapy, pharmaceutical regimens, and exercise. The first line of treatment is the use bronchodilators, including beta 2-agonists such as albuterol and anticholinergics such as ipratropium. Bronchodilators are delivered

Table 8-1 Key Findings on Pulmonary Function Studies in Patients with COPD

Component of PFT	Findings	Comments
FEV_1	decreased	Dyspnea with activities of daily living is noted when FEV_1 falls below 1 L; patients are at risk of hypoxemia, hypercapnia, and cor pulmonale with an FEV_1 below 0.8 L.
$FEV_1\%$ (FEV_1-FVC ratio)	decreased	key indicator of obstructive processes
FVC	decreased	indicative of airway obstruction
RV	increased	due to emphysematous component
TLC	increased	due to emphysematous component
DL_{CO}	decreased	due to emphysematous component

directly to the respiratory system as inhalants. Albuterol is commonly administered using a portable MDI. Ipratropium may be prescribed as a solution for nebulization or as an aerosol for inhalation. The treatment regimen depends on the stage of the disease:

- stage I (mild): treated with short-acting bronchodilators as needed
- stage II (moderate): treated with regular doses of one or more bronchodilators
- stage III (severe): treated with regular doses of one or more bronchodilators and the addition of corticosteroids
- stage IV (very severe): treatment is as in stage III with the addition of long-term oxygen therapy

Patients are instructed in pursed-lip breathing, which slows the rate of breathing. Abdominal breathing exercises are encouraged because they relieve the fatigue caused by using the accessory muscles of respiration. Hospitalized patients may also receive **chest physiotherapy**.

Hypoxemia in patients with COPD can be improved with **low-flow** O_2, and long-term oxygen therapy has been shown to prolong life in patients with a PaO_2 of less than 55 mmHg. Oxygen therapy may be used on a continual, 24-hour basis, or a nocturnal, 12-hour basis. Oxygen comes in several forms, including liquid oxygen (LOX) and portable, compressed gas cylinders. Patients may also use a portable oxygen concentrator that extracts and concentrates oxygen from room air. Patients wear a **nasal cannula** to deliver the oxygen directly into the nares or use a **Venturi mask** (■ **Figure 8-9**). Oxygen is measured in flow rates expressed in liters per minute (L/min).

> Patients on oxygen therapy are often said to be on "home oh-two," meaning oxygen at home. The phrase "home O_2" is often dictated very quickly, is notoriously difficult to hear, and often misunderstood. Speech recognition engines have been known to insert nonsensical phrases such as homo two, homo too, and home oh you.

> This is a 42-year-old man with chronic obstructive pulmonary disease who presented to the emergency department complaining of worsening shortness of breath and respiratory distress. His home oxygen requirement is 2 L by nasal cannula.

 Pause 8-4 Describe nebulization.

Surgical therapy is generally not required, but patients with severe dyspnea due to severe bullous emphysema often benefit from bullectomy, which removes sections of

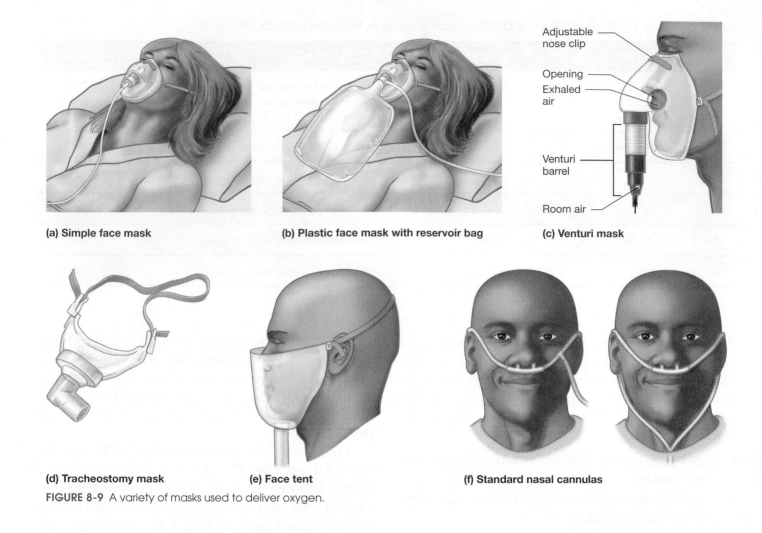

(a) Simple face mask

(b) Plastic face mask with reservoir bag

(c) Venturi mask

Adjustable nose clip

Opening

Exhaled air

Venturi barrel

Room air

(d) Tracheostomy mask   **(e) Face tent**   **(f) Standard nasal cannulas**

FIGURE 8-9 A variety of masks used to deliver oxygen.

the lung that demonstrate no ventilation or perfusion. Under extreme circumstances, patients may benefit from **lung volume reduction surgery (LVRS)**, which reduces the amount of dead air space.

Smoking cessation is extremely important for slowing the progression of COPD, but most patients have little to no success in quitting. Patients using a combination of behavior modification techniques, nicotine replacement therapy, and **nicotine agonists** (eg, Chantix) have the most success quitting, but even the most effective strategies have no more than a 50% quit rate at one year.

Respiratory infections are particularly lethal for patients with COPD, so vaccinations are highly recommended. Vaccinations should include the annual influenza vaccine and vaccination against pneumococcal pneumonia (Pneumovax). Patients may also benefit from prophylactic treatment with antivirals such as amantadine, oseltamivir (Tamiflu), and zanamivir (Relenza).

Although COPD is primarily a lung disorder, it does have systemic ramifications. A more comprehensive assessment of the severity of the disease can be obtained by accounting for the degree of systemic involvement as well as airway obstruction. The **BODE index** (rhymes with toad) is the most widely used prognosticator and consists of four parameters:

B—body mass index

O—degree of airflow obstruction as determined by the FEV_1

D—dyspnea, as measured by the Modified Medical Research Council [MMRC] dyspnea scale

E—exercise capacity as measured by the six-minute walking distance (6MWD), which measures oxygen desaturation during walking and is a good predictor of all-cause and respiratory mortality in patients with COPD

- Airway obstruction may be caused by extrinsic or intrinsic factors.
- Obstructive sleep apnea is caused by mechanical blockage of the airway during sleep with periods of breathing cessation. Poor sleep due to OSA causes hypersomnolence during waking hours and has far-reaching effects on health and cognition. Treatment includes reduction of modifiable risk factors such as weight loss and reduction of alcohol before bedtime. Use of CPAP is highly effective but patient compliance is low. Surgical procedures may include bariatric surgery or UPPP.
- Asthma is a reversible obstructive airway disease caused by inflammation or exercise. Patients self-monitor with peak-flow meters and are treated with fast-acting medications delivered through metered-dose inhalers, as well as oral or inhalant long-acting medications to reduce mast cell response and prevent or counteract bronchoconstriction.
- Chronic obstructive pulmonary disease is a partially reversible obstruction of the airways caused by long-term exposure to inhaled toxins, most commonly cigarette smoke. Chronic inflammation leads to airway remodeling, destruction of alveolar walls, and loss of elastic recoil. Symptoms begin with a cough and progress to dyspnea on exertion, and finally dyspnea with minimal to no activity. Treatment is with bronchodilators, corticosteroids, and home oxygen therapy.

Pleural Disease

Diseases or disorders of the pleural membrane include effusion, pneumothorax, and infection. The pleural membranes are important to the structure and function of the lungs, and disruptions of the membranes can have both painful and catastrophic consequences.

Pleural Effusion

Pleural effusion is an abnormal accumulation of fluid in the pleural space and may be classified as either a **transudate** or an **exudate**. Transudates are caused by a combination of increased hydrostatic pressure and decreased plasma oncotic pressure in the setting of normal capillaries. Transudates are usually ultrafiltrates of plasma. Congestive heart failure is the most common cause of transudative pleural effusions. Hypoalbuminemia associated with cirrhosis and nephrotic syndrome is also a common cause. Iatrogenic transudates may result from misplaced or migrated central venous catheters or nasogastric feeding tubes.

Consider carefully the abbreviation "PE," as this can mean pleural effusion or pulmonary embolism.

Pause 8-5 How does hypoalbuminemia contribute to transudative pleural effusions?

Listen carefully for effusion, diffusion, infusion, suffusion, profusion, and perfusion.

Exudates result from abnormal capillary permeability and decreased lymphatic clearance of fluid from the pleural space. The underlying cause is inflammation mediated by conditions such as pneumonia, cancer, pulmonary embolism, viral infection, or tuberculosis. The fluid is composed of protein, cells, and components of serum. **Parapneumonic pleural effusions** are exudates that accompany bacterial pneumonia. Some parapneumonic effusions form a nonelastic, thick pleural peel that traps the lung and prevents lung expansion.

Mild pleural effusions may be asymptomatic. Larger effusions typically cause dyspnea, usually due to shifts in the diaphragm and chest wall. Patients may also complain of **pleuritic chest pain**, which is a vague discomfort or sharp pain that worsens on inspiration (respirophasic chest pain).

Physical examination reveals **absent tactile fremitus,** dullness to percussion, diminished or absent breath sounds, and **egophony (E-to-A change)** on the side of the effusion. A **pleural friction rub** may be heard as a harsh, grating, creaking, or leathery sound. Massive effusions can cause a shift of the trachea and the mediastinum toward the contralateral side and bulging of the intercostal spaces. Effusions that create a pleural peel entrap the lung and shift the mediastinum toward the side of the effusion. (6)

Diagnosis of pleural effusion is made based on physical examination and chest x-ray. Diagnostic and therapeutic **pleurocentesis**, also called **thoracentesis**, is also performed to withdraw fluid from the pleural space. If the patient is physically able to stand, an upright PA chest x-ray should be performed. On **upright chest radiographs**, effusions may be seen as a **blunting of the posterior costophrenic angle** or **blunting of the lateral costophrenic angle**. Massive effusions opacify large portions of the hemithorax and cause a **mediastinal shift**. **Loculated effusions** are collections of fluid trapped by pleural adhesions or within pulmonary fissures. Additional x-ray views or chest CT scan may be required to differentiate loculations from masses.

Pleurocentesis is performed in the majority of cases of pleural effusion to both relieve symptoms and to obtain fluid for analysis. Withdrawing fluid relieves dyspnea and also provides fluid samples for laboratory evaluation, which is important for determining the underlying cause of the fluid accumulation and for planning the appropriate treatment. Visual inspection of the fluid gives important diagnostic information. Purulent effusions are strongly suggestive of empyema. Bloody fluid is indicative of **hemothorax**, often the result of instrumentation or chest trauma. Milky fluid suggests a **chylous effusion** containing chylomicrons and triglycerides due to traumatic disruption of the thoracic duct. A viscous fluid is suspicious for mesothelioma.

Routine laboratory evaluation of pleural fluid includes cell count (RBC and WBC) and white cell differential, total protein, and LDH. Glucose, cytology, and markers for tuberculosis may also be ordered when appropriate. Specimens should also be sent for Gram stain and culture for both aerobic and anaerobic bacteria. Blood culture bottles may be inoculated during the procedure to culture the pleural fluid. Protein and LDH values similar to those of serum (as compared to a blood sample drawn during thoracentesis) suggest a transudative process. Values that differ significantly from the peripheral blood values suggest an exudative process such as pneumonia or cancer. **Table 8-2** summarizes laboratory values that help distinguish exudative and transudative effusions. An RBC of 10,000 correlates to blood-tinged fluid and an RBC count of 100,000 correlates to grossly bloody fluid. A hematocrit value (ie, a spun hematocrit) should be determined for grossly bloody pleural fluid. A pleural fluid hematocrit value of more than 50% of the peripheral hematocrit level defines a hemothorax. Additional studies such as helical CT scan, thoracoscopy, or thoracotomy may be needed to definitively determine the cause of the effusion.

Table 8-2 Characteristics That Differentiate Transudates and Exudates

Test Name	Transudate	Exudate
appearance	clear	cloudy
protein	less than 3 g/dL	more than 3 g/dl
WBC	few	many
RBC	few	varies
glucose	similar to serum value	less than serum value
LDH	low	high
clot	no	yes

Her pleural fluid was sampled while here. The ratio of ascites to total body protein was 0.5. LDH was consistent with a transudate. Cytology was sent, including flow cytometry for the fluid. She does have a history of breast cancer and this was negative for malignancy.

(6) Tactile fremitus is the palpation of vibrations in the thorax felt while the patient is speaking. An E-to-A change (egophony) occurs when the examiner hears the letter /a/ on auscultation when the patient actually speaks the letter /e/.

Pause 8-6 How does comparing the hematocrit of pleural fluid to peripheral blood help determine the type of effusion?

Effusions can resorb spontaneously, so asymptomatic effusions do not necessarily require treatment, especially if the effusion is responding to treatment of the primary cause. Pleuritic pain can be managed with antiinflammatory medications and analgesics. Therapeutic thoracentesis is used to treat symptomatic effusions and can be repeated as necessary. Chronic, recurrent effusions may require treatment with **tube thoracostomy** (chest tube placement).

Loculated effusions may need to be freed from their fibrous pockets using fibrinolytic agents such as streptokinase or urokinase instilled into the pleural space during thoracoscopy. This procedure allows for the lysis of adhesions and removal of fibrous tissue. If still unsuccessful, thoracotomy with surgical **decortication** is necessary.

> **Pause 8-7** Listen closely for thoracostomy, thoracoscopy, and thoracotomy. These terms are very difficult to differentiate. What key words from the surrounding context might help you distinguish these words when dictated?

A **malignant pleural effusion** is caused by cancer in the region, usually lung cancer or breast cancer, due to direct involvement of the pleura with tumor cells. These pleural effusions tend to be chronic and require repeated thoracentesis for symptomatic control. Patients with a malignant pleural effusion may be treated with indwelling catheters (eg, PleurX or Aspira) that allow the patient to remain at home (instead of hospitalized).

A treatment of last resort for malignant pleural effusions is **pleurodesis** (also known as **pleural sclerosis**). This procedure is used to palliate symptoms in patients with a limited life expectancy. Pleurodesis "fuses" the two pleural membranes by instilling a sclerosing agent into the pleural space. The sclerosing agent causes an inflammatory response resulting in scar tissue that bridges the parietal and visceral membranes, obliterating the pleural space. Commonly used techniques include the placement of sterile, asbestos-free talc by **poudrage** or a talc slurry instilled through a chest tube. Other sclerosing agents include doxycycline, bleomycin sulfate (Blenoxane), zinc sulfate, and quinacrine hydrochloride. Pain associated with pleurodesis is initially quite severe and is treated with anxiolytics and opioid pain medications.

> A pleurocentesis would be helpful in determining whether the effusion is an exudate or a transudate and also would help in determining cytology from the effusion. If this is truly a malignant effusion, he may need pleurodesis for prevention of further effusions and/or consideration of chemotherapy.

Pneumothorax

Pneumothorax is the presence of air or gas in the pleural space resulting in partial or complete collapse of the lung. Normally, the pressure within the pleural space is negative (less than atmospheric pressure) and acts as a counterbalance to the recoil forces of the lung. In the presence of a pleural perforation, air is drawn into the pleural space and disrupts the equilibrium that maintains the lungs in an expanded state. The lung on the affected side recoils (collapses) toward the hilum.

Pneumothorax is classified as spontaneous (primary or secondary) or traumatic (non-spontaneous). Primary spontaneous pneumothorax (PSP) occurs in patients without known underlying lung disease and without a known inciting event. Secondary spontaneous pneumothorax occurs in patients with underlying conditions that predispose them to a pneumothorax. Traumatic pneumothorax is caused by direct injury to the pleural membrane due to penetrating or blunt trauma to the chest or during thoracic procedures.

PSP is most often associated with young, otherwise healthy men with a tall, thin body habitus. Cigarette smoking is a significant risk factor for PSP in this population. The pathophysiology is not completely understood but is thought to be related to the rupture of blebs or bullae on the pleural membrane. The blebs may be a result of smoking or possibly inherited defects of the pleural membrane. PSP may also occur due to atmospheric pressure changes related to diving or high-altitude flying.

Secondary spontaneous pneumothorax (SSP) occurs in patients with underlying parenchymal lung disease. Increased incidence of PSP is seen in patients with COPD, asthma, cystic fibrosis, and tuberculosis. AIDS patients with **Pneumocystis pneumonia (PCP)** are also at risk of SSP. Patients with existing lung disease may also have blebs or bullae that are prone to rupture. The consequences of SSP are usually more severe than PSP due to an already compromised respiratory system.

Non-spontaneous causes of pneumothorax include traumatic pneumothorax and iatrogenic pneumothorax. Trauma may include a penetrating injury such as a bullet or stab wound, a fractured rib that penetrates the pleura, or a blunt injury to the chest wall. Iatrogenic causes include transthoracic needle aspiration, thoracentesis, pleural biopsy, central venous catheter insertion, and positive pressure ventilation.

Tension pneumothorax (■ Figure 8-10) is a potential complication of pneumothorax that occurs when air is trapped in the pleural space under positive pressure. Trauma to the pleural membrane may create a one-way valve that only allows air into the pleural space, but doesn't allow any air to escape. Tension pneumothorax tends to occur most often in the intensive care setting among patients receiving **positive pressure ventilation**. The increased pressure in the pleural space causes the lung to recoil and collapse, shifts the mediastinum, decreases venous return to the heart, reduces cardiac output, and culminates in hypoxemia.

A small pneumothorax may be asymptomatic, but larger lesions cause dyspnea and pleuritic chest pain (pain increasing with inspiration). Depending on the location of the pneumothorax, pain may be referred to the shoulder or to the abdomen. Physical exam may reveal tachypnea, tachycardia, pulsus paradoxus, absent tactile fremitus, hyperresonance to percussion, and decreased breath sounds on the affected side. A large pneumothorax may noticeably shift the trachea to the opposite side (**tracheal deviation**). Patients may also be diaphoretic and cyanotic and demonstrate **splinting** due to pleuritic pain.

Patients suspected of pneumothorax that are capable of sitting up are evaluated with an upright inspiratory chest x-ray. A **visceral-pleural line** with a lack of lung markings peripheral to the line is diagnostic and indicates a collapsed lung. In supine patients, a pneumothorax may appear as an abnormally radiolucent costophrenic sulcus (**deep sulcus sign**), which is seen as a lucent area at the **lateral costophrenic angle** that projects well below the costophrenic angle of the contralateral side. A large tension pneumothorax will show a mediastinal shift, diaphragmatic depression, and rib cage expansion. The size of the pneumothorax is defined by the amount of space within the hemithorax not filled with lung tissue.

> **Pause 8-8** Perform an Internet search for chest radiographs showing the deep sulcus sign. Print out an image for your notes, or sketch a simple diagram.

A small pneumothorax will resolve spontaneously. Patients may be given supplemental oxygen during

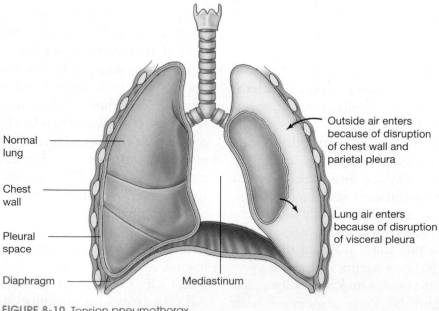

Normal lung

Chest wall

Pleural space

Diaphragm

Mediastinum

Outside air enters because of disruption of chest wall and parietal pleura

Lung air enters because of disruption of visceral pleura

FIGURE 8-10 Tension pneumothorax.

- Pleural effusions are accumulations of fluid within the pleural space and may be classified as transudates or exudates. Detection is by physical examination and chest x-ray. Pleurocentesis and pleural fluid analysis are often required to determine the type of effusion. Symptomatic transudates and almost all exudates require thoracentesis, chest tube drainage, pleurodesis, and/or pleurectomy.

- Pneumothorax is air within the pleural space causing partial or complete collapse of the lung. Pneumothorax may be spontaneous, traumatic, secondary to underlying pulmonary disease, or iatrogenic. Diagnosis is based on physical exam and x-ray findings. A small pneumothorax may resolve spontaneously; larger pneumothoraces may be treated with simple aspiration. Tension pneumothorax, which is life-threatening, must be treated with chest tube placement.

recovery. Patients experiencing more distress may undergo simple aspiration of air (evacuation) using a small-bore catheter attached to a one-way **Heimlich valve**. If unsuccessful, chest tube placement may be required. A tension pneumothorax is considered a medical emergency, and patients are treated with needle aspiration followed by chest tube placement (tube thoracostomy) using a water-seal drainage system and applied suction.

Respiratory Infection

An infection can occur anywhere within the respiratory system. Lower respiratory infections are those infections occurring below the level of the larynx.

Pneumonia

Pneumonia, defined as acute inflammation of the lung parenchyma caused by infection, is the most common cause of death due to infection in the United States. Pneumonia is characterized by consolidation of the affected area and filling of the alveolar airspaces. Pneumonia may also be caused by inhalation of chemicals or trauma to the chest wall, but by far, the most common cause is microbial, including bacteria, viruses, and fungi.

Pneumonia is classified several different ways: by its location and involvement in the lungs as seen on chest radiograph and also by the location of the patient at the time the infection was contracted (ie, within the community or within a healthcare facility). **Lobar pneumonia**, also known as **focal pneumonia** or **nonsegmental pneumonia**, appears as a homogenous consolidation involving one or more lobes of the lung. **Bronchopneumonia** appears as patchy areas of consolidation with **peribronchial thickening** and poorly defined airspace opacities. **Interstitial pneumonia**, caused by infiltrates into the interstitial tissue, appears as focal or diffuse areas of inflammation.

Noting the patient's situation at the time of infection is important in the treatment of pneumonia because the causative agents and, therefore, the treatments differ. **Community-acquired pneumonia (CAP)** develops in patients that have had limited or no contact with healthcare facilities. It is defined as pneumonia that develops in the outpatient setting or within 48 hours of admission to a hospital. **Hospital-acquired pneumonia (HAP)** is contracted while the patient is receiving inpatient care and the symptoms begin more than 48 hours after admission. Patients acquiring pneumonia in a healthcare setting, including nursing homes and long-term care facilities, are at increased risk of being infected with **multiple-drug resistant (MDR) organisms** and must be treated with a different antibiotic protocol. **Ventilator-associated pneumonia (VAP)**, also considered a hospital-acquired pneumonia, is defined as pneumonia that develops more than 48 hours after starting endotracheal intubation or within 48 hours of extubation. VAP is an extremely common complication of mechanical ventilation.

In the immunocompetent patient, the upper airways and oropharynx serve as an important first line of defense in the protection of the lungs. Cilia and mucus help trap organisms before they reach the lower airways. Organisms that reach the alveoli are typically destroyed by alveolar macrophages. Multiple factors can allow the organism to overcome normal host defenses and establish an infection. Organisms may also reach the lungs through hematogenous or contiguous spread. Once infection begins, the host launches an all-out offensive by recruiting white cells and inflammatory mediators, causing the alveolar airspaces and interstitial tissues to fill with exudate, cells, and fibrin. Airspace filling decreases gas exchange, leading to hypoxia.

Patients may also develop a **superinfection** (an infection with more than one agent), most commonly beginning with a viral infection that progresses to a concomitant bacterial infection. **Table 8-3** lists the most common causative agents of pneumonia. Note that many of the species names listed in this table are derived from Latin and end with /ae/. Streptococcus pneumoniae is the most common pathogen affecting all age groups and settings.

The most consistent presenting symptom of pneumonia is cough, usually with the production of sputum. Other symptoms include fever, chills, chest discomfort, dyspnea, fatigue, muscle aches, headache, and nausea. Physical examination often reveals tachypnea with a respiratory rate of 20 or more and a heart rate greater than 100. Auscultation and percussion of the chest reveals crackles, bronchial breath sounds, egophony, and dullness to percussion. Patients may display nasal flaring or use of accessory muscles of respiration.

The diagnosis is suspected based on the patient's complaints and is almost always confirmed on chest x-rays that demonstrate infiltrates. The chest x-ray is a reliable means of diagnosing infection, but it gives very few clues as to the infecting agent. A pattern consistent

Table 8-3 Common Microbial Agents Implicated in Pneumonia

Microbial Agent	Primary Association	Comment
**Streptococcus pneumoniae, often dictated "strep pneumo"	CAP	Classically associated with a cough productive of rust-colored sputum.
**Haemophilus influenzae, often dictated "H flu"	CAP	Encapsulated type B (Hib) is known to be particularly virulent, although routine vaccination (Comvax) has decreased the incidence.
**Chlamydia pneumoniae	CAP	May be referred to as atypical pneumonia or walking pneumonia.
**Mycoplasma pneumoniae	CAP	May be referred to as atypical pneumonia or walking pneumonia.
Legionella pneumophila (Legionnaire disease)	CAP	
Staphylococcus aureus	HAP	Antibiotic selection is important because of the increased prevalence of methicillin-resistant S aureus (MRSA).
Enterococcus (Enterococcus faecalis, Enterococcus faecium)		Group D streptococci is part of gut normal flora; antibiotic selection is important because of the increased prevalence of **vancomycin-resistant Enterococcus (VRE)**.
Pseudomonas aeruginosa	HAP	Characterized by its distinct grape-like odor.
Klebsiella pneumoniae	HAP	Associated with a cough productive of red currant-jelly sputum.
Acinetobacter baumannii	HAP	Commonly associated with VAP.
Listeria monocytogenes		Affects infants age birth to three weeks.
Moraxella catarrhalis	CAP	Seen in patients with chronic bronchitis who develop CAP, requiring hospitalization.
Actinomyces israelii		
Nocardia asteroides		
Pneumocystis jiroveci (formerly P carinii)		Important microbial agent in the immunocompromised patient, especially HIV-positive patients.

Table 8-3 Common Microbial Agents Implicated in Pneumonia (*Continued*)

Microbial Agent	Primary Association	Comment
Fungal Pathogens		
Histoplasma capsulatum (histoplasmosis)		Common fungal agent.
Coccidioides immitis (coccidioidomycosis)		Common fungal agent.
Blastomyces dermatitidis (blastomycosis)		Rare.
Paracoccidioides braziliensis (paracoccidioidomycosis)		Rare.
Candidiasis (usually Candida albicans)		Commonly seen in immunocompromised patients.
aspergillosis (Aspergillus)		Seen in immunocompromised patients.
mucormycosis (Mucorales)		Seen in immunocompromised patients.
Cryptococcus neoformans		Seen in immunocompromised patients.
Viral Agents		
respiratory syncytial virus (RSV)		Common agent in infants and young children.
Adenovirus		
influenza viruses		Very common, may be fatal in the very young and the very old.
metapneumovirus		
parainfluenza viruses		

**most common agents overall

with interstitial pneumonia is most suggestive of mycoplasma or a virus but is not definitive.

Although it is not unreasonable to attempt to identify the pathogen, most infections are treated empirically based on the patient's disposition at the time the infection was acquired (ie, CAP versus HAP). CAP is routinely treated in the outpatient setting. Gram stain, culture, and sensitivity testing of sputum are costly and frequently unsuccessful, so routine use of these tests in CAP is not recommended. However, because of the prevalence of MDR organisms in hospitals and nursing facilities, sputum or bronchial washings from patients with HAP may be cultured to determine the organism's antibiotic sensitivity profile, especially if the patient worsens or fails to respond to empiric treatment in the first 72 hours. In cases of VAP, endotracheal aspirates are cultured.

Primary treatment for bacterial pneumonia is antibiotic therapy with supportive therapy as needed. Outpatients with no other complicating factors are usually treated with monotherapy from the following antibiotic classes: penicillin, respiratory quinolone, tetracycline,

Listen carefully for the difference between mycobacteria, mycoplasma, and other terms such as mycotic and mycosis that begin with the prefix myco (fungus). Even though they begin with the prefix *myco*, mycobacteria and mycoplasma are not actually fungi. Mycobacteria are true bacteria and mycoplasma are obligate intracellular microbes, meaning they live within the host's cells and depend on the cellular functions of the host to replicate.

macrolide, or a beta-lactam. HAP is treated with one or more antibiotics chosen from the following classes: penicillin, carbapenem, monobactam, or cephalosporin. Vancomycin or linezolid are added when MRSA is suspected. Depending on severity of symptoms and comorbid conditions, therapy may include combinations of antibiotics from more than one class. Antibiotics commonly used in the treatment of pneumonia are detailed in the pharmacology section of this chapter.

> RECOMMENDATIONS: Will continue moxifloxacin as ordered and will add cefepime 1 g IV piggyback q.12 h. If the creatinine continues to rise, we may need to adjust the cefepime dose. Will also obtain sputum for culture and sensitivity. Also would like to obtain 2 additional blood cultures 15–30 minutes apart today.

> She has failed Biaxin therapy on an outpatient basis. I would have preferred to use a beta-lactam; however, she is allergic so I will avoid cephalosporins as well as penicillin derivatives. She has a prolonged QT on her EKG of about 510 milliseconds, so I would like to avoid fluoroquinolones. I will choose to give Zithromax by IV.

Vaccination is available for several causative agents of pneumonia. Pneumovax is given to patients at high risk of **pneumococcal pneumonia**, such as the elderly and patients with heart, lung, or immune system disorders. Children under the age of two should be vaccinated against Haemophilus influenzae type B (Hib) and varicella (chickenpox). Annual influenza vaccine, based on the strains predicted to prevail in

(7) A fomite is an inanimate object such as a telephone handset, doorknob, pen, or pencil that can act as a point of transfer between an infected individual and a noninfected individual.

(8) The latent period is the timeframe between inoculation and expression of the disease.

the upcoming flu season, is recommended for patients over 65 years of age and for younger patients at high risk.

> Be careful that you do not transcribe Hib as HIV. Note also that the abbreviation uses two lowercase letters.

Tuberculosis

Tuberculosis (TB) refers to disease caused by Mycobacterium tuberculosis, also referred to as the tubercle bacillus. TB is not currently a prevalent disease in the US, but worldwide, it is the most common cause of mortality related to an infectious disease. The disease is highly contagious and the treatment time is protracted, so the healthcare community must be vigilant to prevent epidemics.

Tuberculosis is spread through inhaled airborne droplets disseminated by patients with active pulmonary disease. Fomites (7) do not appear to be a significant source of spread of the tubercle bacillus. Patients with AIDS are at the greatest risk of contracting TB caused by both M tuberculosis and Mycobacterium avium-intracellulare complex (MAC) because HIV decimates the cell-mediated immune system that is essential for defending against tuberculosis.

Tuberculosis is a slowly progressive disease. Patients may not develop symptoms for weeks or months after initial contact. The disease is also known to have long latent periods. (8) The first symptoms include anorexia, fatigue, and weight loss. Cough, productive of yellow or green sputum, is also a common symptom. Other symptoms include hemoptysis, low-grade fever, drenching night sweats, and dyspnea. Patients co-infected with HIV have extrapulmonary symptoms of disseminated disease.

Diagnosis involves chest x-ray, tuberculin skin test, and sputum culture. Chest x-rays show patchy or multinodular infiltrates. **Cavitation** (areas of cavity formation) is seen with advanced disease. Calcified nodules indicate areas of old infection. Patients with numerous small lesions that resemble millet seeds are said to have **miliary disease**. CT scan may be used to confirm TB or distinguish lesions from malignancy.

Tuberculin skin testing (TST) using the **Mantoux** (man-tū') skin test is the most common test for diagnosing latent TB. To perform the Mantoux test,

- Pneumonia is the most common cause of death due to infection in the United States. Pneumonia is classified according to the patient's disposition at the time of infection: community acquired pneumonia or hospital acquired pneumonia. The most common infecting agent is S pneumoniae. Diagnosis is based on physical exam and areas of consolidation as seen on chest x-ray. Treatment involves antibiotic therapy and supportive therapy as needed.

- Tuberculosis is caused by M tuberculosis, an acid-fast bacillus. In the United States, immunocompromised patients are at the greatest risk of contracting TB. Diagnosis is by chest x-ray, skin testing, and positive sputum culture. Treatment requires antibacterial polytherapy for an extended period of time.

tuberculin **purified protein derivative (PPD)** is injected intradermally to create a wheal, typically in the volar forearm. The wheal is monitored over the next 48–72 hours for signs of induration. The size of the indurated lesion is diagnostic.

Sputum is also tested for the presence of **acid-fast bacilli (AFB)** by smearing a small portion of expectorated sputum on a microscope slide (a sputum smear) and staining using the Ziehl-Neelsen technique. The cell wall and cellular membrane of mycobacterium are different from gram-positive and gram-negative bacteria (9) and therefore do not consistently pick up the dyes used in the Gram stain technique. Rather, mycobacteria are part of a group of bacteria referred to as acid-fast bacilli because they resist decolorization with acid (ie, they retain the stain even when treated with an acid rinse).

Mycobacteria are fastidious and slow growing; laboratory cultures require four to six weeks to grow sufficiently to identify. Because of this lag time, sputum smears stained for AFB (which can be performed in a couple of hours) are an important part of the initial diagnostic workup. Sputum may also be tested using **ribosomal DNA probes** or techniques utilizing DNA polymerase chain reactions (PCR), which allow positive identification within 24 hours.

Treatment of TB requires a multidrug regimen taken over an extended period of time. Drug regimens include the antimycobacterials isoniazid, rifampin, pyrazinamide, and either ethambutol or streptomycin. Noncompliance is common among TB patients, so many are required to undergo **directly observed therapy (DOT)** wherein a healthcare professional observes the patient taking the medications. Inadequate treatment risks recurrence with **multiple-drug resistant TB (MDR-TB)** that requires daily treatment for as long as two years.

Pulmonary Circulation

Disorders of the pulmonary circulation primarily involve blockages due to thromboembolic disease or increased vascular resistance leading to hypertension within the respiratory circulation.

Pulmonary Embolism

Pulmonary embolism (PE) is the occlusion of one or more pulmonary arteries by foreign bodies, air, or thrombi. PE is potentially fatal and is among the top five causes of death among hospitalized patients. PE may present as an acute, imminently (10) life-threatening event or as a slowly evolving condition that worsens over a period of days or weeks. By far, the most common embolus is a clot that has formed elsewhere in the body and passed through the circulation to the lungs. Other types of emboli include air, amniotic

(9) The Gram stain technique uses two different dyes with a decolorization (dye removal) step in between. The components of the bacterial cell wall determine which stain is retained—the red stain (gram-negative) or the purple stain (gram-positive) as shown in Figure 5-4. Gram stain reactions are fundamental to the classification of bacteria because the stain itself gives information about the structure of the cell wall and therefore the DNA content of the bacteria.

(10) Imminent describes an event that is about to occur. Eminent describes a person that is renowned or well-known. (A tip to remember the difference is *imm*inent and *imm*ediate begin with the same letters. Eminent starts with an /e/ like extraordinary.)

fluid, fat from long-bone fractures, parasite eggs, and septic emboli (infectious material). PE involving a clot is actually a complication of an underlying venous thrombosis, most often originating in the deep veins of the leg or the pelvis. Thrombi tend to develop in the valve pockets of veins and other sites of venous stasis. Pieces of the clot break away from the point of formation and pass through the right side of the heart and into the pulmonary circulation.

Microthrombi—tiny aggregates of red cells, platelets, and fibrin—occur frequently within the venous circulation. These tiny clots form in response to local tissue injury and are a natural part of hemostasis. Normally, microthrombi are quickly lysed to prevent uncontrolled propagation of the clot. Thrombosis occurs when clots are allowed to persist and grow larger. Three underlying factors, known as the Virchow triad (venous stasis, hypercoagulability, and vessel-wall inflammation), predispose the patient to thrombosis and thus to PE. Venous stasis may occur during prolonged bedrest or airplane travel. Patients are especially prone to deep venous thrombosis following orthopedic surgery (see also page 142).

> Be careful that you do not confuse the terms hemostasis and homeostasis. Hemostasis refers to the arrest of bleeding. Homeostasis refers to a system that is in balance or equilibrium.

> **Pause 8-9** What is the difference between an embolus and a thrombus? Describe cardiogenic embolism.

Hypercoagulability may be the result of medications, malignancy, or an inherited defect of coagulation. Inherited hypercoagulability defects include dysfunction of **protein C** or **protein S**, deficiency of **antithrombin, prothrombin gene mutation**, and the presence of **antiphospholipid antibodies (lupus anticoagulant)** and/or **anticardiolipin antibodies**. Coagulation disorders are also covered in Chapter 12, page 392.

> Oftentimes, protein C and protein S are dictated together as protein C and S (eg, "Protein C and S activity were normal.") These are distinct proteins and should not be written like the abbreviation for culture and sensitivity (ie, *not* protein C&S).

Pulmonary embolism may involve a single clot or multiple clots. The symptoms as well as the outcomes vary greatly depending on the size and number of clots, location of the clot, the ability of the coagulation system to dissolve the clot, and the underlying condition of the patient's cardiopulmonary system. Small emboli may have no effect and resolve within hours or days without any signs or symptoms. Larger emboli that obstruct a significant portion of the vascular bed can have more catastrophic results due to two important consequences: an increase the pulmonary vascular resistance that raises the pulmonary artery pressure and ischemia of the lung tissue distal to the clot. An increase in the pulmonary artery pressure puts backward pressure on the right side of the heart and reduces cardiac output (acute cor pulmonale). Reduced blood flow to the alveoli causes wasted ventilation with V/Q mismatch, shunting, and hypoxemia. Too little oxygen to support the lung parenchyma causes depletion of surfactant, leading to atelectasis. Reflex bronchospasm may produce wheezing and increased work of breathing.

The clinical presentation of patients with PE may be divided into four scenarios based on the acuity and severity of the occlusion:

- a massive pulmonary embolism caused by a large embolus that leads to circulatory collapse and shock. Symptoms include tachypnea, hypotension, weakness, pallor, diaphoresis, and impaired mentation. Massive PE may be fatal within hours.

- an acute pulmonary infarction of the lung parenchyma. Symptoms include pleuritic chest pain, breathlessness, and hemoptysis.

- an acute embolism without infarction. Symptoms include nonspecific substernal chest pain and dyspnea.

- multiple pulmonary emboli, either as repeated episodes over several years that eventually lead to pulmonary hypertension and cor pulmonale, or as a first-time event that presents with progressive dyspnea, exertional chest pain, and eventually pulmonary hypertension and cor pulmonale.

Pulmonary embolism is notoriously difficult to diagnose, as there is no single symptom, sign, or diagnostic test that definitively diagnoses the presence of a clot in the pulmonary circulation. Clinicians use a scoring system to determine the probability of a pulmonary embolus, and at times, treat the patient empirically based on the prevailing evidence. A very large percentage of patients with pulmonary embolus will have deep venous thrombosis (DVT). A patient with a known DVT and symptoms of PE should be treated for an embolus without further need for diagnostic studies. Common symptoms include dyspnea, tachypnea, and chest pain, but these symptoms occur with many other disorders, making them very nonspecific.

Taken together, an electrocardiogram, arterial blood gases, **D-dimer**, CT imaging studies, and echocardiography can rule out or confirm PE, but only a positive arteriogram can definitively diagnose the presence of an obstruction. Physical examination may reveal hypotension, a **loud second heart sound (S2)** due to a **pulmonic component (P2)**, crackles, and wheezing. An echocardiogram is useful for establishing right ventricular dysfunction which occurs when the pulmonary artery pressure exceeds 40 mmHg. Findings on EKG are typical of right heart strain and might include:

- nonspecific ST-segment and T-wave changes
- right-axis deviation (R greater than S in V1)
- P-pulmonale (tall, peaked P waves in lead II)
- right bundle branch block
- an S1 Q3 T3 pattern on EKG

Arterial blood gas studies may reveal acute **respiratory alkalosis** due to hyperventilation. D-dimer, a degradation product of fibrin, is elevated in the presence of a thrombus. When accompanied by appropriate physical symptoms, D-dimer values greater than 500 ng/mL are highly suspicious for PE.

Chest x-rays are typically normal, which is actually an important finding in the presence of hypoxemia. The ventilation-perfusion scan (**V/Q scan**) showing areas of lung that are ventilated but not perfused gives important but not definitive diagnostic information as well. Results of the V/Q scan are reported as low, intermediate, or high probability of PE. **Pulmonary arteriography** (angiography) provides the most definitive information for diagnosing an embolus, but has been mostly supplanted by CT angiography (helical CT with IV contrast).

Treatment of PE varies depending on severity of symptoms and the cardiopulmonary status of the patient. When a massive PE is encountered, eliminating the clot is paramount. Patients may be given **thrombolytic therapy** or treated surgically with an embolectomy. Clots may also be removed by interventional radiologists using catheters to access the thrombus. When anticoagulation therapy is contraindicated, an inferior vena cava filter (IVCF) may be placed to prevent passage of a clot into the pulmonary circulation.

Thrombolytic therapy uses streptokinase, urokinase, or recombinant tissue plasminogen activator (alteplase) to quickly break down thrombi. Thrombolytic therapy carries the risk of stroke, so it is usually reserved for patients at immediate risk of death.

Anticoagulation therapy is the primary treatment for DVT and PE and should be started immediately. Typically the deep venous clot sheds only a part of itself, with that smaller portion of the clot passing to the lungs. The residual clot must be treated with anticoagulation therapy to prevent it from propagating and embolizing again. Anticoagulants prevent the clot from enlarging, giving the body a chance to remove the clot through normal clearing mechanisms.

There are three major classes of anticoagulants: heparin, warfarin, and fondaparinux. Heparin should be started immediately upon suspicion or confirmed diagnosis of PE. Heparin does not dissolve an existing clot but it does prevent the clot from propagating. Oral warfarin is the drug of choice for long-term therapy, but warfarin typically takes five to seven days to become fully effective. Patients should be given a form of heparin (either unfractionated heparin or low-molecular-weight heparin) or fondaparinux with concomitant oral warfarin until the PT/INR is at least 2 for a minimum of 24 hours. Failure to anticoagulate with heparin before starting warfarin may cause the clot to enlarge and put the patient at risk of another thromboembolic event. Patients are maintained on oral warfarin for three to six months or longer. **Table 8-4** outlines monitoring guidelines for anticoagulants in the setting of DVT and PE.

The activated partial thromboplastin time, abbreviated aPTT, must be distinguished from PT dictated with the preceding article /a/ (a PT vs aPTT). The PT is usually dictated as the PT/INR value, which is a good contextual clue to distinguish aPTT from PT.

Table 8-4 Monitoring Requirements for Anticoagulation Therapy

Anticoagulant	Brand Name	Test Used to Monitor	Target Therapeutic Range
unfractionated heparin	Hep-Lock	activated partial thromboplastin time (aPTT)	1.5 to 2.5 times normal control
low-molecular-weight heparin	Lovenox	no monitoring necessary	
warfarin	Coumadin	PT/INR	2.5 (range of 2–3)

Because pulmonary embolism is extremely difficult to diagnose and the results can be devastating, prevention of DVT is extremely important (see page 142).

Pulmonary Hypertension

Pulmonary hypertension (PH) is characterized by a progressive increase in pulmonary vascular resistance producing increased pressure in the pulmonary circulation. Pulmonary hypertension may be classified as primary or secondary. Primary pulmonary hypertension is rare. No apparent cause can be found and is often referred to as **idiopathic pulmonary arterial hypertension (IPAH)**. **Secondary pulmonary hypertension** constitutes the majority of cases and has underlying causes in other disease processes. Both primary and secondary pulmonary hypertension can be life-threatening and the prognosis is poor, especially for IPAH.

Pulmonary hypertension is defined as a **mean pulmonary arterial pressure** of greater than 25 mmHg at rest or greater than 30 mmHg during exercise. Although PH is defined as pulmonary artery pressures (**PA pressures**) above 25 mmHg, the majority of patients present with pressures of 60 mmHg or higher. The increased pressure within the pulmonary circulation places backward pressure on the right ventricle and overloads the heart, eventually culminating in right ventricular hypertrophy and right heart failure.

The underlying pathophysiologic mechanism of PH is increased pulmonary vascular resistance caused by vasoconstriction of the pulmonary vessels or damage to the pulmonary vascular bed that obstructs circulation. The increased pressure damages the endothelial lining of the vessels and leads to vessel-wall remodeling. The ongoing damage to the vessel walls further increases the pressure, producing more vessel-wall damage, smooth-muscle hypertrophy, proliferation of the intimal lining, and atheromatous changes, creating a self-perpetuating, progressive disorder.

Cardiac disorders and other primary pulmonary disorders, separately or in combination, can produce secondary pulmonary hypertension. Primary respiratory diseases that cause perivascular parenchymal changes (eg, emphysema) increase vascular resistance by creating areas of obstruction. Cardiac diseases involving volume overload damage the pulmonary vascular bed, leading to obstruction. Some of the more common causes of secondary PH include:

- sleep-disordered breathing, such as obstructive sleep apnea
- parenchymal lung disease with hypoxia, such as emphysema
- partial lung resection that removes part of the vascular bed
- vasculitis
- collagen-vascular diseases (autoimmune connective tissue disorders)
- pulmonary embolism
- constrictive pericarditis
- left ventricular failure
- mitral stenosis
- sickle cell disease (distorted red cells become lodged in the vascular spaces)
- polycythemia due to increased blood viscosity
- hepatic cirrhosis and portal hypertension

Another cause of SPH is hepatopulmonary syndrome, which causes microscopic arteriovenous dilations within the lungs, possibly due to loss of hepatic regulation of vasodilators (either increased production or decreased destruction of vasodilators). The dilated vessels cause overperfusion relative to ventilation, leading to hypoxemia. The lesions tend to be more numerous in the lung bases, causing **platypnea** and **orthodeoxia** that improves with recumbency.

Pause 8-10 Rewrite this sentence in layman's terms: The lesions tend to be more numerous in the lung bases, causing platypnea and orthodeoxia that improves with recumbency.

Early detection of SPH is difficult and is often obscured by the underlying disease. As PH progresses, patients experience dyspnea on exertion, fatigue, lethargy, presyncope or syncope with exertion, and chest pain. Patients may also complain of cough or hemoptysis. Hoarseness may be caused by the distended pulmonary artery compressing the recurrent laryngeal nerve.

Physical examination of the patient with advanced disease may reveal a right ventricular heave (11), widely split second heart sound (S2), an accentuated pulmonic component (P2) associated with the second heart sound, a 3rd or 4th heart sound (S3 or S4), systolic ejection murmur, jugular venous distention, and/or peripheral edema. Physical examination and laboratory studies may reveal an underlying collagen-vascular disease or liver disease.

Patients with PH are classified according to functional ability:

class I: no physical limitations

class II: comfortable at rest, slight physical limitations

class III: comfortable at rest, marked limitation in physical activity

class IV: dyspnea and fatigue at rest, inability to perform any physical activity without symptoms

Laboratory studies are performed to rule out underlying causes of SPH. Diagnostic imaging studies and cardiovascular studies are also performed. Patients with moderately advanced PH have distinct findings on chest x-rays, including enlargement of the **central (hilar) pulmonary arteries**, attenuation of peripheral vessels, and oligemic (12) lung fields.

A 2D echocardiogram may show right ventricular hypertrophy, right ventricular dilatation, and right ventricular hypokinesis. Right atrial dilatation and tricuspid regurgitation may also be seen. An echocardiogram with Doppler is the most reliable, *noninvasive* test to estimate the PA pressure. Elevated PA pressure causes tricuspid regurgitation, and the pressure can be calculated by measuring the **tricuspid regurgitant jet**. EKG findings are characteristic of right ventricular hypertrophy with right-axis deviation, **R-to-S wave ratio**

greater than 1 in V1, increased P wave, and right bundle branch block.

A V/Q scan is helpful when chronic pulmonary embolism is suspected. Pulmonary function testing is important for both diagnosis and monitoring of disease. Reduced perfusion decreases the **diffusing capacity for carbon monoxide (DL_{CO})**, so this parameter provides objective evidence of disease progression.

The diffusing capacity of carbon monoxide is usually dictated as the letters d-l-c-o. If subscripts are allowed, the abbreviation CO (carbon monoxide) should be written in capital letters as subscripts. Remember, the O stands for oxygen, not the number zero.

Pause 8-11 Explain why reduced blood flow to the alveoli reduces the diffusing capacity for carbon monoxide.

Right-sided heart catheterization is the gold standard for diagnosing and quantifying PH. This procedure allows for the measurement of pulmonary artery pressure, cardiac output, and left ventricular diastolic pressure. Right-sided O$_2$ saturation is measured to exclude an **atrial septal defect (ASD)**. Catheterization also allows for intraoperative trials of short-acting vasodilators to help with treatment decisions and the selection of oral medications.

It is difficult to access the left atrium with a percutaneous catheter, so the left atrial pressure is assessed by measuring the **pulmonary artery wedge pressure** (■ Figure 8-11). To do this, a catheter is inserted into the right side of the heart and then through the pulmonary artery. The catheter is then wedged into one of the small branches of the pulmonary artery. The pulmonary wedge pressure is within 2–3 mmHg of the actual pressure within the left atrium.

(11) A right ventricular heave is a palpable swell or rise over the right ventricle.

(12) Oligemia is a deficiency of blood in an organ or an area of the body.

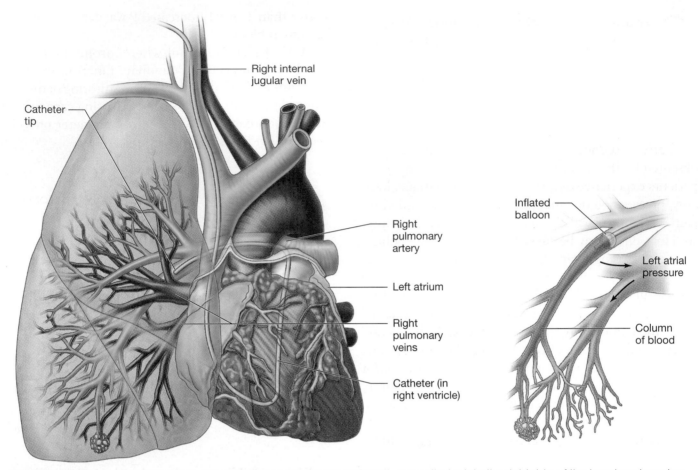

FIGURE 8-11 The pulmonary artery wedge pressure is measured by inserting a catheter into the right side of the heart and passing it through to the pulmonary artery.

 Pause 8-12 Does the right-sided O₂ saturation increase or decrease when there is an atrial septal defect?

Primary or idiopathic PH may be treated with a variety of vasodilators including calcium channel blockers; IV epoprostenol (Flolan); inhaled, oral, or subcutaneous prostacyclin analogs (Ventavis and Remodulin); oral

- Pulmonary embolism results from a thromboembolic event that occurs outside the lungs, usually the deep veins of the legs. Symptoms are widely variable, and outcomes range from imminently life-threatening to a chronic condition.
- PE is notoriously difficult to diagnose. Diagnostic tests include the V/Q scan, HRCT, and D-dimer tests. Treatment is long-term anticoagulation, and in extreme cases, thrombolytic therapy or embolectomy. IVCF may be placed for patients with recurrent PE.

- Pulmonary hypertension is characterized by a progressive increase in the vascular pressure of the pulmonary circulation. The causes of PH may be idiopathic or secondary to cardiac disease, collagen-vascular diseases, hematologic disorders, liver disease, or an underlying pulmonary disorder. Treatment is directed at the underlying disorder. Drugs such as phosphodiesterase inhibitors may also be used to dilate the pulmonary blood vessels.

endothelin-receptor antagonists (Tracleer); and/or oral **phosphodiesterase inhibitors** (Revatio).

Treatment of SPH is primarily directed at controlling the underlying disease. Necessary lifestyle changes include smoking cessation and avoidance of high altitudes. Drugs that promote vasoconstriction, such as **sympathomimetics**, should be avoided. Surgery is indicated for patients with correctable valvular disease. **Pulmonary thromboendarterectomy** may be indicated for patients with chronic thromboembolic disease. Long-term, continuous oxygen therapy has also been proven to be beneficial. Lung transplantation may be considered in severe cases, but transplantation is associated with high morbidity and mortality. This treatment is reserved for patients with **New York Heart Association class IV (NYHA class IV)** disease, defined as dyspnea associated with minimal activity leading to **bed-to-chair limitations.**

Acute Respiratory Failure

Acute respiratory failure (ARF) is a life-threatening syndrome characterized by impaired gas exchange (decreased oxygenation and decreased CO_2 elimination) and/or decreased ventilation (decreased air within the alveoli), resulting in hypoxemia and hypercapnia. Hypoxemia may be severe enough to threaten the function of vital organs. Objective measures for diagnosing ARF include a PaO_2 of less than 60 mmHg on room air or a $PaCO_2$ of more than 50 mmHg. A large number of pulmonary and cardiogenic disorders may lead to ARF.

ARF may originate in any of the components of the respiratory system (airways, alveoli, central nervous system, peripheral nervous system, respiratory muscles, or chest wall) resulting in hypoventilation or hypoperfusion. Mechanical hypoventilation (ie, no inspiratory or expiratory muscle movements) may be caused by depression of the central nervous system due to drugs, neuromuscular diseases that cause weakness or paralysis of the respiratory muscles, or injury to the peripheral nervous system. Hypoperfusion may have pulmonary or extrapulmonary causes. Nonpulmonary causes of hypoperfusion include low cardiac output, hypovolemia, and shock. The underlying pathophysiology of hypoxemia associated with ARF involves hypoventilation, V/Q mismatch, and/or shunt. Areas of the lung that are not receiving proportional amounts of air (V) and blood (Q) are said to have ventilation-perfusion (V/Q) mismatch (as described in Figure 8-4).

Signs and symptoms of ARF include those of the underlying disorder combined with symptoms of hypoxemia or hypercapnia. Untreated, symptoms advance to **obtundation**, respiratory arrest, and death. The most prominent symptoms of hypercapnia include dyspnea and headache as well as peripheral and conjunctival hyperemia, hypertension, tachycardia, tachypnea, impaired consciousness, papilledema, and asterixis. (13)

Hypoxemia is typically first noted on pulse oximetry. Oxygen saturation below 90% that does not respond to O_2 therapy is suspicious for right-to-left cardiac shunting or respiratory failure. Refractory hypoxemia should prompt an arterial blood gas evaluation and further studies to determine the underlying cause. Often the cause is obvious, such as acute myocardial infarction, pancreatitis, or sepsis. Chest x-ray may reveal an increased heart size, **peribronchial cuffing**, pleural effusions, or **perihilar bat-wing distribution of infiltrates**. An echocardiogram is useful if a cardiogenic etiology is suspected.

When treating patients with suspected or proven respiratory failure, the first objective is to address tissue hypoxia, which left untreated inevitably leads to failure of vital organs. To prevent organ failure, the goal of treatment should be a PaO_2 of 60 mmHg or an arterial oxygen saturation (SaO_2) of greater than 90%. Hypercapnia is more easily tolerated than hypoxemia, so restoration of oxygen to the tissues should come first. Hypercapnia leads to acidosis (CO_2 is converted to carbonic acid in the blood, thereby decreasing the pH), therefore the arterial blood pH must be monitored carefully and not allowed to fall below 7.2.

Patients with mild ARF may be able to maintain adequate oxygen saturation using supplemental oxygen with **high flow rates** of 70% to 100% O_2 via **non-rebreather face mask**, but more often, patients have severe hypoxemia that requires **mechanical ventilatory support**.

(13) Asterixis is involuntary jerking movements, especially in the hands, seen primarily with metabolic and toxic encephalopathies.

Patients able to maintain an open airway, cough, and respond to verbal commands may be treated with ventilatory support using **noninvasive positive pressure ventilation (NIPPV)** delivered via full face mask or nasal mask. Tracheal intubation is required if the patient has an upper airway obstruction, an inability to clear secretions on their own, impaired protective reflexes such as a gag or cough, progressive fatigue due to increased work of breathing, or mental status changes.

The first-generation mechanical ventilation devices used *negative* pressure to expand the chest, maintain a patent airway, and expand the alveoli. Patients were placed in an "iron lung" (a metal tube-shaped structure that encased the entire body except the head) with negative atmospheric pressures that "pulled" air out and "drew" air in. Current mechanical ventilation devices use *positive* pressure that *forces* air into the respiratory tree in order to maintain the airway and expand the alveoli. Several modes of positive-pressure ventilation are available:

- controlled mechanical ventilation (CMV) also known as assist-control or A-C
- synchronized intermittent mandatory ventilation (SIMV)
- expiratory positive airway pressure (EPAP)
- positive end-expiratory pressure (PEEP)
- inspiratory positive airway pressure (IPAP)
- pressure support ventilation (PSV)
- pressure control ventilation (PCV)
- continuous positive air pressure (CPAP)

Complications of mechanical ventilation support include **barotrauma (14)** as well as acute respiratory alkalosis caused by overventilation (removal of too much CO_2). Signs of barotrauma include subcutaneous emphysema, pneumomediastinum, subpleural air cysts, pneumothorax, or systemic gas embolism.

(14) Barotrauma is injury from too much pressure. In this case, it is caused by overdistention of the lungs due to excessive tidal volumes. Barotrauma may also occur in the middle ear from scuba diving or flying in over-pressurized airplanes.

Acute Respiratory Distress Syndrome

Acute respiratory distress syndrome (ARDS) is a form of respiratory failure that occurs within hours or days following a systemic or pulmonary insult (acute lung injury) and is characterized by bilateral pulmonary infiltrates and severe hypoxemia. The syndrome is mediated by proinflammatory cytokines that damage capillary endothelial cells and alveolar epithelial cells, causing increased permeability of the alveolar-capillary interface with an influx of fluid, protein, and cellular debris into the alveolar airspaces and interstitium. Damaged alveolar cells are unable to manufacture surfactant, so the alveoli collapse. The collapsed, fluid-filled alveoli cannot exchange gas across the alveolar-capillary membrane, resulting in ventilation-perfusion mismatch, shunting, and pulmonary hypertension. It is important to note that a preexisting lung or cardiac disease does not lead to ARDS; rather it is the result of an aberrant immune system reaction.

The most common risk factor for ARDS is sepsis. Other risk factors include aspiration of gastric contents, burns, shock, lung contusion, trauma, toxic inhalation, drug/alcohol abuse, multiple blood transfusions, and near-drowning episodes. Patients typically present with shortness of breath and rapid respirations. Breathing may be heavily labored with **intercostal retractions**.

The diagnosis of ARDS is based on chest x-ray, arterial blood gas values, and cardiac evaluation. Criteria include:

- acute onset of profound dyspnea
- diffuse, bilateral infiltrates as seen on chest x-ray
- hypoxemia refractory to supplemental oxygen
- normal capillary wedge pressure of less than 18 mmHg
- predisposing clinical finding (eg, sepsis, toxic inhalation, aspiration of gastric contents, long-bone fracture)

Treatment for ARDS is directed toward correcting the underlying condition and providing supportive care in the form of ventilatory support and fluid management. Ventilatory support is necessary to relieve the respiratory muscles of the highly increased work of breathing, which otherwise becomes unsustainable. Mechanical ventilation strategies should include the use of low tidal volumes to prevent pneumothorax and interstitial air. Death from ARDS is most often due to sepsis or multiorgan failure due to hypoxia.

- Acute respiratory failure is a life-threatening syndrome characterized by impaired gas exchange with resultant hypoxemia and organ failure. ARF may be caused by an underlying pulmonary disease, a cardiac disorder, or a neurologic/neuromuscular disorder affecting the muscles of respiration.
- Patients with ARF show ventilation-perfusion mismatch with either dead spaces or shunts, and supplemental oxygen often fails to increase oxygen saturation levels. Mechanical ventilatory support is usually required.
- Acute respiratory distress syndrome is a form of respiratory failure that follows a systemic illness or pulmonary insult and mediated by an overreaction of the immune system. Treatment includes ventilatory support and management of body fluids. The mortality rate is high and cause of death is often sepsis or multiorgan failure due to hypoxia.

Diagnostic Studies

Diagnostic and laboratory tests of significance in pulmonology include bronchoscopy, pulmonary function tests, the chest x-ray, CT imaging, nuclear medicine techniques, arterial blood gas analysis, and coagulation studies (see page 430).

Bronchoscopy

A common procedure for diagnosing and treating lung disorders is bronchoscopy, which is used to visualize the pharynx, larynx, vocal cords, and tracheobronchial tree. The bronchoscope may be flexible or rigid. Both therapeutic and diagnostic procedures can be performed during bronchoscopy. Therapeutic procedures may include removal of foreign bodies, clearing of retained secretions, balloon dilatation, endobronchial laser ablation, brachytherapy, and stent placement. Areas of the trachea and lungs are referenced as shown in ■ Figure 8-12.

A bronchoscopy with or without **endobronchial ultrasound (EBUS)** reveals abnormalities of the bronchial walls including inflammation, swelling, protruding cartilage, ulceration, tumors, and enlargement of mucous gland orifices, or the presence of enlarged submucosal lymph nodes. It may also reveal stenosis, compression, ectasia, irregular bronchial branching, or diverticulum.

Bronchoalveolar lavage (BAL) may be performed during bronchoscopy and involves the instillation of 150–180 mL of saline into a portion of the lung to the level of the alveoli with subsequent aspiration. This procedure can be used to diagnose an infectious or inflammatory process by culturing the aspirated fluid and/or performing cell counts and cytology studies.

Endobronchial biopsy or **transbronchial biopsy** using **transbronchial needle aspiration (TBNA)** may be performed by obtaining a core sample of a lesion using a 19- or 21-gauge cytology needle. A brush biopsy may be performed during a bronchoscopic procedure to diagnose neoplastic diseases. This procedure sweeps a brush repeatedly across a suspected lesion to capture cells for cytologic examination.

Following satisfactory topical anesthesia, the Olympus bronchoscope was passed through the right naris and into the posterior oropharynx. The cords were visualized and moved normally. Following the dripping of 1% lidocaine onto the cords, the bronchoscope was inserted into the trachea and examination of the tracheobronchial tree was begun. The carina was midline. The right upper lobe, right middle lobe, and right lower lobe anatomy appeared normal. The left upper lobe, lingula, and left lower lobe anatomy appeared normal. Under fluoroscopy, the right suprahilar area was identified via the apical segment. Bronchial brushings x2 were obtained for cytology. Bronchial washes were collected for cytology, acid-fast bacilli, and fungus.

Pulmonary Function Tests

Pulmonary function tests measure airflow rates, lung volumes, and gas transfer. PFTs are divided into three major components: spirometry, lung volumes, and diffusion capacity. Airflow rates and lung volumes help distinguish obstructive and restrictive processes and also assess severity of disease. Diffusion capacity assesses the integrity of the alveolar-capillary membrane. Initially, an entire battery of pulmonary function tests may be performed, but after a diagnosis is made, spirometry is used on an ongoing basis to monitor disease and treatment efficacy.

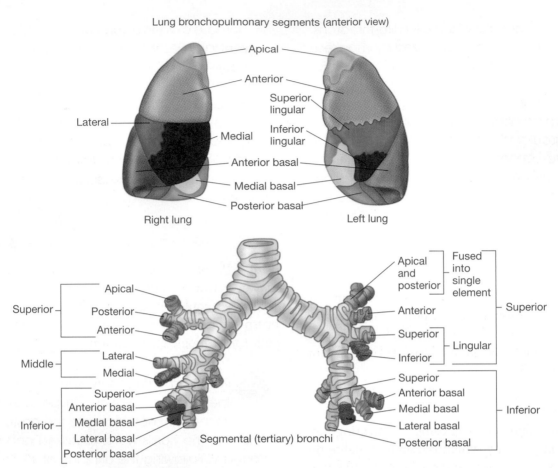

FIGURE 8-12 Bronchopulmonary segments and segmental bronchi.

Spirometry

Spirometry, which measures airflow rates, is a simple and reliable way to determine both the severity and reversibility of airway obstruction as well as restrictive pulmonary dysfunction. To measure airflow rates, the patient is instructed to inhale as deeply as possible and then exhale as forcefully and rapidly as they can through the exhalation port attached to the spirometer. Airflow measurements include:

- forced expiratory volume in 1 second (FEV_1)
- forced vital capacity (FVC)
- forced expiratory flow at 25% to 75% of maximal lung volume (FEF_{25-75})

Lung capacities may also be measured using spirometry:

- vital capacity (VC)
- tidal volume (Vt)

Airflow measurements are expressed as a percentage of the expected values based on the patient's height, age, race, and sex (**Table 8-5**). Obstruction is determined by a reduction in airflow rate as measured by the FEV_1-FVC

ratio. Reduction in FEF_{25-75} is an early indication of mild obstruction and may be detected before other parameters become abnormal. Obstructive processes include asthma, COPD, bronchiectasis, bronchiolitis, and upper airway obstruction. A reduction in lung volume with a normal to increased FEV_1-FVC ratio is indicative of restrictive dysfunction. Restrictive processes, marked by reduced compliance, are seen in fibrotic diseases such as pulmonary fibrosis, pleural disease, or neuromuscular disorders that affect the muscles of respiration.

Table 8-5 FEV_1 Values Characterize the Severity of Obstruction

FEV_1 Percent Reduction	Severity of Airflow Obstruction
<70%	mild
<50% to 69%	moderate
<35% to 49%	severe
<35%	very severe

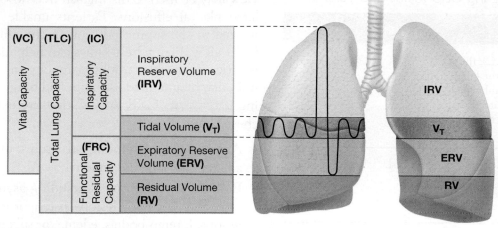

FIGURE 8-13 Lung volumes and capacities.

To determine whether obstruction is reversible, spirometry may be performed after inhalation of a bronchodilator. If the FEV_1 improves more than 12% after administration of the bronchodilator, the obstruction is considered reversible. This test is useful for planning treatment regimens and monitoring the efficacy of the treatment plan.

Bronchoprovocation testing using methacholine is used to diagnose asthma when spirometry tests are normal. Methacholine constricts smooth muscle at lower doses in asthmatic patients. The test is positive for reversible bronchoconstriction if the FEV_1 is reduced by 20% or more after administration of 15 mg/mL or less of methacholine.

A peak-flow meter is a portable device that measures the maximum force of exhaled air (peak expiratory flow). Peak-flow monitoring is a simple method of measuring airflow obstruction that can be used by patients on an ongoing basis to monitor airflow obstruction and to assess the severity of an exacerbation. Peak expiratory flow rate (PEFR), which measures how fast a person can breathe out, can be obtained in the healthcare setting and compared with readings the patient obtains at home with a peak flow meter.

Lung Volumes and Capacities

Lung volumes and capacities are measured to determine the amount of air contained within the lungs during each phase of respiration (■ **Figure 8-13**). Volumes may be determined using the gas dilution method (by inhaling nitrogen or helium) or by plethysmography. (15) Lung volume measurements are outlined in **Table 8-6**. An increased TLC indicates hyperinflation of the lungs, as seen with emphysema.

Increased residual volume indicates air trapping due to obstruction of air during exhalation.

Factors that affect lung volumes include:

- altitude (persons at sea level have smaller lung volumes than people living at higher altitudes)
- height (taller people have higher lung volumes)
- smoking status (smoking reduces lung volume)
- exercise capacity (exercise increases lung volume)
- sex (males have larger capacity than females)

Diffusing Capacity

The ability of the lungs to transfer gas between the alveoli and the blood is called the diffusing capacity and is measured by testing the **single-breath diffusing capacity of carbon monoxide (DL_{CO})**. To perform this test, the patient inhales a small amount of carbon monoxide, holds his or her breath for ten seconds, and then exhales. The amount of CO exhaled is measured and used to calculate the amount of CO that crossed the alveolar-capillary membrane. Since carbon monoxide binds to hemoglobin at the same site as oxygen, the hemoglobin concentration will affect the results of the DL_{CO}. Therefore, this test requires a simultaneous measurement of blood hemoglobin concentration and a corrective calculation of the DL_{CO}. Values

> **(15)** A plethysmograph is an instrument for measuring changes in volume within an organ or the entire body. In pulmonology, plethysmography measures changes in lung volumes.

Table 8-6 Normal Lung Capacities and Volumes

Measurement	Male	Female
total lung capacity (TLC): the total amount of gas in the lungs at the end of maximal inhalation. TLC is not measured directly but is calculated by adding the VC and RV.	6.0 L	4.7 L
vital capacity (VC): the total amount of gas that can be exhaled following a maximal inhalation.	4.6 L	3.6 L
forced vital capacity (FVC): the total volume of air expired with maximal force.	4.8 L	3.7 L
tidal volume (Vt): the amount of gas inhaled and exhaled with each resting breath.	500 mL	390 mL
residual volume (RV): the amount of gas remaining in the lungs at the end of a maximal exhalation.	1.2 L	0.93 L
functional residual capacity (FRC): the amount of air remaining in the lungs after a normal expiration.	2.4 L	1.9 L
inspiratory capacity (IC): the amount of air that can be inhaled after normal expiration.	3.8 L	2.4 L
expiratory reserve volume: the amount of air that can be forcibly exhaled after a normal exhale.	1.0 L	0.7 L

between 75% and 125% of average diffusion capacity in the healthy population are considered normal. The diffusion capacity is especially helpful in diagnosing emphysema and infiltrative lung diseases.

X-Ray Imaging

The chest x-ray (CXR) is one of the most common studies performed in the diagnosis and management of respiratory disease and is typically the first imaging procedure ordered. The most common radiographs are **posteroanterior (PA)** and **lateral views** of the chest. Occasionally **lordotic** and oblique views may be obtained to evaluate nodules, and the **lateral decubitus**

view may be used to distinguish free-flowing and loculated pleural effusions. Patients unable to stand are imaged in the supine position in the **anteroposterior (AP) view**. Plain chest x-rays can help identify abnormalities in the heart, lung parenchyma, pleura, chest wall, diaphragm, mediastinum, and hilum. The following is a list of "CXR ABCs" that are examined on a chest x-ray:

- **A**irways and surrounding structures, including hilar adenopathy or enlargement
- **B**ones and soft tissues, including asymmetry, fractures and lytic bone lesions, osteoporosis, metastatic lesions, foreign bodies, edema, or subcutaneous air
- **C**ardiac silhouette, including cardiac size and shape, presence of calcifications and prosthetic valves
- **D**iaphragm, including position and shape
- **E**ffusions, as indicated by changes in the **costophrenic angles**
- **F**ields (ie, lung parenchyma), including infiltrates, fissures, masses, consolidation, pneumothorax, vascular markings, fibrosis, pleural thickening
- **G**reat vessels, including aortic size and shape and the outlines of pulmonary vessels
- **H**ila and mediastinum, including **hilar lymphadenopathy**, calcifications, masses, and tracheal deviation

Other commonly dictated terms that describe a chest x-ray include:

- Kerley lines: Engorgement or edema of interlobular septa, typically seen when pulmonary capillary wedge pressure reaches 20–25 mmHg. **Kerley A lines** are interlobular septa deep within the lung parenchyma that extend radially from the hilum to the upper lobes. **Kerley B lines** are seen at the lung bases.
- **air bronchograms:** Air-filled bronchi in the periphery of the lungs that can be seen against surrounding alveoli that appear opaque due to an infiltrate or consolidation.

 Pause 8-13 Draw a simple sketch of a lordotic view.

 Be sure to type Kerley lines, not "curly" lines.

The following are excerpts from chest x-ray reports:

Two views of the chest demonstrate larger lung volumes with diffuse emphysematous changes that appear most pronounced in the right upper lobe. There is biapical fibrosis as well as bibasilar subsegmental atelectasis and scarring.

The cardiomediastinal silhouette is enlarged with apparent widening of the mediastinum.

A 2-view chest x-ray demonstrates large lung volumes with elevation of the right hemidiaphragm.

The pulmonary vessels are thinned peripherally.

Focal areas of hyperlucency are noted with no significant attenuation of the pulmonary vessels.

Pleural thickening is seen in the left sulcus.

Lungs are hyperinflated. Diaphragm is flattened. Chest is barrel-shaped. Areas of hyperinflation, with emphysematous and bullous changes noted. Fibrosis is seen.

Chest x-ray performed last night shows volume overload with pulmonary edema and a large right-sided pleural effusion.

Portable chest x-ray shows bibasilar air bronchograms and infiltrates.

Chest x-ray done here showed a rounded mass in his right hilum and right paratracheal areas measuring about 7.3 cm.

Blunting of the costophrenic angle.

There is blunting of the right costophrenic sulcus, most likely due to pleural adhesions.

Pulmonary scarring, particularly in the lingula of the left lung.

There is slight prominence of the pulmonary markings.

Thoracic aorta is calcified.

Mild bronchitis with bilateral perihilar atelectasis, possible viral etiology.

The heart size is normal. No significant airspace opacity, vascular congestion, or effusion.

CT Scans

Computed tomography studies of the chest are quite common and are helpful in the diagnosis of many pulmonary disorders. Several different forms of CT are used. Standard CT imaging of the chest delineates intrathoracic structures more clearly than planar x-rays. CT is also commonly used to guide the placement of biopsy needles. **High-resolution CT (HRCT)** creates much thinner cross-sectional images compared to standard CT and is helpful in the evaluation of interstitial lung diseases.

> **Pause 8-14**   What is the difference between plain x-rays and planar x-rays?

 With CT guidance for localization, a 22-gauge Chiba needle was inserted into the nodule seen in the azygoesophageal recess directly posterior to the right mainstem bronchus. This area was biopsied and material was sent to the pathology lab. No mediastinal, hilar, or axillary adenopathy. There is biapical scarring. Moderate centrilobular and paraseptal emphysema. Moderate centrilobular emphysema, mainly in the upper lobes. Scattered, faint, ground-glass opacities may represent mild pulmonary edema.

Helical (spiral) CT creates 3D images of the chest. The patient must be capable of holding their breath and lying still for 8–10 seconds while the images are generated. CT angiography uses iodinated IV contrast to better visualize the pulmonary arteries and to detect pulmonary emboli. In many cases, CT angiography has replaced V/Q scanning and conventional pulmonary angiography.

> CT angiogram shows an intraluminal filling defect that occludes the anterior basal segmental artery of the right lower lobe. Also present is an infarction of the corresponding lung.
> CT angiography demonstrates a clot in the anterior segmental artery in the left upper lung and a clot in the anterior segmental artery in the right upper lung.

Nuclear Scanning

Nuclear imaging studies used in pulmonology include the PET scan and V/Q scan.

PET Scan

Positron emission tomography (PET) scans use radioactively labeled glucose (FDG) to measure the metabolic activity within the tissues. Focal areas of activity are reported as **hypermetabolic**, and areas of no activity are **hypometabolic**. Areas of activity are quantified and reported using the **standardized uptake value (SUV)**. PET scans are most helpful in the detection and diagnosis of tumors because malignant tissue tends to take up glucose at a higher rate than nonmalignant tissue. A nidus of infection can also be detected on a PET scan because of the increased metabolic activity of white cells at the site of infection. Malignant or infectious areas appear as "bright spots" on the fluoroscopic images. A PET scan can also be used to assess the **paratracheal, tracheobronchial, azygous, and subcarinal lymph nodes** and has largely replaced mediastinoscopy (16) in the diagnosis of mediastinal disease. Metabolically active lymph nodes may indicate metastasis.

Scans through the chest demonstrate small nodes in the lateral aortic space, weakly hypermetabolic, SUV 2.8; in the left paratracheal space 2.9, AP window 3.1. An area of nodularity is noted within the right upper lobe, SUV 4.6, and in the left upper lobe a small nodule is noted, SUV 2.8. On lung window detail, extensive emphysematous and fibrotic changes are seen. Extensive bullous disease noted in the right and left upper lobes in the area of hypermetabolism, seen as an area of parenchymal density adjacent to the right upper lobe bulla and correlates to an 11 mm area of nodularity. This is noncalcified and poorly defined. In the left upper lobe, areas of linear stranding are noted with weak hypermetabolism, as noted. There is no well-defined left-sided pulmonary nodule.

(16) Mediastinoscopy is the introduction of an endoscope into the mediastinum. Mediastinotomy is the surgical opening of the mediastinum.

Ventilation Perfusion Scan

The ventilation-perfusion scan (V/Q scan) is performed in two stages. In the perfusion stage, technetium-99m-labeled macroaggregated albumin (**99mTc-MAA**) is infused into the venous system and acts as a radioactive tracer. Using a gamma camera, the radioactive albumin can be traced as the blood carrying the tagged albumin perfuses the pulmonary capillary bed. The ventilation phase of the test is performed by having the patient breathe a radioactive gas such as **xenon** or **technetium DTPA**. Again, the gamma camera records the pattern of radioactivity as the gas diffuses throughout the lungs. The two images are compared, noting areas that are not equally ventilated and perfused (mismatched). Decreased diffusion of the inhaled radioisotope may be seen with airway obstruction or pneumonia. Decreased circulation within the lungs of the infused radioisotope indicates an obstruction in the pulmonary circulation. A V/Q scan cannot always definitively diagnose pulmonary embolism. The test results are reported as high, intermediate, or low probability of occlusion due to an embolus. A normal chest x-ray with a high-probability V/Q scan provides the most convincing evidence of a PE.

Polysomnography

Polysomnography is the study of sleep and helps classify stages of sleep as well as document apneic and hypopneic periods. During the study, the patient is observed by a technician via video feed. Plethysmography is used to continually monitor breathing effort, and an electroencephalogram (EEG) characterizes sleep architecture. The study also includes airflow sensors at the nose and mouth, oximeters to measure oxygen saturation, electrooculograms to monitor rapid eye movements (REM sleep), and chin electromyography to detect hypotonia. A continuous ECG is performed to monitor for arrhythmias. Limb muscle activity is also monitored to diagnose **restless leg syndrome** or to assess nonrespiratory causes of sleep arousal.

A polysomnography study assesses the following:

- apnea-hypopnea index (AHI): calculated by taking the total number of episodes of apnea and hypopnea and dividing by the hours of sleep
- respiratory disturbance index (RDI): describes the number of times per hour that the oxygen saturation falls greater than three percentage points
- arousal index (AI): the number of arousals per hour as determined by EEG readings

OSA is diagnosed when the AHI is greater than 5. Values between 15 and 30 indicate moderate to severe levels of sleep apnea.

SLEEP ARCHITECTURE: Sleep latency was 40.6 minutes with a total sleep time of 318.9 minutes. Sleep-stage distribution reveals as a percentage of total sleep time: 3.9% stage 1; 73% stage 2, and 23% slow-wave sleep. No REM sleep was achieved.

AROUSAL DATA: The patient's total arousal index was 7.1, of which only 11 were respiratory-related, for an index of 2.1. Her periodic limb movement index, however, was 20.5, and there were no leg movements with respiratory events.

RESPIRATORY ANALYSIS: The patient does not show evidence of abnormal breathing with an apnea-hypopnea index of only 9. The patient had minimal snoring as well.

OXIMETRY DATA: Baseline oxygen saturation was 92.7% with a minimum of 80.6%. Up to 74% of the time was spent with saturations of less than 90%, and she had 41 desaturations greater than 4%. The mean oxygen saturation was 89.2%.

CARDIAC DATA: The maximum heart rate was 91, minimum 70, with a mean of 79. There were occasional PVCs.

LIMB MOVEMENT ANALYSIS: The periodic limb movement index was 20.5, which is elevated. Restless leg syndrome and/or periodic limb movements in sleep may be the cause of difficulty falling asleep, frequent nocturnal awakenings, and/or excessive daytime sleepiness.

IMPRESSION
1. Periodic limb movements in sleep.
2. Moderate arterial oxygen desaturation. There is no evidence of obstructive sleep apnea.

Laboratory Studies

In addition to the basic metabolic profile that provides information on electrolytes and acid-base balance (see page 42), the pulmonologist also depends on arterial blood gas analyses and coagulation studies, particularly D-dimer (see page 431), to diagnose pulmonary disease. Cultures and cytology also play a significant role.

Arterial blood gas analysis (ABG) measures the partial pressures of the respiratory gases, the bicarbonate concentration, and the pH of an *arterial* blood sample (**Table 8-7**). Samples are typically drawn from the radial, brachial, or femoral artery. ABGs assess both the acid-base balance of the body and the pulmonary gas exchange.

Table 8-7 Arterial Blood Gas Measurements

Test Name	Reference Range
pH	7.35 to 7.45
PaO_2	80–100 mmHg
$PaCO_2$	35–45 mmHg
HCO_3^-	22–27 mEq/L
SaO_2	95% to 99%

The total carbon dioxide (CO_2) level may also be determined (**Table 8-8**). Only about 10% of the carbon dioxide produced is present in the blood as actual carbon dioxide. The majority of CO_2 quickly reacts with water in the blood to form carbonic acid that subsequently splits into bicarbonate and hydrogen ions. The total CO_2 level is a measure of all forms of carbon dioxide (as a gas and as bicarbonate ions). CO_2 is measured in *venous* blood and is often reported along with electrolyte values.

Table 8-8 Total Carbon Dioxide

Test Name	Reference Range
CO_2 (total)	22–26 mEq/L

Blood gas done at 11:25 last night shows a pH of 7.35, PCO_2 44, PO_2 53, calculated bicarbonate 24. This was on a nonrebreather mask.

Pharmacology

Pharmaceutical treatments play a major role in the management of pulmonary disorders. Many antimicrobial agents are used as well as bronchodilators, vasodilators, expectorants, immune modulators, smoking cessation aids, and anticoagulants.

Mucolytics and Expectorants

Mucolytics and expectorants (**Table 8-9**) are used to treat cough and congestion caused by thick mucus within the bronchial tree. Mucolytics are used to break up or liquify bronchial secretions to help clear thick, excessive mucus. Expectorants act by increasing the secretion of mucus and reducing the viscosity so it is easier to clear the lungs and bronchi with coughing.

Table 8-9 Mucolytics and Expectorants

Generic	Brand Name	Dose
dornase	Pulmozyme	solution for nebulization 1 mg/mL (2.5 mL)
acetylcysteine	Mucomyst	solution for inhalation 10%, 20%
guaifenesin	Mucinex	600 mg, 1200 mg

Bronchodilators

Bronchodilators help dilate the bronchi and bronchioles by relaxing smooth muscle. The two categories of bronchodilators include beta 2-agonists and anticholinergics. Many of the bronchodilators are delivered as inhalants through small, portable devices. A dose is counted in puffs or **actuations** (the number of times the device is activated). Delivery systems include:

- metered-dose inhaler and metered-dose inhaler with spacer
- Autohaler
- Diskus
- HandiHaler
- Turbuhaler
- Twisthaler
- Flexhaler
- Aerolizer

Beta 2-Adrenergic Agents

Beta 2-adrenergic agents (**Table 8-10**), also called beta 2-agonists, are used to treat reversible bronchospasm. These agents relax bronchial smooth muscle, decrease mast-cell degranulation and histamine release, inhibit microvascular leakage into the airways, and increase mucociliary clearance. Beta 2-agonists come in short-acting (four hours) and long-acting (up to 12 hours) preparations and are delivered as inhalants through inhalers or nebulizers. Short-acting agents are used for exacerbations, and long-acting agents are used on a routine basis for overall control of bronchospasm.

Table 8-10 Beta 2-Adrenergic Agents

Generic	Brand Name	Dose
Short-acting beta 2-adrenergic agonists		
albuterol	Proventil HFA** Ventolin HFA	90 mcg/actuation
levalbuterol	Xopenex Xopenex HFA	45 mcg/actuation
pirbuterol	Maxair Autohaler	200 mcg/actuation
Long-acting beta 2-adrenergic agonists		
salmeterol	Serevent Diskus	50 mcg
formoterol	Foradil Aerolizer	12 mcg/capsule (for inhalation)

**HFA is the abbreviation for hydrofluoroalkane, the propellant used to deliver the medication.

Anticholinergic Agents

Anticholinergic medications (**Table 8-11**) act on bronchial smooth muscle by competitively inhibiting muscarinic cholinergic receptors. Blocking these receptors lessens or prevents constriction of the airways due to acetylcholine. These anticholinergic agents also have antisecretory properties. Anticholinergics are used in conjunction with beta 2-agonists to treat COPD and severe exacerbations of asthma.

Table 8-11 Anticholinergic Medications

Generic	Brand Name	Dose
ipratropium	Atrovent HFA	17 mcg/actuation
tiotropium	Spiriva HandiHaler	18 mcg/capsule (for inhalation)

Corticosteroids

Corticosteroids (**Table 8-12**) are prescribed to reduce airway inflammation. Inhaled corticosteroids are considered the primary drug of choice for control of chronic asthma. They block the late response to inhaled allergens and inhibit leukotriene and cytokine production. Routes of administration include inhalation, IV, and oral. IV and oral treatments work quickly to control an acute exacerbation of asthma but inhalant corticosteroids are only used for long-term control. Inhaled corticosteroids may also be used to treat inflammation associated with COPD.

Table 8-12 Inhaled Corticosteroids

Generic	Brand Name	Dose
budesonide	Pulmicort Flexhaler	90 and 180 mcg per inhalation
fluticasone	Flovent HFA	44 mcg, 110 mcg and 220 mcg per inhalation
	Flovent Diskus	50 mcg
triamcinolone	Azmacort	100 mcg/actuation
Combination Corticosteroids and Beta 2-Agonists		
budesonide and formoterol	Symbicort	80 mcg/4.5 mcg 160 mcg/4.5 mcg
fluticasone and salmeterol	Advair Diskus	100 mcg/50 mcg 250 mcg/50 mcg 500 mcg/50 mcg

Mast Cell Stabilizers

Mast cell stabilizers (**Table 8-13**) prevent mast cells from releasing histamine and other immune system mediators that cause airway inflammation and bronchospasm. These agents reduce airway hyperresponsiveness and block both early and late responses to allergens. They are indicated for maintenance therapy of mild to moderate asthma or prophylaxis for exercise-induced bronchospasm.

Table 8-13 Mast Cell Stabilizers

Generic	Brand Name	Dose
cromolyn sodium	NasalCrom (OTC)	40 mg/mL
nedocromil	Tilade	1.75 mg/actuation

Leukotriene-Receptor Antagonists

Leukotrienes are released by cells of the immune system and are potent mediators of inflammatory reactions. Leukotrienes contribute to the symptoms of asthma by contracting airway smooth muscle, increasing vascular permeability, increasing mucus secretion, and activating other inflammatory cells such as eosinophils. Leukotriene-receptor antagonists (**Table 8-14**) inhibit the action of leukotrienes and thereby reduce inflammation. (17) Unlike many other asthma medications that are inhaled, leukotriene-receptor antagonists are taken orally. They are used for the long-term control and prevention of asthma symptoms and tend to lessen the use of rescue medications. Note the common suffix –*lukast* used for this drug class.

Table 8-14 Leukotriene Receptor Antagonists

Generic	Brand Name	Dose
montelukast	Singulair	4 mg, 5 mg, and 10 mg
zafirlukast	Accolate	10 mg, 20 mg

(17) Systems throughout the body communicate with each other through the use of messenger molecules and cell receptors. Cellular responses are activated by the binding of a specific messenger molecule to a receptor on the target cell's surface. Receptor antagonists work by binding to a given receptor and blocking the biologically active molecule from binding (ie, they "antagonize" the receptor). Even though the antagonist binds to the receptor, it does not provoke a normal response.

Use caution when spelling Singulair; it is easy to spell it Singular. This error will not be detected by spell check software.

A drug closely related to the leukotriene receptor antagonists is Zyflo CR (**Table 8-15**), a leukotriene inhibitor. This particular drug blocks the production of leukotrienes through the inhibition of 5-lipoxygenase.

Table 8-15 Leukotriene Inhibitor

Generic	Brand Name	Dose
zileuton	Zyflo CR	600 mg

Monoclonal Antibodies

Treatment with monoclonal antibodies (**Table 8-16**) is one of the newest approaches to control asthma in patients with elevated levels of IgE antibodies. This treatment consists of a monoclonal IgG antibody that binds selectively to IgE on the surface of mast cells and basophils. This blocks the IgE antibody's normal ability to provoke an allergic response. It is prescribed for patients with moderate to severe asthma in whom symptoms are uncontrolled with corticosteroids. As with other monoclonal antibodies, the generic name for this treatment ends in –*mab* (**m**onoclonal **Ab**).

Table 8-16 IgE Monoclonal Antibodies

Generic	Brand Name	Dose
omalizumab	Xolair	Subcutaneous injections every two to four weeks.

Smoking Cessation Aids

Smoking cessation for patients with respiratory disease is critical yet extremely difficult. Therapies that employ a three-prong approach, including behavior modification techniques, group therapy, and smoking cessation aids (**Table 8-17**), are most successful. Nicotine replacement therapy is available as a gum, transdermal patch, inhaler, lozenge, or nasal spray. The nicotine agonist varenicline (Chantix) blocks the effect of nicotine in the brain and is prescribed orally for one week before attempting to quit smoking and for an additional 12 weeks while the patient abstains from cigarettes. The antidepressant bupropion (Zyban) acts as a nicotinic receptor antagonist and is also prescribed as a smoking cessation aid.

Table 8-17 Smoking Cessation Aides

Generic	Brand Name	Dose
nicotine	Commit (lozenge) Nicorette (gum)	2 mg, 4 mg
	Nicotrol (inhaler, nasal spray)	
	NicoDerm CQ (OTC)	
bupropion	Zyban	150 mg
varenicline	Chantix	0.5 mg, 1 mg

Antimicrobial Therapy

Antimicrobial therapy is widely used in both primary care and acute care for the treatment and prevention of respiratory infection. Therapies include preventative agents such as antivirals and vaccinations as well as antimicrobials to treat acute disease caused by bacteria, fungi, and viruses.

Penicillins

The penicillins represent an important class of antibiotics. The penicillins contain a beta-lactam ring, a configuration of carbon and nitrogen atoms, which contributes to the antibiotics' mode of action. The beta-lactam ring is also a component of other antibiotic classes, including cephalosporins, carbapenems, and monobactams (collectively called the beta-lactam antibiotics). These antibiotics disrupt the assembly of the bacterial cell wall, thereby preventing bacterial replication. The beta-lactam ring is significant because many bacteria have developed resistance to these antibiotics by producing beta-lactamase, an enzyme that destroys the beta-lactam ring and renders the antibiotic ineffective.

Methicillin is classified as a penicillin, but it has been replaced by more stable penicillins and is no longer manufactured. The term methicillin is now used to collectively refer to antibiotics that contain a beta-lactam ring (ie, the penicillins, cephalosporins, carbapenems, and monobactams). Many bacteria have developed resistance to these antibiotics by producing beta-lactamase or by changing the structure of the protein to which these drugs bind. The change in the binding site is the mechanism employed by methicillin-resistant Staphylococcus aureus (MRSA). The number of bacteria that have acquired the ability to resist antibiotics (through either beta-lactamase or a change in the binding protein) is on the rise and presents significant treatment problems.

The most common penicillin-class antibiotics used to treat respiratory infections are piperacillin and amoxicillin (**Table 8-18**). Piperacillin is a broad-spectrum antibiotic that is particularly active against pseudomonas. These antibiotics are combined with tazobactam or clavulanate to inhibit the action of beta-lactamase.

Table 8-18 Penicillins

Generic	Brand Name	Dose
piperacillin and tazobactam sodium	Zosyn	
amoxicillin and clavulanate	Augmentin Augmentin XR	250 mg, 500 mg, 850 mg, 1000 mg

Cephalosporins

The cephalosporins (**Table 8-19**), like the penicillin class of antibiotics, contain a beta-lactam ring and act against organisms by disrupting the structure of the bacterial cell wall. Although there are many antibiotics in the cephalosporin class, only a few are commonly used for respiratory infections. All are given by IV or IM. The cephalosporin class of antibiotics shares the common syllable *ceph* or *cef*.

Table 8-19 Cephalosporins

Generic	Brand Name
ceftriaxone	Rocephin
ceftazidime	Fortaz
cefepime	Maxipime

Macrolides

The macrolides (**Table 8-20**) are a group of antibiotics that inhibit bacterial growth by interfering with protein synthesis. Like the penicillins, the macrolides include a beta-lactam ring and are susceptible to deactivation by organisms that have acquired beta-lactamase or other countermeasures against the beta-lactam antibiotics.

Fluoroquinolones

The fluoroquinolone class of antibiotics (also called quinolones) includes a large number of antibiotics but only a few are used to treat respiratory infections, which are sometimes referred to as the respiratory

Table 8-20 Macrolides

Generic	Brand Name	Dose
azithromycin	Zithromax	250 mg, 500 mg, 600 mg
	Zithromax TRI-PAK	500 mg
	Zithromax Z-PAK	250 mg
erythromycin	E.E.S.	400 mg/5 mL
	Erythrocin	250 mg, 500 mg
clarithromycin	Biaxin	250 mg, 500 mg

quinolones (**Table 8-21**). Levofloxacin (Levaquin) is a popular choice for empiric treatment of community acquired pneumonia. This class of antibiotic uses the suffix *–floxacin*.

Table 8-21 Respiratory Quinolones

Generic	Brand Name	Dose
levofloxacin	Levaquin	250 mg, 500 mg, 750 mg
ciprofloxacin	Cipro	250 mg, 500 mg, 750 mg
	Cipro XR	500 mg, 1000 mg
moxifloxacin	Avelox	400 mg

Vancomycin

Vancomycin is used to treat infections caused by gram-positive bacteria and is effective against MRSA. Vancomycin is administered by IV and levels must be monitored to avoid toxicity. It is recommended that trough levels be drawn one-half hour before the fourth dose. Preventing infection with MRSA is of particular interest to the healthcare community because treatment with vancomycin is expensive and inconvenient.

> Physicians may order a "vanc trough" level. This test measures the concentration of vancomycin in the blood at what should be the lowest concentration point (the nadir) just before the next dose is given.

Tetracycline

The tetracycline class of antibiotics (**Table 8-22**) works by inhibiting protein synthesis. Doxycycline is the most common tetracycline used in respiratory illness and is used to treat the atypical pneumonias, such as chlamydia and mycoplasma.

Table 8-22 Tetracycline

Generic	Brand Name	Dose
doxycycline	Bio-Tab, Doryx, Doxy, Periostat, Vibramycin, Vibra-Tabs	20 mg, 50 mg, 75 mg, 100 mg, 150 mg

Antifungals

The most common antifungal medications used to treat respiratory illness are amphotericin B and fluconazole (**Table 8-23**).

Table 8-23 Antifungals

Generic	Brand Name	Dose
amphotericin B		IV only
fluconazole	Diflucan	50 mg, 100 mg, 150 mg, 200 mg

Antivirals

The antiviral medications used for respiratory illnesses (**Table 8-24**) are used prophylactically as well as therapeutically. Antiviral medications can attenuate a viral illness and should be started within two days of the onset of symptoms. Patients at high risk of succumbing to the yearly flu and patients with underlying respiratory illness such as COPD may be prescribed an antiviral to be taken prophylactically and should be started within 36 hours of exposure.

Table 8-24 Antivirals

Generic	Brand Name	Dose
amantadine	Symmetrel	100 mg
oseltamivir	Tamiflu	30 mg, 45 mg, and 75 mg
zanamivir (effective against both influenza A and B)	Relenza	5 mg

Vaccinations

Vaccinations against influenza and pneumococcal pneumonia are important components of preventive care for patients with underlying respiratory illness. Patients may be vaccinated against influenza and pneumococcal bacteria (**Table 8-25**).

Table 8-25 Vaccinations

Generic	Brand Name
influenza virus vaccine	Fluarix FluMist
pneumococcal pneumonia vaccine	Pneumovax

Anticoagulants

Anticoagulants come in three major forms including warfarin, heparin, and fondaparinux. Anticoagulants work by enhancing the naturally occurring mechanisms that normally prevent the coagulation system from running amok or by slowing the production of coagulation proteins that contribute to clot formation.

Heparin

Heparin augments the activity of antithrombin (an anticoagulant produced in the liver) and prevents conversion of fibrinogen to fibrin (a major component of a clot). Heparin is available as unfractionated heparin (**Table 8-26**) and as low-molecular-weight heparin (LMWH). Unfractionated heparin must be monitored using the **activated partial thromboplastin time (aPTT)**, and the dose should be adjusted until the aPTT value is 1.5 to 2.5 times the control value (as reported by the laboratory). Over-heparinization can be treated with protamine.

Table 8-26 Unfractionated Heparin

Generic	Brand Name	Dose
unfractionated heparin	Hep-Lock Hepflush-10	subcutaneous or IV administration measured in units/kg/hour

Low-molecular-weight heparin (**Table 8-27**) consists of smaller molecules of heparin that are more easily utilized. It has been found to be safer and more effective than unfractionated heparin in treating DVT and PE and does not require monitoring, but the cost of long-term therapy is prohibitive. In the treatment of DVT and PE, LMWH is administered subcutaneously, typically in the abdomen, along with oral warfarin until the warfarin is therapeutic.

Table 8-27 Low-Molecular-Weight-Heparin

Generic	Brand Name	Dose
low-molecular-weight-heparin (enoxaparin)	Lovenox	30 mg, 40 mg (prefilled syringes)

Warfarin

Warfarin interferes with hepatic synthesis of vitamin K-dependent coagulation factors. The first few days of warfarin therapy actually create a hypercoagulable state, so warfarin should always be started with concomitant heparin until the PT/INR value is therapeutic.

Foods high in vitamin K may interfere with the action of warfarin. Patients may need to reduce or eliminate vitamin-K rich foods from their diet, including **cruciferous vegetables** (broccoli, cabbage, brussel sprouts), green tea, asparagus, avocado, liver, soybean oil, peas, spinach, and lettuce.

Warfarin therapy (**Table 8-28**) is administered orally and is monitored routinely using the prothrombin time (PT) expressed as the International Normalized Ratio (INR) (see page 430). PT/INR values are measured daily or every few days until the therapeutic range is reached, and then it is rechecked at weekly or monthly intervals. Physicians often refer patients on chronic Coumadin therapy to the **Coumadin clinic** for ongoing monitoring and adjustment of their Coumadin dose.

> You may hear physicians refer to patients on Coumadin therapy as being "coumadinized." The backformation of the word Coumadin has not been fully accepted as a legitimate word. You should refer to your facility's policy on the use of this word, and if disallowed, recast the sentence when dictated.

Table 8-28 Warfarin

Generic	Brand Name	Dose
warfarin	Coumadin	1 mg, 2 mg, 2.5 mg, 3 mg, 4 mg, 5 mg, 6 mg, 7.5 mg, 10 mg

Fondaparinux

Fondaparinux (**Table 8-29**) inhibits Factor Xa, which plays a part in the activation sequence of thrombin. Thrombin converts fibrinogen to the fibrin strands that hold clots together. Clots that occur in the deep veins consist of red cells held together by fibrin strands, so inhibition of fibrin is one method of preventing deep venous thrombosis. Fondaparinux is used prophylactically in patients who have undergone orthopedic surgery (eg, hip and knee replacement) and also therapeutically in patients with known DVT and PE. Its main advantage over heparin is it is less likely to cause **heparin-induced thrombocytopenia**. It is administered subcutaneously on a daily basis.

Table 8-29 Fondaparinux

Generic	Brand Name
fondaparinux	Arixtra

Phosphodiesterase Inhibitors

Phosphodiesterase inhibitors (**Table 8-30**) are used to treat pulmonary hypertension. They block the action of the phosphodiesterase enzymes (PDE). There are five types of this enzyme, with type 5 being relevant to pulmonology. PDE5 is found in the smooth muscle of arterial walls within the lungs. PDE5 inhibitors increase nitric oxide levels and relax arterial vessel walls, increasing the diameter of the vessels and decreasing intravascular pressure. Sildenafil is the same active ingredient in Viagra, which is used to treat erectile dysfunction. It has the same action on the vessel walls in the corpus cavernosum, allowing more blood to enter the penis.

Table 8-30 Phosphodiesterase Inhibitor

Generic	Brand Name	Dose
sildenafil	Revatio	20 mg

Exercises

Using Context to Make Decisions

1. Add punctuation and edit this excerpt as needed. Insert the names of the ABG values dictated.

   Blood gas at 1130 last night on a nonrebreather was 7.35/44/53 now on BiPAP 100% she is 7.39/43/88.

2. Recast this dictation and correctly punctuate so that no two arabic numbers are transcribed side by side.

   Sleep latency was 40.6 minutes with a total sleep time of 318.9 minutes. Sleep stage distribution reveals as a percentage of total sleep time: 3.9% stage 1.73% stage 2 23% slow wave sleep and no REM sleep was achieved.

3. Complete the following paragraph with the following terms:

   - effusion
   - diffusion
   - infusion
   - suffusion
   - profusion
   - perfusion

   She recently underwent a nuclear stress test that showed normal myocardial _____ with no evidence of myocardial ischemia or prior infarct. The patient is known to have a pleural _____. A recent DL_{CO} showed decreased _____ capacity, possibly due to emphysema. She has a history of breast cancer and receives a monthly _____ of Aredia for bone metastasis. The open wound on her ankle no longer shows a _____ of pus and is beginning to heal after repeated _____ of topical antibiotics.

Use the sample report on page 276 to answer questions 4–16.

4. What word would complete blank #1? _____

5. Match the medications listed under current medications to the items listed in the past medical history. Which medications cannot be directly associated with one of her listed medical problems? _____

   _____

6. What medication did the patient admit to taking that was not listed in the current medications?

   _____

7. What word would complete blank #2?
   a. saturation   c. pressure
   b. concentration   d. diffusion

8. What antibiotic would complete blank #3? _____

   _____

9. Which of the following medications would be appropriate for blank #4?
   a. Flovent   c. Flolan
   b. Flomax   d. Floxin

10. Describe the transcription error under the Laboratory section. _____

    _____

11. What word has been transcribed incorrectly under the Physical Exam? _____

    _____

12. What transcription error occurred in the EKG findings discussed in the Assessment? _____

    _____

13. Which of the following would correctly complete blank #5?
    a. BNP   c. PFT
    b. BMP   d. ABG

14. Which medication chosen from the list of current medications would complete blank #6? _____

_____

15. What medication would complete blank #7? ____

_____

16. Identify the 2 incorrectly transcribed abbreviations in the Assessment and Plan. Correct the errors and then expand *all abbreviations* in this section of the report according to the rules for expanding abbreviations described in the *Book of Style*. _____

_____

Terms Checkup

Complete the multiple choice questions for Chapter 8 located at www.myhealthprofessionskit.com. To access the questions, select the discipline "Medical Transcription," then click on the title of this book, *Advanced Medical Transcription.*

Look It Up

Using the guidelines described on page xvii, complete a research project cystic fibrosis.

Transcription Practice

1. Transcribe the key terms and phrases for Chapter 8.
2. Complete the proofing and transcription practice exercises for Chapter 8.

CHIEF COMPLAINT: Pneumonia.

PRESENT ILLNESS: The patient is a 60-year-old white female who comes in with a 1-week history of low-grade fever of 99.4 degrees with sweats, no chills, an increasing cough with brownish-colored sputum, and increased shortness of breath. She also reports central chest discomfort and describes it as "an elephant sitting on my chest." She denies any chest pain. She was seen 2 days ago and diagnosed with pneumonia and started on Biaxin, which she reports she has been taking faithfully. She comes into the emergency room today for worsening symptoms. She reports 1–3 episodes of pneumonia a year and is __(1)__ dependent, using about 2.5 L per nasal cannula.

PAST MEDICAL HISTORY: 1) Cerebrovascular accident with resultant right-sided weakness. She lives in an assisted living center and uses a motorized wheelchair. She also has seizures status post CVA. 2) Chronic obstructive pulmonary disease. She is on 2.5 L by nasal cannula. 3) Congestive heart failure. She had a dobutamine stress test in May of this year, which was negative for stress-induced ischemia, and the ejection fraction was estimated to be 74%. 4) Chronic low back pain and neck pain. 5) Neuropathy. 6) Depression. 7) Sleep apnea. 8) Osteoporosis. 9) GERD. 10) Dyslipidemia. 11) Frequent UTI with recent vaginal yeast infection secondary to antibiotic therapy.

MEDICATIONS: Aspirin 81 mg p.o. daily, Bactrim DS 1 tablet p.o. b.i.d., Boniva monthly, calcium, Combivent 2 puffs 4 times a day, cyanocobalamin 1000 mcg daily, Demadex 20 mg p.o. daily, Diflucan 150 mg p.o. daily, DuoNeb 1 inhalation 4 times a day by nebulizer, ferrous sulfate 325 mg p.o. daily, Allegra 180 mg p.o. daily, MS Contin 30 mg p.o. b.i.d., Neurontin 800 mg p.o. t.i.d., Nexium 40 mg daily, Dilantin 125 mg p.o. t.i.d., potassium 20 mEq daily, Singulair 10 mg p.o. daily, Spiriva 1 inhalation daily, Zocor 40 mg p.o. daily.

ALLERGIES: Augmentin, Provera.

SOCIAL HISTORY: She has smoked 1 pack per day for more than 35 years.

REVIEW OF SYSTEMS: She reports an intentional 30-pound weight loss in the last year. She notes easy bruising and frequent urinary tract infections.

PHYSICAL EXAMINATION
GENERAL: She looks much older than her stated age and is on nasal cannula at 2.5 L with O_2 __(2)__ in the low 90s.
HEENT: Normocephalic, atraumatic. Pupils are equal and reactive to light and accommodation.
NECK: Supple, no masses.
CHEST: Bilateral wheezes and course crackles are heard.

HEART: Normal heart sounds.

NEUROLOGIC: Right upper extremity is atrophied, with flexion contractures of the fingers.

ABDOMEN: Soft and nontender.

EXTREMITIES: No pedal edema.

LABORATORY: WBC 9.9, hemoglobin 14.6, platelet count 236, normal differential. Sodium 139, potassium 4.2, chloride 102, CO 226, BUN 12, creatinine 0.8, glucose 60; calcium 8.9, slightly elevated alkaline phosphatase at 145. Dilantin level therapeutic at 16.9, TSH normal at 2.9. Chest x-ray shows calcification of her trachea as well as the aorta. Lung fields appear clear; prominent right hilum. The EKG shows sinus rhythm, left axis deviation with T-wave inversions in the inferior as well as anterior leads.

ASSESSMENT AND PLAN

1. COPD with exacerbation. She has failed ___(3)___ therapy on an outpatient basis. I would have preferred to use a beta-lactam; however, she is allergic, so I will avoid cephalosporins as well as penicillin derivatives. She has a prolonged QT on her EKG of about 510 ms, so I will also avoid fluoroquinolones. We will start Zithromax IV. Also, I would have liked to treat her with steroids, but she vehemently refuses this. We will continue bronchodilators for now. She is not on a steroid inhaler either and I will institute ___(4)___-HFA during this admission.

2. CHF. I see no evidence of exacerbation at this time, but I will order a ___(5)___ to confirm. I will continue her ___(6)___ for now as well as potassium supplement.

3. Smoking cessation. We will vigorously pursue smoking cessation during this admission, and I will start her on ___(7)___ 0.5 mg in preparation for that.

4. Chest pressure. This is certainly worrisome for a cardiac etiology. Initial EKG shows no specific changes that do not seem to be new, but we will check serial enzymes.

5. History of CBA with seizure disorder and right hemiparesis. Phenytoin level is therapeutic.

6. DVT prophylaxis with SEDs.

7. GERD. Continue treatment with PPI.

Cardiology

Learning Objectives
After completing this chapter, you should be able to comprehend and correctly transcribe terminology related to:

▶ valvular disease of the heart

▶ cardiac dysrhythmias

▶ hypertensive heart disease

▶ congestive heart failure

▶ atherosclerotic disease

▶ laboratory, imaging, and electrophysiology tests used to diagnose and monitor cardiac disease

▶ drugs used in the treatment of cardiac disease

Introduction

Heart disease in its many forms is the leading cause of death in the United States, and as such, a large number of patient encounters will involve cardiac care. As a transcriptionist, you will encounter terminology related to cardiovascular and cardiopulmonary disorders in many specialties and these terms will form an important part of your foundational knowledge of medical terminology and pathophysiology. Patients with heart disease often have several comorbid conditions, require routine monitoring, and typically take myriad medications, so medical transcriptionists working in cardiology need to be familiar with many pharmacological agents as well as laboratory tests and diagnostic procedures, especially those related to cardiology, pulmonology, diabetes, and renal disease.

Many forms of heart disease share similar symptoms. Rarely will symptoms alone be diagnostic. Common symptoms reported by patients seeking cardiac care include chest pain, **dyspnea at rest** or **dyspnea on exertion**, orthopnea, dizziness, syncope or **near syncope**, fatigue, palpitations, and edema. Patients with heart disease may appear perfectly healthy, but patients suffering from an acute event or those with chronic disease may present with angina, diaphoresis, cyanosis, abnormal heart rate or rhythm, abnormal heart sounds, murmurs, cachexia, **jugular venous pulsations**, edema, and an abnormal pulmonary examination including tachypnea, rales, wheezing, and signs of pleural effusion.

Anatomy

Understanding cardiac anatomy is integral to accurately transcribing cardiology reports. Study ■ **Figure 9-1** to review the arrangement of the chambers, valves, and great vessels as well as the direction of blood flow. It is important to remember that (oddly enough) the base of the heart is proximal to your head and the apex is pointing downward. The heart may also be viewed as two side-by-side pumps; the right heart pumps blood to the lungs and the left heart pumps blood to the body.

Key points to remember include:

- Blood returns to the heart from the general circulation by way of the superior and inferior vena cava that empties into the right atrium.
- The atria fill at the same time during cardiac muscle relaxation (diastole).
- Both ventricles contract and expulse blood at the same time during systole.
- Blood from the left side of the heart enters the general circulation by way of the aorta.
- Blood from the right side of the heart enters the lungs by way of the pulmonary arteries.
- Cardiac muscle contracts due to electrical impulses generated by the pacemaker and propagated throughout the cardiac tissue by the movement of ions across cellular membranes (see also Figure 2-1).
- The kidneys, heart, and lungs must work together to maintain acid-base balance (pH) and total body fluid levels.

Valvular Disease

Valves control the flow of blood through the four chambers of the heart and are integral to the heart's function (see Figure 9-1). When valves malfunction, blood accumulates in the affected heart chamber or vessel and an inadequate amount of blood flows through the heart,

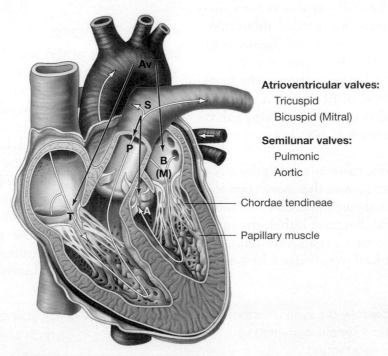

Av

S

P

B
(M)

T

A

Atrioventricular valves:
   Tricuspid
   Bicuspid (Mitral)

Semilunar valves:
   Pulmonic
   Aortic

— Chordae tendineae

— Papillary muscle

FIGURE 9-1 The heart valves, chambers, and supporting structures.

referred to as decreased **cardiac output**. Forms of valvular disease include stenosis, sclerosis, and regurgitation. Also referred to as **retrograde flow**, regurgitation is the backward flow of blood through a one-way valve. A stenotic valve does not open enough to allow sufficient blood to pass through the valve's opening, called the **outflow tract**. In the same way that narrowing the opening of a water hose causes increased pressure within the hose and the jet of water to be smaller yet accelerate faster, stenotic valves have the same effect on the heart and the flow of blood. The back pressure created by stenotic valves causes the affected heart chamber to become enlarged and the muscles in the chamber walls to become hypertrophic. A **sclerotic valve** is stiff and incapable of opening and closing efficiently.

> **Pause 9-1** Compare the terms hypertrophy and hyperplasia. Which of these occurs as the result of increased work (exercise)?

Mild valvular disease may go undetected for the first four or five decades of a person's life, but symptoms may become evident when combined with other forms of heart disease such as atherosclerosis, hypertensive heart disease, ventricular hypertrophy, or endocarditis. Valvular disease may involve any of the four heart valves: mitral, aortic, pulmonic, or tricuspid. Valves may be congenitally malformed or become diseased due to atherosclerosis, myocardial infarction, endocarditis, hypertension, pulmonary disease, connective tissue disease, or the degenerative effects of aging. Valves may also develop **vegetations**, which are clumps or masses composed of fibrin, platelets, and microorganisms that result from infection of the valve. Valvular disease may be classified as stenotic or regurgitant (■ **Figure 9-2**).

In the pre-antibiotic era, rheumatic heart disease, a sequela of strep pharyngitis, was the most common cause of valvular disease. In rheumatic disease, the valve is not actually infected with bacteria; rather, the valve becomes infiltrated with immune complexes (antigen-antibody complexes) that lead to valvular sclerosis.

> **(1)** Holosystolic and pansystolic are synonyms that mean lasting throughout systole, occurring from the first to the second heart sound.

Mitral Valve Disease

Components of the mitral valve include the papillary muscles, **chordae**, **leaflets**, and **mitral annulus**. Malformations or disease of any of these components can cause **mitral valve stenosis** or regurgitation, also called **mitral insufficiency**. Patients with mitral stenosis and **mitral regurgitation (MR)** often have **mitral annular calcification**. The cardinal sign of MR is a holosystolic (1) murmur, heard best at the apex. Severe mitral disease leads to **left-sided heart disease**. Symptomatic mitral stenosis may be treated medically with ACE inhibitors, but progressive disease may require surgical repair or replacement.

Mitral valve prolapse (MVP) is an abnormal bulging of the mitral valve leaflets into the left atrium. MVP may be inherited or it may result from connective tissue disease. MVP may be asymptomatic or cause nonspecific chest pain, dyspnea on exertion, fatigue, and syncope. On examination, MVP may produce a **midsystolic click** and a late systolic murmur. Patients with MVP require antibiotic prophylaxis before undergoing dental procedures. Patients may be treated with betablockers to help with chest pain. Rarely, valve replacement is required.

> **Pause 9-2** Describe mitral annular calcification in layman's terms. List ways this phrase may be misinterpreted when dictated.

Aortic Stenosis

Malformations of the aortic valve are the most common cause of aortic valve disease. Congenital abnormalities include a bicuspid aortic valve instead of the normal tricuspid valve. In addition to congenital malformations, the same atherosclerotic process leading to obstruction of blood vessels has been found to affect the aortic valve as well, leading to **aortic stenosis (AS)**. The narrowed aortic valve places back pressure on the left ventricle and the increased work required to push blood through the valve leads to **left ventricular hypertrophy**. AS may produce a **crescendo-decrescendo murmur**. If medical treatment fails, surgical replacement of the valve is indicated.

> **Pause 9-3** Describe left ventricular hypertrophy in layman's terms.

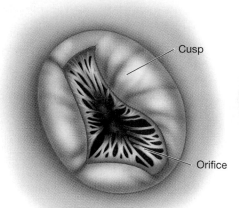

Cusp

Orifice

Normal Valve (open)
Normal valve opens widely and
blood moves through freely.

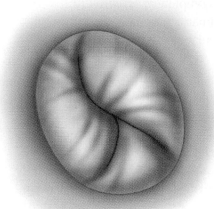

Normal Valve (closed)
Normal valve closes "water tight."

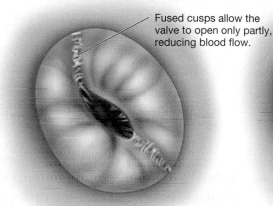

Fused cusps allow the
valve to open only partly,
reducing blood flow.

Stenosis (open valve)
Stenotic valve is thickened and
bound down by scar tissue.

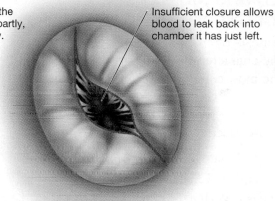

Insufficient closure allows
blood to leak back into
chamber it has just left.

Regurgitation (closed valve)
Valve leaflets are puckered and
pulled apart by scar tissue—
valve cannot close.

FIGURE 9-2 Normal valves compared to abnormal valves showing valvular Stenosis and valvular
regurgitation.

> Examination reveals a crescendo-decrescendo murmur best heard at the base, radiating to the carotids and apex.

Tricuspid Stenosis

Tricuspid stenosis, historically caused by rheumatic fever, is becoming less common in the US due to the efficacy of antibiotic treatment of strep pharyngitis. The tricuspid valve controls the entry of blood returning from the circulatory system into the right atrium. A stenotic tricuspid valve causes back pressure on the vena cava and thus the jugular veins, renal veins, and the hepatic vein, leading to systemic congestion characterized by elevation in the **jugular venous pressure (JVP)**, hepatomegaly, ascites and

dependent edema (2). First-line treatment includes diuretics to reduce fluid volume, but progressive stenosis requires replacement with a bioprosthetic valve.

Tricuspid Regurgitation

Tricuspid regurgitation (TR) is often caused by structural changes in the right ventricle because the valve is controlled by chordae that attach to papillary muscles on the walls of the right ventricle. If the right ventricle becomes enlarged, the chordae are pulled outward, thus pulling the valve open. Note the arrangement of the chordae and the tricuspid valve as shown in Figure 9-1.

> **(2)** Dependent edema is the accumulation of fluid in the extremities (especially the legs) due to gravity.

The greater the ventricular enlargement, the less likely the valve is to close completely. Treatment usually involves treating the primary cause of right ventricular enlargement, but valve replacement may also be required.

Pulmonic Valve Regurgitation

Pulmonary regurgitation (PR) is most often caused by hypertension in the pulmonary arterial vessels that puts backward pressure on the valve. Pulmonic regurgitation is characterized by a **decrescendo diastolic murmur** that radiates toward the midright sternal edge (**Graham Steell murmur**). Treatment most often involves treating the cause of the pulmonary hypertension, not the pulmonary valve itself.

Evaluation and Management of Valvular Disease

Valvular disease is often suspected on physical exam because of the characteristic sounds produced on auscultation. The most common sound is a murmur. Valvular disease may also produce a third or fourth heart sound (S_3 or S_4) or a **split heart sound** (split S_1, split S_2). Murmurs are described by their:

- grade (eg, 2/6, dictated "two over six")
- sound (eg, snap, click, soft, loud, blowing)
- timing relative to diastole and systole (eg, **mid-diastolic, early systolic, pansystolic, holosystolic**)
- anatomic location where they are best heard, such as along the **left sternal border, right sternal border, over the infrascapular area, parasternally, in the upper interscapular area, in the 3rd or 4th intercostal space, over the aorta,** or **at the apex.** Murmurs may also be described as **radiating to the base,** the axilla, the apex, or to the carotids.

(3) The transvalvular gradient is the change in pressure of the blood as it passes from one side of the valve to the other.

> Examination reveals a loud 3/6 pansystolic murmur best heard over the left sternal border and radiating to the axilla.

> **Pause 9-4** According to the *Book of Style*, how would you transcribe "two to three over six systolic ejection murmur"?

Most forms of valvular disease can be diagnosed on echocardiography. **Color flow Doppler** studies performed along with an echocardiogram provide qualitative estimates of the severity of stenosis and regurgitation by estimating the **transvalvular gradient (3). Transesophageal echocardiogram (TEE)** is also useful for diagnosing valvular disease, especially diseases of the aortic valve. In some instances, heart catheterization may be used to visualize the valves and measure gradients and pressures directly. Ventriculography may also be helpful in the diagnosis of valvular disease.

Severe valvular disease may require repair (**valvuloplasty** or **commissurotomy**) or replacement using mechanical valves or xenograft (bioprosthetic) valves made from pig (**porcine**) or cow (**bovine**). Valves may be repaired using a minimally invasive procedure called **percutaneous transluminal balloon valvuloplasty** (■ **Figure 9-3**). Patients with mechanical valves are **chronically anticoagulated** with Coumadin (warfarin) for the rest of their life to prevent the formation of clots (thrombi) and subsequent embolization.

> The patient is status post mechanical valve placement, chronically anticoagulated with Coumadin.

- Valvular disease includes stenosis, sclerosis, regurgitation, and vegetations.
- Valvular disease typically produces a murmur.
- Stenotic valves can cause hypertrophy and edema.

- Valvular regurgitation may cause weakness and fatigue.
- Valvular disease is diagnosed using echocardiography and Doppler studies.
- Severe valvular disease is treated with prosthetic valves.

cross the membrane. Calcium within the muscle fiber causes them to shorten, or contract (systole).

The original electrical impulse is generated by the **sinoatrial node** (SA node), also called the **sinus node**, located near the right atrium (■ Figure 9-4). The SA node is the heart's pacemaker. The electrical impulse travels down the atria to the **atrioventricular node (AV node)** that passes the impulse to the ventricles. Systole and diastole correlate with **repolarization** and **depolarization** of the muscle fibers.

> Resting EKG shows normal sinus rhythm with ST-segment elevation in leads II, III, aVF, V4, V5, and V6, suggestive of early repolarization.

> You may hear dictators refer to repolarization or depolarization as "repol" and "depol," but these terms should be spelled out.

> **Pause 9-5** What is a pacemaker?

The normal resting heart rate, referred to as **normal sinus rhythm (NSR) (4)**, is 60–80 beats per minute (bpm). Dysrhythmias include both rate and rhythm disorders individually or in combination. Rate disorders include **tachycardia** (greater than 100 bpm) and **bradycardia** (less than 50 bpm). Combination disorders include **tachyarrhythmia**, which is a fast, irregular beat, and **bradyarrhythmia**, which is a slow, irregular beat.

Dysrhythmias may be caused by faulty impulse formation or problems conducting the impulse across the heart muscle. The heart's rate and rhythm are also influenced by neurotransmitters and hormones, so not all dysrhythmias are cardiac in origin. These dysrhythmias may be described as **noncardiogenic**.

Patients with dysrhythmias may be asymptomatic, and the disorder may be an incidental finding during routine exam or a workup for another complaint. Symptomatic patients report syncope, near syncope, dizziness, fatigue, and/or palpitations. Dysrhythmias become

(4) Sinus rhythm refers to the heart's rhythm when controlled by the SA node.

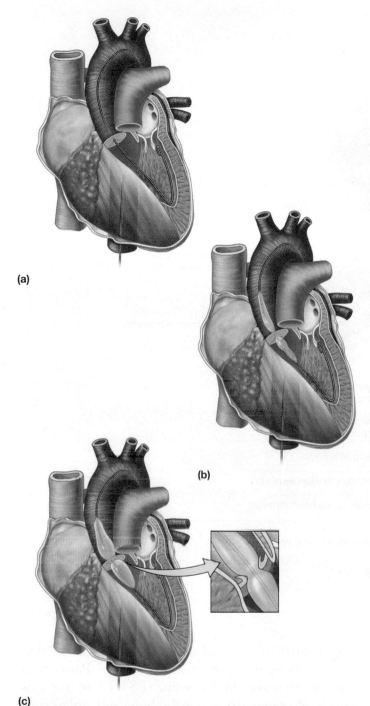

(a)

(b)

(c)

FIGURE 9-3 Percutaneous transluminal balloon valvuloplasty. The guidewire is placed (a) and the balloon is guided over the wire (b). The balloon is inflated to open the stenotic valve (c).

Dysrhythmias

The heart relies on both electrical and mechanical components to pump blood. The electrical aspect causes the muscles to contract, producing the mechanical effect of pushing blood. As an electrical impulse reaches a muscle fiber, the cell membrane becomes polarized and ion channels open to allow calcium to

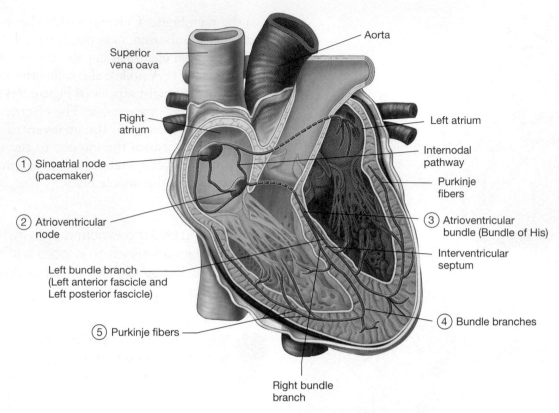

Superior vena oava

Aorta

Right atrium

Left atrium

① Sinoatrial node (pacemaker)

Internodal pathway

Purkinje fibers

② Atrioventricular node

③ Atrioventricular bundle (Bundle of His)

Interventricular septum

Left bundle branch (Left anterior fascicle and Left posterior fascicle)

④ Bundle branches

⑤ Purkinje fibers

Right bundle branch

1. The sinoatrial (SA) node fires a stimulus across the walls of both left and right atria causing them to contract.

2. The stimulus arrives at the atrioventricular (AV) node.

3. The stimulus is directed to follow the AV bundle (Bundle of His).

4. The stimulus now travels through the apex of the heart through the bundle branches.

5. The Purkinje fibers distribute the stimulus across both ventricles causing ventricular contraction.

FIGURE 9-4 Electrical conduction system of the heart.

life-threatening when cardiac output is decreased, leading to cerebral ischemia or myocardial ischemia (ie, the cardiac muscle itself does not receive sufficient oxygen to continue pumping, referred to as **cardiac arrest**).

 Pause 9-6 Why would a dysrhythmia decrease cardiac output?

Normally, the SA node is the heart's pacemaker. A dysrhythmia caused by a malfunctioning sinoatrial node is called **sick sinus syndrome**. Dysrhythmias may also be caused by focal areas of diseased tissue elsewhere in the heart that also act as a pacemaker and generate inappropriate electrical impulses called **ectopic beats**.

Supraventricular arrhythmias result from pacemakers located above the level of the ventricles. **Paroxysmal supraventricular tachycardia (PSVT)** is the most common supraventricular arrhythmia and, unless there is underlying heart disease, does not necessarily require treatment. When indicated, adenosine or calcium-channel blockers may be used to interrupt the episode and return the heart to sinus rhythm. Radiofrequency ablation of the aberrant foci may also be used to prevent future attacks.

Listen carefully so you do not mistake "ectopic" beat for "atopic" beat. The word atopic refers to an inborn allergy.

Pause 9-7 Translate the phrase "paroxysmal supraventricular tachycardia" into layman's terms.

Atrial Fibrillation

Atrial fibrillation (AF) is the most common chronic arrhythmia. Its prevalence rises with age and affects nearly 10% of patients over the age of 80. AF may also be the presenting symptom in thyrotoxicosis (hyperthyroidism) or may be a side effect of alcohol intoxication or other drugs. AF is characterized by rapid ventricular rate and an **irregularly irregular** rhythm. Although chronic AF in and of itself is rarely life-threatening, the increased rate causes a very inefficient pumping action. AF also places the patient at risk for clot formation and subsequent embolization. For this reason, patients with AF are chronically anticoagulated with Coumadin **to a therapeutic INR of 2–3** (see also pages 273 and 430 for additional information on Coumadin and the INR value). Often, AF can be controlled pharmacologically with antiarrhythmic drugs such as sotalol (Betapace) and amiodarone (Pacerone). Patients may also be returned to sinus rhythm using **direct current cardioversion (DC cardioversion)**.

Dictators often refer to atrial fibrillation as "a fib," but you should transcribe the full phrase.

In patients with AF, the heart rate is described as irregularly irregular. It sounds odd to describe a rate as *irregularly irregular*, and it is difficult to distinguish the prefixes when the physician is speaking quickly. A diagnosis of AF will confirm the description of the rate.

The patient is chronically anticoagulated but has a subtherapeutic INR today of 1.5; therefore, we will increase her Coumadin to 5 days a week, up from 3 days a week.

Ventricular Fibrillation

The most lethal arrhythmia is **ventricular fibrillation (VF)**, a common cause of **sudden cardiac death**, which is defined as an unexpected, nontraumatic death in clinically well or stable patients who die within one hour of the onset of symptoms. There is no single cause of VF, but a common cause is myocardial ischemia or infarction. The poorly synchronized and inadequate contractions that result from VF decrease the pumping action of the heart. Cerebral and myocardial ischemias occur or worsen due to the decreased cardiac output. Patients at known risk for episodes of VF or patients who are revived from an episode of sudden cardiac death may elect to have an **automatic implantable cardioverter-defibrillator (AICD)**.

Pause 9-8 Explain why ventricular arrhythmias are so lethal.

Ventricular Tachycardia

Ventricular tachycardia (VT) refers to a heart rate greater than 100 bpm that arises from the ventricle. Ventricular fibrillation is a more disorganized rhythm than VT but the two may be difficult to distinguish. Both VT and VF are major causes of sudden death in patients with cardiovascular disease.

Conduction Disturbances

Arrhythmias may result from a failure to pass the electrical current throughout the heart in the normal pathway at the normal rate. Bradycardia can be caused by conduction disturbances resulting from structural damage to muscle (eg, necrosis or scarring caused by infarction) or by blocks, which are interruptions in the conduction pathways. **Atrioventricular blocks (AV blocks)** are classified as 1st-, 2nd-, or 3rd-degree blocks, and 2nd-degree blocks are subclassified as **Mobitz type I, II or III**. Blocks may also occur in the **bundle of His** (pronounced *hiss*, not *hiz*). The intraventricular conduction system is made of two bundles, designated right and left. A block in the right bundle is referred to as a **right bundle branch block (RBBB)**. The left bundle bifurcates into posterior and anterior **fascicles**, and blocks in these bundles are referred to as **fascicular blocks**. When indicated, conduction defects are treated with permanent pacemaker implantation.

The conduction system is called the *intra*-ventricular conduction system (not *inter*).

 Listen carefully for the sound-alike words fascicular, fasciolar, and follicular.

Some dysrhythmias result when the heart forms accessory, or alternate, pathways for conducting the electrical impulse, as in **Wolff-Parkinson-White syndrome (WPW)**. Asymptomatic patients with WPW do not require treatment. Patients experiencing palpitations, lightheadedness, or syncope may be treated with radiofrequency ablation.

Evaluation and Management of Dysrhythmias

Dysrhythmias are suspected based on a patient's complaints and information gathered on physical exam. Symptoms may include palpitations, syncope, presyncope, dizziness, and fatigue. Patients with dysthymias often have decreased blood pressure, and the force of contractions may be erratic. A **pulse deficit**, which is a difference in the apical and radial pulse rates, may be detected. The radial pulse is taken at the wrist and the apical pulse is measured at the 4th or 5th intercostal space just to the side of the midclavicular line.

Some dysrhythmias can be definitively diagnosed on electrocardiogram, but the challenge arises when the dysrhythmia is sporadic. By their very nature, dysrhythmias are unpredictable and intermittent. To capture an electrical tracing during an actual event, which is required to diagnose a dysrhythmia, an **ambulatory EKG** such as a **Holter monitor** or an **event recorder** is used. Holter monitors record the heart's activity continuously for 24 hours while the patient goes about their activities of daily living. An event recorder, on the other hand, does not monitor continuously. The small device is carried in the patient's purse or pocket or may be attached to the waistband. The patient activates the recording only when they are experiencing symptoms. The recordings are transmitted by phone to a cardiologist for interpretation. **Electrophysiology studies (EP studies)** may be required to diagnose dysrhythmias that are more complex. **Table 9-1** lists rhythm disorders.

Treatment of arrhythmias may simply require lifestyle changes such as decreased alcohol or caffeine intake,

Table 9-1 Cardiac Rhythms

Rhythm	Abbreviation
normal sinus rhythm	NSR
sinus bradycardia	
sinus tachycardia	
sinus arrhythmia	
sinus arrest	
premature atrial contraction	PAC
atrial flutter	
atrial fibrillation	AF (often dictated "a fib")
supraventricular tachycardia	SVT
paroxysmal atrial tachycardia	PAT
Wolff-Parkinson-White syndrome	WPW
wandering atrial pacemaker	
sick sinus syndrome	
junctional escape rhythm	
premature junctional contraction	PJC
junctional tachycardia	
1st-degree AV block	
Mobitz I/Wenckebach	
Mobitz II/1st-degree block	
3rd-degree (complete) heart block	
right bundle branch block	RBBB
premature ventricular contraction	PVC
ventricular tachycardia	VT
torsade de pointes (*tōr-săd də pwant'*) which means a twisting of the points	
ventricular fibrillation	VF (often dictated "v fib")

Table 9-2 Pacemaker Designations

Lead Placement	Chamber Paced	Chamber Sensed	Response to Sensing	Rate Modulation	Multisite Pacing
A	A	T	R	A
V	V	I		V
D	D	D		D
S	S			

Lead placement: A=atrium, V=ventricle, D=dual, S=single
T=triggered, I=inhibited
R=rate modulated

smoking cessation, or treatment for drug abuse when indicated. When lifestyle changes are not sufficient or appropriate, treatments include medications such as digitalis, calcium channel blockers, quinidine, and lidocaine to control or slow down the heart rate. AF is treated medically with rate-controlling medications such as sotalol as well as anticoagulants to prevent clots and embolization. VF and VT are acute, life-threatening events that must be reversed using electrical **defibrillation**.

Conditions that cannot be managed medically may be treated surgically using an implantable pacemaker or an AICD. These devices are described according to their functionality and programming. **Table 9-2** lists the terminology and abbreviations used to describe pacemakers. The chamber refers to the chamber (atrium or ventricle) in which the lead(s) (electrical sensor) is placed. These single-letter designations are combined into abbreviations such as DDIR (dual paced, dual sensed, inhibited response, rate modulated), DDDR, and VVI. Only the relevant or applicable letter is dictated, so the abbreviation may be three, four, or five characters long.

Once a pacemaker is implanted, patients must routinely undergo **pacemaker interrogation**. This procedure, often performed by a representative (often dictated "rep") of the pacemaker's manufacturer, tests the pacemaker for proper function and battery life.

 Terms you may hear dictated in reference to a pacemaker interrogation include:

battery life
impedance (measured in ohms)
sensed or sensing (v-sensed or ventricular sensed)
paced or pacing (A-paced, atrial-paced)
mode
mode switches

Physicians often will dictate the type of pacemaker by brand name and model as well as a description of its programming using coded nomenclature, which unfortunately produces abbreviations using the letters D and V that are impossible to distinguish.

Be sure to flag any dictated abbreviation that you cannot distinguish with absolute certainty. Do not guess or assume.

She has a biventricular Medtronic pacemaker InSync III. Battery voltage is 3.039 V and estimated longevity is 7½ years. Her P wave measured 2.80 mV. R wave to the RV lead was 5.6 mV and R wave to the LV lead was 11.2 mV. Atrial-lead impedance was 498 ohms. RV-lead impedance was 505 ohms and LV-lead impedance was 513 ohms. Atrial threshold was 0.5 V at 0.4 msec. RV threshold was 0.5 V at 0.4 msec and the LV was 1 V at 1 msec. No reprogramming changes were made.

EKG shows A sensing with V pacing with appropriate capture.

Table 9-3 AICD Designation Codes

Location of Lead	Shock Chamber	Antitachycardia Pacing Chamber	Tachycardia Detection	Antibradycardia Pacing Chamber
O	O		E	O
A	A		H	A
V	V			V
D	D			D

Lead location: O (the letter O) = none, A=atrium, V=ventricle, D=dual (atrium and ventricle)
E=electrical, H=hemodynamic

An AICD is used in patients that have survived an episode of sudden cardiac death or those at risk of experiencing VF or VT. The nomenclature for AICDs is similar to that used in pacemakers (**Table 9-3**). AICDs may be set to detect an event based on a drop in blood pressure (hemodynamic detection) or a change in the electrical activity of the heart. An example of an AICD description would be VVED (ventricular shock, ventricular pacing, electrical detection, dual chamber detection of bradycardia). Like pacemakers, AICDs are also interrogated routinely.

> **AICD INTERROGATION DATA:** The patient has a St. Jude Medical Current VR RF 1207-36. Battery voltage is 3.2 volts. R wave measured 12 mV. Threshold in the ventricle is 0.25 V at 0.4 msec and the impedance is 490 ohms. High-voltage lead impedance is 40 ohms. Estimated longevity is 8 years. There have been no episodes of VT or VF. He is 100% sensed in the ventricles.
>
> The patient has not had any VT or VF. No reprogramming changes made. He is paced in the atrium 94% of the time and in the ventricles less than 0.1% of the time.

Pause 9-9 What is the difference between a permanent pacemaker and an implantable cardioverter-defibrillator? Can you see a purpose for a combination device?

Arrhythmias resulting from faulty impulse formation (aberrant pacemakers) or conduction errors may be treated with **radiofrequency catheter ablation (RFCA)**, which destroys the focal point of tissue producing the

- The SA node is the heart's normal pacemaker.
- Dysrhythmias may be caused by rogue pacemakers, typically caused by damaged heart tissue outside the SA node.
- Bradycardia may be caused by conduction delays, such as damaged tissue that does not transmit the electrical signal quickly or efficiently.
- Dysthymias may be caused by blocks in the normal conduction pathways.

- An EKG tracing is required to accurately diagnose a dysrhythmia. EP studies may be performed to diagnose arrhythmias that are more complex.
- Implantable pacemakers and AICDs are used to treat arrhythmia when medical management has failed. Aberrant pacemaker nodes may be ablated using cardiac catheterization and radiofrequency techniques.

arrhythmia. A catheter is threaded from the groin or the neck into the heart, and focal points of tissue are ablated (destroyed) using radio waves that superheat the tissue, producing a very controlled area of necrosis. Success rates are high in patients with more common forms of SVT and idiopathic VT. RFCA may also be used for WPW, atrial tachycardia, and atrial flutter. Patients with AF refractory to rate-controlling medications may also be treated with radiofrequency ablation.

Congestive Heart Failure

Congestive heart failure (CHF) is characterized by the heart's inability to pump sufficient blood to meet the body's needs, leading to fluid overload (congestion). Incidence of CHF continues to rise in the US, with age being the most significant risk factor. As many as 75% of cases occur in individuals over age 65. There are many causes of CHF, but the underlying factor is the heart's inability to maintain adequate circulation. This may be due to a weak heart's inability to adequately pump blood, a normal heart muscle's inability to cope with a valvular disorder, or the increased workload necessary to overcome systemic or pulmonary hypertension. The heart muscle may become weak from age, chronic hypertension, infection, or decreased functioning muscle tissue due to ischemia or infarction. A normal heart may progress to heart failure if it must constantly pump blood into blood vessels with a lot of resistance (hypertension) or narrowing due to atherosclerosis.

 Pause 9-10 Explain how chronic, severe ischemia can eventually lead to CHF.

Edema is one of the cardinal symptoms of heart failure. Edema in the abdomen (ascites), hepatic congestion, and dependent edema are caused by the right heart's inability to keep pace with the volume of blood returning from the venous system. The increased pressure due to congestion in the venous system forces fluids across the vascular membrane into the interstitial spaces, resulting in edema. Likewise, left heart failure causes congestion in the lungs due to the heart's inability to keep pace with the volume of blood returning from the lungs, resulting in pleural effusion.

Symptoms of CHF include dyspnea on exertion, progressing to dyspnea even at rest, cough, orthopnea, and fatigue. Clinical findings include edema (manifest as ascites, dependent edema, **pitting edema**, and jugular venous pulsations), rales, gallop rhythm, pleural effusion, and cardiac enlargement. Patients with hepatic congestion may display a **hepatojugular reflux** (elicited by placing moderate pressure on the liver and noting increased pressure in the jugular vein). Patients with long-standing disease may appear cachectic or cyanotic.

 Note the phrase is hepatojugular reflux (not reflex).

The degree of heart failure is rated using the **New York Heart Association (NYHA)** functional classification system:

class I: no symptoms and no limitation of ordinary physical activity (eg, no shortness of breath when walking or climbing stairs)

class II: mild symptoms such as shortness of breath or angina with slight limitation during ordinary activity

class III: comfortable only at rest; marked limitation in activity due to symptoms, even during activities such as walking short distances

class IV: severe limitations, mostly bedbound; symptoms even while at rest

Laboratory findings may include electrolyte imbalances (hyponatremia, hyperkalemia, or hypokalemia), renal insufficiency, and azotemia. **Brain natriuretic peptide (BNP)** is released into the peripheral blood when the left ventricular filling pressure is high; this test is used as a marker for CHF.

The abbreviation BNP cannot be distinguished from BMP when dictated. Use context to determine which abbreviation was dictated. BMP is a panel of six tests, so more than one result is typically dictated. BNP is a single value and is dictated when CHF is suspected or confirmed.

Treatment of CHF involves correction of the underlying cause, including valvular lesions, myocardial ischemia, and hypertension. When treating the underlying cause is not possible or satisfactory, treatment focuses on reducing fluid volume with the use of

- The most common symptoms of CHF are dyspnea, cough, and edema, often with sudden weight gain.

- CHF is characterized by the heart's inability to adequately pump blood and may be caused by an underlying cardiac disease or by other diseases that put too much strain on the heart.

- The severity of CHF is rated according to the patient's functional status using the NYHA classification.

- CHF is treated with diuretics to reduce the body's fluid volume and antihypertensive medications to lower blood pressure.

diuretics such as hydrochlorothiazide (HCTZ) or furosemide (Lasix). Patients being treated for CHF need to monitor their weight carefully to detect any sudden increases in weight (eg, several pounds in one to two days) due to retained fluid. Treatment also includes ACE inhibitors and vasodilators to lower blood pressure and decrease vascular resistance.

Atherosclerotic Diseases

Atherosclerotic disease is characterized by plaques formed by the deposition of lipid in the **intima (5)** of large- and medium-sized arteries. Lipid deposition causes a local, chronic inflammatory reaction, so the plaques also contain white cells and platelets. Over time, these plaques become hardened and calcific due to fibrosis and calcium deposition that is associated with inflammatory responses. Calcium can be detected on **electron-beam computed tomography (EBCT)** and reported as a **coronary calcium score.** Dyslipidemia has an established role in the pathophysiology of atherosclerosis (see page 38). The plaques are significant for two reasons: first, they physically obstruct the flow of blood and cause the blood vessels to be less capable of dilating and constricting as needed to adjust blood pressure. Secondly, the plaques may "burst," releasing their gruel-like substance, which can embolize and occlude smaller vessels downstream and/or invoke the body's coagulation response, recruiting platelets and fibrinogen to form a clot at the site of the plaque. These clots are the most lethal, as they often completely occlude an already narrowed vessel. When these events take place in a coronary artery, a **myocardial infarction** occurs. A similar event in the cerebrovascular system produces a cerebral infarction, also called a **cerebrovascular accident (CVA).**

Coronary Artery Disease

The leading cause of death in the US is coronary heart disease (coronary artery disease, atherosclerotic heart disease). More than one in five deaths is attributable to cardiovascular disease. Risk factors for CAD include **premature family history (6),** dyslipidemia, obesity, diabetes mellitus, hypertension, physical inactivity, and cigarette smoking. Many risk factors are related to lifestyle and diet, referred to as **modifiable risk factors,** the most significant being cigarette smoking.

In order for the heart to pump continuously, the muscular walls must be **perfused** with oxygen-rich blood. Occluded arteries prevent adequate **perfusion** of the muscle cells causing weakness, fatigue, and pain. Exertion, such as climbing stairs or running, can cause an episode of **angina pectoris** (chest pain due to ischemia) in patients suffering from coronary artery disease. Chest pain may be described as tightness, squeezing, burning, pressing, choking, aching, bursting, gas, indigestion, or an ill-characterized discomfort.

Pause 9-11 Compare the definitions of perfuse and profuse.

(5) The intima is the innermost layer of the arterial vessel wall. Listen carefully so you do not confuse this term with intimate.

(6) A patient is said to have a premature family history of coronary artery disease if a cardiovascular event occurs in a primary family member before the age of 50.

Patients suffering from angina undergo tests to determine the severity of the occlusions. A treadmill stress test with electrocardiogram and echocardiography are **noninvasive tests** to determine if CAD is severe enough to warrant surgical treatment versus medical therapy. After walking on a treadmill, the heart is examined with ultrasound (echocardiogram) to look for changes in wall motion. Areas of the heart receiving inadequate oxygen will show less movement (**hypokinesis**) or no wall motion (**akinesis**), often dictated as **regional wall motion abnormalities**. Patients may also undergo a **nuclear stress test** using radionuclides such as **technetium 99c sestamibi** or **thallium 201**.

> **Pause 9-12** Explain the term regional wall motion abnormality. Why do you think the abnormalities are "regional"?

> A nuclear stress test showed normal myocardial perfusion with no evidence of myocardial ischemia or prior infarct. Her left ventricular ejection fraction was normal at 70%.

A positive stress echocardiogram is typically followed by **cardiac catheterization** and **angiography**, which allows the physician to directly observe the individual coronary arteries and determine the exact amount of occlusion. The coronary arteries are shown in ■ **Figure 9-5**, and **Table 9-4** lists the coronary arteries and their abbreviations. Ischemia typically occurs when an artery is about 70% occluded. Angiographic procedures use catheters that are inserted into the femoral artery, threaded up to the aorta and into

the coronary arteries. If occlusion is seen on angiography, **percutaneous coronary intervention (PCI)** may be performed at the same time (7). **Balloon angioplasty**, a form of PCI, uses a balloon tip on the end of a catheter to "squish" the plaques against the arterial walls, increasing the diameter of the arterial lumen. To maintain the opening, a stent may be placed in the artery at that same time. Many patients receive **drug-eluting stents**, which slowly release drugs such as sirolimus or paclitaxel at the site of the stent. It is not unusual for the stent to eventually become occluded, referred to as **in-stent restenosis**.

> Be careful that you do not transcribe "instant restenosis." The correct phrase is "in-stent restenosis."

> The correct term is drug-eluting stent. These stents have medication *ad*sorbed to the surface of the stent. Elute means to move from an adsorbent into solution.

> **(7)** Another term used for balloon angioplasty is PTCA, percutaneous transluminal coronary angioplasty.

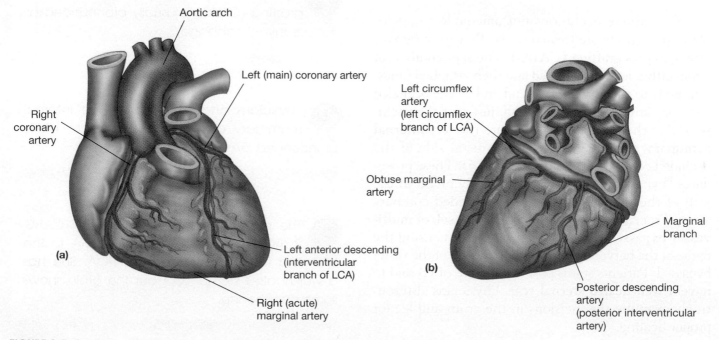

FIGURE 9-5 Coronary arteries from (a) anterior view and (b) posterior view of the heart.

Table 9-4 The Coronary Arteries

Artery	Abbreviation/ Acronym
left (main) coronary artery	LCA
left circumflex artery (left circumflex branch of LCA)	LCX
obtuse marginal arteries (obtuse marginal branches of LCX)	OM1, OM2
left anterior descending (interventricular branch of LCA)	LAD
diagonal branch (of the LAD)	
right coronary artery	RCA
right (acute) marginal artery	RMA
posterior descending artery (posterior interventricular artery)	PDA

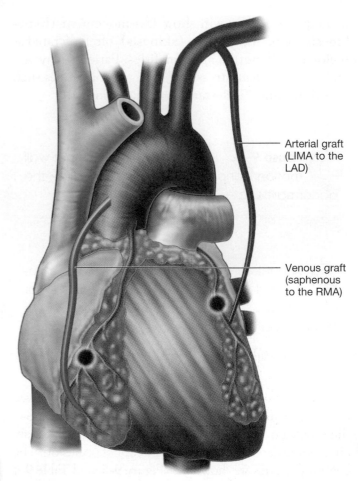

FIGURE 9-6 Coronary bypasses using the LIMA and the saphenous vein.

Arterial graft (LIMA to the LAD)

Venous graft (saphenous to the RMA)

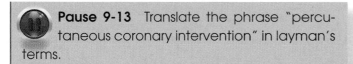

Pause 9-13 Translate the phrase "percutaneous coronary intervention" in layman's terms.

More severe occlusions not amenable to angioplasty or stenting are treated surgically with **coronary artery bypass grafting (CABG)**. The **saphenous vein** (from either leg) is **harvested** and then attached (anastomosed) to the aorta at one end and to the occluded coronary artery on the other end, just past the occlusion. Another method is to reroute the **left internal mammary artery (LIMA)** to the distal side of the occluded coronary artery (■ Figure 9-6). These procedures "bypass" the blockage and supply blood to the wall of the heart affected by the occluded coronary artery. Procedures include **2-vessel, 3-vessel,** or **multi-vessel bypasses**. Physicians describe grafts using the name of the harvested vessel and the name of the vessel bypassed. Patients status post CABG are often said to have a **well-healed sternal scar**. Physicians also routinely examine the incisions in the groin and leg for proper healing.

The abbreviation for coronary artery bypass grafting (CABG) is usually pronounced as the acronym "cabbage."

Physicians often dictate the left internal mammary artery as the acronym LIMA, pronounced *lēmə*.

The patient underwent a 2-vessel CABG 2 months ago, including the LIMA to the LAD and the saphenous to the RCA. She has a well-healed sternal scar but the groin shows some dehiscence.

Myocardial Infarction

A myocardial infarction is caused by the interruption of blood flow to the heart muscle. Symptoms include sudden chest pain, often radiating to the left arm or left side of the neck and the jaw, shortness of breath, nausea, vomiting, palpitations, diaphoresis, and a sense of impending doom. Symptoms often crescendo as opposed to occurring suddenly and all at once. A significant number of MIs are silent, in that they produce no symptoms. MI is diagnosed based on symptoms, EKG findings, and serial blood tests. An MI that causes ST-segment elevation, as seen on an EKG, is referred to as an **ST-segment elevation myocardial infarction (STEMI)**. An actual infarction causes muscle cells to die and release their contents into the bloodstream. **Troponin I** (the letter I, not the roman numeral) and **CK-MB (8)** are specific to heart muscle and can be detected in the blood after a myocardial infarction. Levels begin to appear in the blood within four to six hours and continue to rise over the ensuing 24 hours, so **serial enzymes** (a series of blood samples) are drawn in order to document the increasing levels. EKG changes and a serial rise in troponin I and CK-MB are diagnostic for acute MI. Chest pain has many causes, and patients seeking emergency care due to chest pain must be evaluated to **rule out myocardial infarction (ROMI)**.

An MI caused by a blockage in a major coronary artery causes muscle damage that penetrates the full thickness of the heart muscle (**transmural**). The MI may be further classified as anterior, posterior, or inferior. A more focal decrease in blood supply may result in a **subendocardial MI** (■ Figure 9-7). Immediate treatment involves aspirin, nitroglycerin, and oxygen. Pain may be treated with morphine. Further treatment involves fibrinolysis using fibrinolytics or percutaneous coronary intervention. Damaged tissue is less capable of conducting electrical impulses, leading to lethal arrhythmias, and sudden death may result from ventricular fibrillation.

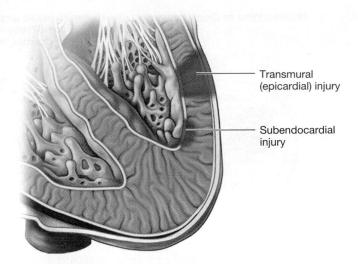

FIGURE 9-7 Transmural and subendocardial injury following myocardial infarction.

> Be careful that you do not transcribe "interior MI" instead of "inferior MI." Although it is extremely difficult to hear the difference in these two terms, it should not present a problem since there is no such entity as an "interior MI."

Patients presenting with one of the **acute coronary syndromes (ACS)**, which includes **unstable angina (9)** and **non-ST-segment elevation myocardial infarction (NSTEMI)**, are at risk of life-threatening cardiac events (■ Figure 9-8). The **Thrombolysis in Myocardial Infarction (TIMI)** study group has developed a **TIMI score** for estimating 30-day mortality associated

(8) CK is the abbreviation for creatine kinase. This enzyme has two forms, called isoenzymes. The CK-MB fraction is mostly found in cardiac tissue whereas CK-MM is found in muscle tissue throughout the body.

(9) Unstable angina is anginal pain occurring at rest and lasting more than 15 minutes. Episodes of angina tend to increase in severity over a period of weeks and often herald a true myocardial infarction. Unstable angina is thought to be due to transient platelet aggregation or coronary artery spasms.

> You may hear a physician dictate ROMI as an acronym (*rō' mē* or *ră'-mē*). Some may even say the patient was ROMI'd (romied), meaning they underwent testing to rule out a myocardial infarction. When "romied" is dictated, recast the sentence to avoid using this term.

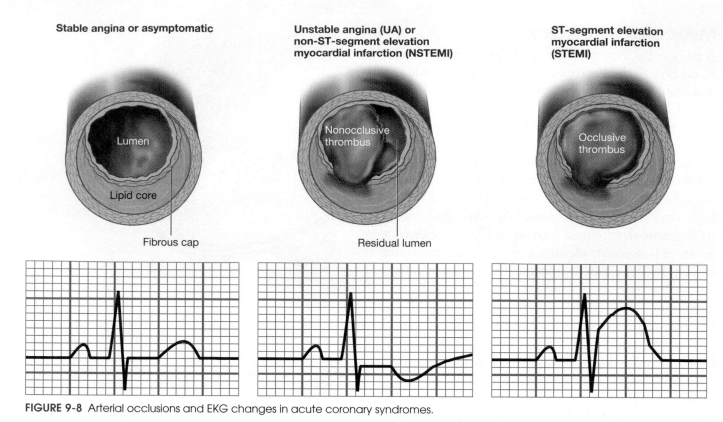

Stable angina or asymptomatic

Lumen

Lipid core

Fibrous cap

Unstable angina (UA) or non-ST-segment elevation myocardial infarction (NSTEMI)

Nonocclusive thrombus

Residual lumen

ST-segment elevation myocardial infarction (STEMI)

Occlusive thrombus

FIGURE 9-8 Arterial occlusions and EKG changes in acute coronary syndromes.

with acute coronary syndromes. The score is based on the following criteria:

- age over 65
- greater than three coronary risk factors
- prior coronary stenosis of 50% or more
- evidence of ST-segment deviation
- at least two episodes of angina in the preceding 24 hours
- use of aspirin in the preceding seven days
- elevation of cardiac enzymes

Each risk factor is assigned a value of 1 for a maximum score of 7. The higher the score, the higher the estimated risk of mortality in the next 30 days.

The abbreviation STEMI is pronounced as the acronym *stem-ē* and NSTEMI is also pronounced as the acronym *en-stem-ē*. The acronym TIMI is pronounced *tĭ-mē*. Listen carefully and use context to distinguish these three terms.

Because CAD carries significant morbidity and mortality, preventative measures are very important. Patients at risk are prescribed medications to control dyslipidemia, lower blood pressure, and reduce platelet activity (**antiplatelet therapy**) using platelet inhibitors such as clopidogrel. Lifestyle changes such as **smoking cessation**, weight loss, and routine exercise are stressed. Patients with diabetes mellitus carry a significantly higher risk of CAD, and blood sugar and insulin control are imperative to prevent cardiac complications.

 Pause 9-14 Why is antiplatelet therapy used to prevent heart attack?

Cerebrovascular Disease

The same atherosclerotic processes that occur in the coronary arteries can also occur in the cerebrovascular system. A CVA (commonly known as a stroke) is an acute ischemic event occurring in the cerebral vasculature. Strokes may be caused by blockage of blood flow or hemorrhage (eg, cerebral aneurysm). A blockage may be due to an embolus or a thrombus. Common causes of cardiogenic embolus include atrial fibrillation, myocardial infarction, valvular vegetations, and prosthetic heart valves. A common cause of noncardiogenic embolus is **carotid artery disease**.

Symptoms of cerebrovascular ischemia include sudden-onset numbness, paresthesias, weakness, or paralysis of the contralateral limbs and the face; aphasia; confusion; visual disturbances in one or both eyes (eg, transient **monocular blindness**); dizziness or loss of balance and coordination; and headache. Neurologic symptoms lasting less than one hour and not causing long-term effects are termed **transient ischemic attacks (TIA)**.

The right-sided **common carotid artery (CCA)** originates from the **innominate artery** and the left-sided common carotid artery originates directly from the aortic arch. The arteries enlarge in the midneck, forming a carotid bulb (■ **Figure 9-9**). The bulb bifurcates (10) into the **external carotid artery (ECA)** and the **internal carotid artery (ICA)**.

The carotid arteries are particularly prone to forming atherosclerotic plaques, especially in areas of turbulent flow such as the **carotid bifurcation**. **Concentric plaques** narrow the lumen, leaving a central space for the blood to flow. **Eccentric plaques** form on one or two sides of the vessel wall and cause blood to flow around them. Eccentric plaques cause **turbulence** that

is heard as a **bruit**. These plaques may cause carotid artery stenosis leading to cerebrovascular ischemia, or these plaques may produce emboli that pass directly to the intracerebral circulation.

 Do not confuse parotid and carotid. There is no such thing as "parotid arteries."

Pause 9-15 Compare the terms concentric and eccentric. Why do you think eccentric plaque causes turbulence?

Significant occlusion of the carotid arteries, often detected on physical examination as a bruit, may cause confusion, lapses in memory, or frank blackouts. Doppler studies of the carotid arteries (carotid duplex studies) are commonly performed to assess patients for

(10) Bifurcate means to split into two; in this case, two branches.

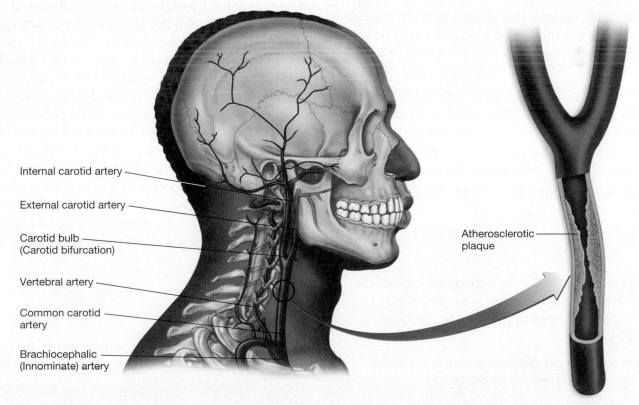

FIGURE 9-9 Anatomy of the carotid arteries (right side of neck). The right common carotid artery originates from the innominate artery. The left common carotid artery originates directly from the aortic arch.

carotid artery disease. **Magnetic resonance angiography (MRA)** may also be performed on the extracranial carotid arteries using either 2D time-of-flight (2D TOF) or optimization of multiple overlapping thin slab acquisition (MOTSA) techniques.

Carotid Doppler (**carotid duplex ultrasound**) studies estimate the degree of carotid artery stenosis based on the velocity of blood flow through the carotid arteries as well as the appearance of stenosis as seen on ultrasound. Velocities reported include the **peak systolic velocity (PSV)** and the end diastolic velocity, measured in centimeters per second (cm/s). Values may also be reported as a ratio of ICA peak velocity to CCA peak velocity (ICA PSV/CCA PSV). Normal velocity through the ICA is less than 125 cm/s. Accelerated velocity is indicative of stenosis, and the velocity is used to estimate the degree of stenosis. A peak velocity in the range of 125–230 cm/s in the ICA corresponds to 50% to 69% stenosis. Turbulence indicates a disruption in the path of the blood flow. The vertebral artery is also examined for antegrade flow.

> The right common carotid artery was well visualized with approximately 20% plaque along the common carotid course. No plaque appeared occlusive. Velocities from the ostium to the distal common carotid were commensurate with mild stenosis of 20% to 39%. The right internal carotid artery had occlusive plaque just past the ostium. There was no evidence of flow either with color flow or Doppler modality. The external carotid had plaque but had normal velocity flow.

Symptomatic patients with greater than 70% occlusion in one or more carotid arteries may undergo endovascular therapy including **carotid angioplasty and stenting (CAS)** or **carotid endarterectomy (CEA)**. Endarterectomy is the excision of atheromatous deposits and endothelium.

Peripheral Vascular Disease

Patients with coronary artery disease and carotid artery disease often have **peripheral vascular disease (PVD)** as well. PVD may also be called **peripheral artery disease (PAD)** or **peripheral artery occlusive disease (PAOD)**. Symptoms include **intermittent claudication,** (12) slowly healing wounds of the lower extremities, and decreased hair growth on the calves. Legs and feet are often cool to the touch. Pedal pulses are also reduced or absent. Peripheral vascular disease is diagnosed using Doppler studies of the lower extremity arteries as well as measuring the **ankle-brachial index (ABI)**. A suspicious Doppler exam may be confirmed with MRA. Significant lower extremity occlusion may be treated surgically with an **aortobifemoral bypass** or **femoropopliteal bypass (fem-pop bypass)** procedure (■ Figure 9-10).

> **FINDINGS**
> 1. Mild to moderate, diffuse atherosclerotic plaque noted in the right carotid system. The peak velocity in the right internal carotid artery is 121 cm/s. There is an estimated 50% to 60% **(11)** diameter stenosis involving the proximal portion of the right internal carotid artery.
> 2. The left carotid artery has similar mild to moderate, diffuse plaque throughout its course. The peak velocity in the left internal carotid artery is 167 cm/s. There is a 60% to 70% diameter stenosis involving the left internal carotid artery.
> 3. Both vertebral arteries have normal antegrade flow.

(11) Percentages written as a range should include the percent sign with each quantity in the range separated by the word "to" (a range of 20% to 39%).

(12) Intermittent claudication is pain in the calves after walking two to four city blocks.

> ABI sounds like AVI when dictated. Be sure to use context to distinguish abbreviations.

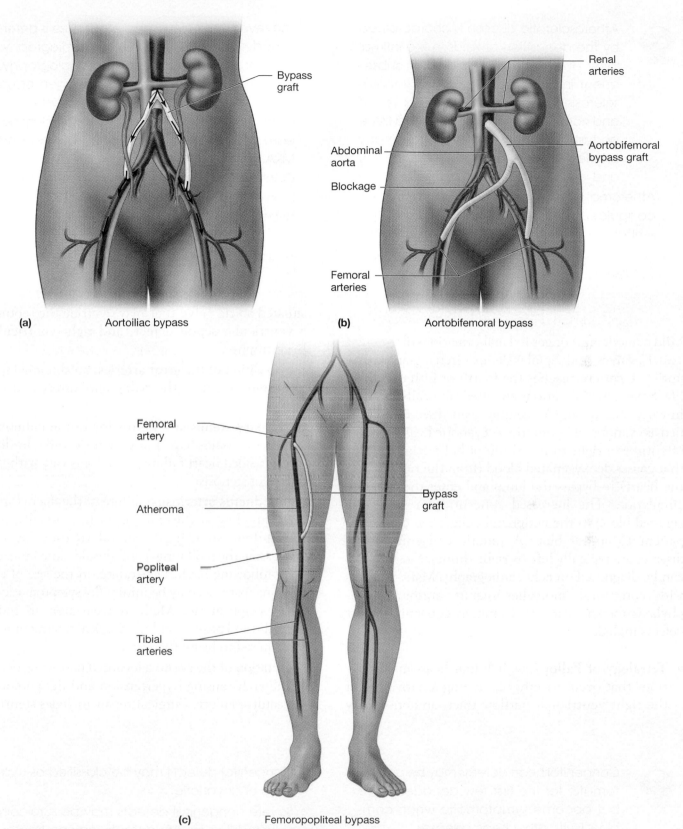

(a) Aortoiliac bypass

(b) Aortobifemoral bypass

(c) Femoropopliteal bypass

FIGURE 9-10 (a) Aortoiliac bypass, (b) aortobifemoral bypass, and (c) femoropopliteal bypass.

- Atherosclerotic disease is characterized by the deposition of lipids in the intimal layer of the arterial vessels with subsequent inflammatory reactions. Atherosclerosis causes vessels to become stiff and narrowed, resulting in reduced tissue perfusion. Atherosclerosis affects many arteries including the coronary, carotid, and lower extremity arteries.
- Atheromatous plaques may burst, inciting the coagulation cascade and producing an embolus or thrombus with subsequent MI or CVA.

- The severity of coronary artery disease is determined using EKG, stress echocardiography, nuclear perfusion studies, and angiography. Heart muscle with decreased oxygen or no oxygen shows abnormal wall movement.
- Carotid artery disease and peripheral artery disease are assessed using Doppler studies and MRA.
- Occluded arteries may be treated with balloon angioplasty, stenting, endarterectomy, or bypass surgery.

Congenital Heart Disease

Mild to moderate congenital malformations of the great vessels, valves, and septal walls are often asymptomatic until the patient reaches the fourth or fifth decade of life. Severe malformations are often surgically repaired in early childhood. Congenital heart disease is classified as cyanotic or acyanotic. A cyanotic heart defect is oftentimes a **right-to-left shunt** or bidirectional shunt that causes deoxygenated blood (from the right side of the heart) to bypass the lungs and enter the systemic circulation. The increased concentration of deoxygenated blood in the peripheral circulation causes the patient to appear blue. Acyanotic congenital heart diseases are typically **left-to-right shunts**. Most defects can be diagnosed on echocardiography. Many patients with congenital anomalies require antibiotic prophylaxis for endocarditis. Common congenital heart defects include:

- **Tetralogy of Fallot** (*fahl-ō'*): four heart malformations that occur together including a narrowing of the right ventricular outflow tract, an abnormally situated aortic valve that may override the septum, a ventricular septal defect, and right ventricular hypertrophy.

- **transposition of the great arteries:** an abnormal spatial arrangement of the pulmonary artery and the aorta.

- **pulmonary stenosis:** a narrowing of the pulmonic valve or a dome-shaped or dysplastic valve leading to right-sided heart failure. Symptoms vary with the degree of stenosis.

- **patent ductus arteriosus:** failure of the ductus arteriosus to close at the time of birth. Normally, this duct allows shunting of blood to the placenta (bypassing the fetal lungs) and should close immediately following birth. Depending on the size of the opening, patients may be minimally symptomatic or very symptomatic. Medical treatment includes NSAIDs and prostaglandins. Surgical treatment may be required to ligate the lesion.

- **coarctation of the aorta:** a localized narrowing of the aortic arch causing hypertension and the potential for cardiac failure. Surgical repair includes stenting

- Congenital heart defects may be asymptomatic for the first few decades of life but become symptomatic when combined with other heart diseases.

- Congenital defects may be classified as cyanotic or acyanotic.
- Severe congenital defects may be surgically repaired; less severe defects may be treated medically.

or resection of the narrowed area with end-to-end anastomosis.

- **ventricular septal defect:** a defect in the ventricular septum causing a left-to-right shunt, creating a murmur. Small shunts are asymptomatic but larger shunts should be surgically repaired.

- **patent foramen ovale (PFO)** and **atrial septal defect (ASD):** failure of the foramen ovale to close in utero. PFO is a type of atrial septal defect caused by a failure of the atrial septum to properly form and close, forming a path between the right and left atria. Large ASDs are typically repaired early in life. Small ASDs are typically asymptomatic until the fourth decade of life and may be associated with strokes and transient ischemic attacks, requiring chronic anticoagulation.

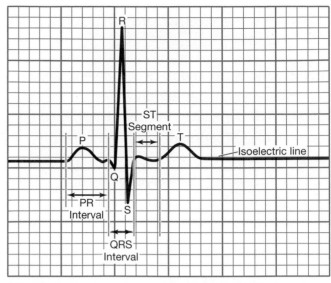

FIGURE 9-11 ST segment, PR interval, and the QRS interval (also called the QRS complex) on a normal EKG tracing.

Diagnostic Studies

Diagnostic procedures in cardiology focus on structure and electrical function. Laboratory tests are mostly performed on blood and measure levels of enzymes and lipids. Both imaging tests and laboratory tests are performed either to evaluate the patient's risk for coronary disease or to diagnose a specific coronary event.

Imaging and Electrocardiography

The two most common technologies employed in the field of cardiology include electrocardiograms (electrical impulses) and echocardiography (sound waves). Cardiology also takes advantage of nuclear imaging techniques as well as invasive procedures (angiography) using fluorescent imaging techniques.

Electrocardiogram

The **electrocardiogram (EKG or ECG)** is the most common noninvasive cardiac test. The test is performed by attaching electrical leads to specific areas of the body to detect and graph electrical activity of the heart. An EKG can be diagnostic for dysrhythmias, but otherwise provides important screening information in suspected myocardial ischemia, infarction, heart failure, and other forms of heart disease. A **12-lead EKG** uses six **precordial leads**, three **limb leads**, and three **augmented limb leads**.

The leads may also be referred to in groups based on the area of the heart being detected: anterior, inferior, and lateral. Electrical impulses, described as peaks, waves, segments, and intervals, are recorded on graph paper marked in 1 mm increments. The *waves* are designated P, T, Q, R, and S. *Intervals* are designated PR and QT (■ **Figure 9-11**). *Segments* are designated PR and ST. Changes in the height of the peaks or shapes of the waves provide important diagnostic information.

 Areas of the heart are described as in**f**erior and anterior, never *int*erior.

Pause 9-16 Using the *Book of Style*, write out the correct format for the various leads used in an EKG:

Standard bipolar leads: _____
Augmented limb leads: _____
Precordial leads: _____

Phrases heard on electrocardiogram reports include:

nonspecific ST (segment) and T-wave changes

1 mm ST-segment depression

ST-segment depression, ST-segment elevation

downsloping ST segment

inverted T wave

right-axis deviation, left-axis deviation

long-QT syndrome, short-QT syndrome

poor R-wave progression over the precordium

When dictated, the word "nonspecific" often sounds like "no specific," which can have the opposite meaning. The correct phrasing in the context of an EKG is "nonspecific ST changes."

Providers usually dictate "S T T wave changes" even though the ST is a segment (not a wave). They are actually inferring "ST-segment and T-wave changes." An acceptable way to transcribe this would be "ST and T-wave changes."

Echocardiogram

An **echocardiogram** uses sound waves (ultrasound) to visualize the heart as well as internal structures and wall movements. Echocardiographic techniques include transthoracic and transesophageal (the transducer is placed in the esophagus). The echocardiogram produces actual images of the heart, as opposed to representations of activity as in the electrocardiogram. When combined with color flow Doppler technology, an echocardiogram also allows visualization of the movement of blood through the chambers and valves in order to diagnose valvular stenosis and/or sclerosis. An echocardiogram also measures the **left ventricular ejection fraction (LVEF)**, which is the percentage of blood contained in the ventricle that passes through the valve at the end of systole. An echocardiogram is often performed immediately following a treadmill stress test (**stress echocardiogram**) in order to visualize the heart's response to increased oxygen demands. The **anterior wall** (not

interior wall) of the heart can be observed for decreased motion, indicating ischemia. Wall thickness is measured to indicate hypertrophy, and chamber sizes are also measured. Changes in valve area, measured in centimeters squared (cm^2), may indicate valvular disease.

 Common phrases used in echocardiography reports:

concentric left ventricular hypertrophy

no regional wall motion abnormalities

segmental wall motion abnormalities

negative for inducible myocardial ischemia

no valvular vegetations seen

ejection fraction

anterolateral severe hypokinesis

anterior wall akinesis

no intracardiac masses

no intramural thrombi

diastolic filling

right ventricular systolic pressure (RVSP)

global hypokinesis

valve area

Pause 9-17 An echocardiogram does not visualize the coronary arteries. How does an echocardiogram contribute to the diagnosis of coronary artery disease?

Stress Test

A **stress test** is performed to assess the patient's response to exercise. The patient walks on a treadmill for a specific amount of time, speed, and elevation. The most common treadmill protocol used is the **Bruce protocol**. An EKG is performed simultaneously to look for changes during exertion. Patients unable to walk on a treadmill due to disability or musculoskeletal pain undergo a **pharmacological stress test** which uses adenosine or dobutamine to simulate a physiologic response similar to exercise in order to stress the heart.

Nuclear Stress Test (Myocardial Perfusion Study)

A nuclear stress test, also called a **myocardial perfusion study**, is performed to assess **myocardial perfusion** and **inducible myocardial ischemia**. The patient is injected with a radionuclide (technetium 99m sestamibi or thallium 201), which acts as a tracer molecule, and then walked on a treadmill. Adenosine may be used to simulate the stress of exercise if the patient is unable to walk on a treadmill. The tracer molecule, which can be seen using a gamma camera, attaches to red blood cells. Images are taken before and after exercise and compared. Areas of the heart that are obstructed due to coronary artery disease, and therefore receiving decreased blood, show less evidence of tracer molecules. These areas are referred to as **perfusion defects**.

 Pause 9-18 What is meant by "inducible myocardial ischemia"?

Cardiac Catheterization

Cardiac catheterization is an invasive test for definitively diagnosing many disorders of the heart. Catheterization may be used to diagnose and treat coronary artery disease, dysrhythmias, and valvular disease. Catheterization allows for hemodynamic evaluation including intracardiac pressure, oxygen saturation, and cardiac output. Catheterization with coronary angiography remains the criterion standard for diagnosing coronary artery disease. Percutaneous *arterial* access is used for coronary angiography and left-heart procedures. Percutaneous *venous* access is used for right-heart catheterization. These procedures may be performed intraoperatively, but most often they are performed in the catheterization lab (**cath lab**). Physicians that perform these studies are called interventional cardiologists.

Right-Heart Catheterization

Accessing the right heart allows for the measurement of oxygen saturation, cardiac output, and pressures within the right atrium and right ventricle. The pulmonary artery pressure and the pulmonary capillary wedge pressures, which can be extrapolated to determine the left atrial pressure, can also be measured (see page 257). These measurements aid in the diagnosis of valvular disease and intracardiac shunts and are used to differentiate cardiac and pulmonary diseases. A **Swan-Ganz catheter** is used to measure right-heart pressures, oxygen saturation levels, and cardiac output.

Left-Heart Catheterization

Left-sided catheterization allows for the assessment of the mitral and aortic valves as well as left ventricular function (**ventriculography**). Coronary angiography is also performed with this approach. Interventions include **plain old balloon angioplasty (POBA)**, stenting of occluded coronary arteries, balloon valvuloplasty for pulmonic or mitral valve stenosis, stenting of coarctation of the aorta, or branch pulmonary artery stenosis. Repair of congenital defects such as ASD, PFO, and PDA may also be accomplished using left-heart catheterization. The most common approach to the left side of the heart is through the common femoral artery. A J-tipped guidewire is threaded up through the femoral artery, into the aorta, through the aortic arch, through the aortic valve, and into the left ventricle. Once the guidewire is placed, the catheter is threaded over the guidewire. Various catheter tips are placed to accomplish a variety of diagnostic and therapeutic procedures.

Coronary Angiography

Coronary angiography is used to visualize the coronary anatomy and to identify occluded coronary arteries. Access is typically obtained by threading a catheter through the common femoral artery, up to the aorta and over the aortic arch. From the aortic arch, the catheter is directed into the left main coronary artery or the right coronary artery. Commonly used catheters include the Judkins and pigtail catheters. Once the catheter is in place, radiopaque dye is injected into the arteries (■ **Figure 9-12**). **Intravascular ultrasound (IVUS)** may also be used to visualize the lumen of the arteries.

Blood flow across a stenotic region can be measured using guidewires with sensors. The amount of blood passing through the stenotic region is expressed as a **fraction flow reserve (FFR)**, which is the ratio of maximal flow through the stenotic area compared to normal maximal flow. An FFR of less than 0.75 is considered abnormal. If clinically significant occlusions are identified, angioplasty and/or stenting are performed to open the occlusion (■ **Figure 9-13**).

Stents may be bare metal or coated with a polymer that elutes a drug that reduces neointimal hyperplasia and reduces in-stent restenosis. Drug-eluting stents include the sirolimus-eluting stent (**Cypher**), the

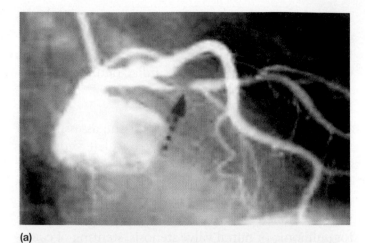

(a)

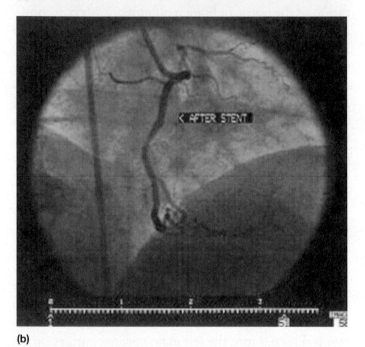

(b)

FIGURE 9-12 Coronary artery with contrast media (a) before stent placement and (b) after stent placement. *Source:* Courtesy of Dr. Walt Marquardt, Mercy Hospital.

paclitaxel-eluting stent (**Taxus**), (**13**) and the newer generation zotarolimus-eluting stent (**Endeavor**), and everolimus-eluting stent (**Xience V**). Angioplasty and stenting cause damage to the intimal wall of the arteries and are prone to reocclusion by platelet plugs that form in response to arterial-wall injury. During the procedure, patients are given glycoprotein IIb/IIIa receptor

(13) The manufacturers of TAXUS and CYPHER have trademarked the stent names using all uppercase. It is acceptable to transcribe trademarked names that use idiosyncratic capitalization with standard capitalization.

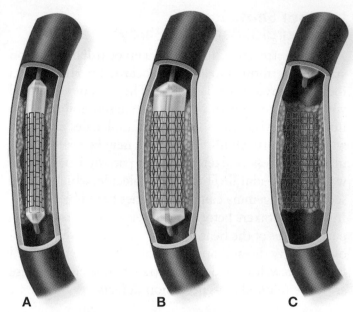

A   B   C

FIGURE 9-13 Stent placement. (a) The stent is fitted over a balloon-tipped catheter and moved into position at the site of the blockage; (b) the balloon is inflated and then (c) deflated, leaving the stent in place.

inhibitors (eg, abciximab, trade name ReoPro) that prevent platelet aggregation and thrombus formation. Following percutaneous intervention, patients are given antiplatelet therapy (clopidogrel, trade name Plavix) for several months, or in some cases indefinitely to prevent restenosis of the stented artery.

PTCA is commonly used to treat an acute ST-segment elevation myocardial infarction. Patients suffering a heart attack are often rushed to the cath lab for immediate treatment of the occluded arteries to restore blood flow to the ischemic muscle tissue. The **door-to-balloon time** refers to the amount of time that transpires from the time the patient is received at the ER to the time the guidewire approaches the occlusion. The Joint Commission considers 90 minutes or less to be a core quality measure in the care of acute coronary events.

The **TIMI grade flow** is a widely used scale to report coronary blood flow assessed during PTCA.

- TIMI 0 flow (no perfusion) refers to the absence of any antegrade flow beyond a coronary occlusion
- TIMI 1 flow (penetration without perfusion) is faint antegrade coronary flow beyond the occlusion, with incomplete filling of the distal coronary bed
- TIMI 2 flow (partial reperfusion) is delayed or sluggish antegrade flow with complete filling of the distal territory
- TIMI 3 flow (complete perfusion) is normal flow that fills the distal coronary bed completely

Electrophysiology Studies

Electrophysiology studies are invasive tests that use catheters to access the heart and perform diagnostic and therapeutic procedures for arrhythmias. The right atrium or right ventricle is approached through an incision in the central venous system, typically in the internal jugular vein, subclavian vein, or common femoral vein. Many arrhythmias can be treated by catheterizing the right atrium because the SA node is located in the right atrium, as are most of the common re-entrant pathways associated with atrial flutter. Catheter tips placed in the right ventricle allow the measurement of conduction through the bundle of His and aids in the diagnosis of bundle blocks. Ectopic nodes causing arrhythmias, especially supraventricular arrhythmias, are treated with radiofrequency ablation.

Laboratory Studies

Serum blood tests used in the area of cardiology assess risk for CAD or diagnose a current event. See page 43 for an explanation of lipid profiles and triglycerides.

High-Sensitivity C-Reactive Protein

Inflammation is known to play a role in the development of atherosclerosis. The high-sensitivity C-reactive protein (hsCRP, also called a super-sensitive CRP [ssCRP]) assay (**Table 9-5**) is a serum blood test used as a marker of low-grade vascular inflammation. It is used to assess a patient's risk for developing atherosclerosis. This test is a more sensitive indicator of vascular inflammation than the traditional C-reactive protein (CRP) test.

Table 9-5 High-Sensitivity CRP

hsCRP Value (mg/dL)	Interpretation of Cardiovascular Risk
<0.06	low
0.06 to 0.09	mild
0.10 to 0.16	moderate
0.17 to 0.32	high
>0.32	highest

Brain Natriuretic Peptide

The brain natriuretic peptide (BNP) blood test is used to assess damage to the left ventricle (**Table 9-6**). Values vary slightly by age and gender. A cutoff point of

100 pg/mL may be used as the highest value of the reference range for the majority of patients. Moderate to severe CHF may produce BNP values greater than 400 pg/mL. Values may also be elevated between 100 and 400 pg/mL in right-heart failure with cor pulmonale, pulmonary hypertension, and acute pulmonary embolism.

Table 9-6 Brain Natriuretic Peptide

BNP Value (pg/mL)	Reference Range
0–100	normal
100–199	compensated CHF
200–400	moderate CHF
>400	moderate to severe CHF

Troponin I

Troponin I (**Table 9-7**) is a protein found in cardiac muscle tissue that appears in the blood after myocardial damage. Serial elevations are indicative of myocardial infarction.

Table 9-7 Troponin I

Troponin I Value (ng/mL)	Interpretation
0.00 to 0.07	normal
0.08 to 0.50	increased risk of cardiac muscle damage
>0.50	myocardial infarction

Creatine Kinase

Creatine kinase MB fraction (CK-MB), an enzyme found predominantly in cardiac tissue, appears in the blood following myocardial damage. Serial elevations are indicative of myocardial infarction. Creatine kinase (**Table 9-8**) should not be confused with creatinine. See also Table 5–9.

Table 9-8 Creatine Kinase-MB Fraction

Test Name	Reference Range
creatine kinase (CK-MB)	0–5 ng/mL

Pharmacology

Cardiac patients are usually treated medically with a battery of pharmaceuticals before attempting surgery or other invasive procedures. Many medications used in the treatment of cardiac disease sound similar, so it is important to pay special attention to the dose to make sure you are transcribing the correct medication. Always correlate medications with their available doses as a form of "checks and balances" to ensure accuracy in your transcription. The following sections include the most commonly used classes of medications in the practice of cardiology.

Refer to page 47 for a list of statin drugs for controlling cholesterol, page 47 for nutritional derivatives for hyperlipidemia, pages 49 and 224 for a list of diuretics, and page 48 for a list of antihypertensive medications.

Nitrates

Nitrates (**Table 9-9**) act as a vasodilator. Vasodilation decreases vascular resistance and lowers blood pressure. Nitrates should not be confused with nitrites, which are found in the urine of patients with bacterial cystitis. Nitrates are delivered as nitroglycerin, administered as a tablet, transdermal patch, transdermal ointment, translingual solution, or sublingual tablet. Ointments are applied to the skin using a guide that is marked off in inches for measuring the dose.

 Note: The spelling of nitroglycerin does not end with an /e/.

Calcium Channel Blockers

Calcium channel blockers (**Table 9-10**) prevent the transfer of calcium across the muscle membrane thereby decreasing the strength of muscle contractions. It also acts on the blood vessels to relax the vessel walls and decrease vascular resistance. Several generic forms of calcium channel blockers have the ending *–ipine*.

Table 9-9 Nitroglycerin

Generic	Brand Name	Dose
sublingual nitroglycerin	NitroQuick	0.3 mg, 0.4 mg, 0.6 mg
nitroglycerin ointment	Nitro-Bid	2% (prescribed in inches)
transdermal nitroglycerin	Nitro-Dur	0.1 to 0.8 mg per hour
isosorbide dinitrate	Isordil	5 mg, 40 mg
isosorbide mononitrate	Imdur	30 mg, 60 mg, 120 mg

Table 9-10 Calcium Channel Blockers

Generic	Brand Name	Dose
amlodipine	Norvasc	2.5 mg, 5 mg, 10 mg
nifedipine	Procardia Procardia XL	10 mg 30 mg, 60 mg, 90 mg
verapamil	Calan Calan SR	40 mg, 80 mg, 120 mg 120 mg, 180 mg, 240 mg
	Verelan	120 mg, 180 mg, 240 mg, 360 mg
diltiazem	Cardizem Cardizem LA	30 mg, 60 mg, 90 mg, 120 mg 120 mg, 180 mg, 240 mg, 300 mg, 360 mg, 420 mg

Antiplatelet Drugs

Antiplatelet drugs (**Table 9-11**) reduce platelet activity and reduce the likelihood of a clot forming at the site of atheromatous plaque. Aspirin is often prescribed in small daily doses of 81 mg (baby aspirin) for this purpose. **Enteric-coated aspirin** is typically recommended because this form of aspirin is less likely to cause stomach upset. Clopidogrel (Plavix) is also prescribed, especially following infarction and/or stent placement. ReoPro is used intraoperatively during PTCA to prevent clots.

Rate-Controlling Medications

Antiarrhythmic drugs (**Table 9-12**) act by altering the membrane ion conductance. Class I agents interfere with sodium channels, and class II agents, which act on the sympathetic nervous system, mostly consist of beta-blockers. Class III agents affect potassium movement across the membrane, and class IV agents act on calcium channels. Class V is a catch-all grouping of agents that are known to help control heart rates but the mechanisms are not known. Beta-blockers with the suffix -olol are listed on page 48.

Table 9-11 Antiplatelet Drugs

Generic	Brand Name	Dose
clopidogrel	Plavix	75 mg
aspirin		81 mg
abciximab	ReoPro	

(14) Digoxin is often dictated in the slang form as "dig" (*dij*), but the term should always be spelled out. Therapeutic levels may be monitored, and many physicians dictate a "dig level" or a "dig trough" to measure the patient's serum levels of the medication.

Table 9-12 Rate-Controlling Medications

Generic	Brand Name	Dose
amiodarone (class III)	Pacerone	100 mg, 200 mg, 400 mg
sotalol (class III)	Betapace	80 mg, 120 mg, 160 mg, 240 mg
dofetilide	Tikosyn	125 mcg, 250 mcg, 500 mcg
disopyramide	Norpace	100 mg, 150 mg
lidocaine (class I)		IV bolus
flecainide (class I)	Tambocor	50 mg, 100 mg, 150 mg
propafenone (class I)	Rythmol Rythmol SR	150 mg, 225 mg, 300 mg 225 mg, 325 mg, 425 mg
digoxin (14)	Lanoxin	125 mcg, 250 mcg

Exercises

Using Context to Make Decisions

Use the sample report 9A on page 477 of Appendix B to answer the following questions:

1. List five of the patient's cardiovascular risk factors.
   _____

2. Why is the patient on Coumadin therapy? _____
   _____

3. Match each of this patient's medications to one of the items listed under the Past Medical History.
   a. Triamterene/HCTZ 75/50 mg daily_____
   b. Mobic 7.5 mg b.i.d._____
   c. atenolol 50 mg daily_____
   d. Synthroid 0.088 mg daily_____
   e. TriCor 145 mg daily_____
   f. Januvia 100 mg daily_____
   g. Coumadin daily_____
   h. hydrocodone p.r.n._____
   i. aspirin 81 mg daily_____

4. Why was an adenosine nuclear stress test ordered instead of a nuclear stress test using a treadmill?
   _____

5. What evidence is there that this patient has a premature family history of heart disease? _____
   _____

Use the following excerpt to answer questions 6 and 7.

   Physical exam reveals a 2/6 holosystolic _____ heard best in the 3rd and 4th intercostal space, radiating to the axilla.

6. Which of the following would complete the sentence?
   a. bruit   c. murmur
   b. pleural effusion   d. rub

7. Where is the 3rd and 4th intercostal space?
   a. between the ribs
   b. between the shoulder blades
   c. in the sternum
   d. in the thoracic spine

Use the sample report on page 308 to answer questions 8–14.

8. Which list item (not a numbered blank) under the Assessment and Plan contains a transcription error? (hint: not a punctuation error)
   a. Assessment and Plan #3
   b. Assessment and Plan #1
   c. Assessment and Plan #7
   d. No errors

9. What word should be transcribed in blank #1? ____
   _____

10. Which of the following terms would be appropriate for blank #2?
    a. epistaxis   c. edema
    b. headaches   d. hip pain

11. What word should be transcribed in blank #3?
    _____

12. What word should be transcribed in blank #4?
    _____

13. What word should be transcribed in blank #5?
    _____

14. What word should be transcribed in blank #6?
    _____

15. Look up the word commissurotomy and describe how this term is applied to the repair of heart valves.
    _____

Terms Checkup

Complete the multiple choice questions for Chapter 9 located at www.myhealthprofessionskit.com. To access the questions, select the discipline "Medical Transcription," then click on the title of this book, *Advanced Medical Transcription*.

Look It Up

Using the guidelines described on page xvii, complete a research project on myocarditis and endocarditis.

Transcription Practice

1. Transcribe the key terms and phrases for Chapter 9.

2. Complete the proofing and transcription practice exercises for Chapter 9.

HISTORY OF PRESENT ILLNESS: The patient came to the office for a followup visit today. She has a known history of dyslipidemia and coronary artery disease and had an acute anterior myocardial infarction last December. She underwent percutaneous intervention of the LAD and the large diagonal branch. The left circumflex artery had borderline stenosis and that was left alone. Her RCA was nondominant. The patient denies any recent symptoms of angina. No shortness of ____(1)____ on mild exertion, orthopnea, or paroxysmal nocturnal dyspnea. She was diagnosed recently with type 2 diabetes mellitus and was started on metformin. Since then she has followed a more restricted diet and has lost weight. She has had recurrent ____(2)____ recently; therefore, her aspirin was discontinued. Her blood pressure has been suboptimally controlled, and her Diovan was changed to Benicar HCT. Her blood pressure remains elevated however.

ASSESSMENT AND PLAN

1. No history of coronary artery disease status post ____(3)____ intervention of the LAD and the diagonal branch following an ____(4)____ myocardial infarction 10 months ago.
2. Previous history of ischemic cardiomyopathy with normalization of her left ventricular ____(5)____ fraction.
3. Dry cough with ACE inhibitor.
4. Hypertension. This has remained poorly controlled on her current regimen. I asked her to increase Coreg to 12.5 mg b.i.d.
5. ____(6)____, on Lipitor and Zetia.
6. Because of her complaint of nosebleed, her aspirin has been discontinued. However, she is to continue Plavix indefinitely.
7. Recent diagnosis of type 2 diabetes mellitus with subsequent weight loss.

PEARSON
myhealthprofessionskit™

To access the transcription practice exercises for this chapter, go to www.myhealthprofessionskit.com. Select the discipline "Medical Transcription," then click on the title of this book, *Advanced Medical Transcription*.

Immunology

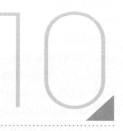

Preview Terms
Before studying this chapter, make sure you understand the following terms. Definitions can be found in the glossary.

allergy
antibody
antigen
autoimmune
differentiation
immune complex
mediators (cell mediators)

Learning Objectives

After completing this chapter, you should be able to comprehend and correctly transcribe terminology related to:

▶ immune hypersensitivity disorders

▶ autoimmune diseases

▶ inborn and acquired immunodeficiency

▶ organ transplantation and organ rejection

▶ laboratory and imaging tests used to diagnose and monitor diseases of the immune system

▶ drugs used in the treatment of immune disorders and organ transplantation

Introduction

The immune system is a complex network of cells, organs, and lymphatic vessels that protects the body from infection and malignancy. The field of immunology is expanding rapidly, and the increased understanding of the immune system has led to treatments for many seemingly unrelated disorders and diseases including hemolytic disease of the newborn, immune deficiency, and many forms of cancer. The development of monoclonal antibodies as a therapeutic modality has changed the course and severity of many such diseases. Going forward, it will be important for MTs to have a solid understanding of the immune system, including the major histocompatibility complex, as well as the use of monoclonal antibodies, immune stimulants, and immune suppressants for the prevention and treatment of disease.

Physiology of the Immune System

The immune system includes the bone marrow, spleen, thymus, lymph nodes, and the lymphatic circulation. The thymus and liver play a role in the maturation and differentiation of immune cells. The spleen filters out old cells and sequesters red and white cells. The bone marrow produces stem cells, which are also known as pluripotent cells because they have the potential to produce one of the several types of leukocytes. The white cells are divided into two major categories: myelocytes (including granulocytes and monocytes) and lymphocytes.

Granulocytes include neutrophils, basophils, and eosinophils. The cytoplasm of the granulocytes contain granules (hence their name). The granulocytes are also called polymorphonuclear leukocytes (PMNs) because the mature form of these cells contains nuclear material that is cleaved into many shapes (■ Figure 10-1). The subclasses of granulocytes are differentiated by their appearance using Wright stain. The neutrophils are so named because they stain in a "neutral" pattern (compared to basophils and eosinophils).

The basophils contain large granules that stain with basic dye (hence the name). Eosinophils, on the other hand, contain granules that take up eosin (red) dye. Basophils migrate from the peripheral blood into the tissues and mature into mast cells. Basophils are filled with granules of histamine and other immune mediators. When provoked, mast cells release histamine that initiates the release of a cascade of biological chemicals resulting in a hypersensitivity (allergic) reaction. Eosinophils are associated with both allergic reactions and parasitic infections.

Monocytes appear in the peripheral blood and also migrate into the tissues to become macrophages. As their name suggests, macrophages are rather large cells whose primary function is to phagocytize foreign materials as well as the cellular debris left in the wake of an immune response.

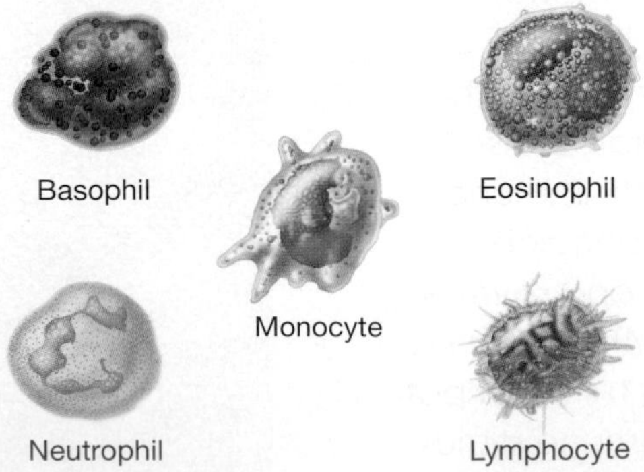

Mature lymphocytes are released into the peripheral blood and migrate into tissues and lymph nodes. They are an extremely important component of the immune system, as they play key roles in both the upregulation and downregulation of the entire system. Although all lymphocytes appear the same under the microscope, they are differentiated into two main classes: T cells and B cells. They can be identified in the laboratory by the presence of cell-surface markers called **clusters of differentiation (CD)**. B lymphocytes complete their maturation and take on their specific role of producing antibodies within the bone marrow. Non-B lymphocytes leave the bone marrow and pass through the thymus where they complete their maturation and become differentiated into T cells (T for thymus).

The immune system has an extensive network of lymph tissue and vessels. The system of lymph vessels parallels the veins and arteries and carries milky-appearing lymph fluid, called chyle, comprised of serous fluid, white cells, and fatty acids. Chyle circulates throughout the lymphatic system and drains into the thoracic and lymphatic ducts in the mediastinum. From the mediastinum, chyle drains into the superior vena cava where it is returned to the main circulation.

Lymph nodes are masses of lymphoid tissue, each node about the size of a pea, that are found in clusters throughout the body. Lymph nodes filter debris left from the breakdown of cells, bacteria, viruses, and fungi. Two-thirds of the body's lymph nodes are found in the abdomen surrounding the intestinal tissue (called gut-associated lymphoid tissue or GALT). These clumps of nodes are called Peyer patches. They are important to the protection of the body as a whole because the GI tract can easily serve as an entry point for microorganisms or foreign material. A large number of lymph nodes are also found in the lungs because the lungs are vulnerable to organisms and foreign material that enter through the airways. Macrophages are also found in the alveoli to help protect the lungs.

Cell-Mediated Immunity

T lymphocytes are the regulatory cells of the immune system, and collectively their functions are referred to as cell-mediated immune responses. T cells leave the bone marrow and go through a preprocessing stage in the thymus where they develop the ability to react against a specific antigen. There are literally millions

FIGURE 10-1 White blood cells found in the peripheral blood.

of T-cell lines, each with the ability to react to only one antigen. Once the T cell has become differentiated, it leaves the thymus and lodges in lymphoid tissue throughout the body, awaiting activation. This preprocessing of T cells occurs in the last few months of gestation and the first few months of life.

T cells are further differentiated into specific roles within the immune system and can be identified by the types of CD proteins expressed on their cell surface. These proteins are actually receptor molecules on the surface of lymphocytes and contribute to the function of the cell. T cells that express CD4 on their surface (CD4$^+$) are called T helper cells (T$_H$ cells) and are the most numerous type of T cell. As their name implies, they help the immune system in nearly all its functions. Much of their helper activity is mediated through lymphokines. **(1)** In addition to stimulating B cells to produce antibodies (as described in the following section), T helper cells secrete lymphokines that upregulate and downregulate immune activity and secrete chemotactic cytokines that draw more white cells to the site of infection or injury. T cell mediators include **interleukins, interferons,** and **colony stimulating factor (CSF)**. **Table 10-1** lists cytokines and their functions.

Another type of T cell, called a natural killer (NK) cell, is capable of a direct attack on microorganisms and virus-infected cells. NK cells latch onto invaders and secrete proteins that cause holes to form in the offending cell's membrane. The cell fills with fluid and bursts. Natural killer cells also have the ability to recognize and destroy tumor cells and are a key component of the body's immunosurveillance of cancer.

Activation of T cells is accomplished by a complicated interplay of immune cells and foreign materials. Macrophages are embedded in the lymph tissues and are often the first cells to encounter a foreign substance such as a bacteria or fungus as it passes through the lymph tissue. Macrophages ingest microorganisms, partially digest them, and pass "pieces" of the foreign material to the T and B lymphocytes lying adjacent to them in the lymph tissue. For this reason, macrophages are sometimes referred to as professional antigen-presenting cells (APCs). When a T lymphocyte recognizes the antigen (based on its antigen specificity determined in the preprocessing phase described above), the T cell becomes

(1) Lymphokines are polypeptide messengers produced by lymphocytes that affect other cells by instigating or inhibiting immune responses. Cytokines are also biological chemicals that act on cells to produce a given reaction. Both lymphokines and cytokines are a form of cell-to-cell communication. A chemotactic cytokine is a polypeptide that causes cells of the immune system to move toward the site of an immune response.

Table 10-1 Cytokines and Their Functions

Cytokines	Names and Types	Comments
interleukin (IL)	up to 30 known interleukins, written IL-1, IL-2, etc	Interleukins communicate and coordinate the immune response. For example, IL-1 and IL-6 are pro-inflammatory and IL-12 slows the immune inflammatory response.
interferons (INF)	3 types, designated alpha, beta and gamma (INF-α, INF-β, INF-γ)	Interferons are released by T cells in response to viral invasion. They inhibit the production of the virus within infected cells, prevent the spread of the virus to other cells, and enhance the activity of macrophages, natural killer cells, and cytotoxic T cells. Interferons also inhibit the growth of certain tumor cells.
tumor necrosis factor (TNF)	2 types, designated alpha and beta (TNF-α, TNF-β)	TNF plays a critical role in the stimulation of macrophages and granulocytes and initiates programmed cell death (apoptosis).
colony stimulating factors (CSF)	granulocyte (GCSF) granulocyte-macrophage (GM-CSF) erythropoietin	Stimulates the bone marrow to produce and release more granulocytes, macrophages, and red cells.

activated. The macrophages release interleukin-1 (IL-l) that causes the T cell to proliferate.

Humoral Immune Response

The immune response mounted by antibodies and the lymphocytes that produce them is called the humoral immune system. The primary role of the humoral system is to provide long-term protection from bacterial, viral, and fungal antigens. Antibodies are produced by B cells, and the exact antibody produced by any single B cell is determined very early in the person's life in a preprocessing stage similar to T cells. This maturation process determines the type of antibody the cell will produce, so that early in a person's life millions of B-cell lines are created in an attempt to anticipate every possible antigen that the person may encounter over a lifetime. These millions of "naïve" B cells inhabit the lymphoid tissue and await activation, which occurs when the B cell comes into contact with its antigen.

Like the T cells, B cells become activated when presented with an antigen by a professional antigen-presenting cell (eg, a macrophage or T cell). The "presentation of antigens" occurs when macrophages and T cells physically come into contact with the B cell. Once activated, the B cell begins to clone itself in preparation to secrete antibodies that correspond to the "presented" antigen. Once activated, B cells transform into lymphoblasts and create two cell lines: memory cells and antibody-secreting **plasma cells**. Plasma cells immediately begin to secrete the B cell's predetermined antibody. Memory cells do not begin secreting antibodies right away; they await a subsequent exposure to the same antigen, at which point they can immediately respond by manufacturing their antibody. It takes several days for the plasma cells to manufacture significant numbers of antibodies, but the memory cells are capable of responding immediately on any subsequent

exposure to the same antigen. This process is exploited by vaccinations that prompt the immune system to create memory cells using a harmless form of the antigen (eg, live, attenuated viruses; attenuated or dead bacteria). When the person is exposed to the actual organism, the memory cells quickly manufacture sufficient antibodies to counteract the infection before the organism can cause illness.

> **Pause 10-1** Research the terms humeral and humoral and give the definitions.

Antibodies, also called immunoglobulins (Ig), have a Y-shaped structure made of two heavy amino acid chains and two light amino acid chains. (2) There are five types of heavy chains (alpha, gamma, mu, delta, and epsilon), and these heavy chains determine the antibody class (A, G, M, D, and E). There are two types of light chains, designated **kappa** and **lambda**. (3) The upper arms of the Y shape are the points at which the antibody molecule binds to its specific antigen (■ **Figure 10-2**). This portion of the antibody is called the hypervariable region, meaning this portion of the molecule differs from all other antibodies and makes the antibody unique and specific for a given antigen.

Antibodies may be secreted into the blood and lymph and circulate freely or they may be bound to the surface of T and B cells. Antibodies are intended to have a one-to-one relationship with an antigen, but some antibodies cross-react with other antigens that share similar epitopes. (4) This is oftentimes the basis of autoimmune disorders.

There are five classes of immunoglobulins: IgA, IgE, IgD, IgG, and IgM. As mentioned above, the type of heavy chain determines the antibody class. Each type of immunoglobulin plays a distinct role, although the exact role of IgD is not completely understood. IgA is called the secretory immunoglobulin because it is found in secretions such as saliva and tears and also on mucous membranes. IgE is found on the surface of mast cells and is associated with hypersensitivity responses. IgM is produced when the immune system encounters an antigen for the first time. IgM is a large antibody complex consisting of five individual IgM antibodies bound together. The multiple binding sites of the IgM molecule make this class of antibody more efficient, which is important since it is a "first-responder." IgG is produced later in the immune response and also reappears when the immune system is confronted with the same antigen weeks, months, or years later.

---

(2) The descriptive terms heavy and light refer to the molecular weight of the amino acid chains that make up the antibody molecule.

(3) Immunoglobulin light chains are also called **Bence Jones proteins** when they appear in the urine.

(4) An epitope is a specific, identifiable site on an antigen molecule that can be recognized by an antibody. A single antigen may have more than one epitope.

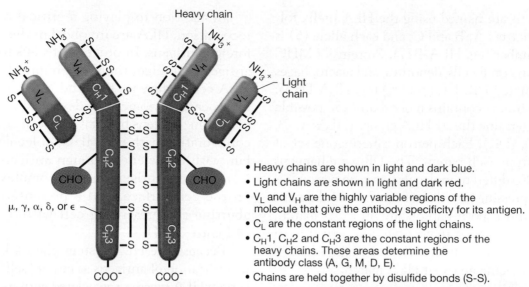

Heavy chain

Light chain

- Heavy chains are shown in light and dark blue.
- Light chains are shown in light and dark red.
- V_L and V_H are the highly variable regions of the molecule that give the antibody specificity for its antigen.
- C_L are the constant regions of the light chains.
- C_H1, C_H2 and C_H3 are the constant regions of the heavy chains. These areas determine the antibody class (A, G, M, D, E).
- Chains are held together by disulfide bonds (S-S).

FIGURE 10-2 Structure of an immunoglobulin showing two light chains (red) and two heavy chains (blue).

The distinct roles of IgG and IgM can be used to construct a timeline of the immune system's response and to determine the chronicity of an infection. For example, the presence of IgM antibodies indicates an ongoing infection or a recent infection (because they are secreted first). The presence of IgG antibodies signifies a past infection and indicates immunity (ie, the ability to resist a subsequent infection from the same organism). The laboratory reports the amount of antibody directed against a *single antigen* in titers (see page 333) or units. Concentrations of each *class* of immunoglobulin (regardless of their antigen specificity) are reported in grams per deciliter.

An immune complex is formed when an antibody and its corresponding antigen are bound together (■ Figure 10-3). The antibody, in and of itself, does not destroy the antigen or the cell that is attached to the antigen. The immune complexes formed by the antigen-antibody pair cause antigens to agglutinate (stick together) or precipitate (fall out of solution) and make them more amenable to phagocytosis. Antibodies attached to cells act as "tags" that mark the cell for destruction by other components of the immune system. Immune complexes attached to cells fix complement (see below), causing the cell to lyse. In some cases, antibodies can neutralize an antigen by preventing the antigen from attaching to its target.

Major Histocompatibility Complex

Much of the immune system's response is based on the ability of the body to recognize foreign molecules and to selectively destroy the molecule and/or the cell associated with the molecule. To recognize a foreign object, the body must first be able to recognize "self." The **major histocompatibility complex (MHC)** is a system of cell surface proteins that allow an organism to recognize "self" and to differentiate foreign cells and foreign proteins. In humans, cell surface proteins associated with the MHC are called **human leukocyte antigens (HLA)**. HLA are expressed on the surface of all nucleated cells.

There are hundreds of unique MHC proteins expressed on the surface of cells, and they are divided into three classes. Class I and class II proteins are significant to immunology. Proteins of MHC class I are found on the surface of all nucleated cells and platelets.

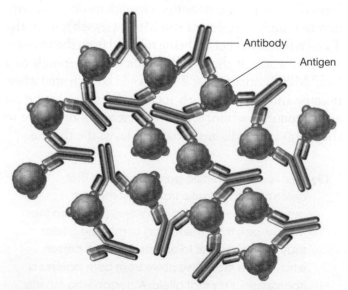

Antibody

Antigen

FIGURE 10-3 Multiple antibody molecules attached to numerous antigen sites to create an immune complex.

Class I antigens are named using the HLA prefix followed by the letters A, B and C, and each allele (5) is assigned a number (eg, HLA-B27). Proteins of MHC class II are found on B cells, dendrites, and macrophages and are designated DR, DP, and DQ (eg, HLA-DR3). The human genome contains more than 1250 possible alleles that determine the six HLA groups (HLA-A, -B, -C, -DP, -DQ, -DR). Each person inherits one set of HLA alleles from each parent. The DR gene happens to expresses two different molecules, so each person has 14 alleles (expressing anywhere from 7 to 14 different antigens—seven if both parents are an exact match, which would be next to impossible, fourteen if both parents are completely different), and siblings have a 25% chance of being an exact HLA match.

> She was negative for factor V Leiden mutation, prothrombin mutation, positive for 1 copy of the C677T mutation and 1 copy of the A1298C mutation. She is also positive for 2 copies of the 4G allele of the PAI-1 gene.

As described above, perinatal preprocessing of T cells assigns an antibody to each T-cell line. During preprocessing, T-cell antigen specificity is determined by a random rearrangement of several genes that results in the creation of millions of different T-cell lines capable of matching up to the multitude of antigens that a person may potentially come into contact with over their lifetime. But before a T cell can leave the thymus, it is "tested" to make sure its antigen specificity does not happen to match antigens of the MHC (ie, self); if so, the T cell is destroyed before being released from the thymus. In other words, if the T-cell specificity corresponds to a "self" MHC antigen, that T cell would be activated when it came into contact with its own cells, producing an autoimmune reaction; only cells that are nonreactive to the body's own cells are allowed to leave the thymus.

> **(5)** An allele is a specific gene sequence that determines a genetic trait. A trait may be determined by one pair of alleles (one from the mother, one from the father) or multiple alleles may work together to express a trait. A person who inherits the same allele from both parents is homozygous for that allele. A person who inherits different alleles for the same gene is heterozygous.

In addition to playing a critical role in cellular recognition, HLA are involved in the recognition of foreign antigens. In order for T cells to recognize an antigen as foreign, the antigen must be bound to an HLA cell-surface protein and "presented" to T cells for processing. Some have described the presentation of foreign antigens by MHC molecules as a "hot dog" configuration with the MHC molecule acting like a bun with the wiener (foreign antigen) sandwiched inside. These antigen-antigen complexes are located on the cell surface, and a presentation occurs by abutting the presenting cell with a T helper cell (■ Figure 10-4).

Because the HLA system plays a key role in the identification of antigens as either "self" or "non-self," certain HLA types are associated with increased susceptibility to infection as well as increased incidence of autoimmune diseases such as type 1 diabetes mellitus (HLA-DR3), ankylosing spondylitis (HLA-B27), and systemic lupus erythematosus (HLA-DR3).

Complement

The **complement** system is a group of 20 proteins (designated C1, C2, etc) made in the liver. These proteins participate in a cascade of chemical reactions that result in the lysis of an antibody-tagged cell. The complement system is activated by either immune complexes or antibodies attached to cell membranes. When complement is "fixed" to an antigen-antibody complex, the attached cell wall is lysed. Complement can also promote phagocytosis, cause the agglutination of organisms, and neutralize viruses. Complement components are **acute-phase reactants** (proteins that become elevated in the blood during an inflammatory reaction). CH50 is a functional assay (performed in the laboratory) to test levels of all the complement components as a whole. CH50 is decreased in autoimmune disorders such as systemic lupus erythematosus and disorders involving increased numbers of immune complexes because these proteins are constantly consumed. The individual complement components C3 and C4 can also be measured; decreased levels are indicative of chronic immune disorders.

> Note the spelling of complement (not compliment). It takes this spelling because it "completes the actions" of the T cells and antibodies.

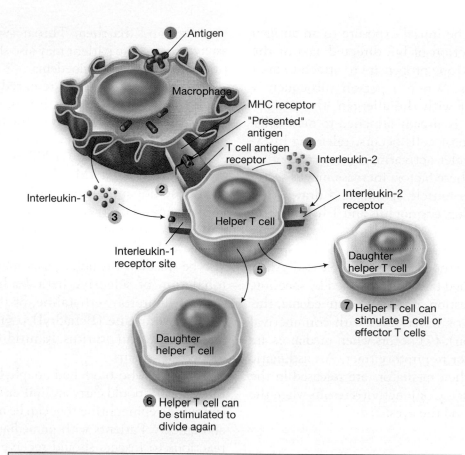

KEY:

1 Antigen processing cell such as a macrophage ingests a pathogen and displays its antigen on the macrophage's cell membrane.

2 "Presented" antigen is recognized by helper T cell.

3 The macrophage secretes a cytokine called interleukin-1.

4 Interleukin-1 stimulates the helper T cell to secrete interleukin-2 which combines with interleukin receptors.

5 When interleukin-2 binds to the receptor site the helper T cell divides.

6 The daughter cell produced can divide again if exposed to the same antigen. This greatly increases the number of helper T cells which can even further divide proportionate to the antigen exposure.

7 As helper T cells continue to divide they can stimulate B cell activation and produce effector T cells.

FIGURE 10-4 The macrophage presents the foreign antigen to the T cell by binding with the CD4 antigen on the T helper cell and using MHC antigens for identification. The binding causes the release of cytokines, which act on the macrophage.

Hypersensitivity

Hypersensitivity, also called allergy, refers to an abnormal or exaggerated response by the immune system. Allergic reactions can occur as immediate reactions, late-phase reactions, or chronic allergic inflammation. An example of a late-phase reaction is the rash caused by poison ivy. Chronic allergic inflammation is caused by continuous or repeated exposure to an allergen (eg, pollens, cat dander). Long-standing inflammation causes structural and functional changes in the affected tissue.

Immediate or acute-phase reactions occur within seconds to minutes of allergen exposure and are mediated by IgE. **Atopy** is the genetic predisposition to make IgE antibodies in response to antigen exposure. Patients prone to IgE-mediated allergic reactions are said to be atopic. The initial exposure to an antigen prompts the production of IgE directed against the antigen. IgE has a strong propensity to attach to mast cells and basophils. When a person subsequently comes into contact with the allergen, the antigen binds with IgE that is already attached to mast cells. Degranulation of mast cells occurs, releasing histamine, heparin, platelet-activating factors, and other leukotrienes (6). These factors increase mucus secretion, cause smooth-muscle spasm, and draw other inflammatory cells (eg, eosinophils and T helper cells) to the area.

The symptoms of a hypersensitivity response depend on the where the mediators are released. Allergic rhinitis (also called hayfever), marked by sneezing, itching, nasal congestion, nasal turbinate edema, rhinorrhea, and itchy or watery eyes with conjunctival hyperemia (**injection**), (7) occurs when mediators are released in the upper respiratory tract. An asthmatic attack can result when mediators are released in the lower respiratory tract. Conjunctivitis results when the reaction occurs around the eyes.

Anaphylaxis

Anaphylaxis is a widespread, immediate hypersensitivity reaction that results from mast-cell degranulation. Histamine released into the circulatory system causes body-wide vasodilation as well as increased permeability of the capillaries with a significant loss of plasma from the circulation (hypotension), culminating in **anaphylactic shock**. Common causes of anaphylaxis are insect venoms (**envenomization**) and foods (eg, peanuts, shellfish). An immediate anaphylactic response may also be followed by a late-phase reaction that occurs 6–24 hours later. These reactions are mediated by T cells, not antibodies.

Symptoms of anaphylaxis include hypotension, dysrhythmia, and respiratory distress caused by laryngeal edema and bronchospasm. The GI system can also be affected with resultant nausea, abdominal cramping, bloating, and diarrhea. Throat swelling can cause asphyxiation. The patient may also show flushing, pruritus, urticaria, and angioedema.

Emergent treatment is required, especially when the patient is in respiratory distress or is hypotensive. Laryngeal edema requires endotracheal intubation or a tracheostomy to prevent death by asphyxiation. Aqueous epinephrine 1:1000 in a dose of 0.2 to 0.5 mL is injected IM. Vasopressor drugs such as high-dose dopamine, norepinephrine, and phenylephrine may be given to increase blood pressure. Fluid resuscitation using saline, **lactated Ringers**, plasma colloid solutions, or **plasma expanders** may also be needed. Bronchospasm may be treated with inhalation of selective beta 2-adrenergic agonists such as albuterol, terbutaline, or IV aminophylline. Diphenhydramine (Benadryl) is given for urticaria, angioedema, and pruritus. Ranitidine (Zantac) helps reduce GI spasms.

Patients who have had anaphylactic reactions or those at risk should carry an **EpiPen**, a prefilled syringe containing epinephrine that can be administered easily and quickly. Patients with immediate hypersensitivity reactions to insects should receive venom immunotherapy for prophylaxis.

Angioedema

Angioedema is a form of anaphylaxis that occurs in the subcutaneous tissues. It may be accompanied by urticaria (local wheals and erythema). Angioedema may be acute or chronic (lasting more than six weeks); the acute form is mediated by IgE and histamine released in response to drugs, venom, or ingested foods. Angioedema is characterized by locally diffuse and painful soft-tissue swelling, especially around the eyelids, lips, face, and tongue. Swelling may also occur in the hands or feet. Patients may also have symptoms of respiratory distress. Treatment is with oral prednisone and possibly subcutaneous epinephrine or IV antihistamines.

---

(6) Leukotrienes are also cytokines that contribute to immune responses, especially hypersensitivity responses.

(7) Injection is another term to describe swelling or inflammation and is often used to describe the conjunctivae.

Be sure to distinguish wheals (a raised, erythematous skin reaction) and wheels. Another commonly confused term is whelp and welt. A welt is another term for wheal. A whelp is a newborn puppy.

- T and B lymphocytes can be differentiated using cell-surface markers called clusters of differentiation (CD).
- B cells produce antibodies and play a central role in the humoral response. T cells play a key role in cellular immune responses as well as regulation of the immune system. Antibody specificity of B cells and T cells is determined early in a person's life.
- Cytokines such as interleukin, interferon, and colony stimulating factors are immune mediators that allow for cell-to-cell communication.
- There are five classes of immunoglobulins (antibodies) composed of heavy chains and kappa or lambda light chains. The heavy chain determines the antibody class: IgG, IgM, IgA, IgE, and IgD.
- IgM antibodies are produced first followed by IgG. These two antibody titers can be used to create a timeline of an infection.

- Antigens tag cells for destruction or facilitate the removal of antigens by agglutination, precipitation, or complement fixation.
- Cell surface proteins of the HLA system help the immune system distinguish self from nonself and also participate in the presentation of antigens that activates an immune response. HLA antigens are designated with the letters A, B, C, DR, DP, and DQ.
- Complement is a system of proteins that adds to the effectiveness of the cellular and humoral immune systems. Immune complexes fix complement, causing cell lysis and increasing phagocytosis.
- Hypersensitivity is an exaggerated response by the immune system. The most severe form of hypersensitivity is anaphylactic shock. More common forms include allergic rhinitis and angioedema.

Autoimmune Disorders

Immune tolerance is the ability of the immune system to recognize self-antigens while retaining the ability to mount a response against nonself antigens. Autoimmune diseases result when the immune system fails to tolerate self-antigens. Autoimmunity may be mediated by T cells or by antibodies. Cell-mediated autoimmune diseases may be caused by cells that have become immunized to autologous tissues. Autoimmunity may also be caused by disordered immune regulation due to diminished activity of T-suppressor cells that normally prevent overreactivity. Several autoimmune diseases are known to be mediated solely by antibodies. Examples include hemolytic anemia, **idiopathic thrombocytopenic purpura (ITP)**, and Goodpasture syndrome. In these autoimmune diseases, antibodies attach directly to cells or platelets and fix complement with ensuing cell destruction. Autoimmune disorders are known to attack many tissue types, including vital organs. Patients diagnosed with autoimmune disorders are monitored carefully, and they routinely receive extensive physical examinations as well as cardiopulmonary and renal assessments to detect visceral involvement.

Another type of antibody-mediated autoimmune disease is caused by antibodies that compete with or mimic physiologic agonists. For example, in Graves disease, antibodies bind to thyroid cells, mimicking thyroid stimulating hormone, and stimulate the thyroid to produce more thyroid hormone. In patients with myasthenia gravis, antibodies bind to acetylcholine receptors and block neurotransmitters, resulting in muscle weakness. **Table 10-2** lists common autoimmune disorders and their associated antibodies.

Rheumatoid Arthritis

Rheumatoid arthritis (RA) is an autoimmune inflammatory disease affecting the synovial membranes of the peripheral joints. RA has systemic manifestations as well. RA leads to joint destruction with significant morbidity and disability. Although RA itself is not fatal, patients typically have a shorter lifespan compared to patients without RA. Onset is typically between 35 and 50 years of age, but it can also begin in childhood. The exact etiology is unknown; many factors are thought to contribute to the development of the autoimmune reaction, including a viral or bacterial infection as the inciting event. There is a known

Table 10-2 Common Autoimmune Disorders and Associated Antibodies

Autoimmune Disorder	Primary Associated Antibodies	Target Organ/Tissue
immune thrombocytopenic purpura (ITP)	antibodies directed against platelet surface	platelets
Goodpasture syndrome	antibodies directed against basement membrane of alveoli and glomerulus	lung and kidney
systemic lupus erythematosus (SLE)	ANA, anti-dsDNA, anti-Sm	joints, muscles, skin, kidney, heart, lung
rheumatoid arthritis (RA)	RF, ANA, anti-CCP	joints
Sjögren syndrome	ANA, RF, anti-SS-A (Ro), anti-SS-B (La)	exocrine glands, mucous membranes
scleroderma	anti-Scl-70	skin and joints, multiple organs
Graves disease	antibodies against TSH receptors	thyroid (metabolic defects)
insulin-dependent diabetes	antibodies against islet cells, insulin, and insulin receptors	pancreas (metabolic defects)
Addison disease	antibodies against adrenal gland cells	adrenal gland
primary myxedema	antibodies against microsomes	thyroid

genetic predisposition in individuals with the class II HLA shared epitope. (8)

The disease typically begins as an inflammatory reaction in the peripheral joints with hyperplasia of synovial lining cells (**pannus formation**). The early stages of the disease show articular effusions and other manifestations of inflammation. The hyperplastic synovial lining releases inflammatory proteins and excessive enzymes that erode cartilage, bone, ligaments, and tendons. Plasma cells within the joints produce antibodies that form immune complexes in the synovial space, causing macrophages and T cells to migrate to the inflamed joints and release proinflammatory cytokines and chemokines (eg, tumor necrosis factors [TNF], granulocyte-macrophage colony-stimulating factor [GM-CSF], and various interleukins). Release of these immune-system mediators destroys local tissue and also produces the systemic manifestations of fatigue and malaise. Vessel walls become inflamed (vasculitis) and granulomatous nodules (**rheumatoid nodules**) form, especially in the subcutaneous tissue over the

affected joints but also in organs. In the later stages of the disease, fibrous tissue replaces inflamed joint tissue, resulting in fibrous ankylosis of the affected joints.

The course of RA follows an unpredictable progression. A few patients actually experience remission, but the majority of patients continue to progress. The onset of the disease is typically insidious. Patients may experience **prodromal symptoms** of malaise, weight loss, and vague joint pain or stiffness. Patients may also note generalized weakness and fatigue, anorexia, and in some cases low-grade fever. Symmetric joint swelling with stiffness, erythema, warmth, tenderness, and limited range of motion are the most common symptoms. The hallmark of RA is joint stiffness and pain upon awakening that improves as the day progresses. The affected joints cause difficulty with activities of daily living, such as dressing, standing, and any activity involving dexterity.

The joints are almost always affected symmetrically. The most commonly involved joints are the middle metacarpophalangeal (MCP) joints, wrists, proximal interphalangeal (PIP) joints, knee, and metatarsophalangeal (MTP) joints. Less commonly, the hips, shoulders, elbows, and cervical spine are involved. Patients typically hold the joints in flexion to minimize pain, resulting in flexion contractures. Deformation of the joints, tendons, and cartilage lead to joint instability,

(8) The class II HLA shared epitope is a sequence of amino acids shared by several HLA class II molecules.

synovial cysts, and ruptured tendons. Entrapment syndromes, especially carpal tunnel syndrome due to entrapment of the median nerve, are common. **Ulnar deviation** of the fingers, swan-neck and **boutonniere deformities** (hyperextension of the DIP with hyperflexion of the PIP joint), and **hammertoes** are classic findings in patients with RA. Valgus deformity of the knee and Baker cyst (popliteal cyst) may also be seen. Deformities with difficulty using the hands lead to atrophy of the interosseous muscles of the hands.

Extraarticular manifestations of RA (■ **Figure 10-5**) include dryness of the eyes (**keratoconjunctivitis sicca**) due to vascular changes in the eyes. Dry mouth and dry mucous membranes are also common. Later in the disease, a number of patients will develop rheumatoid nodules at sites of pressure or chronic irritation, especially on the extensor surface of the forearm and over the MCP joints. Involvement of the cervical spine can cause **atlantoaxial subluxation** and spinal cord compression, especially when the neck is extended. These patients must be evaluated carefully before undergoing endotracheal intubation. Patients with severe cases of RA tend to develop these same rheumatoid nodules in the heart.

Other symptoms include vasculitis with purpura and ulcer formation. Pulmonary involvement may cause pleural effusions, interstitial fibrosis, pulmonary nodules, or **bronchiolitis obliterans-organizing pneumonia (BOOP)**. A subset of patients may also develop **Felty syndrome** characterized by splenomegaly and neutropenia with severe destructive arthritis. Most patients have **anemia of chronic disease** and thrombocytosis. RA patients are also more prone to infection, especially patients taking immunosuppressive treatment to lessen the effects of RA. Periarticular osteoporosis results from localized inflammation, and generalized osteoporosis may develop from long-term corticosteroid use.

The diagnosis of RA is based on clinical findings, serological markers, and x-ray findings. Patients with bilateral articular pain, especially in the hands, should be evaluated for RA. The American College of Rheumatology has developed a list of criteria for diagnosing rheumatoid arthritis. The presence of at least four of the following criteria supports the diagnosis of RA:

- morning stiffness that lasts at least one hour
- arthritic pain of three or more joints with soft-tissue swelling or fluid. Affected joints should include the proximal interphalangeal (PIP), metacarpophalangeal (MCP), wrist, elbow, knee, ankle, and/or metatarsophalangeal (MTP) joints

- arthritis of hand joints
- symmetric arthritis (simultaneous involvement of the same joint areas on both sides of the body)
- rheumatoid nodules
- positive rheumatoid factor (see below)
- radiographic changes typical of RA, including erosions or bony calcification in or adjacent to affected joints of the hands or wrists

Rheumatoid factor (RF), which is an antibody directed against other antibody molecules, is present in about 70% of patients with RA. The titer may be low or undetectable early in the disease but rises as the disease progresses. RF is highly suggestive of RA but cannot be used solely and definitively to diagnose RA, as this same antibody may be found in lower titers in patients with other autoimmune diseases, viral hepatitis, TB, cancer, and even a small percentage of the general population with no specific diagnosis. The most specific serological test for RA is the **anticyclic citrullinated peptide (anti-CCP)**. An RF titer measured by latex agglutination of greater than 1:80 or a positive anti-CCP test supports the diagnosis of RA. The presence of both anti-CCP and RF is highly specific for RA. Patients may also be positive for anti-RA33 and **antinuclear antibodies (ANA)**. Early in the disease process, HLA typing showing the presence of HLA-DR4 (a shared epitope) may be helpful in differentiating RA from other forms of autoimmune disease. Other tests included in the diagnostic workup include nonspecific markers of generalized inflammation:

- elevated acute-phase reactants such as erythrocyte sedimentation rate (ESR) and C-reactive protein
- elevated immunoglobulins (specifically IgM and IgG)
- moderate anemia and thrombocytosis

Synovial fluid analysis may also be performed. Results correspond to a noninfectious, inflammatory response, as outlined in **Table 10-3**.

Radiographic findings are very helpful in the diagnosis of RA, although x-rays taken in the first six months of the disease process are often negative. Early signs of change include soft-tissue swelling and **juxtaarticular demineralization** (osteoporosis) in the wrists and feet. As the disease progresses, joint-space narrowing and **marginal erosions** develop. Subluxation at C1-2 (atlantoaxial subluxation) occurs late in the disease process. MRI of the knee may show **abnormal bone signals** indicating bone marrow lesions or **bone marrow edema**.

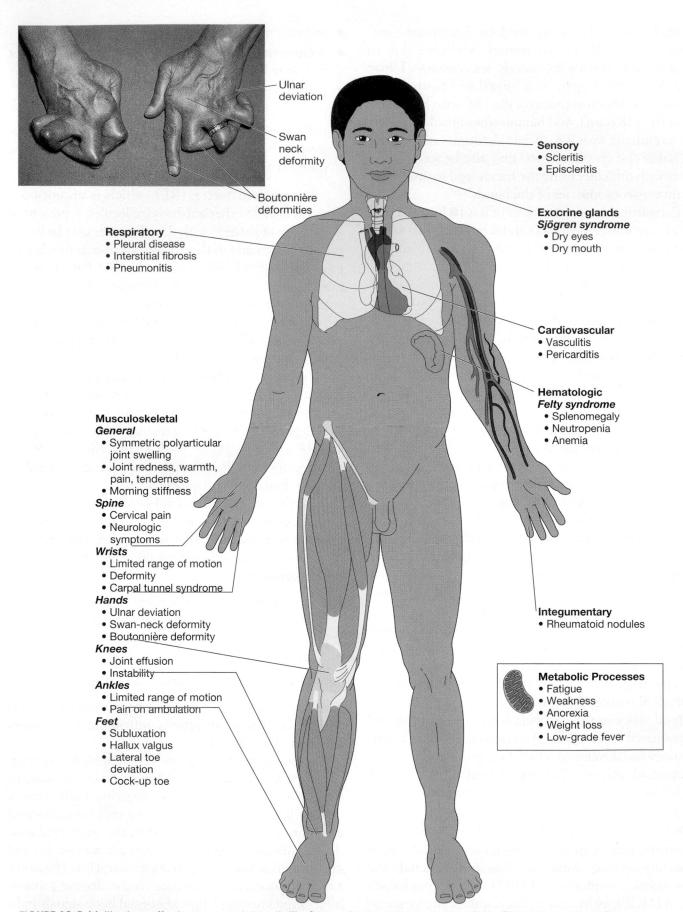

Ulnar deviation

Swan neck deformity

Boutonnière deformities

Sensory
• Scleritis
• Episcleritis

Exocrine glands
Sjögren syndrome
• Dry eyes
• Dry mouth

Respiratory
• Pleural disease
• Interstitial fibrosis
• Pneumonitis

Cardiovascular
• Vasculitis
• Pericarditis

Hematologic
Felty syndrome
• Splenomegaly
• Neutropenia
• Anemia

Musculoskeletal
General
• Symmetric polyarticular joint swelling
• Joint redness, warmth, pain, tenderness
• Morning stiffness
Spine
• Cervical pain
• Neurologic symptoms
Wrists
• Limited range of motion
• Deformity
• Carpal tunnel syndrome
Hands
• Ulnar deviation
• Swan-neck deformity
• Boutonnière deformity
Knees
• Joint effusion
• Instability
Ankles
• Limited range of motion
• Pain on ambulation
Feet
• Subluxation
• Hallux valgus
• Lateral toe deviation
• Cock-up toe

Integumentary
• Rheumatoid nodules

Metabolic Processes
• Fatigue
• Weakness
• Anorexia
• Weight loss
• Low-grade fever

FIGURE 10-5 Multisystem effects of rheumatoid arthritis. *Source:* Photo © Biophoto Associates/Photo Researchers, Inc.

Table 10-3 Typical Synovial Fluid Analysis Results in Patients with RA

Test Name	Reference Range
volume	>3.5 mL
clarity	translucent to opaque
color	yellow to opalescent
WBC	3000 to 50,000
PMNs	50% or more of white cells
culture	negative
glucose	>25 g/dL but lower than serum
crystals	absent

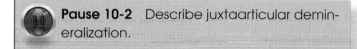

Pause 10-2 Describe juxtaarticular demineralization.

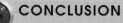

CONCLUSION

1. Arthropathic changes most conspicuous at the base of the right thumb.

2. Extensive arthropathic changes and remodeling of the distal 2nd metacarpal noted at the metacarpophalangeal joint. Distribution of arthropathy consistent with rheumatoid arthritis.

Treatment for RA primarily involves physical measures and medications. Patients are counseled on good nutrition and general well-care. Patients are encouraged to rest, although extended bedrest is discouraged. Exercise is also encouraged, especially passive range of motion exercises during acute exacerbations to prevent **flexion contractures** as well as routine range of motion exercises performed in warm water. Exercise also helps prevent atrophy. Splinting affected joints for a short period may also be helpful. Orthopedic shoes with good support and metatarsal supports help relieve pain during weightbearing. Occupational therapy may also be prescribed to help patients adapt to limitations and learn to use assistive devices to perform activities of daily living.

There is a wide range of medications used to treat rheumatoid arthritis. The goals of pharmaceutical treatment are to reduce pain, reduce inflammation, and to slow the progression of disease. The following categories of medications are used:

- analgesics
- NSAIDs
- corticosteroids
- **disease modifying antirheumatic drugs (DMARDs)**

Analgesics (eg, acetaminophen/paracetamol, tramadol, codeine, and opiates) help relieve pain, but they do not affect inflammation or slow the progression of disease. NSAIDs are also helpful for treating pain and swelling, but also do not alter the course of the disease. NSAIDs are used as **bridging therapy** until DMARDs take full effect. Aspirin is no longer recommended due to GI side effects associated with long-term, high-dose aspirin use. Celecoxib is typically recommended due to its reduced GI toxicity, but other NSAIDs (ibuprofen, naproxen, ketoprofen, piroxicam, and diclofenac) are equally as effective. All NSAIDs are associated with adverse events such as renal toxicity, increased hypertension, edema, and decreased platelet function.

DMARDs is dictated as the acronym *dee mards.*

Glucocorticoids are potent antiinflammatory drugs and are commonly used in patients with RA. Because of the serious side effects, low-dose systemic steroids such as prednisone are used only in the short term for extreme exacerbations. Corticosteroids in the form of intraarticular depot injections may be used for isolated joints, but injections are limited to four times a year.

The mainstay of pharmacologic treatment for RA is the DMARDs. Although these medications take weeks or even months to be fully effective, they are worthwhile because they actually alter the course of the disease. DMARDs slow the progression of joint destruction and reduce the need for analgesics and steroids. The DMARDs are separated into two categories: xenobiotic and biologic. Xenobiotics were the first DMARDs used and include gold salts, D-penicillamine, chloroquine and hydroxychloroquine, sulfasalazine (SSZ), methotrexate (MTX), azathioprine, and cyclosporin A.

The newest DMARD, considered an antiinflammatory, is leflunomide (Arava). Methotrexate is usually the treatment of choice and is initially given 7.5 mg per week, up to a maximum of 25 mg per week. Liver function must be monitored every three to six months.

> **Pause 10-3** Explain why some drugs are classified as DMARDs. What is the difference between a DMARD and an NSAID?

The biologic DMARDs include the **TNF blockers** etanercept, infliximab, adalimumab, and golimumab. TNF, a cytokine, activates lymphocytes and leukocytes and mediates the release of other cytokines. Blocking this key agent of the immune system reduces the destructive effects of an otherwise out-of-control immune reaction. Because TNF also plays a key role in fighting infection, TNF inhibitors cause a mild immune suppression. It is important to screen patients for latent TB (with chest x-ray and PPD testing) before starting TNF-inhibition therapy. TNF inhibitors are also contraindicated in patients with acute or chronic infections, demyelinating disorders, and recent malignancy.

> **HISTORY OF PRESENT ILLNESS:** The patient is here for PPD placement in preparation for anti-TNF, which we discussed last visit. PPD was placed on the left forearm. Continue for now the methotrexate 10 tablets every week; sulfasalazine 3 in the morning, 3 at night. If the PPD is negative, we will apply for anti-TNF.

Other biologic DMARDs include immunomodulators that block IL-1 (anakinra, trade name Kineret), T-cell inhibitors (abatacept, trade name Orencia), IL-6 inhibitor (tocilizumab, trade name Actemra), and antibodies directed against B cells (rituximab, trade name Rituxan).

At times, surgery may be indicated to reconstruct or replace joints, especially when damaged joints severely limit function. Hip and knee replacements are the most successful. Excision of MTP joints can improve walking and balance, and thumb fusions can increase functionality of the hand. Neck fusions may be required for subluxation of C1 on C2. Synovectomy may be used to relieve joint inflammation but the results are only temporary.

Systemic Lupus Erythematosus

Systemic lupus erythematosus (SLE), also called **disseminated lupus erythematosus**, is an autoimmune disorder that affects multiple organ systems. It occurs predominantly in females of childbearing age. Remissions and exacerbations are common and the overall clinical course is unpredictable. The severity ranges from very mild to rapidly fulminant with life-threatening complications. Infection is the most common cause of death early in the disease, and cardiovascular complications are the most common causes of death late in the disease process.

The exact cause of SLE is unknown, but it is believed that a genetic predisposition combined with environmental triggers precipitate autoimmune reactions and immune-system dysregulation. Many of its clinical manifestations are the result of antigen-antibody complexes that become trapped in the capillaries of the skin and visceral structures (eg, the kidneys and lungs), leading to complement activation and tissue destruction. Autoantibody-mediated destruction of platelets and red cells also occurs. Antibodies directed against nuclear components, called antinuclear antibodies (ANA), and antibodies directed against **double-stranded DNA (anti-dsDNA, also called anti-native DNA)** are found in almost all patients with active SLE. Several drugs are known to produce a lupus-like syndrome, which is reversible with complete withdrawal of the offending drug.

The signs and symptoms of SLE vary greatly. In some patients, the symptoms develop abruptly with fulminant manifestations, and with others, the course is indolent and more insidious. SLE should be suspected in persons with multisystem complaints and positive serology. Since almost any organ system can be affected, with a wide range of severity, the list of possible symptoms and manifestations is long. A brief description of symptoms by body system is given here:

- Constitutional: fever, anorexia, malaise and weight loss, lymphadenopathy and splenomegaly.
- Ophthalmologic: conjunctivitis, photophobia, blurred vision, and monocular blindness.
- Dermatologic: **malar rash** (also called the butterfly rash due to its shape) is the most classic sign of SLE. A plaque-like discoid rash that develops in sun-exposed areas may also be seen in patients with discoid lupus (a separate entity from SLE). Other signs include **periungual erythema**, nail-fold infarcts, palmar erythema, alopecia, purpura, petechiae, mucous membrane lesions, and Raynaud phenomenon. Photosensitivity (rash following sun exposure) is also common.

- Respiratory: serositis, recurrent pleurisy, pleural effusion, bronchopneumonia, and restrictive lung disease. Alveolar hemorrhage may be seen in severe flare-ups. Patients may also have pulmonary emboli, pulmonary hypertension, or shrinking lung syndrome.

- Cardiac: pericarditis with chest pain, pericardial effusions, myocarditis, valvular involvement, coronary artery vasculitis, and arrhythmias. Patients with SLE are known to have accelerated atherosclerosis that increases the risk of coronary events.

- Neurologic: psychosis, organic brain syndrome, seizures, neuropathies, transverse myelitis, and strokes caused by involvement of the central nervous system. Mild cognitive impairment is common.

- Renal: glomerulonephritis (histological types include mesangial, focal proliferative, diffuse proliferative, and membranous) is common with resultant hypertension, peripheral and periorbital edema.

- Musculoskeletal: polyarthritis involving the small joints of the hands, wrists, and knees (usually non-destructive and nondeforming). Patients with long-standing disease may develop **Jaccoud arthritis** of the MCP and interphalangeal joints with **ulnar drift** and swan-neck deformities but no bony erosions.

- Hematologic: **autoimmune hemolytic anemia**, leukopenia, thrombocytopenia, recurrent arterial and venous thromboses.

- Obstetric: early and late fetal demise, especially in patients with antiphospholipid antibodies (probably due to thromboses).

- Gastrointestinal: nausea, vomiting, and abdominal pain from bowel vasculitis, impaired bowel motility, bowel perforation, pseudoobstruction, pancreatitis, and serositis.

Patients experiencing neurologic symptomatology, systemic vasculitis, profound thrombocytopenia, rapidly progressive glomerulonephritis and/or diffuse alveolar hemorrhage should be treated emergently and aggressively.

The diagnosis of SLE is based on clinical criteria as well as serological studies. A patient must show at least four of the following symptoms:

- malar rash (distribution over the cheeks and nasal bridge with sparing of the nasolabial fold)
- discoid rash
- photosensitivity
- oral ulcers
- arthritis
- serositis
- renal disease (proteinuria or cellular casts)
- neurologic disease (seizures, psychosis)
- hematologic abnormalities (hemolytic anemia, leukopenia, lymphopenia, thrombocytopenia)
- serologic abnormalities (positive **LE cell prep, anti-dsDNA, anti-Smith [anti-Sm], anticardiolipin IgG or IgM** or lupus anticoagulant, false-positive syphilis test)
- positive ANA

Laboratory evaluation is especially helpful in the differentiation of SLE from other autoimmune disorders. Laboratory evaluation should include serological studies to detect autoantibodies, a CBC, urinalysis, and chemistry profile. Patients with SLE may have any number of the following abnormalities:

- anemia, leukopenia, thrombocytopenia
- positive antiphospholipid antibodies (lupus anticoagulant, anticardiolipin antibody), **positive direct Coombs, hypocomplementemia,** ANA, anti-dsDNA, anti-Sm
- proteinuria, hematuria

Additional studies that may be useful include:

- erythrocyte sedimentation rate (ESR) and C-reactive protein (CRP), which are typically elevated
- complement levels; C3 and C4 are typically depressed in active disease due to overconsumption and are useful assays to monitor disease severity
- liver function studies, which may be slightly elevated
- creatinine kinase, which is elevated in myositis
- other autoantibody assays (Ro [SS-A], La [SS-B], **ribonucleoprotein [RNP]**)

X-rays of the affected joints may show periarticular osteopenia and soft-tissue swelling, but destructive arthritis is uncommon in SLE. Chest x-rays and CT scans of the chest are useful for monitoring lung disease associated with SLE.

> ASSESSMENT: Systemic lupus erythematosus with secondary Sjögren's based on patient presenting with photosensitivity, serositis, pericardial effusion, dry eyes, dry mouth, and low complement. SS-A and SS-B were negative.

Treatment for SLE is based on the severity of the disease. Little or no therapy may be needed for intermittent or mild disease. Arthralgias may be treated with NSAIDs. Patients suffering fever, serositis, skin and joint manifestations may find relief with hydroxychloroquine (Plaquenil) or other antimalarial medications. Low to moderate dose steroids may be used for acute flares. Patients with moderately severe disease may be treated with MTX, azathioprine, or mycophenolate mofetil (CellCept).

Patients with severe disease, including hemolytic anemia, thrombocytopenic purpura, massive pleural and pericardial involvement, renal damage, acute vasculitis, and/or florid CNS involvement, are treated with corticosteroids as first-line therapy. Immunosuppressants are typically added to the corticosteroid regimen, including azathioprine (Imuran) and cyclophosphamide (Cytoxan). Patients with renal involvement may be treated with IV Cytoxan together with mesna (Mesnex) on a monthly basis. Mesna is given to protect the bladder mucosa from the effects of cyclophosphamide.

Severe exacerbations of SLE often require 4–12 weeks for recovery. Thromboembolic events, including emboli in placental vessels during pregnancy, require treatment with heparin and long-term Coumadin. Patients who are positive for anticardiolipin antibodies should be treated with heparin or low-dose aspirin during pregnancy. Patients with recurrent thromboses and positive antiphospholipid antibodies should be treated lifelong with **Coumadin with a target INR of 3**.

Patients with SLE experience accelerated levels of atherosclerosis and should be closely monitored. Lifestyle changes should be instituted to modify all possible risk factors for coronary artery disease.

Recent lab studies showed the G6PD to be normal, aldolase negative, dsDNA negative. Sm and RNP negative. SS-A is greater than 8. SS-B negative. Vitamin D 21. CCP negative. ANA is 1:1280, both the speckled and Ro pattern.

Recheck the CBC, CMP, ESR, CRP, C3, and C4. Continue the Plaquenil and for now continue artificial tears, increase oral fluid intake, avoid sweetened candy.

(9) Raynaud phenomenon is a blanching of the fingers due to vasospasm and subsequent decreased blood flow.

Sjögren Syndrome

Sjögren syndrome (SS) is an autoimmune disorder affecting the exocrine glands. It may be primary or associated with other autoimmune disorders such as rheumatoid arthritis, SLE, **primary biliary cirrhosis**, scleroderma, Hashimoto thyroiditis, polyarteritis, or interstitial pulmonary fibrosis. Primary SS is associated with HLA-DR2 and HLA-DR3.

The pathologic mechanism, as with other autoimmune disorders, is not entirely understood. Salivary, lacrimal, and other exocrine glands become infiltrated with CD4-positive T cells and B cells that produce inflammatory cytokines. The chronic inflammatory response damages secretory epithelium and decreases tear production, saliva, and other protective and lubricating fluids. A decrease of tears results in keratoconjunctivitis sicca with possible corneal damage. Severe cases may cause epithelial strands on the corneal surface (**keratitis filiformis**). Diminished saliva (**xerostomia**) causes dysgeusia and dysphagia, especially for dry foods such as crackers. Xerostomia predisposes patients to dental caries and thrush. The **parotid glands** become enlarged in about a third of patients with SS. The skin and mucous membranes of the respiratory, gastrointestinal, and urogenital tracts may also be affected.

 Be sure you do not transcribe carotid glands instead of parotid glands.

A number of patients also experience a nondestructive, nondeforming arthritis. Other extraglandular manifestations include generalized lymphadenopathy, **Raynaud phenomenon,** (9) parenchymal lung involvement, and vasculitis. The kidneys may also be affected, resulting in mild renal impairment. Patients with SS show an increased risk of developing non-Hodgkin lymphoma.

Diagnosing primary Sjögren syndrome can be problematic, as there is much overlap in symptoms with RA, scleroderma, and other autoimmune disorders. SS should be suspected in patients with dry eyes or dry mouth, enlarged salivary glands, peripheral neuropathy, purpura, or unexplained renal tubular acidosis. Diagnosis is made based on serological tests, ophthalmologic examination, and biopsy of the lip.

The **Schirmer test** is a simple test that measures the quantity of tears secreted. It is performed by placing a

- Rheumatoid arthritis is a systemic autoimmune disorder that affects the synovial membranes of the peripheral joints. Symptoms include pain and stiffness with destruction of the joints primarily in the hands and feet, hips, and knees. Systemic symptoms include malaise, weakness, fatigue, and weight loss. Diagnosis is based on x-ray studies and serological studies, including elevated titers of anti-CCP and RF. Treatment includes analgesics, NSAIDs, and DMARDs.

- Systemic lupus erythematosus is an autoimmune disorder that affects multiple organ systems. Antigen-antibody complexes form in the skin, capillaries, and organs causing the activation of complement and subsequent tissue destruction. Symptoms and severity of disease vary widely. Diagnosis is based on symptoms and serological studies, including anti-dsDNA, anti-Sm, anticardiolipin antibodies, positive ANA, and positive lupus anticoagulant. Treatment includes NSAIDs, antimalarial medications, and immunosuppressants.

- Sjögren syndrome is an autoimmune disorder affecting the exocrine glands. Symptoms include dry mouth, dry eyes, arthritis, lymphadenopathy, and Raynaud phenomenon. Diagnosis is based on positive serological studies including anti-SS-A and anti-SS-B. Treatment is primarily symptomatic with eyedrops and strategies to moisten the mouth.

piece of filter paper under the lower eyelid and noting the degree of saturation after five minutes. A more specific test places a drop of rose Bengal or lissamine green solution on the eye. Devitalized areas of the cornea will take up the stain. Biopsy of the lip showing lymphocytic infiltration of the **accessory salivary glands** is diagnostic for Sjögren's.

Patients with SS may be **seropositive** for rheumatoid factor, antinuclear antibodies, and the cytoplasmic antibodies **SS-A (Sjögren syndrome antigen A)** and **SS-B (Sjögren syndrome antigen B)**. SS-A and SS-B are also called Ro and La respectively.

Treatment is primarily symptomatic. Artificial tears applied several times a day relieves dry eyes. Sipping water, chewing gum, or sucking on hard candies helps with xerostomia. Pilocarpine or cevimeline may be prescribed as well.

ASSESSMENT: Sjögren's based on a positive ANA, dsDNA, with dry eyes and dry mouth. Biopsy is positive with positive Schirmer test. Need to rule out underlying systemic lupus erythematosus.

Mixed Connective Tissue Disease

Mixed connective tissue disease (MCTD) is diagnosed when symptoms of lupus, systemic sclerosis, rheumatoid arthritis, and polymyositis overlap. Cardinal features of MCTD include Raynaud phenomenon, swollen hands, arthritis and arthralgia, acrosclerosis, esophageal dysmotility, myositis, and pulmonary hypertension. Patients must have antibodies against RNP and **small nuclear ribonucleoprotein (snRNP)**. Treatment is similar to that of SLE but the prognosis is less favorable than SLE. Infection is a major cause of death.

Immunodeficiency

Immunodeficiency disorders may be primary or secondary. In all cases, they predispose patients to infection. Primary immunodeficiencies are genetically determined. The majority of primary immunodeficiencies are caused by B-cell defects that decrease antibody titers. These patients are at increased risk of infection from encapsulated gram-positive bacteria. The most common B-cell disorder is **selective IgA deficiency**.

T-cell disorders make up 5% to 10% of primary immunodeficiencies. Defects in T cells increase a patient's susceptibility to opportunistic infections as well as many common pathogens. Since plasma cells are dependent upon T cells for stimulation, many T-cell disorders also cause immunoglobulin deficiencies. Examples of T-cell disorders include DiGeorge syndrome, ZAP-70 deficiency, X-linked lymphoproliferative syndrome, and chronic mucocutaneous candidiasis.

About 20% of primary immunodeficiencies are classified as combined B- and T-cell defects, the most common of which is **severe combined immunodeficiency (SCID)**. Primary defects may also be found in the complement system and NK cells, but these are rare. Defects in phagocytic cells (monocytes, macrophages, and granulocytes) are found in about 15% to 20% of immunodeficient patients and predispose patients to cutaneous staphylococcal and gram-negative infections. The most common phagocytic cell defects include chronic granulomatous disease, leukocyte adhesion deficiency, and Chédiak-Higashi syndrome.

Secondary, or acquired, immunodeficiencies are more common than primary. There are many causes for secondary immunodeficiency, including undernutrition or malnutrition, and immunosuppressive treatments such as chemotherapy and radiation therapy. Chronically or critically ill patients as well as elderly patients may also have impaired immune responses. The most significant secondary immunodeficiency is AIDS.

AIDS

Acquired immunodeficiency syndrome (AIDS) is caused by infection with the **Human immunodeficiency virus (HIV)**. AIDS is distinguished from inborn causes of immunodeficiency because it is an *acquired* deficiency (ie, not genetically determined). There are two forms of HIV (HIV-1 and HIV-2), but HIV-1 is predominant. Both are **retroviruses**, meaning their chromosomal material is stored in the form of RNA (instead of DNA). RNA viruses use **reverse transcriptase** to convert their RNA to DNA once they have infected a host cell. This is an important distinction in both the pathophysiology and the treatment of HIV infection.

Viruses are very simple organisms. Generally, they consist of an envelope surrounding genetic material. They must incorporate their genetic material into the

(10) Opportunistic pathogens are organisms that normally do not cause disease. These organisms take the opportunity to thrive when the immune system is too debilitated to keep them under control. Most opportunistic organisms are a normal part of the environment and may even be a part of the body's normal flora.

host cell's genetic material and use the manufacturing capabilities of the host to replicate. HIV attaches to CD4+ lymphocytes and penetrates the T cell's membrane. Once inside the host cell, reverse transcriptase converts the RNA to DNA that is then incorporated into the host's DNA (■ Figure 10-6). The transcription from RNA to DNA actually results in many "errors," creating mutations, and this variability creates challenges for the host to control the virus. These mutations increase the chances of producing strains resistant to both host immunity and drugs and make effective vaccinations against the virus an elusive target.

HIV infection of CD4+ lymphocytes causes depletion of this important T-cell subtype. The normal CD4+ count is about 750 cells/mcL. When the CD4+ count drops below 200 cells/mcL, a variety of opportunistic pathogens (10) escapes control of the immune system and produces disease. Because CD4+ cells play an integral role in the initiation, propagation, and termination of an immune response, a reduction in these cells has a profound effect on the entire immune system, including the humoral immune system. Without the normal controls imposed on B cells by the T helper cells (CD4+), B cells become dysregulated and secrete excess antibodies to previously encountered antigens, resulting in **hyperglobulinemia**. Also, without the assistance of T helper cells, B cells are unable to produce sufficient antibodies to any *newly* encountered antigens, including vaccines. Both the humoral and cell-mediated responses are affected, but the cell-mediated immune response is affected more so, leading to a predominance of nonbacterial infections (mostly fungal and viral). HIV also infects nonlymphoid cells, including dendritic cells in the skin, macrophages, and brain microglia, as well as the heart and kidneys.

HIV infection displays three clinical stages: acute seroconversion, asymptomatic infection, and AIDS. Seroconversion occurs within weeks to months of the initial infection. The patient may experience a flu-like illness with fever, lymphadenopathy, and rash. This stage is often attributed to mononucleosis or a nonspecific viral infection. Following this, the patient enters an asymptomatic phase that can last as long as ten years. Before symptoms of AIDS develop, the patient is described as being HIV-positive. A patient is diagnosed with AIDS when their CD4+ T-cell count falls to 200 cells/mcL or less and they develop clinical

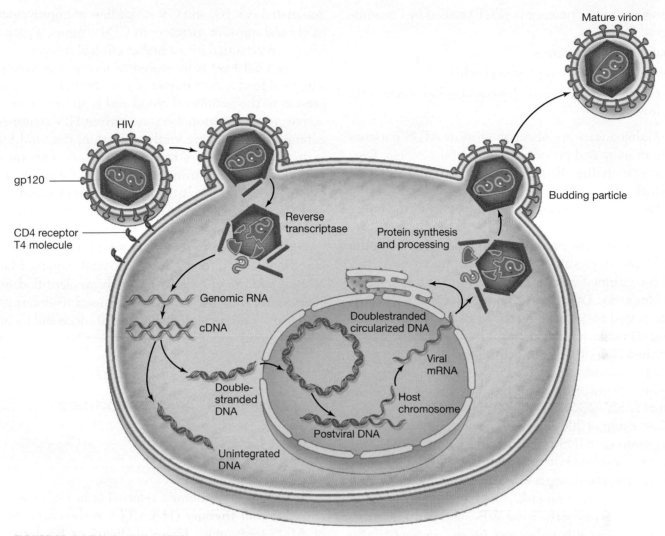

FIGURE 10-6 HIV infecting a CD4+ cell.

signs of the disease, including opportunistic infections, **Kaposi sarcoma**, lymphoma, and/or neurologic dysfunction.

The average interval between initial HIV infection and progression to AIDS is eight to ten years. Often, patients present with generalized lymphadenopathy. A CBC typically reveals mild-to-moderate **cytopenias** (leukopenia, anemia, and/or thrombocytopenia). AIDS manifests as recurrent and severe infections caused by opportunistic organisms as well as malignancies. AIDS may also cause dementia, encephalopathy, and **wasting syndrome** marked by weight loss and loss of muscle mass. Common symptoms include painful mucosal lesions and white plaques caused by candida, painful rash due to herpes zoster (VZV), diarrhea, fatigue, and fever. The following opportunistic infections are seen in immunocompromised patients, especially in AIDS patients:

- candidiasis anywhere in the upper respiratory tract
- coccidioidomycoses (Coccidioides immitis)
- cryptococcosis (Cryptococcus)
- cryptosporidiosis (Cryptosporidium)
- cytomegalovirus (CMV)
- herpes simplex virus (HSV)
- histoplasmosis (Histoplasma)
- isosporiasis (Isospora)
- mycobacterial infection (Mycobacterium avium-intracellulare complex [MAC], Mycobacterium kansasii, Mycobacterium tuberculosis)

- pneumocystis pneumonia (PCP) caused by Pneumocystis jiroveci
- salmonella septicemia
- toxoplasmosis (Toxoplasma gondii)
- progressive multifocal leukoencephalopathy (JC virus)

Malignancies are also common in AIDS patients with an increased prevalence of Kaposi sarcoma, lymphoma, including **Burkitt lymphoma**, and invasive cervical cancer.

Patients with recurrent, serious opportunistic infections should be evaluated for HIV infection. Serology tests can detect the presence of antibodies to HIV using ELISA techniques as a screening test. A positive ELISA test is confirmed with a more sensitive test, the **Western blot assay**. Laboratory tests for detecting the actual virus as well as quantifying the virus are also available using **reverse transcription-PCR (RT-PCR)** or branched DNA (bDNA) technology.

CD4$^+$ counts are used as a diagnostic tool and for ongoing monitoring. The reference range for CD4 counts is 500–2000 cells/mcL. For statistical tracking, a CD4$^+$ count of 200 cells/mcL is the defining cutoff for a diagnosis of AIDS in the United States. The CD4$^+$ count is considered the best indicator of risk for opportunistic infection, with counts below 200 cells/mcL presenting the highest risk. The CD4$^+$ count is determined by measuring the total WBC and multiplying by the percentage of lymphocytes (as determined by the CBC differential). That value is multiplied by the percentage of lymphocytes that are CD4$^+$.

Once diagnosed, patients are staged into one of three categories. The stage is based on clinical presentation as well as CD4$^+$ cell counts:

- category A: positive HIV serology without a history of symptoms of AIDS
- category B: HIV infection with symptoms directly attributable to a defect in T-cell-mediated immunity
- category C: HIV infection characterized by manifestations of opportunistic infections (as listed above)

Patients may be classified into a subcategory based on their CD4$^+$ T-cell count. Subcategories A1, B1, and C1 are characterized by CD4$^+$ counts greater than 500 cells/mcL. Categories A1, B2, and C2 are marked by CD4$^+$ counts between 200 cells/mcL and 400 cells/mcL. Patients with counts less than 200 cells/mcL are

designated A3, B3, and C3. Regardless of improvement in clinical status or increases in CD4$^+$ counts, a patient is never reclassified into a higher clinical category.

The viral load is measured to monitor treatment. The viral load is the number of virus particles (virions) present in the peripheral blood and is an indication of active viral replication. Because current HIV treatment is targeted at reducing viral replication, the viral load is the best indicator of treatment efficacy. Laboratory methods for determining the viral load measure the quantity of viral RNA using **nucleic acid sequence-based amplification (NASBA)**, reverse transcription PCR (RT-PCR), or similar technologies.

HIV is known to mutate at a high rate, and these mutations lead to resistance to antiviral therapy. Many of these patterns of resistance have been identified, and **genotyping** the viral RNA can be used to determine which antiviral therapies will be most successful for any given patient.

Pause 10-4 Describe genotyping.

Antiretroviral therapy, referred to as **highly active antiretroviral therapy (HAART)**, is the cornerstone of AIDS treatment. These medications hinder viral replication and have significantly increased patient longevity. No treatment is curative; the goal is to reduce the **plasma HIV RNA level** and increase the CD4$^+$ count in order to prevent opportunistic infections. Despite therapy, AIDS is eventually fatal. Causes of death often include refractory opportunistic infections, cancer, and liver failure due to hepatitis B or C. Therapy typically includes a combination of two or three drugs from different antiviral classes.

HISTORY OF PRESENT ILLNESS: The patient is a 46-year-old right-handed male with a history of HIV, on HAART, with CD4 count greater than 300, who recently was discharged after a 42-day course of antibiotics for MRSA secondary to an abscess in his right groin.

The classes of antiviral drugs include:

- nucleoside reverse transcriptase inhibitors (NRTIs)
- nucleotide reverse transcriptase inhibitors (nRTIs)
- non-nucleoside reverse transcriptase inhibitors (NNRTIs)
- protease inhibitors (PIs)
- entry inhibitors (EIs)
- integrase inhibitors

The efficacy of the treatment regimen is assessed by measuring plasma HIV RNA levels every four to eight weeks. The goal is to achieve a viral load of less than 50 copies/mL. Therapy should be monitored closely and adjusted as necessary, as some virions develop resistance to one or more of the drugs. Several classes of anti-retrovirals are given concomitantly to provide maximum coverage. Patients may also require intermittent or long-term prophylaxis for opportunistic infections such as PCP and toxoplasmosis. Common antibiotics include TMP-SMX, dapsone (Aczone), pentamidine, or atovaquone. Azithromycin is used to prevent Mycobacterium avium complex (MAC). Fluconazole (Diflucan) is commonly given to prevent or treat fungal infections, especially candidiasis and cryptococcal infections.

Transplantation

Transplantation is the transfer of cells, tissues, or organs (called a graft). Cellular transplants include **hematopoietic stem cells (HSC)**, lymphocytes, and pancreatic islet cells for the treatment of diabetes. Skin grafts are also used, either from donor banks or from autologous skin transferred from another area of the patient's body. Whole organs, such as liver, kidney, heart, lung, and pancreas may be transplanted, and in some cases, segments of organs (eg, lung or liver lobes) may be transplanted. Organ grafts may be placed in the anatomically normal position, called an **orthotopic transplant** (eg, the heart). Alternatively, organs may be transplanted in a different location, such as a kidney transplanted to the iliac fossa, referred to as a **heterotopic transplant**. Several types of grafts are routinely performed:

- **autograft:** a graft consisting of the patient's own tissue (eg bone, bone marrow, skin)
- **isograft:** a graft consisting of syngeneic (genetically identical) donor tissue
- **allograft:** a graft consisting of genetically dissimilar donor tissue

- **xenografts:** a graft consisting of tissue from a different species (eg, heart valves from pigs)

The majority of transplants, especially organ transplants, are allografts from **living related donors**, **living unrelated donors**, or cadaveric donors. Kidneys and hematopoietic stem cells (ie, bone marrow) are commonly derived from living donors. It is becoming more common for living donors to donate segments of liver, pancreas, or lung.

The immune system's ability to detect and destroy foreign tissue presents a formidable barrier to transplantation as a routine medical treatment. The degree of immune response depends on the degree of **histocompatibility**, or genetic disparity, between the graft and the host. Destruction of the graft following transplantation is referred to as **rejection**. Some organs or tissues are less prone to rejection than other tissues. For example, the eye is immunologically privileged, meaning it has minimal immune system cells and can tolerate a mismatched graft.

To decrease the risk of rejection, recipients and donors are screened for compatibility and presensitization. In many cases, it is imperative to match donors and recipients for **ABO (blood group) antigens**. HLA typing may be performed to match as many histocompatibility (MHC) antigens as possible, although time constraints do not typically allow for HLA typing of cadaveric organ transplants. In the US, only two of six antigens on average are matched between kidney donors and recipients. Recipients are screened for the presence of **presensitization antibodies** that develop against HLA and ABO antigens as a result of prior transfusions, multiple pregnancies, or a previous transplant. These antibodies may react with the new graft, causing immediate rejection. Compatibility screening is called **tissue typing** or **crossmatching**, and includes the following tests:

- ABO blood group compatibility
- **lymphocytotoxicity assay**, which tests the recipient's sera against donor lymphocytes. A positive reaction indicates the recipient already has antibodies to antigens on the donor's cells and is a contraindication for transplantation.
- **panel-reactive antibody (PRA)**, which tests the recipient's sera against a panel of common lymphocyte antigens for the presence of presensitization antibodies

In addition to screening for incompatibility, both donor and recipient must be tested for active and latent infections including cytomegalovirus (CMV), Epstein-Barr virus (EBV), herpes simplex virus (HSV), varicella-zoster virus (VZV), hepatitis B and C viruses, HIV, West Nile virus (if exposure is suspected), and TB.

Rejection of transplanted tissue is carried out by both cellular and humoral arms of the immune system, although the T cells are the central component in graft rejection. Natural killer (NK) cells also play a role in graft rejection through direct cytolytic effects on graft cells. In addition, the transplanted organ carries with it "passenger" interstitial dendritic cells with a high density of MHC molecules. These passenger donor cells are a major source of recipient immune stimulation and play a significant role in organ rejection.

> **Pause 10-5** Explain in layman's terms the role of passenger dendritic cells in organ rejection.

Immunosuppression is the primary approach to protecting the graft and prolonging graft survival. Unfortunately, immunosuppressant drugs quash many immune functions and cause most posttransplantation complications, including life-threatening infections. Immunosuppressants are typically taken for the remainder of the patient's life. Classes of immunosuppressants include:

- corticosteroids
- **calcineurin inhibitors** (cyclosporin, tacrolimus)
- **antiproliferative agents** (azathioprine, mycophenolate mofetil)
- **rapamycin** (sirolimus, everolimus)
- **immunoglobulin therapy** (antilymphocyte globulin [ALG], antithymocyte globulin [ATC], monoclonal antibodies [basiliximab, daclizumab])

Rejection may be hyperacute, accelerated, acute, or chronic. Hyperacute rejection, which has become quite rare with improved pretransplant screening, occurs in the first 48 hours following transplantation. It is caused by preexisting antibodies that form antigen-antibody complexes and activate the complement system, causing massive small-vessel thrombosis and graft infarction. When this occurs, the only course of action is to remove the graft.

Acute rejection is mediated by lymphocytes that have been activated by donor dendritic cells (passenger leukocytes). Donor tissue shows hemorrhage, edema, and necrosis. This type of rejection accounts for about half of all rejections and occurs within the first six months following transplantation. Acute rejection may be reversed by intensifying immunosuppressive therapy.

Accelerated rejection occurs three to five days following transplantation. It is also caused by preexisting antibodies against the graft, but these antibodies do not fix complement. Treatment is with high-dose corticosteroids and antilymphocyte preparations.

Chronic rejection occurs months or even years after transplantation and is mainly manifest as fibrosis and graft dysfunction. Causes include **periprocedural ischemia**, **reperfusion injury**, infection, hypertension, hyperlipidemia (a common side effect of immunosuppressive therapy), or immune-mediated rejection by both antibodies and T cells. Proliferation of neointima leading to transplantation atherosclerosis eventually occludes blood vessels, resulting in patchy ischemia and fibrosis of the graft. Heart transplants show accelerated coronary artery atherosclerosis. Transplanted lungs may develop **bronchiolitis obliterans**. Liver transplants show **vanishing bile duct syndrome**. Kidneys display glomerulopathy (**chronic allograft nephropathy**). Currently, there is no treatment to stall or reverse chronic rejection.

> **Pause 10-6** Explain this statement in layman's terms: Proliferation of neointima leading to transplantation atherosclerosis eventually occludes blood vessels, resulting in patchy ischemia and fibrosis of the graft.

Infection due to immunosuppression is a major threat to both the transplanted tissue and to the host. In the postoperative period, transplant patients may contract the same **nosocomial** infections as other surgical patients, including Pseudomonas species and gram-positive bacteria that are prone to infect wounds. Early infection of the graft, the graft's vascular supply, or suture sites can cause mycotic aneurysms or dehiscence. Opportunistic infections may occur after one to six months of immunosuppression. Common pathogens are the same as those affecting AIDS patients: CMV, EBV, VZV, hepatitis B or C, listeria, nocardia, aspergillus, cryptococcus, Pneumocystis, toxoplasma, strongyloides,

- Immunodeficiency disorders may be inherited or acquired, the majority of which are acquired (secondary). Common causes of acquired immunodeficiency include undernutrition or malnutrition, immunosuppressive treatment such as chemotherapy and radiation, and advanced age. HIV infection is a significant cause of acquired immunodeficiency.

- AIDS is caused by an infection with HIV. The virus affects CD4+ lymphocytes, which leads to a severe crippling of the immune response. Manifestations include frequent infection by opportunistic organisms, malignancies, cachexia, and neurologic disorders. Diagnosis is based on serological studies and CD4+ cell counts. The cornerstone of treatment includes HAART and antimicrobial therapy. Therapy is monitored using CD4+ cell counts and viral load.

- Transplantation is the transfer of cells, tissues, or organs. A transplant may be classified as an autograft, isograft, allograft, or xenograft. When possible, donors and recipients are matched for ABO and HLA compatibility. Immunosuppressant drugs are given to protect the graft from rejection, but these drugs also place the patient at risk of infection. Graft vs host disease may also occur when leukocytes are transferred from donor to recipient.

and leishmania. After six months, the risk of infection returns to baseline for the majority of patients.

Other potential complications of transplantation include viral-induced cancers such as hepatocellular carcinoma (hepatitis B or C), lymphoproliferative disorders such as B-cell non-Hodgkin lymphoma, cervical cancer, Kaposi sarcoma, and basal cell carcinoma. Side effects of long-term use of immunosuppressive therapy also include hyperlipidemia, failure to grow (children), and osteoporosis.

Graft vs host disease (GVHD) is caused by donor T cells that act on the host's cells. GVHD is most common in bone marrow transplants (HSC recipients). It may also be caused by passenger lymphocytes in liver and small-bowel transplant recipients.

Laboratory Studies

The laboratory plays a significant role in the diagnosis and management of immune-system disorders.

Serology

Serological assays measure the level of antigens and antibodies in serum, which is the watery portion of the blood that is obtained after the sample has clotted and has been separated from the cells and platelets. Several methods are used to measure antigens and antibodies:

Western blot: an assay that first separates proteins using electrophoresis and then identifies bands of proteins using monoclonal antibodies. Electrophoresis uses an electrical current applied to a special gel, causing molecules to move toward a positively or negatively charged pole. Proteins travel across the gel in response to electrical current, and the distance traveled is determined by the molecular weight and positive or negative charge of the protein molecule. The exact distance traveled can be used to identify proteins. The Western blot technique is most known for its use as a confirmatory test for HIV.

Agglutination assays: tiny latex beads are coated with a specific antigen and then suspended in the patient's serum. If antibodies are present in the patient's serum, the antibodies bind to the antigens on the surface of the beads and cause the beads to clump or agglutinate and fall out of solution. The clumps can be visualized, indicating a positive test.

Enzyme-linked immunosorbent assay (ELISA, pronounced $\bar{e}$ $l\bar{\imath}'z\partial$): Purified antigens are fixed to the surface of a tiny test tube (called a microtiter well) or to beads. The patient's serum is then added and antibodies present in the serum will attach to the fixed antigens. A second antihuman antibody (with an enzyme attached) is added to the test well. This antibody will recognize the patient's antibodies that are attached to the fixed antigen, creating a "sandwich" (antigen-antibody-antibody). Finally, an enzyme substrate is added that reacts with the enzyme attached to the antibody (■ **Figure 10-7**). The enzyme creates a color reaction that can be measured with a spectrophotometer. The intensity of the color is proportional to the amount of antibody being assayed. This test can also be reversed by affixing a specific antibody to the microtiter well and measuring a specific antigen. The results may be reported as a titer or as units. The antibody titer can be converted to units per milli-liter using a conversion

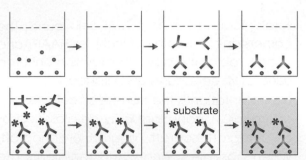

FIGURE 10-7 An ELISA test uses antigens fixed to a microtiter well to bind serum antibodies. A second antibody with enzyme attached is added followed by a substrate that creates a color change. The test is performed in a tray containing many small microtiter wells.

factor (based on the results of a known concentration of antibody).

Immunofluorescence antibody (IFA): This test is most commonly used to detect antibodies against cellular components such as the nucleus, centromeres, and mitochondria. A thin layer of cells is affixed to a microscope slide. The patient's serum is added to the slide and allowed to incubate. Next, antihuman antibodies with Fluorescein attached is added. These antibodies will react with any antibodies attached to the layer of cells. The slide is examined under a fluorescent microscope for the pattern of fluorescence.

Patterns reported by the lab include **speckled, homogeneous, centromere, nucleolar,** and **nucleolar/ cytoplasmic.**

Complement fixation: A known antigen, patient serum, and complement are added to a test container and allowed to react. Next, sheep red blood cells coated with antigen are added. If complement has not been fixed and consumed (ie, a negative reaction between the known antigen and the patient serum), the sheep red blood cells will lyse in the presence of complement. If complement has been consumed by the first reaction, the sheep cells will not lyse.

The following antigens, antibodies, and complement levels are commonly measured in the laboratory for the diagnosis and management of autoimmune disorders.

Autoantibodies

Antibodies are normally produced against "foreign" antigens (microorganisms, foods, pollens, etc), but the immune system is also known to erroneously create antibodies against the body's own cellular components. Certain autoimmune antibodies can be detected in the serum of patients with autoimmune hepatitis, primary biliary cirrhosis, primary sclerosing cholangitis, and other autoimmune diseases (**Table 10-4**).

Table 10-4 Autoantibodies Associated with Autoimmune Diseases

Test	Abbreviation	Reference Range
rheumatoid factor	RF	0–15 units/mL
anticyclic citrullinated peptide	anti-CCP	0–30 units/mL
antinuclear antibodies	ANA	1:40 borderline positive >1:160
anti-ribonucleoprotein	anti-RNP	negative
anti-double-stranded DNA	anti-dsDNA	0–4 units/mL
anti-Smith	anti-Sm	negative
Sjögren syndrome A antibody	anti-SS-A (Ro)	negative
Sjögren syndrome B antibody	anti-SS-B (La)	negative
anti-ribonucleic acid protein	anti-RNP	negative
anti-SCL-70	anti-SCL-70	negative
anti-smooth muscle	ASMA	<1:20 (<20 units)

29

Table 10-4 Autoantibodies Associated with Autoimmune Diseases (*Continued*)

Test	Abbreviation	Reference Range
thyroid peroxidase antibody	anti-TPO	<35 units/mL
anticardiolipin antibodies (antiphospholipid antibodies)	ACA	IgG 0–20 GPL units/mL IgM 0–10 MPL units/mL
lupus anticoagulant	LA	Actual antibody levels not assayed. Negative results based on prolongation of the aPTT without correction and prolonged Russell viper venom time. See also page 394.
68 kd antibody (HSP-70)		negative
ribosomal P antibody		negative (<1.0 unit/mL)
beta 2-glycoprotein I antibody		IgA ≤ 20 SAU IgG ≤ 20 SGU IgM ≤ 20 SMU
Coombs test		negative (see also page 425). Positive test indicates presence of antibodies attached to RBCs.
classic antineutrophil cytoplasmic antibody, also called PR3 ANCA	c-ANCA	0–20 units/mL
perinuclear antineutrophil cytoplasmic antibody, also called MPO ANCA	p-ANCA	0–20 units/mL
parietal cell antibodies		negative (positive results reported in titers)
antimitochondrial antibody	AMA	<1:20 (<1.0 unit/mL) weak positive 1:20 to 1:80 (1.0 to 1.3 units/mL) positive >1:160 (>1.3 units/mL)
F actin		<20 units/mL weak positive 20–30 units/mL positive >30 units/mL

Antibodies may be reported in titers or in units. The titer represents the highest dilution of the serum at which the antibody is still detectable. For example, in the ELISA test described above, the serum is serially diluted (eg, 1:2; 1:4; 1:8; 1:16 and so on). Each dilution of the serum is added to a test well in the microtiter tray. Eventually, the serum will become so dilute that there will be too few antibodies to be detected. The last positive (detectable) dilution is reported as the titer. The higher the dilution, the higher the titer, the more antibodies are present in the serum. Therefore, a titer of 1:4 represents a smaller number of antibodies than a titer of 1:16. More recently, tests have been developed using enzyme immunoassays that report antibody levels in units.

The prefix *anti–* is added to the name of the antigen to signify an antibody directed against that antigen. Dictators do not always dictate "anti"; sometimes when dictating the serology results, they will simply give the name of the antigen with the assumption that they are referring to the antibody against that antigen.

Markers of Inflammation

Two general markers of inflammation are the erythrocyte sedimentation rate (ESR) and the C-reactive protein (CRP) tests (**Table 10-5**). Neither of these tests indicates the cause or the location of the inflammation, but both are used as screening and monitoring tests to assess the degree of inflammation.

The ESR, also called the **sed rate**, is a measure of how quickly red cells fall out of solution. It is determined by allowing a narrow column of blood, which is marked off in millimeters, to stand for one hour, allowing the red cells to settle (sediment). At the end of the hour, the level of the blood cells is noted. Inflammatory reactions change the composition of proteins in the blood and cause red cells to agglutinate. The clumped red cells fall faster, increasing the sedimentation rate (■ **Figure 10-8**).

Table 10-5 Markers of Inflammation

Test Name	Reference Range
erythrocyte sedimentation rate (ESR) Westergren method	female: 0–20 mm/h male: 0–15 mm/h
C-reactive protein (CRP)	<0.5 mg/dL

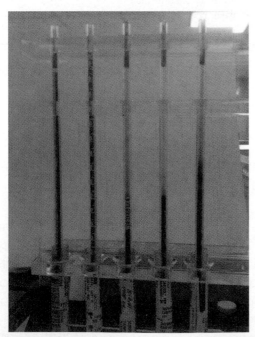

FIGURE 10-8 Samples being tested for erythrocyte sedimentation rate using the Westergren method. The two samples on the left have a low sed rate. The three samples on the right show an elevated sed rate. *Source:* Courtesy of Rebecca Ardoin.

> Dictators may dictate either "sed rate" or the initials ESR. The number is dictated, but the units (mm/h) are almost never dictated. It is acceptable to simply type the value (eg, The sed rate today is 15).

Complement

Components of the complement system (**Table 10-6**) may be measured to help diagnose a chronic immune disorder such as SLE, RA, and glomerulonephritis. Total complement levels are decreased over time as these proteins are consumed by disorders that produce immune complexes. CH50 measures total complement activity and is decreased when all of the components are being consumed. Complement may be activated in several ways, and depending on the activation path, consumes different components of the complement system. The individual components C3 and C4 are measured to determine which pathway is being activated. Relative values of C3 and C4 are indicative of specific disorders.

Table 10-6 Complement Levels

Test Name	Reference Range
CH50	142–279 units/mL
C3	83–172 mg/dL
C4	14–40 mg/dL

Immunoglobulin Assays

The amount of any single *class* of immunoglobulin may be measured (**Table 10-7**). These tests are used to determine specific deficiencies or gammopathies within a single class of immunoglobulins.

Table 10-7 Immunoglobulin Classes

Test Name	Reference Range
IgG	650–1700 mg/dL
IgA	40–350 mg/dL
IgM	40–350 mg/dL
IgD	0–8 mg/dL
IgE	1–120 mg/dL

The immunoglobulins are part of the total serum protein concentration, so the immunoglobulin values (in part or in total) should never exceed the reported value of total protein.

Allergy Testing

Allergy may be tested using skin tests or serum tests. Skin testing uses standardized concentrations of a given antigen injected directly into the skin (percutaneous prick or intradermal injection). A positive reaction is indicated by a wheal or flare. The most commonly used antigens are pollens (tree, grass, and weed), molds, house dust mites, animal danders and sera, insect venom, foods, and beta-lactam antibiotics. False positives occur in dermatographism (a wheal and flare reaction provoked by stroking or scraping the skin).

Serological tests include **radioallergosorbent testing (RAST)**. This test detects the presence of allergen-specific IgE in serum. To perform the test, a known allergen is mixed with the patient's serum. ^{125}I-labeled anti-IgE antibody is then added, which reacts with the patient's IgE. The amount of IgE can be quantified by measuring the amount of radioactivity in the test well.

Immunotherapy

Immunotherapy is used to desensitize an individual to an antigen (ie, induce tolerance), especially when the antigen cannot be avoided and drug treatment is inadequate. Desensitization is used to treat allergies for generally unavoidable antigens such as pollens, dust mites, molds, and insect venoms. The exact mechanism is not understood, but it is a widely used technique for lessening the effects of hypersensitivity responses. Immunotherapy consists of repeated injections of gradually increasing doses of antigen. Doses may also be placed under the tongue. The therapy requires repeated exposure (injections) given weekly, advancing to biweekly, and then monthly. The dose typically starts at 0.1 to 1.0 biologically active unit (BAU), depending on initial sensitivity, and is increased weekly or biweekly with each injection until a maximum tolerated concentration is reached.

Pharmacology

Treatment of allergic and immune disorders relies heavily on pharmaceutical agents, including antibiotics, immune suppressants, and biologically derived treatments such as monoclonal antibodies and cytokine antagonists.

DMARDs

The disease modifying antirheumatic drugs (DMARDs) do more than reduce symptomatology; they actually slow the progression of disease. The biologic DMARDs are those that are derived from biological molecules such as monoclonal antibodies. These agents are injected on various schedules ranging from several times weekly to every few weeks. They may be combined with other nonbiologic DMARDs such as methotrexate. The TNF-alpha blockers listed here (**Table 10-8**), also called TNF-alpha antagonists, block the action of tumor necrosis factor and lessen the inflammatory reaction in autoimmune disorders.

In addition to targeting TNF-alpha (as above), other biologic DMARDs (**Table 10-9**) target interleukin receptors or interfere with the stimulation of T cells.

Table 10-8 Biologic DMARDs—TNF-Alpha Blockers

Generic	Brand Name	Dose
adalimumab	Humira	40 mg subcutaneously every one to two weeks
etanercept	Enbrel	25 mg to 50 mg subcutaneously once or twice weekly
infliximab	Remicade	IV at weeks zero, two, and six; then every four to six weeks
golimumab	Simponi	50 mg subcutaneously monthly

Table 10-9 Other Biologic DMARDs

Generic	Brand Name	Dose
rituximab (anti-CD20)	Rituxan	IV infusions given two weeks apart, may be repeated every six months
abatacept (prevents stimulation of T cells)	Orencia	IV at weeks zero, two, and four; then every four weeks
tocilizumab (IL-6 receptor antagonist)	Actemra	monthly intravenous infusions
anakinra (IL-1 receptor antagonist)	Kineret	100 mg daily subcutaneously

The traditional DMARDs, also called xenobiotics (**Table 10-10**), are those treatments aimed at reducing the progression of rheumatic diseases but are not based on biological molecules. This group of medications includes two antimetabolites (methotrexate and leflunomide), the antimalarial drug hydroxychloroquine, and an antiprostaglandin (sulfasalazine).

Methotrexate is known to inhibit folate production that is needed for DNA, RNA, and protein synthesis, but its exact mode of action in inflammatory disorders is not fully understood. Because it inhibits synthesis of DNA, methotrexate is also considered an antimetabolite and an antineoplastic. Leflunomide interferes with an enzyme involved with pyrimidine metabolism, resulting in reduced inflammation.

Sulfasalazine, also used as an antibiotic, inhibits prostaglandin synthesis and thereby reduces inflammatory reactions. Hydroxychloroquine has been used to treat malaria as well as mild rheumatic disorders. It acts in inflammatory disorders by inhibiting dendritic cells.

Table 10-10 Xenobiotic DMARDs

Generic	Brand Name	Dose
methotrexate (MTX)	Rheumatrex	2.5 mg (tablets)
sulfasalazine	Azulfidine Azulfidine EN-tabs	500 mg
hydroxychloroquine	Plaquenil	200 mg
leflunomide	Arava	10 mg, 20 mg

Allergy Medications

Hypersensitivity reactions are treated with antihistamines, decongestants, and nasal corticosteroids.

Antihistamines

Antihistamines are given to counteract the effects of histamine (**Table 10-11**). First generation antihistamines work by blocking the effects of histamine on H_1 (histamine) receptors. This class of medication is known for causing drowsiness. The second-generation antihistamines are less sedating and have a longer half-life, with once-a-day dosing. Drugs in this class end in —*ine*.

Table 10-11 Antihistamines

Generic	Brand Name	Dose
First Generation		
diphenhydramine	Benadryl	12.5 mg, 25 mg, 50 mg
Second generation		
fexofenadine	Allegra	30 mg, 60 mg, 180 mg
cetirizine	Zyrtec	5 mg, 10 mg
desloratadine	Clarinex	2.5 mg, 5 mg
loratadine	Claritin	5 mg, 10 mg
azelastine	Astelin nasal spray	0.1% and 0.15% solutions

Intranasal Corticosteroids

Intranasal corticosteroids (**Table 10-12**) are used to treat allergic rhinitis. These medications decrease local inflammation, swelling of tissues, and irritation of mucosa.

Table 10-12 Intranasal Corticosteroids

Generic	Brand Name	Dose
fluticasone	Flonase	50 mcg/inhalation
mometasone	Nasonex	50 mcg/spray

Decongestants

Decongestants (**Table 10-13**) stimulate alpha-adrenergic receptors in the sympathetic nervous system causing nasal passages to constrict, which lessens swelling and congestion. They also dry mucous membranes and decrease drainage.

Table 10-13 Decongestants

Generic	Brand Name	Dose
pseudoephedrine	Sudafed Sudafed 12-Hour	30 mg, 60 mg 120 mg
phenylephrine	Neo-Synephrine	

Antiretroviral Therapy

Antiretroviral therapy (**Table 10-14**) for HIV takes several approaches. The entry inhibitors (EIs) block the CD4$^+$ receptor and prevent the virus from binding and entering the T cell. The reverse transcriptase inhibitors (NRTIs and NtRTIs) are nucleoside and nucleotide analogs that interfere with the transcription of the virus's RNA into DNA. The nonnucleoside inhibitors (NNRTIs) block the enzyme that transcribes the RNA into DNA. The protease inhibitors interfere with the maturation of the virus. HAART uses combinations of antiretrovirals (**Table 10-15**) to interfere with HIV replication at several key points.

Table 10-14 Antiretroviral Therapy

Generic	Brand Name	Dose
Reverse Transcriptase Inhibitors		
abacavir (ABC)	Ziagen	300 mg
lamivudine (3TC)	Epivir	100 mg, 150 mg, 300 mg
Protease Inhibitors		
darunavir (DRV)	Prezista	300 mg, 600 mg
tipranavir (TPV)	Aptivus	250 mg
ritonavir (RTV)	Norvir	100 mg
atazanavir (ATV)	Reyataz	100 mg, 150 mg, 200 mg, 300 mg
fosamprenavir (f-APV)	Lexiva	700 mg
lopinavir and ritonavir (LPV/r)	Kaletra	100/25 mg, 200/50 mg
NNRTIs		
efavirenz (EFV)	Sustiva	600 mg
nevirapine (NVP)	Viramune	200 mg
Fusion Inhibitor		
enfuvirtide	Fuzeon	108 mg
Integrase inhibitor		
raltegravir (RAL)	Isentress	400 mg

Table 10-15 Combination Drugs for HIV

Generic	Brand Name
abacavir and lamivudine	Epzicom
abacavir, lamivudine and zidovudine	Trizivir
efavirenz, emtricitabine and tenofovir DF	Atripla
emtricitabine and tenofovir DF	Truvada
lamivudine and zidovudine	Combivir

Immunosuppressive Therapy

There are several classes of immunosuppressive drugs:

- NSAIDS (Chapter 5, page 153)
- corticosteroids
- calcineurin inhibitors (cyclosporin, tacrolimus)
- antiproliferative agents (azathioprine, mycophenolate mofetil)
- rapamycin (sirolimus, everolimus)
- immunoglobulin therapy (antilymphocyte globulin [ALG], antithymocyte globulin [ATC], monoclonal antibodies [basiliximab, daclizumab])

Corticosteroids

Corticosteroids are the cornerstone of immunosuppressive drugs. They are still widely used but they have many side effects, especially with long-term use. Newer, more targeted drugs have been developed to achieve immunosuppression without the side-effect profile of steroids. Steroids still have value in treating acute episodes of inflammation. Oral and systemic steroids are listed in **Table 10-16**. Intraarticular injectable steroids are discussed in Chapter 5, page 152.

Table 10-16 Oral and Systemic Corticosteroids

Generic	Brand Name	Dose
prednisone		1 mg, 2.5 mg, 5 mg, 10 mg, 20 mg, 50 mg
methylprednisolone	Medrol	2 mg, 4 mg, 8 mg, 16 mg, 32 mg
	Medrol Dosepak	4 mg
hydrocortisone	Cortef	5 mg, 10 mg, 20 mg
dexamethasone	Decadron	0.5 mg, 0.75 mg, 1 mg, 1.5 mg, 2 mg, 4 mg, 6 mg

Calcineurin Inhibitors

Calcineurin inhibitors (**Table 10-17**) are potent immunosuppressants used to suppress an immune response following organ transplantation. These drugs block T-cell transcription processes required for production of IL-2. This effectively inhibits T-cell proliferation and activation.

Table 10-17 Calcineurin Inhibitors

Generic	Brand Name	Dose
cyclosporine	Neoral Sandimmune	25 mg, 100 mg
tacrolimus	Prograf	0.5 mg, 1 mg, 5 mg

Antiproliferative Agents

Antiproliferative agents (**Table 10-18**) inhibit DNA replication and suppress B- and T-cell proliferation. These agents are used in both autoimmune disorders and following organ transplantation.

Table 10-18 Antiproliferative Agents

Generic	Brand Name	Dose
azathioprine	Imuran	50 mg
mycophenolate mofetil	CellCept	500 mg

Rapamycin

Rapamycin, also called an mTOR inhibitor, blocks the action of IL-2 and causes the T-cell and B-cell cycle to stop at the G1-S phase of mitosis. These drugs are used in organ transplantation to prevent rejection (**Table 10-19**).

Table 10-19 Rapamycin Drugs

Generic	Brand Name	Dose
sirolimus	Rapamune	1 mg, 2 mg
everolimus	Zortress	0.25 mg, 0.5 mg, 0.75 mg

Immunosuppressive Immunoglobulins

Immunoglobulins directed against human lymphocytes (**Table 10-20**) are used to disable T cells, thereby suppressing cell-mediated immune reactions following organ transplantation. Antilymphocyte globulin (also called antithymocyte globulin and lymphocyte immune globulin) consists of polyclonal antibodies produced in either horses or rabbits. Because these antibodies are derived from other animals, they differ slightly from human antibodies, and the immune system may create neutralizing antibodies directed against the unique epitopes derived from the horse or rabbit.

Table 10-20 Antilymphocyte Globulin

Generic	Brand Name
ATG/ALG (lymphocyte immune globulin)	Atgam

Monoclonal Antibodies

Antibodies may also be directed against a specific receptor on the T-cell surface (**Table 10-21**). The monoclonal antibodies basiliximab and daclizumab are directed against IL-2 receptors on T cells. These antibodies deplete circulating T cells and inhibit cell-mediated and humoral immune responses. These particular agents are also given pretransplant as induction agents to reduce the number of T cells before the donor organ is placed.

OKT3, the first monoclonal antibody to be put into commercial use in 1986, is still used to prevent organ transplant rejection. This particular monoclonal antibody is directed against the T-cell CD3 antigen.

Table 10-21 Anti-T-Cell Monoclonal Antibodies

Generic	Brand Name
basiliximab	Simulect
daclizumab	Zenapax
OKT3 (muromonab)	Orthoclone OKT3

Exercises

Using Context to Make Decisions

Use the following excerpt to answer question #1.

> ANA has been done 3 times. The first in August, 20XX, was 1:320. Followup in January, 20XX, was 1:160, and repeat a week later was 1:80.

1. Based on this excerpt, the patient's antibody level is

    a. increasing

    b. decreasing

Use the following excerpt to answer question #2.

> MEDICATIONS
> 1. Sulfasalazine 500 mg 2 in the morning, 2 at night.
> 2. Prednisone once every 8 days.
> 3. Methotrexate 10 tablets every week.
> 4. Humira 40 mg every 2 weeks.
> 5. Folic acid 1 mg daily.
> 6. Calcium and vitamin D twice a day.

2. The most likely diagnosis for this patient is

    a. RA   **c.** AIDS

    b. SS   **d.** SLE

Use the following excerpt to answer questions 3–5.

> DIAGNOSTIC DATA
> The ANA was positive; however, the titer was not ordered. Labs drawn 2 years ago were negative for CCP, RNP, dsDNA, and SS-A antibodies. SS-B is 1.5. Smith negative, snRNP, and scleroderma centromere negative.
>
> ASSESSMENT
> 1. Sjögren's with positive ANA, dry eyes, dry mouth, and alopecia. Rule out underlying ____(1)____.
> 2. Acanthosis nigricans.

> PLAN
> As the patient is on intermittent chronic steroids, I would start the patient on calcium, vitamin D, and proceed with bone density. Will repeat the blood work including the CBC Chem 20 ESR CRP specific antibodies C3 and C4 UA double-stranded DNA hepatitis B and C TSH vitamin D rheumatoid factor anti-CCP.

3. Which of the following would most likely complete blank #1?

    a. atopy   **c.** RA

    b. SLE   **d.** hypersensitivity

4. The last sentence of the Diagnostic Data section is referring to

    a. antigens

    b. antibodies

    c. proteins

    d. abnormal cellular components

5. Which of the following is correctly punctuated?

    a. Will repeat the blood work including the CBC, Chem-20, ESR, CRP-specific, antibodies C3 and C4, UA, double-stranded DNA, hepatitis B and C, TSH, vitamin D, rheumatoid factor, anti-CCP.

    b. Will repeat the blood work including the CBC, Chem-20, ESR, CRP, specific antibodies, C3 and C4, UA, anti-dsDNA, hepatitis B and C, TSH, vitamin D, rheumatoid factor, anti-CCP.

    c. Will repeat the blood work including the CBC, Chem-20, ESR, CRP-specific antibodies, C3 and C4, UA, double-stranded DNA for hepatitis B and C, TSH, vitamin D, rheumatoid factor, anti-CCP.

    d. Will repeat the blood work including the CBC, Chem-20, ESR-CRP, specific antibodies, C3 and C4, UA double-stranded DNA, hepatitis B and C, TSH, vitamin D, rheumatoid factor, anti-CCP.

Use the following excerpt to answer questions 6 and 7.

ASSESSMENT

1. Rheumatoid arthritis. Positive for ___(1)___. and rheumatoid factor.

2. Parathyroid hormone is down again to 9.3.

3. History of kidney stone.

4. Anemia.

PLAN

Because of the increasing pain and synovitis, would add ___(2)___ 500 mg daily for the 1st week, twice a day in the 2nd week, 3 times a day in the 3rd week. Continue the methotrexate. Okay to use the prednisone 2.5 daily. Return visit in 6 weeks.

6. Which of the following goes in blank #1?

    a. anti-SS-A   c. anti-CCP

    b. anti-SS-B   d. anti-Smith

7. Which of the following goes in blank #2?

    a. Rheumatrex   c. Enbrel

    b. Rituxan   d. Sulfasalazine

Use the following excerpt to answer question #8.

HISTORY OF PRESENT ILLNESS: He is now taking the vitamin D 50,000 units daily. He still complains of significant pain in his back and neck. He has been given NSAIDs by his primary doctor. He takes ibuprofen p.r.n. and has been on multiple medications without much response. I explained to the patient that he really needs to be on an anti-TNF. His PPD and QuantiFERON-TB were negative.

8. What is the significance of the underlined comment?

    a. The patient was suspected to have active M tuberculosis.

    b. These are biologic markers for RA.

    c. The patient is being evaluated for immunodeficiency.

    d. These tests are necessary before initiating adalimumab.

Use the excerpt on page 342 to answer questions 9–11.

9. Which of the following completes blank #1?

    a. RA   c. SLE

    b. SS   d. HIV

10. Which of the following completes blank #2?

    a. antibiotic   c. monoclonal antibody

    b. HAART   d. steroid

11. Which of the following completes blank #3?

    a. antiretroviral

    b. immunosuppressive

    c. DMARD

    d. immunoglobulin

Terms Checkup

Complete the multiple choice questions for Chapter 10 located at www.myhealthprofessionskit.com. To access the questions, select the discipline "Medical Transcription," then click on the title of this book, *Advanced Medical Transcription*.

Look It Up

Using the guidelines described on page xvii, complete a research project on allergic rhinitis.

Transcription Practice

1. Transcribe the key terms and phrases for Chapter 10.

2. Complete the proofing and transcription practice exercises for Chapter 10.

HISTORY OF PRESENT ILLNESS: This is a 48-year-old black male with stage IV chronic kidney disease secondary to _____(1)_____ nephropathy. The patient's history of renal insufficiency dates back 3 years. At that time, he had a baseline creatinine between 3.2 and 3.3. When he was initially diagnosed with renal insufficiency, he had been noncompliant with his _____(2)_____ regimen. But since that time, he has been very compliant with his 3-drug _____(3)_____ therapy. His last CD4 count was 350.

MEDICATIONS
1. Kaletra daily.
2. Epivir 1 daily.
3. Ziagen 2 daily.
4. Lasix 20 mg b.i.d.
5. Valsartan 20 mg b.i.d.
6. Ambien 10 mg at bedtime.

Obstetrics and Gynecology

11

Preview Terms
Before studying this chapter, make sure you understand the following terms. Definitions can be found in the glossary.

Learning Objectives

After completing this chapter, you should be able to comprehend and correctly transcribe terminology related to:

▶ menstrual disorders including amenorrhea, dysfunctional uterine bleeding, and polycystic ovary syndrome

▶ pelvic disease including infection, leiomyoma, and endometriosis

▶ pregnancy, labor, and delivery

▶ therapeutic procedures used in gynecology

▶ laboratory and imaging studies used to diagnose and monitor gynecologic disorders

▶ laboratory and imaging studies used to monitor pregnancy

▶ drugs used in the treatment of gynecologic disorders

▶ drugs used in pregnancy, labor, and delivery

adrenarche
amenorrhea
aneuploid
dysmenorrhea
dyspareunia
hirsutism
karyotype
menarche
menometrorrhagia
menorrhagia
menstruation
metrorrhagia
oligomenorrhea
puberty
thelarche

Introduction

A large number of patient encounters in both the outpatient and inpatient settings involve gynecologic evaluations. Visits may involve an annual **well-woman exam** or evaluation for breast or pelvic disease. Obstetrical visits, including prenatal care and labor and delivery, also account for a significant number of patient encounters. Transcriptionists working in both acute care and ambulatory care will encounter many reports that involve gynecologic or obstetric terminology.

Anatomy and Physiology

The female reproductive system includes the breast tissue, external genitalia, and internal genitalia. Major components of the external genitalia are noted in ■ Figure 11-1.

The cervix is the neck of the uterus that connects the uterine body to the vagina. The cervix has an external os that opens to the vagina and an internal os that opens to the uterus. The area between the internal and external os is called the endocervix. The lower, narrower portion of the uterus is the isthmus. The central portion is referred to as the body and the upper portion is the fundus (■ Figure 11-2). The cornua are the horn-shaped areas projecting from the fundus that form the junction with the fallopian tubes. The uterine wall consists of several layers. The innermost layer is the endometrium. Under the endometrium is the myometrium, a layer of smooth muscle. The surrounding tissue is the perimetrium.

> **(1)** Adnexa is the plural form of adnexum. In reference to the uterine adnexa, the term is always plural because it refers to the fallopian tubes, ovaries, and related structures.

> Note the spelling of cornua/cornual. This term should not be confused with cornea and corneal.

The adnexa **(1)** include the ovaries, fallopian tubes, and structures of the broad ligaments. The fallopian tubes, also called the uterine tubes, extend laterally from the cornua of the uterus and end near the ovaries. Tubes are 10–14 cm in length and vary in diameter from about 1–3 cm. The tubes are suspended in the abdominal cavity by the mesosalpinx, a portion of the broad ligament. The fallopian tubes are divided into four anatomic regions: **infundibulum**, **ampulla**, **isthmus**, and **intramural** sections. The infundibulum (the tunnel-shaped end of the tube) has 20–30 fingerlike projections (**fimbriae**) that spread over the surface of the ovary to trap the ovum at the time of ovulation and sweep the ovum into the ampulla. The ampulla is about 4–6 cm in length and is the widest region of the tube. Fertilization typically takes place in this part of the tube. The isthmus is the

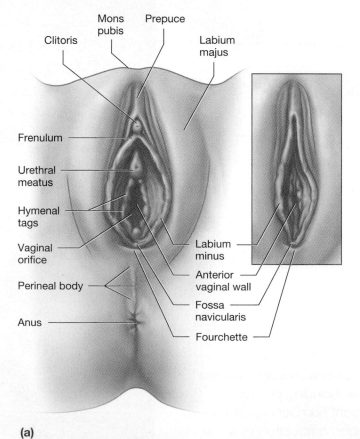

(a)

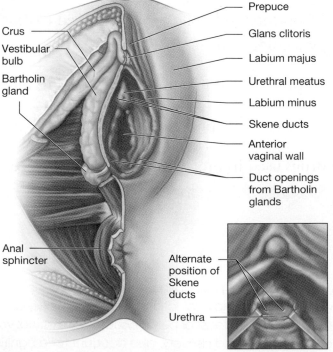

(b)

FIGURE 11-1 Female external genitalia.

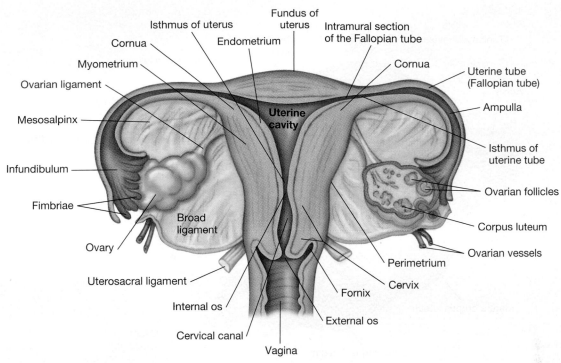

FIGURE 11-2 Anatomy of the uterus and adnexa.

shorter, narrower section of the tube that connects the ampulla to the intramural section of the tube. The intramural section extends through the wall of the uterus at the cornua and opens into the uterine cavity.

Physiology

The reproductive system is under the control of the hypothalamus-pituitary-ovary (HPO) axis. Hormonal changes are regulated using negative-feedback loops that help these three components communicate and control the reproductive cycle. The hypothalamus releases **gonadotropin-releasing hormone (GnRH)** that stimulates the pituitary to produce the gonadotropins **follicle stimulating hormone (FSH)** and **luteinizing hormone (LH)**. FSH initiates follicular growth and LH triggers ovulation.

The primary female sex hormones are the estrogens and **progestins**. There are three forms of estrogen: **estrone, estradiol** (also called **E2**), and **estriol**. The ovaries primarily secrete estradiol, which is by far the most potent of the three forms of estrogen. Estrogen acts on the endometrium, causing it to proliferate (thicken). In addition to their role in reproduction, the estrogens have widespread effects on other aspects of physiology including bone metabolism, fat and protein metabolism, skin texture, and the distribution of body hair.

There are two progestins: progesterone (also called P4) and **17-hydroxyprogesterone, (2)** but their effects are almost identical and can be considered together. The most important function of the progestins is to promote changes in the endometrial lining in order to support gestation (thus their name progestins).

> **Pause 11-1** A common abbreviation for progesterone is P4. The abbreviation E2 is often dictated for estradiol. Looking carefully at the name of the three types of estrogen, why do you think estradiol is called E2?

With each ovulatory cycle, FSH and LH cause 6–12 primordial follicles (immature follicles each

(2) A hydroxyl chemical group is made up of an oxygen atom and a hydrogen atom (OH). Compounds that contain a hydroxyl group may use OH as part of their abbreviation, such as OHP for hydroxyprogesterone. You may also hear 17-OHP called 17-alpha-hydroxyprogesterone.

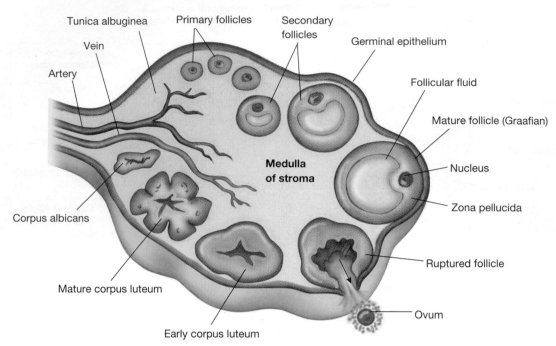

FIGURE 11-3 An ovary showing stages of ovulation.

containing a single ovum) to begin to mature; this process is called **follicular recruitment**. As the follicles enlarge and mature, an antrum (room) forms within the follicle and fills with fluid containing a high concentration of estrogen (■ Figure 11-3). These slightly immature follicles are called **antral follicles**. During each cycle, only one follicle completes the maturation process and the others involute in a process called atresia. The mature follicle, called a **graafian follicle**, reaches about 1–1.5 cm in diameter. LH is required for the final stages of follicular maturation. An **LH surge** occurs about 16 hours before ovulation (■ Figure 11-4), which is the point at which the follicle ruptures and the ovum is released into the **fimbriated end** of the fallopian tube.

> A common mistake is to transcribe annual follicles or astral follicles instead of antral follicles.

(3) The trophoblast is the outer layer of cells that surrounds the embryo and eventually becomes part of the placenta.

After release of the ovum, the graafian follicle begins the transformation to a **corpus luteum**. Under the influence of luteinizing hormone, the corpus luteum secretes a large amount of progesterone as well as estrogen, which cause the proliferation of the endometrial lining and the accumulation of blood. The corpus luteum begins to degenerate into a corpus albicans and involutes on the 12th day after ovulation, which corresponds to the 26th day of the menstrual cycle. This degeneration causes a sudden drop in estrogen and progesterone that triggers the beginning of menstruation approximately two days later. If fertilization occurs, the trophoblast (3) of the developing embryo secretes **human chorionic gonadotropin**, which prevents the involution of the corpus luteum. Instead of degenerating, the corpus luteum begins to secrete even larger quantities of progesterone and estrogen and continues to do so for the first few months of the pregnancy. After about the 12th week of pregnancy, the placenta secretes sufficient hormones to maintain the pregnancy, and the corpus luteum regresses.

The endometrium varies throughout the menstrual cycle. During menses, the **endometrial stripe** is thin and patchy. On days four to six, the endometrium is at its thinnest and is uniform and **homogeneous**

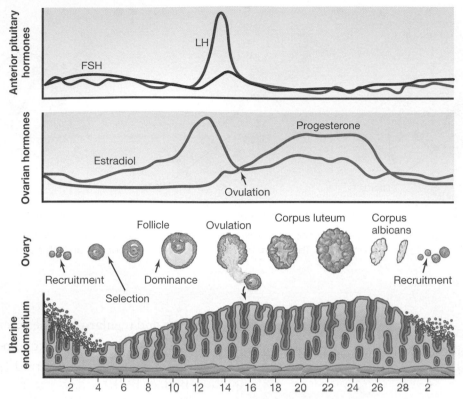

FIGURE 11-4 The menstrual cycle.

when viewed on a sonogram. During the proliferative phase (leading up to menstruation), the endometrial stripe develops a multilayer or **trilaminar** appearance and becomes 12–14 mm thick.

The Gynecologic Exam

The gynecologic exam is an important part of the well-woman exam and aids in the diagnosis of breast and pelvic disorders. To perform the pelvic exam, the patient is placed in the **lithotomy position** (lying on her back with knees flexed and legs spread apart). The pattern of hair growth is noted. **Hirsutism** may be evaluated using the **Ferriman-Gallwey score**. An abnormal amount of pubic hair, more typical of a male pattern that extends upward toward the abdomen, is called an **escutcheon**. The external genitalia are examined for lesions, vesicles, and genital warts. The **introitus** (external entry of the vagina) is palpated for cysts or abscesses in the **Bartholin** and **Skene glands**. The vaginal opening is examined for signs of pelvic relaxation (prolapsed uterus), cystocele, or rectocele.

A speculum is inserted into the vagina to visualize the cervix and to perform a **Papanicolaou (Pap) test**. The cervix should be pink and shiny without discharge. The cervical os will be small and round in a **nulliparous cervix;** the parous or multiparous os has a fish-mouth shape (see page 361 for definitions of nulliparous and multiparous). The vaginal canal is examined and should appear pink with rugae.

The pelvic structures are assessed using the bimanual exam (ie, an exam using both hands). Two fingers are inserted into the vagina. The other hand is placed above the pubic symphysis and gently palpates the uterus and adnexa. The uterus is normally about 4 × 6 cm and tilts anteriorly (**anteverted**), although a posterior tilt (**retroverted**) is not uncommon (■ **Figure 11-5**). The uterus may also be bent at an angle toward the front (**anteflexed**) or toward the back (**retroflexed**). The uterus should be slightly mobile and smooth. The cervix should be slightly mobile (from side to side) without **cervical motion tenderness**. The ovaries are typically about 2 × 3 cm in young women, but are not palpable in postmenopausal females.

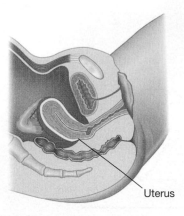

(a) Retroversion

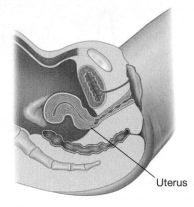

(b) Retroflexion

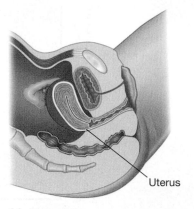

(c) Anteversion

FIGURE 11-5 The uterus may be described as (a) retroverted (tilted posteriorly), (b) retroflexed (bent at a posterior angle) or (c) anteverted (tilted anteriorly). The uterus may also be anteflexed (bent at an anterior angle).

> Stay engaged while transcribing! It is easy to accidentally transcribe "by manual exam" instead of "bimanual exam."

> Skin: Acne and increased hair growth on the upper lip, sideburns, chin, mustache, and lower back, with a Ferriman-Gallwey score of 28. No acanthosis nigricans.
>
> Abdomen: Soft, nontender, without organomegaly. Male escutcheon noted.
>
> Pelvic: Normal external female genitalia. Vagina clean, well-rugated and without discharge. Normal-appearing exocervix with a parous os. Bimanual exam reveals a slightly retroverted uterus that is nontender and not enlarged, with no adnexal mass. No nodularities.

Disordered Menses

The menstrual cycle is a complex physiological process that involves the interplay of various glands and organs. Many women experience some type of menstrual abnormality at some time in their life. An assessment of a menstrual disorder begins with a complete menstrual history that includes:

- age at menarche
- average number of days of menses
- length and regularity of the interval between cycles
- start date of the last menstrual period (LMP)
- dates of the preceding period (previous menstrual period, or PMP)
- color and volume of flow
- symptoms that accompany menstruation (eg, cramping, loose stools)

Most menstrual disorders involve a hormonal abnormality within the HPO axis or a structural disorder within the pelvis (eg, fibroids, tumors, congenital malformations). Some women with coagulopathies experience problems with heavy menstrual bleeding. Oftentimes, hormonal disruptions interfere with ovulation. During an anovulatory cycle, the corpus luteum does not form, progesterone is not secreted, and menses do not begin. The endometrium continues to proliferate until it outgrows its blood supply and then begins to bleed, sometimes profusely. Cycles that last less than 21 days are most likely anovulatory cycles. Ovulatory bleeding, which is a single episode of spotting between cycles, is common.

Amenorrhea

Amenorrhea is an absence of menses. Amenorrhea is classified as primary or secondary. Primary amenorrhea is a failure of menses to occur by age 16 with otherwise normal growth and the presence of secondary sex characteristics. Secondary amenorrhea is cessation of menses for more than six months. Most causes of secondary amenorrhea are related to anovulation, but some causes are anatomical due to structural changes that cause **outflow tract obstruction**. The most common causes of amenorrhea are outlined in the following sections.

Structural Defects

Structural anomalies that obstruct the outflow tract account for approximately 20% of primary amenorrhea cases. Hormonal development is normal and menses begin, but the menstrual flow is obstructed. These girls experience cyclic pelvic pain. Causes include **imperforate hymen** and **transverse vaginal septum**. **Hematocolpos** may cause a vaginal bulge or a perirectal mass. **Hematometra** causes uterine distention. **(4)**

    Vaginal agenesis, or **müllerian dysgenesis** (also known as Mayer-Rokitansky-Kuster-Hauser [MRKH] syndrome), is caused by agenesis or partial agenesis of the müllerian duct system. Secondary sex characteristics are normal but the upper two-thirds of the vagina and the uterus are aplastic. Amenorrhea is often the first sign of this congenital disorder. Acquired anatomic abnormalities such as endometrial scarring (**Asherman syndrome**) following uterine instrumentation or postpartum hemorrhage may cause secondary amenorrhea.

> **Pause 11-2** Research the term müllerian. To what does this term refer?

Hormone Alterations

Alterations in hormones may manifest as a cessation of menses. **Functional hypothalamic amenorrhea** is characterized by abnormal hypothalamic GnRH secretion, which may be caused by congenital disorders, eating disorders, excessive exercise, psychiatric disorders, or prolonged mental or physical stress. A thorough social history is necessary to determine whether eating disorders, excessive exercise (eg, marathon runners, gymnasts), or stress are contributing to menstrual irregularities.

    Kallmann syndrome is a congenital GnRH deficiency marked by failure of normal pubertal development, anosmia, midline facial defect, renal agenesis, and neurologic deficit. It is an X-linked recessive disorder. Amenorrhea may also be caused by pituitary tumors such as **prolactinomas**, which cause **hyperprolactinemia**. Symptoms of pituitary tumor include **galactorrhea** (milk production not associated with pregnancy

or breastfeeding), headaches, and reduced peripheral vision (**visual field cuts**, also called visual field defects) due to impingement on the optic tract. **Cushing disease**, also caused by a pituitary tumor, results in amenorrhea by suppressing gonadotropin secretion. Pituitary tumors, diagnosed by MRI, are classified as **microadenomas** (less than 10 mm in size) or **macroadenomas** (greater than 10 mm in size). Other pituitary causes include **empty sella syndrome** and pituitary infarct.

    Turner syndrome (karyotype 45,X) is an example of a hereditary disorder that leads to gonadal dysgenesis. The gonads of patients with Turner syndrome show accelerated loss of germ cells and a depletion of ovarian follicles that result in early amenorrhea. The ovaries usually contain only fibrous tissue (called streak gonads). Patients with Turner syndrome also show an array of physical anomalies and metabolic disorders.

    Primary ovarian insufficiency (POI), also known as **premature ovarian failure (POF)** or **hypogonadotropic hypogonadism**, is marked by menopausal symptoms before the age of 40. Patients experience estrogen deficiency and its associated symptoms including hot flashes, vaginal dryness, dyspareunia, and insomnia. Endocrine disorders that result in androgen excess, such as polycystic ovary syndrome (POS), also manifest as amenorrhea.

> Listen carefully and use context to distinguish the abbreviations POF and POS.

Other Causes of Amenorrhea

Too much or too little body fat affects the reproductive system. Too little body fat (BMI less than 18.5), especially when caused by excessive exercise and decreased caloric intake, may result in amenorrhea through suppression of GnRH and low estradiol levels. Eating disorders such as anorexia nervosa or binging-and-purging disorders (bulimia) may lead to amenorrhea as well. Excessive weight with a BMI greater than 30 may also cause amenorrhea due to excess extraglandular production of estrogen.

    Amenorrhea may also result from chronic disease, hypothyroidism, hyperthyroidism, immunodeficiency,

> **(4)** Hematocolpos is the accumulation of menstrual blood in the vagina. Hematometra is the accumulation of blood in the uterus.

autoimmune disorders, liver failure, renal failure, diabetes, and psychiatric disorders including depression, obsessive-compulsive disorder, or schizophrenia. Medications known to cause amenorrhea include oral contraceptives, antipsychotics, antidepressants, antihypertensives, H_2-receptor blockers, opiates, and cocaine.

Diagnosis and Treatment

Teenage girls who have no signs of puberty by age 14 or in whom menarche has not occurred by age 16 should be evaluated for causes of primary amenorrhea. Patients with hypothalamic pituitary failure do not show **thelarche** or **adrenarche**. Women of reproductive age should be evaluated for secondary amenorrhea if they have missed more than three consecutive menses or have less than nine menses per year. Of course, pregnancy should be ruled out first.

The patient's history and physical exam is extremely important to the diagnostic process and provides information to guide the selection of laboratory studies. A detailed history should include inquiries concerning recent weight change, change in diet, exercise intensity, and recent gynecological procedures. Recent and current medications should also be evaluated.

The physical examination should look for evidence of pubertal delay, anatomic abnormalities, **virilization**, and **defeminization**. Signs of virilization include hirsutism, temporal balding, acne, voice deepening, increased muscle mass, and **clitoromegaly** (an enlarged clitoris). Defeminization in postpubertal females includes a decrease in previously normal secondary sexual characteristics, such as decreased breast size and vaginal atrophy. Young girls should be evaluated for secondary sexual characteristics including breast and pubic hair development. Pubertal delay is assessed using **Tanner staging** (■ Figure 11-6). Tanner stages I through V, based on breast development

and pubic hair distribution, describe the level of sexual maturation.

The breasts should be examined for galactorrhea, a sign of possible hyperprolactinemia. Expressed fluid from the nipples can be identified as milk (as opposed to a discharge) by visualizing fat globules under a low-power microscope.

Overall hair distribution should also be assessed. **Panhypopituitarism** decreases androgen levels, causing sparse pubic and axillary hair. Hirsutism is a sign of adrenal and ovarian androgen secretion. Hirsutism should be distinguished from **hypertrichosis**, which is excessive growth of hair on the extremities, head, and back that is commonly a family trait. Other dermatologic signs of androgen excess include **acanthosis nigricans** (dark, velvety patches) and acne.

Anatomical abnormalities may be evident on physical exam. A pelvic examination may reveal a transverse vaginal septum or an imperforate hymen. A bulging hymen may be caused by hematocolpos, suggesting an outflow obstruction. Examination of the vaginal canal may suggest estrogen deficiency; in postpubertal females, a thin, pale vaginal mucosa without rugae indicates estrogen deficiency. The presence of cervical mucus with **spinnbarkeit** (a stringy, stretchy quality) usually indicates adequate estrogen. Clitoromegaly may indicate increased androgen effect. A **clitoral index (CI)**, determined by measuring the **glans of clitoris**, greater than 35 mm^2 indicates increased androgens, and an index greater than 100 mm^2 is evidence of virilization (normal CI is less than 35 mm^2).

 Note the spelling of glans of clitoris; it is spelled like glans penis (not glands).

The following laboratory values are useful in the diagnosis of amenorrhea:

- thyroid function studies
- prolactin
- total testosterone
- **dehydroepiandrosterone sulfate (DHEA-S)** (5)
- FSH
- karyotype evaluation

Amenorrhea with high FSH levels (**hypergonadotropic hypogonadism**) suggests ovarian dysfunction, and low FSH levels (hypogonadotropic hypogonadism)

(5) DHEA, DHEA sulfate (DHEA-S), and androstenedione are precursors of androgens and estrogens. DHEA is secreted from the adrenal cortex and is rapidly conjugated with sulfate to form DHEA sulfate. Measurement of plasma DHEA-S levels is useful in the investigation of hirsutism and amenorrhea and the diagnosis of androgen-secreting adrenal tumors. Reference ranges are variable and are based on age and gender.

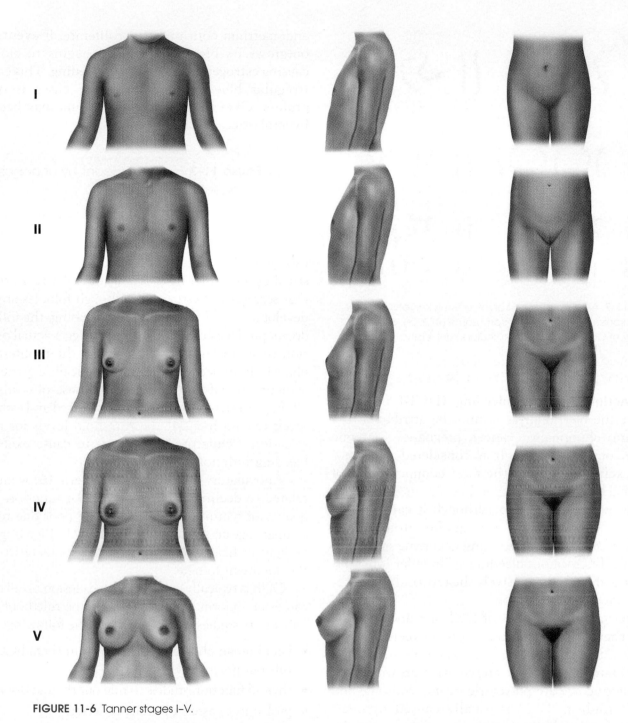

FIGURE 11-6 Tanner stages I-V.

suggest hypothalamic or pituitary dysfunction. A brain MRI helps diagnose pituitary tumors. Patients with suspected genetic disorders may be evaluated for chromosomal abnormalities using karyotype evaluation (■ Figure 11-7).

Treatment for amenorrhea is generally directed at the underlying cause. Primary amenorrhea due to outflow tract obstruction almost always requires surgical repair. Secondary amenorrhea in the absence of significant hormone abnormalities may be treated with a **progestin withdrawal bleed** (also called a **progesterone challenge test**) using Provera 5–10 mg per day for 7–10 days. A positive withdrawal bleed (ie, bleeding occurs) indicates hypothalamic pituitary dysfunction, ovarian failure, or estrogen excess. A negative withdrawal bleed (ie, no response to progesterone) may warrant investigation of an endometrial lesion or outflow tract obstruction.

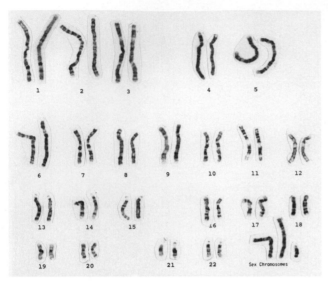

FIGURE 11-7 An example of a karyotype. This karyotype shows two X chromosomes and a Y chromosome (47,XXY). *Source:* Courtesy of Catherine G. Palmer, Indiana University.

Dysfunctional Uterine Bleeding

Dysfunctional uterine bleeding (DUB) is abnormal uterine bleeding that cannot be attributed to a structural abnormality, cancer, pregnancy, systemic disease, or medications. It is considered a diagnosis of exclusion. DUB is the most common cause of abnormal uterine bleeding and occurs most often in women over the age of 45, although it can occur at any age. DUB should be distinguished from menorrhagia, which is heavy bleeding occurring at regular intervals. DUB causes bleeding at irregular intervals. Bleeding may be excessively heavy or light, prolonged, frequent, or random.

The majority of cases of DUB are anovulatory. When there are fewer than 21 days between bleeding episodes, the cycles are most likely anovular. The most common causes for anovulation in women of reproductive age are polycystic ovary syndrome and hypothyroidism. DUB is usually caused by overgrowth of the endometrium due to estrogen stimulation without adequate **opposing progesterone**, a pattern seen in anovulatory cycles. During an anovulatory cycle, the corpus luteum does not form, so progesterone levels never rise. The **unopposed estrogen** continues to stimulate the endometrium. As the endometrium continues to proliferate, it eventually outgrows its blood supply and begins to slough, causing **estrogen breakthrough bleeding**. This causes irregular bleeding that in some cases is quite profuse. Over time, the endometrium may become hyperplastic.

 Pause 11-3 What is meant by unopposed estrogen?

Patients approaching menopause may experience **estrogen withdrawal bleeding** and a shortened menstrual cycle caused by aberrant follicular recruitment that secretes less estradiol. Although follicles are still developing and FSH levels are increasing, the follicles do not produce enough estrogen to trigger actual ovulation (ovarian failure). In this case, the proliferative phase is shortened and bleeding is typically experienced as light, irregular spotting. In the case of ovulatory DUB, progesterone secretion is prolonged and estrogen levels remain low—at the threshold levels for menstruation. Ovulatory DUB tends to cause excessive bleeding with normally timed cycles.

Anovulatory bleeding in **climacteric (6)** women is related to declining ovarian follicular function. The quality of recruited follicles may be poor due to the woman's age and varying estradiol levels. Bleeding may be light or heavy depending on the characteristics of the dominant follicle.

DUB is typically a diagnosis of exclusion, so all other causes of abnormal bleeding should be ruled out first. Laboratory studies typically include the following:

- beta human chorionic gonadotropin (beta hCG) to rule out pregnancy
- thyroid function studies to rule out thyroid disorders
- prolactin to assess pituitary function
- FSH and estradiol levels if premature ovarian failure is suspected
- testosterone and DHEA-S levels if polycystic ovary syndrome is suspected
- liver function studies to rule out liver disease
- coagulation studies if bleeding is excessive
- CBC to rule out anemia and establish baseline hemoglobin and hematocrit levels
- serum progesterone levels, drawn during the luteal phase (after day 14) to determine if ovulation occurred. Levels above 3 ng/mL are indicative of ovulation.

(6) Climacteric refers to endocrine and other changes occurring during the transition to menopause (not to be confused with climactic).

Imaging studies such as **transvaginal ultrasound (TVUS)** and diagnostic procedures such as **hysteroscopy, dilation and curettage (D&C)**, or **endometrial biopsy** may also be needed to further delineate the cause. Endometrial biopsies often show a proliferative or **dyssynchronous endometrium**.

DUB is most often treated hormonally. Acute, heavy bleeding may require infusion of IV crystalloid fluid or blood products to restore blood volume. Extremely heavy bleeding may also require insertion of a bladder catheter into the uterus, inflated to 30 mL of water to tamponade the bleeding. Prolonged bleeding is treated with conjugated estrogens (Premarin) given by IV every four to six hours for four doses followed by combination (estrogen-progestin) oral contraceptives. Estrogen therapy alone cannot be used for long periods without opposing with a progestin or the endometrial lining will proliferate and begin to bleed again.

For active bleeding (not requiring IV treatment), treatment consists of **oral contraceptive pills (OCPs)** given four times daily for one to two days followed by two pills daily through day five and then one pill daily through day 20. OCPs are continued for at least three cycles.

Chronic DUB may be managed with a progestin (medroxyprogesterone acetate or norethindrone acetate) for 12 days per month, a progestin-secreting **intrauterine device (IUD)** such as Mirena or Plan B (levonorgestrel), or daily OCPs. Surgery is indicated when hormonal therapy fails. Options include **endometrial ablation** and hysterectomy. Leuprolide (Lupron) may be used as pretreatment to thin the endometrium before the ablation procedure.

Polycystic Ovary Syndrome

Polycystic ovary syndrome (POS), also called polycystic ovarian syndrome (PCOS), is characterized by mild obesity, irregular menses or amenorrhea, and excess androgens. The syndrome is associated with infertility and increased risk for metabolic syndrome, leading to diabetes mellitus and heart disease. Although many women with this syndrome have polycystic ovaries, the disease itself is not defined by the presence of cysts. Ovaries may be enlarged or normal in size. The exact mechanism is not fully understood, but women with PCOS are known to have altered androgen and estrogen metabolism with increased production of androgenic hormones (**androstenedione**, testosterone, and DHEA-S). Increased circulating androgens are believed to be the basis of many of the symptoms.

Increased estrogen levels increase the risk of endometrial hyperplasia, and in the long run, endometrial cancer. PCOS is also associated with peripheral insulin resistance and hyperinsulinemia, and it is thought that elevated insulin augments the effects of gonadotropins on ovarian function. Obesity is known to amplify the symptoms of PCOS, and weight loss is an integral part of the treatment.

Symptoms of PCOS usually begin during puberty and worsen over time. Typical manifestations of PCOS are virilization (acne, androgenic alopecia), hirsutism, obesity, and amenorrhea, oligomenorrhea, or irregular menses. Hair is commonly seen on the upper lip, chin, around the nipples, and along the **linea alba** of the lower abdomen. Some women have darkened skin (acanthosis nigricans) in the axillae, on the nape of the neck, and in skinfolds due to high levels of insulin. Infertility is a common consequence of PCOS due to decreased or absent ovulation.

Obesity is present in nearly half of all women with PCOS. Those with normal weight may be described as having **thin PCOS**. Patients are also more likely to have diabetes mellitus or impaired glucose tolerance. Metabolic syndrome (see page 40) is also more common among patients with PCOS. Treatment for PCOS is important to prevent other chronic and debilitating diseases.

Diagnosis of PCOS is based on the presence of at least two of the following three features:

- oligoovulation or anovulation
- clinical or biochemical evidence of hyperandrogenism
- polycystic ovaries as seen on ultrasound

Physical examination shows hirsutism, abdominal obesity with a waist circumference of greater than 35 inches (88 cm), acanthosis nigricans, hypertension, and other signs of metabolic syndrome. Abundant cervical mucus may be noted, reflecting high levels of estrogen. A transvaginal ultrasound can be used to evaluate the ovaries. Polycystic ovaries are defined as having greater than 10–12 antral follicles (also called **resting follicles**) measuring 2–9 mm in diameter.

Laboratory evaluation includes total testosterone or **free testosterone**, FSH, LH, prolactin, and TSH. Women with clinical evidence of androgen excess should also have DHEA-S and 17-OHP measured. **Sex hormone binding globulin (SHBG)** may also be measured and is typically low. An oral glucose tolerance test (OGTT) may also be performed to evaluate impaired glucose tolerance and rule out diabetes.

- Most menstrual disorders involve a hormonal abnormality within the HPO axis or a structural disorder within the pelvis (eg, fibroids, tumors, congenital malformations).
- Primary amenorrhea is a failure of the menses to start, and secondary amenorrhea occurs after menses have been established. Amenorrhea may be due to hormonal abnormalities in the HPO axis, structural abnormalities that prevent the outflow of menses, or premature ovarian failure.
- Dysfunctional uterine bleeding is uterine bleeding of varying amounts and duration that occurs at irregular intervals. The most common cause is anovulation but ovulatory DUB is also possible. Treatment is with oral hormonal therapy, endometrial ablation, or hysterectomy.
- Polycystic ovary syndrome is characterized by mild obesity, disordered menses, hirsutism, and excess androgens. PCOS is associated with decreased fertility and metabolic syndrome. Treatment includes weight loss, diet, exercise, and medications to treat hyperinsulinism. Women not desiring pregnancy may be treated with OCPs.

A two-hour post-load glucose of less than 140 mg/dL indicates normal glucose tolerance. Values above 140 mg/dL are indicative of impaired glucose tolerance and above 200 mg/dL indicate diabetes mellitus. A fasting lipid profile is also important to assess for dyslipidemia.

Patients are treated medically to reduce androgen levels, promote ovulation, and to improve metabolic derangements. Overweight patients are encouraged to lose weight and implement a moderate exercise program. Patients are encouraged to follow a diet designed for type 2 diabetics. Weight loss is associated with improved endocrine-metabolic parameters as well as decreased hirsutism, return of ovulation, increased SHBG levels, and a decrease in free testosterone.

> **Pause 11-4** What is the role of sex hormone binding globulin? How does SHBG play a role in PCOS?

Metformin is commonly prescribed to address insulin sensitivity and hyperinsulinemia and is known to induce ovulation in a substantial number of patients with PCOS. Patients desiring pregnancy are given metformin and clomiphene citrate. Metformin treatment for PCOS and infertility is considered an **off-label use**. (7)

Women who do not wish to become pregnant can be treated with OCPs such as Yaz. Contraceptives can help with hirsutism and restore normal menses. Resumption of normal estrogen-progestin cycles with monthly bleeds prevents endometrial hyperplasia and reduces the risk of cancer. A withdrawal bleed can be induced with medroxyprogesterone (Provera) given for 5–10 days before the start of oral contraceptive therapy. Additional treatment for hirsutism may include spironolactone, which is actually a diuretic with antiandrogen effects. Eflornithine (Vaniqa), a topical cream, may be applied to slow hair growth in unwanted areas. Unwanted hair may also be treated with **depilation** or electrolysis.

Pelvic Disorders

Pelvic disorders encompass a wide array of benign and malignant diseases. The most common diseases of the pelvis include infection, masses (benign and malignant), and endometriosis.

Sexually Transmitted Diseases

Sexually transmitted diseases (STDs), also called **sexually transmitted infections (STIs)**, are caused by a variety of microorganisms (**Table 11-1**). STDs are

(7) The off-label use of a drug is the practice of prescribing a drug for a given indication for which the FDA has not given its approval. The drug itself has been approved for other indications.

often classified as gonococcal, nongonococcal, and viral. In many clinical environments, patient compliance and followup is poor, so infections are treated empirically based on the most likely causative agent. Although laboratory tests are available for definitive identification, patients often do not return to the clinic for more specific treatment based on testing results. For this reason, point-of-care testing is used whenever possible and antibiotics are prescribed empirically.

Table 11-1 Causes of Sexually
Transmitted Infections

Bacterial/Fungal	Viral	Parasitic
syphilis, gonorrhea, chancroid, lympho-granuloma venereum, granuloma inguinale, chlamydia, myco-plasma, Ureaplasma	genital and anorectal warts (HPV), genital herpes, and HIV infection	Trichomonas

Nongonococcal STI

Nongonococcal infections are most often caused by Chlamydia trachomatis, an intracellular bacterium, but may also be caused by **Mycoplasma genitalium**, **Ureaplasma urealyticum**, or Trichomonas vaginalis (8). Symptoms include vaginal discharge, dysuria, urinary frequency and urgency, and urethritis. Symptoms may be similar to gonococcal infection and can be distinguished by a urine WBC count of greater than five cells per high-power field. Exudates may also be tested specifically for chlamydia using nucleic-acid based tests. Treatment includes single-dose azithromycin or a week-long course of ofloxacin, levofloxacin, erythromycin, or a tetracycline. Oftentimes patients are co-infected with gonorrhea as well. When gonorrhea is suspected, the treatment regimen should also include a cephalosporin.

Left untreated, chlamydial infections may become asymptomatic over the course of several weeks, although patients are still infected. Long-term infection results in chronic endometritis, salpingitis, or peritonitis with subsequent pelvic pain, infertility, and increased risk of ectopic pregnancy.

Gonorrhea

Gonococcal (GC) infection is caused by Neisseria gonorrhoeae. GC usually infects the urethra and cervix but may also infect the rectum, pharynx, and conjunctivae.

GC often causes cervicitis with dysuria, vaginal discharge, and inflammation of Skene ducts and Bartholin glands. Untreated, GC may progress to pelvic inflammatory disease (see below).

Identification tests may be done on genital, rectal, or oral swabs. Urine may be tested using **nucleic acid amplification tests (NAAT)**. GC is treated with a single dose of ceftriaxone IM or cefixime administered orally.

Trichomonas

Trichomonas vaginalis is a flagellated protozoan. (9) Symptoms include a copious, yellow-green, frothy vaginal discharge with soreness of the vulva and perineum accompanied by dyspareunia and dysuria. The vaginal walls and surface of the cervix may show punctate, red spots. A **KOH preparation (KOH prep)** is performed using vaginal secretions placed on a slide with potassium hydroxide. This will produce the characteristic "fishy odor" when sniffed (called the **whiff test**). A **saline wet mount** (vaginal secretions placed on a slide with saline and a cover slip) can be examined for motile trichomonads. Treatment is with metronidazole (Flagyl).

 Pause 11-5 KOH prep is pronounced *k-o-h*. How does this test get its name?

Human Papilloma Virus

Genital warts, also called venereal warts, are caused by the **Human papilloma virus (HPV)**. There are over 70 serotypes of HPV. Types 6 and 11 are known to cause benign genital warts (**condylomata acuminata**). Types 16 and 18 are associated with intraepithelial neoplasia (see page 357) and carcinoma. Infection causes soft, moist, minute pink or gray, raised lesions. Patients may complain of itching or burning. The diagnosis may be confirmed using NAAT for HPV. Warts are treated with cryotherapy, electrocauterization, laser, or surgical excision. HPV is the only STD for which there is a vaccine, marketed under the name **Gardasil**.

---

(8) The slang name for Trichomonas vaginalis is "trich," but the full name should be transcribed when dictated.

(9) Flagellated means the organism has a long whip-like structure that helps it move about.

Herpes Simplex Virus

Herpes simplex viruses (Human herpesviruses 1 and 2) cause recurrent infections of the eyes, lips, mouth, and genitalia. **Herpes simplex virus type 2 (HSV-2)** is most commonly associated with genital herpes and is spread through sexual contact. Vesicles form that eventually erode to produce ulcers. Lesions may be found on the labia, clitoris, perineum, vagina, and cervix. Urinary symptoms may also be present. Lesions typically heal but the recurrence rate is 80%. Infants born vaginally to an infected mother may be infected with HSV, causing a severe, life-threatening infection. Genital herpes is treated with antiviral medications including acyclovir (Zovirax), valacyclovir (Valtrex), and famciclovir (Famvir). These medications only reduce symptoms; there is no cure.

 HSV causes small blisters called vesicles (not vesicals).

Pelvic Inflammatory Disease

Pelvic inflammatory disease (PID) is an infection of the upper genital tract (above the cervix, including the uterus and adnexa). The disease typically begins as a sexually transmitted infection that ascends from the vagina and cervix. PID is the most common gynecologic cause of emergency department visits in women of reproductive age. Prompt treatment is necessary to prevent sequelae, including chronic pelvic pain and infertility. The primary risk factor is sexual promiscuity, especially without barrier protection. An untreated bacterial vaginosis also increases the risk of PID. Use of an IUD carries an increased risk of PID, but only in the first few weeks following placement. Rarely PID may be iatrogenic following endocervical procedures such as endometrial biopsy, curettage, and hysteroscopy.

PID commonly occurs in women under the age of 35 and almost never affects prepubertal or postmenopausal females. Often, PID is polymicrobial. The most common causes are Neisseria gonorrhoeae and Chlamydia trachomatis. As inflammation progresses, other organisms, which may be part of the normal flora, also become involved. Polymicrobial infections may include aerobic and anaerobic bacteria such as **Gardnerella vaginalis**, Ureaplasma urealyticum, Trichomonas vaginalis, Haemophilus influenzae, Streptococcus agalactiae, or enteric gram-negative rods. Viral infections such as HSV-2 and cytomegalovirus (CMV) may also be involved. **Actinomycete** species have been identified almost exclusively in those patients with IUDs.

The course may begin as vaginitis or **cervicitis** with mucopurulent discharge. Often, these infections are asymptomatic and go untreated. The infection then spreads to the endometrium (**endometritis**), the fallopian tubes (**salpingitis**), and possibly the ovaries (**oophoritis**). Inflammation may extend to **parametrial** structures, including the bowel. Infection may spread to the peritoneum through purulent materials spilling from the fallopian tubes with subsequent peritonitis and perihepatitis (**Fitz-Hugh-Curtis syndrome**). Opening of the cervix during menstruation may facilitate the upward movement of microorganisms, especially since patients often become symptomatic in the first few days following menses.

Patients typically present with lower abdominal pain, fever, cervical discharge, and abnormal uterine bleeding. Pain may be described as dull, aching or crampy, bilateral, constant, and aggravated by motion. Patients may complain of dyspareunia and dysuria.

On examination, the cervix shows a mucopurulent discharge, appears red, and bleeds easily. Cervical motion tenderness, uterine or adnexal tenderness are common. Guarding and rebound tenderness may also be observed. Right upper quadrant tenderness suggests Fitz-Hugh-Curtis syndrome. A **tuboovarian abscess (TOA)** with peritoneal signs may also develop. Abscesses, hydrosalpinx, and pyosalpinx may be detected as a palpable adnexal mass. Rupture of the abscess or the fallopian tube may lead to septic shock. Even after resolution of the infection, patients may experience chronic pelvic pain and recurrent infections. Patients are also more likely to have difficulty conceiving.

The diagnosis is based on history and clinical symptoms. There is no single finding on physical examination that definitively points to PID, but patients suspected of having PID should be treated immediately and aggressively to prevent serious sequelae. Diagnostic tests include cervical specimens to test for N gonorrheae and C trachomatis with PCR, **DNA probes**, or routine culture. Cervical discharge may also be examined using a saline wet mount (also called saline microscopy). Cervical leukorrhea (more than 10 WBCs per high-power field or more than one WBC per epithelial cell seen) and/or the presence of **clue cells** are highly suspicious for PID.

A **rapid protein reagin (RPR)** test should be run to rule out syphilis. Ultrasound may also be performed to rule out ectopic pregnancy, **ovarian torsion**, hemorrhagic cyst, endometrioma, or appendicitis. Findings on ultrasound may include thickened, fluid-filled fallopian tubes and **free pelvic fluid**. Laparoscopy can provide a definitive diagnosis and may be required if patients do not respond to empiric medical treatment within 48–72 hours.

Treatment is primarily with broad-spectrum antibiotics given empirically to cover N gonorrheae and C trachomatis. Most patients are treated as outpatients, but some circumstances require inpatient care. Tuboovarian abscesses may require ultrasound-guided or CT-guided percutaneous or transvaginal drainage. A ruptured abscess requires emergent laparotomy. Antibiotic therapy may include a combination of two medications selected from the following: cephalosporin (cefoxitin, ceftriaxone, ceftizoxime, or cefotaxime), probenecid, doxycycline, clindamycin, gentamicin, and metronidazole. Sexual partners should also be treated with antibiotics. Ultimately, **salpingo-oophorectomy** (removal of fallopian tube and ovary) or hysterectomy may be required.

Salpingitis

Salpingitis is inflammation of the fallopian tube, most commonly caused by an infection. **Pyosalpinx** is defined as pus in the fallopian tube, which usually results from acute salpingitis. Acute salpingitis is often used synonymously with pelvic inflammatory disease because it is the most common form of PID. Salpingitis is believed to begin as an infection that ascends from the endocervix to the endometrium and then the fallopian tube. Untreated gonorrhea or chlamydial disease is a common cause of salpingitis. Tuboovarian abscess is a serious complication of acute salpingitis and PID. The abscess begins with a collection of pus within a space created by adhesions in and around the fallopian tubes, ovaries, uterus, and intestines.

A sequela of pyosalpinx is **hydrosalpinx**, which is characterized by fimbrial obstruction with a collection of watery fluid inside the fallopian tube. The tube appears dilated and is filled with clear, colorless fluid. Hydrosalpinx adversely affects fertility due to occlusion of the fimbriated end as well as destruction of the normal cellular architecture within the tube. Other unknown factors associated with hydrosalpinx also affect fertility, and **salpingectomy** (10) of a hydrosalpinx has been shown to increase pregnancy rates with in vitro fertilization.

Cervical Intraepithelial Neoplasia

The precursor to cervical cancer is **cervical intraepithelial neoplasia (CIN)**. Cellular changes (dysplasia) occur at the squamocolumnar junction of the cervix where squamous cells encroach on the mucosal epithelium of the vagina, (the transitional zone). Untreated, this dysplasia leads to cancer. CIN and cervical cancer are highly associated with HPV infection.

There are no specific symptoms of CIN. Detection is by routine screening using Pap smears taken from the cervix and endocervix. Widespread use of Pap smears has dramatically decreased the incidence of cervical cancer in the US. The results of the Pap smear are reported by the pathology lab using the CIN system or the **Bethesda system (Table 11-2)**.

Table 11-2 Classification of Histological Findings on Pap Smear

Description	CIN System	Bethesda System
benign	benign	normal
benign with inflammation	benign with inflammation	normal, ASC-US*
mild dysplasia	CIN I	low-grade SIL*
moderate dysplasia	CIN II	high-grade SIL
severe dysplasia	CIN III	
carcinoma in situ		
invasive cancer	invasive cancer	invasive cancer

*ASC-US atypical squamous cells of undetermined significance, SIL squamous intraepithelial lesion

A Pap smear showing **atypical squamous cells of undetermined significance (ASC-US**, pronounced ăsk-ŭs) should prompt a test for HPV. If HPV is negative,

(10) Salpingectomy is the removal of a fallopian tube and salpingostomy is a surgical incision into a fallopian tube, typically performed to remove an ectopic pregnancy or to repair the tube.

the patient should be followed with a repeat Pap smear. Patients with CIN I/SIL or positive HPV should undergo **colposcopy** using **5% acetic acid** to identify actively proliferating squamous epithelium. In addition, a **Schiller test** using **Lugol solution** applied to the cervix will stain normal squamous epithelium, allowing selection of nonstaining cells for punch biopsy. CIN II and III are treated with **cone biopsy (conization)**.

Leiomyoma

Leiomyomas, also known as fibroids, are benign uterine tumors arising from smooth muscle and connective tissue in the uterus. Leiomyomas are discrete, round, and firm. Fibroids have estrogen receptors, so they tend to enlarge during the reproductive years and regress after menopause. The majority of leiomyomas occurs in the uterine corpus, but occasionally they may be found in the cervix, vaginal canal, or on the broad ligaments or ovaries. Fibroids are classified according to their location (■ Figure 11-8):

- **submucosal:** located just beneath the endometrium; may become pedunculated
- **intramural:** located wholly within the uterine wall
- **subserosal:** located at the serosal surface (outer surface of the uterus) and may become pedunculated
- **intracavitary:** project into the uterine cavity
- **intraligamentous:** attached to the broad ligaments

Depending on their size or location, fibroids may or may not produce symptoms; many leiomyomas are asymptomatic and are found incidentally. Typical symptoms include menorrhagia, menometrorrhagia, and pelvic pain. Large fibroids pressing on the bladder may cause urinary frequency or urgency. Fibroids can cause

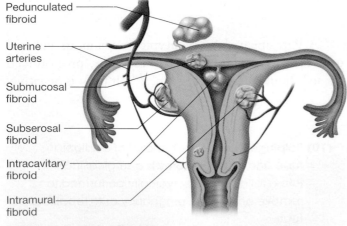

Pedunculated fibroid

Uterine arteries

Submucosal fibroid

Subserosal fibroid

Intracavitary fibroid

Intramural fibroid

FIGURE 11-8 Uterine fibroids.

infertility if they interfere with ovulation or implantation, or they may cause spontaneous abortion. A **pedunculated fibroid** that becomes twisted can be acutely painful. Fibroids that outgrow their blood supply and degenerate become necrotic and may be quite painful.

Large fibroids may increase the size of the uterus sufficiently to be detectable on bimanual exam. The size of an enlarged uterus is described in terms of comparable weeks of gestation. An enlarged uterus due to fibroids may be described as a nine-week uterus (for example), meaning the uterus is the same size as a gravid uterus at nine weeks' gestation. Fibroids can be diagnosed easily by ultrasound or **sonohysterogram (saline-instilled sonogram)**.

Hormone therapy offers temporary relief and may be used to shrink fibroids or to reduce bleeding until the patient's hematocrit recovers sufficiently for definitive surgery. Medications used to shrink fibroids include **GnRH analogs** (leuprolide) and progestins (medroxyprogesterone). Surgery may be offered to patients with a rapidly enlarging pelvic mass or to those with persistent pain or who are refractory to hormone therapy. Patients desiring to become pregnant may need surgical removal of fibroids that interfere with fertility. Patients wishing to preserve fertility opt for **myomectomy** (removal of the fibroid). Fibroids tend to recur, so the only definitive treatment is hysterectomy.

The surgical approach taken for a myomectomy depends on the location of the fibroid; options include laparoscopy, laparotomy, and hysteroscopy. Women who wish to become pregnant should be informed about the type of surgery required to remove their fibroids. Patients who have procedures that require **hysterotomy** or procedures that **enter the myometrium** to remove fibroids should not be allowed to labor due to the risk of uterine rupture at the incision site; these patients will require cesarean delivery. A newer approach for fibroids that are not easily accessible is **uterine artery embolization**. This procedure blocks the blood supply to the fibroid, leading to infarction and degeneration.

Endometriosis

Endometriosis is the aberrant growth of endometrial tissue (glands and stroma) outside the uterus, particularly the dependent parts of the pelvis and around the ovaries. The disease is poorly understood and extremely debilitating, although it is benign. Endometriosis is a common cause of infertility and is the most common cause of secondary dysmenorrhea.

Endometriosis affects 7% to 10% of women. The disease is driven by estrogen, so it typically affects women during their reproductive years. The exact mechanism that causes endometrial cells to migrate to other parts of the body is not well understood. **Endometriotic tissue** is most commonly found in the peritoneal or serosal surface of pelvic organs, especially the ovaries, broad ligaments, posterior **cul-de-sac**, and **uterosacral ligaments**. Less commonly, lesions may be found in the small and large intestine, ureters, bladder, vagina, cervix, pleura, and pericardium. The transplanted tissue contains estrogen and progesterone receptors, just like intrauterine endometrial tissue, and therefore responds to hormonal stimulation. The lesions proliferate, bleed, and digress with hormonal fluctuations. Bleeding from these ectopic sites is thought to initiate inflammation within the peritoneal cavity, causing scarring in the form of adhesions. These adhesions can be painful, as they distort the peritoneal surface and pelvic anatomy.

Endometriosis is known to reduce fertility. **Peritubal and periovarian adhesions** can interfere with ovum transport through the fallopian tube. Peritoneal endometriosis is also known to cause **subfertility** (reduced fertility). Patients desiring pregnancy may require fertility treatment in the form of intrauterine insemination (IUI), **superovulation**, or in vitro fertilization (IVF). See page 363 for a discussion of infertility treatments.

Pelvic pain typically starts two to seven days before the onset of menses and becomes increasingly severe until flow starts to abate. The pain tends to worsen over time and some women experience continual pain. Patients may also complain of dyspareunia and midline pelvic pain, which is typically more painful than **lateral disease**. Pain may be experienced in various locations depending on the location of the implants. An endometrioma in the large intestine may cause abdominal bloating, pain during defecation, or rectal bleeding. Implants in the bladder manifest as dysuria, hematuria, and suprapubic pain. An endometrioma on the ovary may form a cystic mass that causes severe, acute pain if it ruptures. Severe, acute abdominal pain may also be due to chemical peritonitis from a **ruptured endometriotic cyst**.

Physical examination during a menses tends to reveal more areas of pain. Examination may show induration or tender nodules in the cul-de-sac and **rectovaginal septum**. The uterus may be retroverted with decreased uterine mobility (**fixed uterus**) due to adhesions. Bimanual exam may elicit cervical motion tenderness or adnexal tenderness. Adnexal masses as well as nodules on the uterosacral ligament may be palpable. Symptom severity does not correlate with the physical exam findings; some women even have a normal pelvic exam.

The diagnosis is suspected based on clinical presentation. A biopsy using a laparoscope is the most reliable way to diagnose endometriosis and is considered the primary diagnostic modality. Lesions may appear clear, red, brown, or black, and the size varies depending on the menstrual-cycle day. Areas of endometriosis on the peritoneum tend to be punctate, greater than 5 mm, and look like **powder-burn lesions**.

Imaging tests are not optimal for diagnosing endometriosis but may be helpful in ruling out other disorders and for monitoring treatment. Transvaginal ultrasound is useful for identifying **chocolate cysts** on the ovary. These cysts contain a low-level homogenous internal echo consistent with old blood. MRI may be helpful in identifying rectal lesions.

Staging the disorder is helpful for treatment planning and evaluating response to therapy. Endometriosis is staged as I (minimal), II (mild), III (moderate), and IV (severe). Staging is based on the number, location, and depth of implants, and the presence of adhesions.

Treatment is based on suppression of ovulation to reduce hormone levels, thereby inhibiting growth and activity of endometriotic implants. Endometriosis usually recurs after hormonal suppression therapy is stopped, so **bilateral salpingo-oophorectomies (BSO)** are the only definitive treatment. Medical treatment uses **combination oral contraceptive pills (COCPs)**, progestational agents, and GnRH analogs. One of several treatment regimens may be prescribed based on the patient's age, symptoms, and desire to preserve fertility:

- GnRH analogs for six months with **add-back therapy** with norethindrone to treat bone demineralization, vaginal dryness, and vasomotor symptoms caused by a lack of estrogen. GnRH analogs induce hypogonadotrophic hypogonadism by down-regulation of the pituitary gland.

- COCPs, hormone patch, or vaginal ring for 6–12 months. Skipping the placebo tablets (for three to four cycles) prevents menstruation and decreases painful episodes.

- Provera 100 mg IM twice a week for four weeks then 100 mg every four weeks. Breakthrough bleeding is treated with oral estrogen or **estradiol valerate**.

- Levonorgestrel intrauterine system (LNG-IUS) inserted during laparoscopy.

- Sexually transmitted infections are caused by bacteria, fungi, protozoa, and viruses. Infections are typically classified as gonococcal, nongonococcal, or viral. Symptoms vary depending on infecting agent and may include vaginal discharge, genital warts, and vesicles. All but the viral STIs are treated with antibiotics.

- Left untreated, an STI may progress to pelvic inflammatory disease. Viral STIs cannot be cured, but symptoms may be reduced using antiviral medications.

- Pelvic inflammatory disease is an infection of the upper genital tract that typically starts as an ascending infection of the vagina or cervix. Symptoms include lower abdominal pain, fever, discharge, and vaginal bleeding. Examination may reveal pyosalpinx, hydrosalpinx, or tuboovarian abscess. Treatment includes broad-spectrum antibiotics.

- Salpingitis is inflammation of a fallopian tube, usually caused by infection. Pyosalpinx and hydrosalpinx are associated with salpingitis. Hydrosalpinx often results in subfertility requiring salpingectomy.

- Cervical intraepithelial neoplasia represents precancerous changes in the cervix. CIN is highly associated with HPV infection and is detected by routine Pap smears. Treatment includes conization or LEEP.

- Leiomyoma, commonly known as fibroids, are benign tumors of the muscle and connective tissue of the uterus. Symptoms depend on the size, number, and location of the fibroids and range from asymptomatic to severe pelvic pain. Treatment includes myomectomy, uterine artery embolization, or hysterectomy.

- Endometriosis is the aberrant growth of endometrial tissue outside the uterus. Endometriotic tissue, which may implant anywhere in the pelvic cavity, responds to hormonal fluctuations in the same way as entopic endometrial tissue. Symptoms include pelvic pain, especially during menses. Treatment is with hormonal suppression with OCPs, progestins, or GnRH analogs. Surgical treatment may include ablation of lesions and lysis of adhesions. Definitive treatment is bilateral oophorectomy.

Any of the above regimens can be followed with long-term, low-dose OCPs.

Always confirm the word/spelling of drug forms such as estradiol valerate. Many of the chemical forms sound alike (eg, maleate, fumarate, hydrate, citrate, butyrate, and tartrate).

Conservative surgical treatment may include ablation or excision of implants and lysis of peritubal and periovarian adhesions. This approach is often used for women desiring to preserve fertility. Ablation techniques include electrodiathermy (bipolar diathermy) or lasers. **Semiconservative therapy** involves hysterectomy and **cytoreduction** of pelvic endometriosis. This approach is used for women who no longer desire to conceive but do not want to go through **surgical menopause**. Ovarian endometriomas can be removed, leaving as little as a tenth of the ovarian tissue to maintain hormone production. Radical surgery, which is a **total abdominal hysterectomy and bilateral oophorectomies (TAH-BSO)** with cytoreduction of visible endometriosis, provides definitive treatment. **Adhesiolysis** (lysis of adhesions) is also performed to allow intrapelvic organs to return to their normal anatomic positions.

Obstetrics

Obstetrics is the care of women during pregnancy, parturition, and the puerperium (the period following labor until complete involution of the uterus, typically 42 days). A women's obstetrical history is an important component of her overall health history. The obstetrical history includes dates and outcomes of all pregnancies.

The obstetrical history is described in terms of **gravidity** and **parity**. Gravidity is the number of confirmed pregnancies. Parity is the number of deliveries after 20 weeks of gestation. A **multifetal pregnancy** (twins, triplets, etc) is counted as one in terms of gravidity and parity. **Abortus** refers to the number of losses prior to 20 weeks of gestation. Abortions may be spontaneous, therapeutic, or elective, but all are counted under abortus. The sum of parity and abortus should always equal gravidity. Parity may be broken down into more detailed information and written in this order:

- the number of term deliveries (after 37 weeks)
- the number of premature deliveries (occurring between 20 and 37 weeks)
- the number of abortions
- the number of living children

An obstetrical history may be written two different ways:

gravida 2, para 1, abortus 1

gravida 2, para 1-0-1-1

This represents the history of a woman who has been pregnant twice, delivered one at full term, and had one abortion (type of abortion not indicated). A woman who is currently pregnant and has had one term delivery, one set of twins, and one delivered at 34 weeks would be gravida 4, para 3, or gravida 4, para 2-1-0-4. Other terms used to describe a woman's pregnancy status include:

- **gravid:** a woman who is currently pregnant
- **nulligravida:** a woman who has never been pregnant
- **primigravida:** a woman in her first pregnancy
- **secundigravida:** a woman in her second pregnancy
- **multigravida:** a woman who has been pregnant more than once
- **nulliparous:** a woman who has never delivered a pregnancy (may also describe the cervix if deliveries have been by C-section)
- **primiparous:** describes a woman who has delivered one pregnancy
- **multiparous:** describes a woman who has delivered more than one pregnancy

 It is very easy to mistype gravidity as gravity.

Pregnancy is suspected in all females of reproductive age who have missed a menstrual period. Urine and blood tests can be used to detect the **beta unit of human chorionic gonadotropin hormone (beta hCG)** produced by trophoblasts very early in the pregnancy and later by the placenta. Levels of beta hCG can be detected in the blood as early as 8–11 days after conception. Most pregnancy tests have a sensitivity of approximately 25 milliunits/mL. In a **normal singleton pregnancy**, beta hCG levels double about every 1.4 to 2.1 days during the first 60 days (or 7½ weeks) then begin to decrease between the 10th and 18th week. Beta hCG tests may be qualitative (positive or negative) or quantitative (measuring the exact level). In a normal pregnancy, **quantitative serum hCG** levels correlate with gestational age. Abnormally high levels or an accelerated rise in beta hCG should prompt investigation for a molar pregnancy (see page 365), multiple gestation (**multifetal pregnancy**), or chromosomal abnormalities. A slow rise or a leveling off of beta hCG may indicate an ectopic pregnancy or herald a miscarriage.

Physical examination will show changes indicative of early pregnancy. On bimanual exam, the cervix feels softer and larger (**Hegar sign**) and the **gravid uterus** is enlarged and softer. The cervix may appear bluish or purple due to increased blood supply (**Chadwick sign**). Around 12–15 weeks from the LMP, the uterus can be palpated above the pubic symphysis and by 20–22 weeks the uterus reaches the umbilicus. At 36 weeks, the upper pole approaches the xiphoid process. Fetal movements are usually felt by an examiner at about 20 weeks. **Quickening** refers to the first movements felt by the mother.

Ultrasonography is also used to diagnose and monitor pregnancy. The earliest structure identifiable by transvaginal ultrasound is the **gestational sac**. The sac can be visualized at about five to six weeks from LMP and corresponds to a beta hCG level of about 100 milliunits/mL. The **yolk sac**, seen as a small sphere with a hypoechoic center, can be recognized within the gestational sac at about five weeks until approximately ten weeks' gestation. A gestational sac of 10 mm or larger without an identifiable yolk sac is a **blighted ovum** and will not progress. The **fetal pole** should also be visualized on TVUS at approximately five to six weeks' gestation.

The fetal pole is a linear, hyperechoic structure that grows approximately 1 mm/d. With a **viable intrauterine pregnancy, fetal heart motion** can be seen as early as five to six weeks. **Fetal heart tones** can be heard using Doppler ultrasound at about 8–10 weeks.

Physiology of Pregnancy

Normal physiologic changes occur in the pregnant woman to accommodate the growing fetus. To support the placenta during the first trimester, the cardiac output is greatly increased and the heart rate increases from a normal of about 70 beats per minute to about 90 beats per minute. The stroke volume also increases. During the second trimester, the blood pressure drops somewhat and usually returns to normal in the third trimester. Functional murmurs and heart sounds are typically accentuated during pregnancy and premature atrial and ventricular beats are common.

Red cell mass and plasma volume also increase during pregnancy, but the plasma volume increases more, so a dilutional anemia results with a drop in the hemoglobin from 13 g/dL to about 12 g/dL. WBC count increases to 9–12 with a marked leukocytosis (up to 20) during and immediately following labor. Iron requirements also increase in order to support the fetus and the placenta. Increased progesterone levels cause smooth muscles to relax and decrease GI motility. This leads to gastroesophageal reflux and delayed gastric emptying with heartburn and belching. The placenta produces a hormone similar to TSH, leading to a mild hyperthyroid-like state. Changes in adrenal hormones lead to increased edema and an increased need for insulin (insulin resistance). This may exacerbate preexisting diabetes or lead to **gestational diabetes.**

The placenta also produces melanocyte-stimulating hormone (MSH) that causes skin pigmentation changes late in pregnancy. **Melasma** (also called the **mask of pregnancy**) appears as blotchy, brownish pigment over the forehead and across the face as well as the areolae, axillae, and genitals and at times creates a **linea nigra,** a dark line that runs down the midabdomen.

Prenatal Visits

Prenatal visits occur at four-week intervals for most of the pregnancy. Intervals are reduced to two weeks and then one week as the due date approaches. The **fundal height**, which is the distance from the pubic symphysis to the top of the uterus, is measured at each obstetrical visit to assess fetal growth. Ultrasonography may be performed to determine the exact fetal size and position and to investigate any abnormalities. Sonography can also detect a multifetal pregnancy, hydatidiform mole (see page 365), **polyhydramnios,** or abnormalities involving the placenta.

In the first trimester, transvaginal ultrasound measurements help determine the accuracy of the due date, also called the **estimated date of confinement (EDC),** by comparing the **crown-rump length** to expected lengths based on gestational age. The **gestational age** refers to the length of the pregnancy based on the first day of the last menstrual period. The **sonographic age** should correlate to the gestational age. The conceptual age is the true fetal age and refers to the length of the pregnancy from the time of conception. In the second trimester, gestational age may also be calculated using the **head circumference** or the **biparietal diameter (BPD).** The median length of pregnancy is 280 days (40 weeks) from the first day of the last period. Infants born prior to 37 weeks are considered preterm and infants born after 40 weeks are considered postterm.

> ▶ Patient is a 42-year-old gravida 4, para 0 with an EDC of 05/11/20XX. She has a singleton viable pregnancy with size not compatible with dates. Fetus measures 2.7 mm, compatible with 5 weeks and 6 days; she is 6 weeks and 5 days according to dates.

Evaluating the mother's current medications is also important. The FDA classifies drugs into categories of safety for use during pregnancy: **Categories A, B, C, D, and X.** Category A drugs are considered safe during pregnancy. Categories B and C have not been adequately studied and the risk of harm is unknown. Category D drugs are known to have some fetal risk but the risks and benefits must be evaluated. There may be greater harm to the mother by withdrawing or not administering the drug. Category X drugs have proven fetal risks that outweigh any possible benefit and should never be given during pregnancy.

Drugs administered in the first 20 days following fertilization may have an all-or-nothing effect on the embryo—either the potential to kill the embryo or have no effect at all. **Teratogenesis** (malformation of the fetus) is most likely to occur during **organogenesis,** which occurs between days 20 and 56 following fertilization. Teratogenesis is unlikely to occur during the 2nd and 3rd trimesters but some drugs may affect the growth of the fetus or the function of fetal organs. All pregnant women are encouraged to take prenatal vitamins that contain supplemental iron and 400 mcg of **folate (folic acid)** to prevent anemia and reduce the risk of **neural tube defects**. (11)

Prenatal Testing

Early in the pregnancy, a series of physical assessments and laboratory tests should be performed. Clinical **pelvimetry** assesses the pelvic type (**android, gynecoid, platypelloid,** and **anthropoid**) and may help in the management of dystocia or cephalopelvic disproportion at the time of delivery.

Routine laboratory evaluations include urinalysis (UA), urine culture, and CBC. Serological studies include tests for infectious diseases including syphilis (RPR), rubella, varicella (VZV), hepatitis (HBsAg), and HIV. Blood type is determined, including Rh type (see below under erythroblastosis fetalis). Pap smear is performed (if not already up to date) and cervical cultures are taken for gonorrhea and chlamydia. At about 35–37 weeks, the vagina and anorectum are cultured for colonization by **group B streptococci (GBS)**. Although group B strep is typically harmless to the mother, it can infect the infant during delivery, causing a life-threatening newborn sepsis. Mothers positive for group B strep are treated prophylactically with penicillin, cefazolin, erythromycin, or clindamycin.

Women of certain ethnic backgrounds may be tested for inherited blood disorders known to cause anemia. Women of African descent are tested for **sickle cell trait** (see page 390), and women of African, Asian, or Mediterranean descent may be evaluated for abnormal hemoglobin (eg, **hemoglobin S, C, or F; alpha or beta thalassemia**). Learn more on page 387. Genetic screening tests to determine carrier states of genetically transmitted diseases may be offered to newly pregnant woman or women planning to be pregnant, especially those with specific ethnic backgrounds. Ashkenazi Jews may elect to be tested for **Tay-Sachs** and **Canavan disease**. All women are offered a screening test for the cystic fibrosis gene.

Fetal tests for genetic or metabolic disorders may also be offered. Pregnant women over age 35 may elect to have **chorionic villus sampling (CVS)** or **genetic amniocentesis** to detect fetal chromosomal abnormalities. Noninvasive **nuchal translucency testing** (also called **nuchal fold test**) may be performed to assess for **Down syndrome (trisomy 21)** and congenital heart

defects. Decreased serum levels of **pregnancy-associated plasma protein A (PAPP-A)** has been associated with **aneuploidy**. Between 16 and 20 weeks, maternal serum may be tested for elevated levels of alpha-fetoprotein (AFP, also abbreviated MSAFP to indicate maternal serum), which may indicate a neural tube defect. A **triple screen** for Down syndrome includes alpha-fetoprotein, estriol, and hCG; the **quad test** for Down syndrome includes the triple screen plus **inhibin A**.

> ▶ Recommend nuchal cord translucency and quad test for the patient. We discussed prenatal testing including chorionic villus sampling and amniocentesis.

Infertility

Infertility is defined as the inability to conceive after one year of unprotected intercourse. **Assisted reproductive technology (ART,** usually dictated as an acronym) is used to assist couples in conception. Techniques include:

- **ovulation induction (OI):** use of clomiphene citrate to induce ovulation.
- **intrauterine insemination (IUI):** placement of sperm directly into uterine cavity using a catheter inserted through the cervix.
- **in vitro fertilization (IVF):** involves **egg retrieval** to be combined with sperm in the laboratory. Fertilized eggs are cultured three to five days to the **blastocyst** stage, after which they are transferred to the uterus. Transfer may be back to the biological mother or to a surrogate (one who will carry the pregnancy). **Two-embryo transfer** is commonly used, which may result in a singleton or twin pregnancy. This technique is used to treat infertility due to oligospermia, sperm antibodies, tubal dysfunction, endometriosis, and unexplained infertility.
- **controlled ovarian hyperstimulation (COH):** administration of clomiphene citrate and/or gonadotropins followed by hCG to induce ovulation of more than

> **(11)** Neural tube defects are those caused by incomplete closure or functional incompetence of the neural tube, the embryonic origins of the brain and spinal cord.

one egg. This technique is used to harvest multiple eggs prior to IVF.

- **intracytoplasmic sperm injection (ICSI,** pronounced *ik-sē*): procedure performed along with in vitro fertilization that injects sperm directly into eggs. This technique is used when there is a **male factor** such as very low sperm counts.

Patients over the age of 35 typically have **decreased ovarian reserve**. Ovarian reserve may be tested by measuring **antimüllerian hormone (AMH)** levels. Decreased antimüllerian hormone and decreased FSH levels are indicative of decreased ovarian reserve. Patients may also be tested using a **clomiphene challenge test** whereby they are given clomiphene citrate 100 mg on days five to nine of the menstrual cycle. A dramatic increase in FSH and estradiol levels from day 3 to day 10 of the cycle is indicative of decreased ovarian reserve.

Male partners may also be evaluated for abnormalities that may lead to infertility. A semen analysis should be performed to confirm an adequate sperm count with normal morphology and normal motility. FSH values may also be evaluated in males. **Table 11-3** lists normal sperm parameters.

Table 11-3 Normal Semen Analysis Parameters

Parameter	Reference Range
volume	2–6 mL
concentration	greater than 20 million/mL
motility	greater than 50% of sperm should show motility
morphology	greater than 14% of sperm should show normal morphology using strict criteria outlined by the World Health Organization (WHO)

(12) In a medical context, the term abortion does not carry the same connotation or inference as the societal use of the term. Medically, the term abortion simply means the pregnancy ended before 20 weeks' gestation with no implication as to the cause.

(13) The products of conception consist of the gestational sac, embryonic or fetal tissue, placenta, and any other tissues associated with a pregnancy.

Pregnancy Loss

A pregnancy can end prematurely for many different reasons, a few of which are outlined in the following sections.

Abortion

Abortion (Ab) is the termination of a pregnancy before 20 weeks' gestation (or prior to viability). **(12)** Abortions may be spontaneous or therapeutic. A **therapeutic abortion (TAb)** is an **elective (induced) abortion**. The decision may be based on a desire to not have children or for medical reasons related to the health of the mother or the condition of the fetus. A **spontaneous abortion (SAb)** is embryonic or fetal death before 20 weeks' gestation that is not induced by medical treatment. Recurrent spontaneous abortions are also known as **recurrent pregnancy loss**. A spontaneous abortion may result in a complete loss of the **products of conception (POC), (13)** or some or all of the tissues may be retained. The following are categories of spontaneous abortions:

- **threatened Ab:** bleeding or cramping but the pregnancy continues; no dilation of the cervix
- **inevitable Ab:** the cervix is dilated and membranes may be ruptured, passage of the POC have not yet occurred but the loss is considered unavoidable; bleeding and cramping persist
- **complete Ab:** the fetus and placenta are completely expelled
- **incomplete Ab:** some portion of the POC remain in the uterus; only mild cramps are reported but bleeding is persistent
- **missed Ab:** the pregnancy stops developing with a disappearance of previously detected embryonic cardiac activity, but the POC have not been expelled. Symptoms of pregnancy are no longer experienced, but there may be a brownish vaginal discharge.

Incomplete and missed abortions require uterine evacuation to remove products of conception. At less than 12 weeks' gestation, this can be performed using

The abbreviation for abortion (Ab) is usually dictated as two letters, a-b. A spontaneous abortion is dictated s-a-b, and therapeutic abortion is dictated t-a-b.

suction curettage. Dilation or medical induction may be required for second-trimester abortions. Dilation of the cervix can be accomplished using **laminaria,** misoprostol (Cytotec) or mifepristone (Mifeprex, also called RU486). A paracervical block may be used for anesthesia.

After 20 weeks' gestation, fetal death is no longer considered an abortion but a **stillbirth.** A live birth that occurs between 20 and 37 weeks is considered a **preterm birth.** Maternal causes of stillbirth include uncontrolled diabetes mellitus, preeclampsia or eclampsia, sepsis, substance abuse, or trauma. Placental causes of stillbirth include **placental abruption** (detachment of the placenta from the uterus), **chorioamnionitis** (infection in the amniotic fluid), fetomaternal hemorrhage, twin-twin transfusion, umbilical cord accidents (eg, prolapse, knots), **uteroplacental vascular insufficiency,** and **vasa previa.** Fetal karyotype analysis and autopsy may be performed to determine cause of death.

Ectopic Pregnancy

An **ectopic pregnancy** is one in which the embryo implants in a location other than the endometrial lining of the uterine cavity. The most common sites for ectopic pregnancy are the fallopian tubes and the cornual area of the uterus. Other sites include the peritoneum, abdominal viscera, the ovary, and the cervix. A **heterotopic pregnancy** is a simultaneous implantation of two embryos, one ectopic and one intrauterine. Women with a history of infertility, PID, ruptured appendix, abdominal surgery, or prior tubal surgery are at increased risk of ectopic pregnancy. IUD use also carries an increased risk of ectopic pregnancy. Ectopic pregnancies cannot be carried to term.

> **Pause 11-6** Why do you suppose that women with a history of a ruptured appendix or previous abdominal surgery are at increased risk of ectopic pregnancy?

An ectopic pregnancy may be suspected when the quantitative beta hCG levels do not rise appropriately or rise and then begin to fall. The gestational sac of an ectopic pregnancy typically ruptures anywhere from six to 16 weeks into the pregnancy. Rupture of an ectopic pregnancy causes severe lower quadrant pain that is sudden and lancinating. Depending on the size of the gestational sac and the location, bleeding may be severe enough to cause hemorrhagic shock. An ectopic pregnancy may also rupture less dramatically and cause blood to leak over a period of days. Vaginal spotting may occur and a mass may be palpable on examination. Ruptured ectopic pregnancies must be treated emergently with a **salpingostomy** or salpingectomy.

Early ectopic pregnancies (less than 3 cm in diameter with no fetal heart activity detected) that are diagnosed before they rupture may be treated medically using methotrexate given intramuscularly. Beta hCG and sonogram are repeated several days later and a second dose of methotrexate is given if the beta hCG level has not decreased by 15%.

Trophoblastic Disease

Gestational trophoblastic disease includes **complete and partial moles, choriocarcinomas,** and **invasive moles.** A **mole** is a mass of tissue formed by the degeneration of the products of conception. Complete and partial moles are also called **hydatidiform moles** or **hydatid moles.** A complete mole contains no fetal tissue; a partial mole contains some fetal tissue. The majority of moles express only the paternal chromosomes—sometimes two copies of the paternal chromosomes and sometimes only a single copy of paternal chromosomes. Most show a chromosomal composition of 46,XX. A hydatidiform mole may become malignant and invade the myometrium or metastasize.

A **molar pregnancy** with a complete mole typically enlarges faster than a normal embryo, produces more hCG, and is more likely to become malignant. Maternal symptoms are often more severe due to the extremely high levels of hCG (serum greater than 40,000 milliunits/mL or urine greater than 100,000 milliunits per 24 hours). High levels of hCG can produce a thyrotoxicosis.

Treatment is surgical removal (suction) of the molar tissue. Chemotherapy is indicated if pathology studies indicate malignancy. Patients should be monitored for two years for a gradual decline and continued negative hCG level.

Vanishing Twin

Vanishing twin syndrome describes an initially multifetal pregnancy with the subsequent **demise** of one or more of the fetuses. The pregnancy continues because at least one fetus remains viable. There may be complete reabsorption of the vanishing twin, development of a cyst-like abnormality, or formation of a **fetus papyraceus** (pressed, paper-like fetal tissue). Chromosomal analysis of the fetal tissue often shows chromosomal abnormalities such as **diploidy** or **triploidy**. Fetal demise early in the pregnancy typically has little or no consequences on the remaining fetus, but a vanishing twin late in the pregnancy may lead to complications in the remaining fetus or the mother, including preterm labor, infection, hemorrhage, coagulopathy, or difficulty with labor.

Recurrent Pregnancy Loss

Recurrent pregnancy loss is defined as the loss of three or more viable pregnancies. A **hysterosalpingogram (HSG)** or sonohysterogram may be performed to check for structural uterine abnormalities that may cause recurrent losses. Coagulopathies are common maternal causes of recurrent pregnancy loss due to arterial and venous thromboses (see also Chapter 12 for more detailed information on coagulopathies). Coagulopathies affecting pregnancy include:

- positive Lupus anticoagulant (antiphospholipid antibody)
- activated protein C resistance
- protein S or protein C deficiency
- antithrombin deficiency
- hyperhomocysteinemia caused by mutations (C677T and A1298C) in the gene that encodes for **methylenetetrahydrofolate reductase (MTHFR)**
- anticardiolipin antibody
- **factor V Leiden**

Patients with the above coagulopathies are treated with heparin (8000 to 20,000 units two or three times a day), LMWH, or low-dose aspirin throughout the pregnancy and during the postpartum period.

Chromosomal abnormalities of the fetus, such as a **translocation** or aneuploidy, can cause pregnancy loss. A **balanced translocation** occurs when parts of two different chromosomes switch places with each other without any loss or duplication of chromosomal information. An **unbalanced translocation** causes the loss or addition of chromosomal information. The cause of multiple miscarriages may be determined by performing a karyotype on the products of conception.

Abnormalities of Pregnancy

The degree to which pregnancy is monitored is indicative of the wide range of problems that may be encountered during gestation and parturition. Many abnormalities can be life-threatening to the mother and/or the fetus.

Hyperemesis Gravidarum

Many pregnant women experience nausea, especially in the first trimester. Some women may experience extreme nausea and vomiting, called **hyperemesis gravidarum**. Poor fluid intake combined with vomiting leads to dehydration, ketosis, and weight loss. Treatment is inpatient admission for IV fluids. An ultrasound should be performed to rule out hydatidiform mole or multifetal pregnancy. Persistent nausea may be treated with antiemetics including vitamin B_6, doxylamine, promethazine (Phenergan), ondansetron (Zofran), metoclopramide (Reglan), or prochlorperazine (Compazine).

Erythroblastosis Fetalis

Erythroblastosis fetalis, also called **hemolytic disease of the newborn (HDN)**, is caused by blood-group incompatibility between the mother and fetus. At the first prenatal visit, women should be tested for ABO blood type and Rh blood type, as well as the presence of blood-group antibodies with an **indirect Coombs** test (see page 425). If Rh negative, the mother should have **reflex antibody screening** for the presence of antibodies against $Rh_0(D)$, the most clinically significant Rh antigen. An Rh-negative mother with Rh-positive partner may have offspring that are Rh positive. An Rh-negative mother exposed to an Rh-positive fetus is likely to form antibodies against the Rh antigen, especially if there is a significant **fetomaternal hemorrhage** (10–150 mL of fetal blood crossing into the maternal blood stream).

To test for a fetomaternal bleed, a **rosette test** (a qualitative test for the presence of a bleed) and a **Kleihauer-Betke test** (a quantitative test to measure the volume of the bleed) are performed on maternal blood samples. Fetomaternal hemorrhage can occur following trauma, obstetrical procedures, or during **parturition**, including abortion and ectopic pregnancy. **Anti-$Rh_0(D)$ antibody titers** are also monitored; a titer greater than 1:16 indicates a significant number of antibodies have formed and the fetus is at risk. Antibodies formed during the first pregnancy can affect any subsequent Rh-positive fetuses to an even greater degree.

Rh antibodies directed against the fetal red blood cells will cause red cell lysis, resulting in fetal anemia with high-output heart failure, pleural effusion, and edema (**hydrops fetalis**). Increased cardiac output in the fetus increases flow velocity and can be detected by measuring the fetus's **middle cerebral artery flow** (velocity) using Doppler ultrasound. If the middle cerebral artery flow is elevated, **percutaneous umbilical blood sampling (PUBS)** can be performed to analyze the fetal blood for anemia and **erythroblastosis**, which is the presence of nucleated (immature) red blood cells caused by increased pressure on the fetal bone marrow to compensate the anemia.

To prevent the formation of anti-Rh_0(D), Rh-negative mothers are given **anti-Rh_0(D) IgG injections (RhoGAM)**. These antibodies bind to the Rh antigens on fetal red blood cells that happen to cross into the maternal blood stream. By blocking the antigens on the fetal red blood cells, the maternal immune system is not stimulated to create antibodies. Anti-Rh_0(D) injections are given at 28 weeks' gestation and within 72 hours of parturition. Additional doses are given following amniocentesis, chorionic villus sampling, or if a fetomaternal bleed of greater than 30 mL occurs. The injection is also administered after ectopic pregnancy or abortion (spontaneous or therapeutic). If the pregnancy terminated at or before 12 weeks' gestation, a smaller dose of anti-Rh_0(D) IgG can be given (**MICRhoGAM**).

Other blood group antigens (besides the Rh group) can also cause hemolytic disease of the newborn. Mothers who have received prior blood transfusions or have had multiple pregnancies may have antibodies directed against other RBC antigens such as **Kell, Duffy, Kidd,** and **Lewis**. There is no prophylactic treatment for these blood-group antigens.

Incompetent Cervix

The cervix should remain firm and closed throughout the first and second trimesters. Cervical dilation with minimal uterine contractions occurring between 15 and 28 weeks' gestation is considered an **incompetent cervix** and often results in miscarriage. Treatment is with **cervical cerclage** using the **McDonald** or **Shirodkar** method. The patient is also placed on restricted activities. Cerclage is usually performed at the end of the first trimester of pregnancies that follow a miscarriage due to an incompetent cervix. The stitch is removed around the 37th week.

Placenta Previa

Placenta previa is implantation of the placenta over or near the internal cervical os. Placenta previa may be total, partial, or marginal. Total placenta previa entirely covers the cervical os. Partial placenta previa covers part of the os, and marginal is at the border of the os. An early placenta previa may resolve if the placenta migrates away from the os as the pregnancy progresses. Placenta previa or a low-lying placenta (very near the os) may cause poor fetal growth, premature delivery, or a difficult delivery.

Patients typically experience painless vaginal bleeding with bright red blood beginning mid to late pregnancy. Patients may also experience uterine contractions. The diagnosis is made by ultrasound. Massive hemorrhage is the most common complicating factor in placenta previa, and obstetricians should anticipate the need for transfusion and possible **cesarean hysterectomy**.

Preeclampsia and Eclampsia

Preeclampsia is characterized by new-onset hypertension and proteinuria occurring anywhere from 20 weeks of gestation up to six weeks postpartum. **Eclampsia** is defined as generalized seizures (grand mal seizures) in a patient with preeclampsia. The exact etiology of preeclampsia is not understood. The syndrome affects the central nervous system, the hematologic and vascular systems, the kidneys, liver, fetus, and placenta. Early signs include nondependent edema, especially in the face and hands, and sudden weight gain. Right upper quadrant pain indicates capsular swelling around the liver, and increased reflex activity is a sign of neuromuscular irritability that may progress to seizures.

Activation of the coagulation system causes decreased platelet count and possibly **disseminated intravascular coagulation** (see page 394). **HELLP syndrome** (hemolysis, elevated liver function tests, and low platelet count) develops in a significant number of patients with severe eclampsia. HELLP syndrome is marked by **microangiopathic** findings such as petechiae, low platelet count, **schistocytes** and **helmet cells** (see page 429) seen on peripheral blood smears. Liver enzymes are also elevated.

The diagnosis of preeclampsia is based on an elevated blood pressure exceeding 140/89 mmHg with proteinuria greater than 300 mg per 24 hours or 1+ on random dipstick urine. Hospitalization is usually required. The goal is to prolong pregnancy until the fetal lungs are mature. The only definitive treatment is delivery, but symptom management is attempted for as long as possible. **Magnesium sulfate ($MgSO_4$)** is administered for the prevention and treatment of seizures. Hypertension may be treated with antihypertensive medications.

Preterm Labor

Preterm labor is defined as contractions causing cervical change (effacement and dilation) before the 37th week of gestation. Risk factors include premature rupture of the membranes, infection, cervical incompetence, multi-fetal pregnancy, and placental abnormalities. Infection may include chorioamnionitis, pyelonephritis, or a sexually transmitted infection. Group B streptococci is a common cause of infection leading to preterm labor.

Treatment of preterm labor depends on the gestational age. Generally, patients are put on bedrest and increased hydration. If known, the underlying cause of the preterm labor is addressed. Antibiotics are prescribed for a known infection or for GBS prophylaxis. **Tocolytics** (medications to stop contractions), such as magnesium sulfate, indomethacin, and nifedipine are given if bedrest and hydration do not control the contractions. Indications for tocolytics include six or more contractions per hour with cervical changes. Tocolytics do not significantly extend a pregnancy and are not effective enough to stave off delivery long enough for a 20-week (or less) gestation to become viable. Viability is considered highly unlikely before 24 weeks, so tocolytics are not recommended before 24 weeks' gestation. If the pregnancy is between 24 and 34 weeks' gestation and the cervix continues to dilate, corticosteroids (betamethasone) are given to induce fetal lung maturity and reduce the risk of neonatal respiratory distress syndrome. Tocolytics may be able to delay labor for 48 hours, the time required for steroids to accelerate fetal lung maturity.

 Magnesium sulfate may be dictated "mag sulfate."

Patients in preterm labor may be evaluated to determine if the fetal lungs are mature enough for delivery to proceed. The ratio of lecithin to sphingomyelin (**L/S ratio**) increases as the fetal lungs mature. These levels can be measured in the amniotic fluid. An L/S ratio of two or more indicates low risk for respiratory distress syndrome.

Premature Rupture of Membranes

Leakage of amniotic fluid before the onset of labor is called **premature rupture of membranes (PROM)**. Fluid may be felt as a sudden gush or a steady trickle. Amniotic fluid can be distinguished from urine using Nitrazine paper,

- A woman's obstetrical history is described using the terms gravidity and parity. It may also include the number of term deliveries, premature deliveries, number of abortions, and the number of living children.
- Pregnancy produces many physiologic changes in the mother, including changes in pulse, cardiac output, blood pressure, blood volume, and white cell counts.
- Pregnancy is monitored with routine prenatal visits, sonographic examinations, blood and urine analyses. Women may choose to be screened for genetic diseases or have the fetus tested for genetic abnormalities including neural tube defects and aneuploidy.
- Infertility is the inability to conceive after one year of unprotected intercourse. Assisted reproductive technology is used to treat infertility, including OI, COH, IUI, IVF, and ICSI. Both female and male factors may be implicated in infertility.

- Pregnancy loss may be due to abortion (spontaneous or therapeutic), ectopic implantation, trophoblastic disease, chromosomal abnormalities of the embryo, or structural or metabolic disorders of the mother. The etiology of many pregnancy losses is unknown.
- Recurrent pregnancy loss is the loss of three or more viable pregnancies. Common causes of recurrent pregnancy loss include coagulopathies in the mother or chromosomal abnormalities. Serology studies and karyotyping are performed to help diagnose the causes of recurrent pregnancy loss.
- Abnormalities of pregnancy include hyperemesis gravidarum, HDN, preeclampsia, infection, incompetent cervix, abnormal placentation, and premature rupture of membranes. A pregnancy extending beyond 40 weeks also places the mother and baby at risk.

which turns deep blue at a pH greater than 6.5. Amnionic fluid has a pH of 7 to 7.6. Alternatively, a sample of secretions taken from the **posterior vaginal fornix** or cervix can be placed on a slide and examined for **ferning** (crystallization pattern that looks like a palm leaf), which is indicative of amniotic fluid. A sonogram may demonstrate **oligohydramnios** (decreased or deficient amniotic fluid). After rupture, the majority of women go into labor spontaneously within the ensuing 24 hours.

Postterm Pregnancy

A **postterm pregnancy** is one that exceeds 40 weeks. A postterm pregnancy increases risks for both the mother and the fetus. Complications include:

- **macrosomia** (large infant or enlargement of the head due to hydrocephalus, encephalocele, hydrops, or other abnormality)
- dysmaturity syndrome
- oligohydramnios
- **meconium staining** and **meconium aspiration (14)**
- dystocia

At 41 weeks, an assessment of the fetus includes amniotic fluid volume, fetal movements, and fetal heart rate. Evidence of fetal compromise or oligohydramnios is indication for immediate delivery.

Labor

Often, the first sign of impending labor is the **bloody show**, a small plug of mucus and blood that is released from the cervical os. It may appear up to 72 hours before contractions begin. Labor is divided into three stages. The first stage begins with the onset of labor and ends with full dilation of the cervix. During pregnancy, the cervix is firm and retains the fetus in the developing uterus. As delivery approaches, the cervix begins to soften and thin out in a process called **cervical ripening**. With the cervix softened and relaxed, uterine contractions are able to pull the cervix open. **Effacement** describes the thinning and shortening of the cervix. Dilation describes the opening of the cervical os. The cervix must be 100% effaced and dilated to 10 cm for a vaginal delivery to proceed.

The first phase of stage 1 is the latent phase. During this phase, contractions become more coordinated and the cervix effaces and dilates to 4 cm. The latent phase is followed by the active phase, during which the cervix becomes fully dilated and the fetus descends into the midpelvis. If not already ruptured, **amniotomy** (purposeful rupture of the membranes) may cause labor to progress more quickly. A prolonged latent phase occurs when more than 20 hours in a nullipara or 14 hours in a multipara is required to reach 3–4 cm of cervical dilation and begin the active phase.

The second stage of labor begins with full cervical dilation and ends with delivery of the fetus. This stage typically requires the mother to bear down hard to push the fetus through the cervical opening. The third stage of labor begins with the delivery of the infant and ends with delivery of the placenta.

The position of the fetus is also described as labor progresses. **Station** describes the position of the presenting part of the fetus relative to the maternal ischial spines. Station 0 corresponds to a level even with the spines, and at this level the baby is said to be **engaged**. The five positions above (positive numbers) and below (negative numbers) the spines are measured in 1 cm increments and noted as +1 through +5 (above) or −1 through −5 (below). **Fetal lie** describes the relationship of the long axis of the fetus relative to the mother. If the two are parallel, the fetal lie is longitudinal. If the two are at 90-degree angles, the fetal lie is transverse. Fetal attitude describes the way the fetus's body parts are arranged. The normal fetal attitude is called the fetal position, with the knees bent and tucked inward toward the chest and the arms folded toward the center of the chest. Abnormal fetal attitudes include positions with the head extended back or the arms behind the back.

Presentation describes the part of the infant abutting the cervical opening (eg, head, shoulder, buttocks, or feet) and therefore the part that will deliver first. A **cephalic presentation** means the head will deliver first. **Vertex** refers to the crown of the head toward the cervix and is the most desirable presentation. A **breech presentation** is buttocks first; **complete breech** is a sitting position with hips and knees flexed; **frank breech** is buttocks first with hips flexed, legs straight, and the feet close to the face. A shoulder presentation may present the shoulder, arm, or trunk first. One foot first is **single footling** and two feet completely extended is a **double footling** presentation.

Attitude describes the relationship of the infant's head relative to its spine; normally, the chin should be

---

(14) Meconium is the initial tar-like stool consisting of mucus and bile. It is normally released after birth, but may be released in utero, in which case it stains the amniotic fluid green.

close to the chest. **Asynclitism** is malposition of the fetal head within the pelvis with the head being flexed, neutral, or extended. **External cephalic version**, which involves gentle manipulation of the mother's abdomen, may be attempted to move the fetus to a vertex presentation before labor begins.

Position describes the relationship of the presenting part relative to the mother's pelvis. A vertex (head down) presentation may be described as vertex, left occiput anterior (**vertex, left occipitoanterior, [LOA]**), meaning the back of the baby's head (occiput) is resting on the left anterior portion of the mother's pelvis. If the baby is lying straight, without any turn to the left or right, the position is **occipitoanterior (OA)** or **occipitoposterior (OP)**. An occipitoposterior presentation presses the back of the baby's head on the mother's back and causes **back labor** (contractions felt in the back more than the abdomen). A breech presentation may be described as **right sacrum posterior (RSP)**, meaning the infant's buttocks (sacrum) face anteriorly and toward the right. The most common and preferable presentation is vertex, LOA. An abnormal presentation is called a **malpresentation**. Table 11-4 describes the various fetal presentations.

Contractions must be of sufficient power to produce active labor. The power of the contractions is expressed in **Montevideo units (MVU)**, which is the strength of the contractions (measured in millimeters of mercury) multiplied by the number of contractions in 10 minutes (eg, three contractions at 70 mmHg is 210 MVUs). Adequate labor is considered to be at least 200 MVUs per 10 minutes.

Analgesia

The most common type of analgesia offered during labor is a **lumbar epidural** that provides regional anesthesia. A local anesthetic such as ropivacaine or bupivacaine is continuously infused into the epidural space. An opioid such as fentanyl (Duragesic, Sublimaze) may be added. Analgesic may also be administered by IV. Choices include fentanyl, meperidine (Demerol), or morphine sulfate. Narcan can be used as an antidote if toxicity occurs.

Local forms of anesthesia include **pudendal block**, **perineal infiltration**, and **paracervical block**. Local anesthesia is used much less often now with the increased use of lumbar epidurals. A pudendal block involves injecting a local anesthetic such as lidocaine (Xylocaine) through the vaginal wall to deaden the pudendal nerve. This anesthetizes the lower vagina, perineum, and posterior vulva. Paracervical blocks are performed by injecting lidocaine at the 3-o'clock and 9-o'clock positions of the cervix.

Table 11-4 Fetal Presentations

Position	Abbreviation	Description
left occipitoanterior	LOA	head down, occiput toward the mother's left front quadrant
right occipitoanterior	ROA	head down, occiput toward the mother's right front quadrant
left occipitoposterior	LOP	head down, occiput toward the mother's back left quadrant
right occipitoposterior	ROP	head down, occiput toward the mother's back right quadrant
occipitoanterior	OA	head down, body straight, occiput toward the mother's front, no tendency toward left or right
occipitoposterior	OP	head down, body straight, occiput toward the mother's back, no tendency toward left or right
left sacrum anterior	LSA	buttocks down, toward the mother's front left quadrant
right sacrum anterior	RSA	buttocks down, toward the mother's right front quadrant
left sacrum posterior	LSP	buttocks down, toward the mother's left back quadrant
right sacrum posterior	RSP	buttocks down, toward the mother's right back quadrant

General anesthesia is generally not used for routine deliveries because it affects both the mother and the fetus. A general anesthetic such as thiopental along with succinylcholine may be used for an emergency cesarean delivery.

Fetal Monitoring

Fetal status monitoring is an important component of managing labor. Monitoring includes the fetal heart rate (HR) and the heart rate variability, especially in relation to uterine contractions and maternal movements. External heart rate monitors are placed on the mother's abdomen. If amniotic membranes have ruptured, infants may be monitored internally by placing a lead on the fetal scalp. The infant may also be monitored with oximetry using an internal sensor placed directly against the infant's skin.

Fetal status is described as **reassuring** or **nonreassuring**. A reassuring pattern is 120–160 beats per minute at baseline with a variation of 6–25 beats with movement or contractions and without **decelerations** (decreasing heart rate). A nonreassuring pattern shows late decelerations (gradual decrease in HR following the peak of a contraction), variable decelerations, tachycardia, severe bradycardia (less than 110 beats per minute), or a loss of normal variability.

Correlating fetal HR with fetal movements is called a **nonstress test**. A nonstress test is nonreassuring if no accelerations occur in a 40-minute period. A **contraction stress test** monitors fetal movements and HR during contractions. When problems are detected, **intrauterine fetal resuscitation** is attempted by giving the mother O_2 by facemask, a rapid IV infusion, and repositioning her on her side. Emergency cesarean may be performed if the fetal heart pattern is not improved.

Induction of Labor

Induction of labor is the administration of uterine stimulants (**oxytocics**) to cause contractions. An **elective induction** is performed to control the delivery date. An L/S ratio may be performed to assure fetal lung maturity. Misoprostol (Cytotec) vaginally is commonly used. Another common choice is prostaglandin E2 (dinoprostone) given intracervically or as an **intravaginal pessary**. Mechanical methods of dilation may use laminaria or transcervical balloon catheters. Once the cervix has begun to open and efface, contractions may be induced using a constant IV infusion of oxytocin (Pitocin).

Dystocia

Dystocia is difficult, abnormally slow, or nonprogressing labor. Dystocia may also be described as dysfunctional labor or **failure to progress**. Common causes of dystocia include small maternal pelvis causing **cephalopelvic disproportion (CPD)**, also called **fetopelvic disproportion**, fetal macrosomia, and abnormal presentation.

A breech presentation may be problematic because the buttocks are not a good dilating wedge; after the body is delivered, the head tends to become trapped during delivery. The umbilical cord is also more likely to be compressed during the delivery of a breech presentation, resulting in fetal hypoxemia. Shoulder dystocia occurs when the **head is delivered onto the perineum** but the shoulder is lodged behind the symphysis pubis. The **McRoberts maneuver** (hyperflexing the maternal thighs while applying suprapubic pressure) may be attempted to dislodge the shoulder. The **Woods screw maneuver** involves inserting the hand into the posterior vagina and rotating the fetus. These maneuvers risk fracturing the fetal humerus or clavicle, although at times the clavicle may be fractured on purpose. If attempts to reposition the infant fail, the infant's head is pushed back into the vagina or uterus (**Zavanelli maneuver**) and then a cesarean delivery is performed.

Protracted Labor

Protracted labor is a type of dystocia characterized by abnormally slow cervical dilation (**arrest of dilation**) or a lack of fetal descent during active labor (**arrest of descent**). Active labor typically begins after the cervix dilates to 4 cm or more and cervical dilation normally proceeds at approximately 1 cm/h. The head also descends at approximately 1 cm/h. A multipara may advance more quickly than a nullipara. In a nulliparous woman, a prolonged labor is defined as a lack of progress for three hours with a regional anesthetic or two hours without an anesthetic. In multiparous women, a lack of progress for two hours with a regional anesthetic or one hour without constitutes prolonged labor. Abnormal presentation or CPD can cause labor to slow or fail to progress (**arrest of labor**). Hypotonic (weak) or hypertonic (overly strong or closely spaced) contractions may also affect the active phase.

Treatment of protracted labor depends on the cause, but options include administration of oxytocin, cesarean delivery, or operative delivery. Hypotonic contractions may respond to oxytocin. Hypertonic uterine dysfunction may result from the use of oxytocin, and discontinuing oxytocic stimulation and giving analgesics may help. Cesarean delivery may be needed for CPD, which often occurs when the infant weighs more than 5000 g. Delivery that stalls during the second stage of labor may require operative delivery using forceps or vacuum extraction.

Delivery

A woman who goes into labor without being induced and delivers vaginally is said to have had a **normal spontaneous vaginal delivery (NSVD)**. Many obstetric units now offer a combined **labor, delivery, recovery, and postpartum (LDRP)** room that allows the mother to labor, deliver, and recover in the same room. Other arrangements may use a traditional labor room with a separate area for delivery. Upon admission to the obstetrical unit, the pregnant woman should be examined using the **Leopold maneuver** to estimate the size of the fetus and determine the fetal position and presenting part.

The second stage of delivery is marked by full dilation of the cervix. At this point, the mother can begin to bear down to push the infant through the vaginal area. An **episiotomy** (an incision in the perineum) may be performed to prevent tearing of the perineal tissues. The most common is a **midline episiotomy**, which is made from the midpoint of the **fourchette** directly back toward the rectum. Alternatively, a **mediolateral episiotomy** may be made by cutting at a 45-degree angle from either side of the fourchette. If no episiotomy is performed, the infant is said to be delivered over an **intact perineum**.

The infant's nose, mouth, and pharynx are aspirated with a bulb syringe as soon as the head is delivered. After complete delivery, the cord is clamped and cut. If the baby is in distress, a segment of the cord may be doubly clamped and a sample of blood withdrawn from the cord to be analyzed for blood gases. Normal arterial blood pH is 7.15 to 7.2. The baby may be warmed in a **resuscitation bassinet**. The placenta is delivered following delivery of the infant. The placenta should be inspected to make sure no fragments have been retained in the uterus. Oxytocin may be administered after delivery of the placenta to help the uterus contract. The mother should be carefully monitored for hemorrhage in the postpartum period.

An **operative vaginal delivery** involves the use of **forceps** or a **vacuum extractor** to facilitate delivery. Instrumentation is used when the second stage of labor is prolonged, if fetal compromise is suspected, or if the mother is distressed or exhausted. Complications of operative delivery include hemorrhage, perineal trauma, neonatal bruising, **cephalohematoma**, and retinal bleeding.

Cesarean delivery is a surgical procedure to remove the infant through an abdominal incision. The most common reasons for performing a cesarean delivery are protracted labor, dystocia, and **nonreassuring fetal status** (fetal distress). Genital herpes infection is also an indication for cesarean delivery, as the risk of transmitting the virus to the infant as it passes through the vaginal canal is quite high. **Abnormal placentation** (eg, placenta previa) is also an indication for cesarean birth. Women with uterine scars from a **transmural incision** for myomectomy are typically delivered by cesarean.

> She spontaneously delivered a girl over an intact perineum, with Apgar scores of 9 at one minute and 9 at five minutes. The placenta was delivered by gentle traction and appeared to be complete. The estimated blood loss was 300 mL, and the patient was recovered in the LDR.

> **Pause 11-8** Describe a transmural incision for myomectomy.

> **Pause 11-7** You may hear phrases such as "she spontaneously delivered an Apgar nine slash nine girl," but it is best to recast this phrase as in the previous example. Look up the rules for transcribing Apgar scores in the *Book of Style*.

A cesarean delivery typically uses a transverse incision through the lower abdomen. Incision types include **Maylard, Joel Cohen**, or, more commonly, a **Pfannenstiel** incision. After entering the fascia and peritoneum, a bladder flap is formed by incising the **vesicouterine peritoneal reflection**.

A lower-segment incision into the uterus is the most common approach; a vertical incision on the anterior wall of the uterus may be used in cases of abnormal placentation or malpresentation. Lower-segment incisions are made in the thinner, elongated portion of the uterus under the **bladder reflection**. Patients that have had one cesarean birth may elect to have repeat cesarean as there is some concern for uterine rupture in women attempting a **vaginal birth after cesarean delivery** (**VBAC**, *vē-băk*). VBAC is considered safe if the preceding cesarean delivery used a **lower uterine transverse incision**.

After delivery of the infant, the placenta is removed. Gentle traction may be applied to the placenta to facilitate removal. The uterus may be **externalized (15)** for inspection and suturing. The endometrial cavity should be clean and free of any traces of placenta. It should also feel firm and contracted. Following delivery, oxytocin may be administered to help contract the uterus, and if unsuccessful, the prostaglandin Hemabate may be given. The **incision-to-delivery time** should be as short as possible, as long intervals between incision and delivery of the infant are associated with worsening neonatal outcomes.

Complications of Delivery

The most common complications during delivery involve fetal presentation, the umbilical cord, and abnormal placentation.

Umbilical Cord Prolapse Umbilical cord prolapse occurs when the cord becomes positioned in front of the fetal presenting part and is compressed as the infant descends into the birth canal. Compression constricts blood flow to the infant, causing fetal hypoxemia, bradycardia, or severe variable accelerations. An **occult prolapsed cord** is contained within the uterus and an **overt prolapsed cord** protrudes into the vagina. An overt prolapse may occur if the membranes rupture before the head is engaged. Changing the mother's position may relieve pressure on the cord, or administering a tocolytic such as terbutaline may slow contractions and allow manipulation of the presenting part and the cord. If the heart rate remains depressed, emergency cesarean must be performed. The cord may become looped around the infant's neck, called a **nuchal cord**, but typically does not require intervention and is not associated with an adverse perinatal outcome.

Placenta Accreta Placenta accreta, **placenta increta**, and **placenta percreta** are characterized by an abnormally adherent placenta that is difficult to deliver. This occurs when the villi penetrate the uterine myometrium. Risk factors for placenta accreta include advanced maternal age, **increased parity**, prior cesarean delivery or myomectomy, endometrial defects (Asherman syndrome), and placenta previa. Placenta accreta is suspected when the placenta has not been delivered within 30 minutes following delivery of the infant. It may also be diagnosed before delivery by ultrasonography.

Attempts to remove the placenta with placental traction may cause a large hemorrhage. Hysterectomy is the most definitive treatment, but if future childbearing is important, resection of the abnormal site may be attempted. Incomplete expulsion of the placenta increases the risk of postpartum hemorrhage and infection. Methotrexate treatment may also be attempted if all or part of the placenta is left in situ and the patient is otherwise stable.

Puerperium

Puerperium is defined as the time from the delivery to about six weeks following birth. During this time, most of the changes of pregnancy, labor, and delivery resolve and the body has reverted to the nonpregnant state. Immediately after delivery, a large amount of red blood flows from the uterus until the uterine contraction phase occurs. Thereafter, the volume of vaginal discharge (**lochia**) rapidly decreases. The duration of this discharge, known as **lochia rubra**, is variable. The red discharge progressively changes to brownish red, with a more watery consistency (**lochia serosa**). Over a period of weeks, the discharge continues to decrease in amount and color and eventually changes to yellow (**lochia alba**).

The Neonate

The newborn infant is immediately evaluated for respiratory effort, heart rate, color, muscle tone, and reflex irritability. The infant is assessed at one minute

---

(15) Externalized means the uterus is brought outside the abdominal cavity through the abdominal incision. Some physicians dictate exteriorize and some dictate externalize, but in this context, they have the same meaning.

and again at five minutes following birth and assigned an **Apgar score**. (16) The Apgar score is based on five parameters and each parameter is given a score of 0–2, for a maximum score of 10. A score between 8 and 10 is ideal and indicates the infant is making a good transition to the extrauterine environment. Scores below seven at five minutes indicate a degree of fetal distress.

(16) The mnemonic APGAR (appearance, pulse, grimace, activity, and respiration) is used to help remember the five components of the Apgar score, but Apgar is actually an eponym, not an acronym, so it is written in title case.

She spontaneously delivered a girl from the OA position over a small, second-degree laceration at the fourchette. Apgar scores were 8 at one minute and 9 at five minutes.

In the immediate postdelivery period, neonates are examined, weighed, and observed. An antimicrobial agent (eg, erythromycin or 1% silver nitrate) is placed directly in the eyes to prevent gonococcal and chlamydial ophthalmia. Vitamin K 1 mg IM is administered to prevent hemorrhagic disease of the newborn.

If necessary, the gestational age may be determined by a careful physical examination of the neonate and calculated using the **Ballard score**. The Ballard score is based on characteristics of skin, hair (**lanugo**), breasts and genitals, eyes and ears as well as neuromuscular signs.

- Labor is divided into three stages: dilation and effacement of the cervix, delivery of the fetus, and delivery of the placenta. The position of the infant relative to the mother's pelvis during labor is described as station, fetal lie, and presentation.
- The most common form of analgesia used during labor and delivery is a lumbar epidural. IV analgesics and local anesthetics may also be used. General sedation is only used in emergencies requiring cesarean delivery.
- Fetal monitoring is often performed during labor to detect accelerations and decelerations in fetal heart rate. Fetal status is described as reassuring or nonreassuring.
- Induction of labor uses oxytocics to initiate contractions and dilate the cervix.
- Dystocia is difficult, slow, or nonprogressing labor. A failure to progress may be caused by CPD, fetal macrosomia, or abnormal presentation. CPD and macrosomia usually require cesarean delivery. An abnormal presentation may be addressed with maneuvers to reposition the baby or cesarean delivery.
- Protracted labor is characterized by abnormally slow cervical dilation or lack of fetal descent. Treatment options include oxytocics to promote cervical dilation, operative delivery to assist with fetal descent, or cesarean delivery.
- An operative vaginal delivery involves the use of forceps or a vacuum extractor.
- A cesarean delivery is a surgical procedure to remove the infant through an incision in the abdominal wall. Indications for cesarean delivery include CPD, nonreassuring fetal status, abnormal placentation, history of genital herpes, or vaginal colonization with group B strep.
- Common complications of delivery include umbilical cord prolapse, abnormal fetal presentation, and placenta accreta.
- Puerperium is the time from delivery of the placenta to approximately the 6th week postpartum. During this time, the lochia gradually decreases and the uterus returns to its prepregnancy state.
- The neonate is immediately assessed using the Apgar score. The newborn is weighed, measured, and assessed for appropriate gestational age. The infant is given a vitamin K injection, and an antimicrobial ointment is placed in the eyes to prevent microbial ophthalmia.

Procedures

Obstetrical and gynecologic procedures are performed both in the ambulatory setting and in the surgical suite. Many obstetricians and gynecologists are also surgeons and perform many of these procedures.

Dilation and Curettage

A dilation and curettage (D&C) involves dilation of the cervix with curettage of the entire endometrial cavity using a curette or suction. A D&C may also involve the use of forceps to remove polyps and may be performed in the office or in an outpatient surgical setting.

Hysteroscopy

A hysteroscopy is a visual examination of the uterine cavity using an endoscope inserted through the cervix. Biopsies and excision of polyps, endometriomas, or fibroids may also be performed. This procedure may be an in-office or outpatient surgical procedure.

Saline-Instilled Sonohysterogram

A saline-instilled sonohysterogram is performed with the endometrial cavity filled with saline. The saline helps to visualize submucous myomas or endometrial polyps using transvaginal ultrasound. This procedure is performed in the office with oral analgesia.

Hysterosalpingogram

A hysterosalpingogram is the study of the uterine cavity and fallopian tubes using radiopaque dye injected through the cervix. This procedure is mainly used in the investigation of infertility and to evaluate the patency of the fallopian tubes. The dye is noted to fill the fallopian tube and then spill into the abdominal cavity. A patent tube is said to show **fill and spill** of the dye.

Laparoscopy

A laparoscopy is the visualization of the abdominal and pelvic cavity using an endoscope passed through an abdominal incision. This procedure is used to diagnose pelvic disease and for therapeutic procedures (eg, tubal ligation, removal of fibroids). Laparoscopy is usually performed under general anesthesia.

Colposcopy

A colposcopy is an in-office procedure that utilizes a microscope to visualize the cervix and vaginal tissues using 5X and 50X magnification. This procedure may be used with acetic acid to differentiate tissues that are rapidly proliferating (eg, CIN). Colposcopy may be used to guide treatment with electrocautery, cryosurgery, CO_2 laser, or loop resection.

Conization

A conization is the removal of the entire transformation zone and endocervical canal using a scalpel, CO_2 laser, or **loop electrical excision procedure (LEEP)**, cold knife, needle electrode, or large-loop excision.

 LEEP is usually dictated as the acronym. Do not transcribe it as leap or LEAP.

Endometrial Ablation

An endometrial ablation destroys the endometrial layer of the uterus and is used to treat dysfunctional uterine bleeding. Techniques include laser, rollerball, resectoscopy, or thermal destruction (hyperthermia or cryotherapy).

Diagnostic Studies

The majority of diagnostic studies used in obstetrics and gynecology involve evaluations of pituitary and gonadal hormones and ultrasound imaging techniques. Cultures and DNA studies for STDs are also widely used.

Ultrasound

Ultrasound techniques are the most widely used imaging modality in gynecology and obstetrics. Ultrasound transducers may be moved over the abdomen (transabdominal) or placed intravaginally (transvaginal). Sonograms may be used to screen for pelvic abnormalities that can be further studied using other imaging procedures. Ultrasound is preferred over plain x-ray and CT because ultrasound does not involve ionizing radiation that can damage ova or the developing fetus.

Laboratory Studies

Laboratory studies in obstetrics and gynecology identify infectious agents, clarify hormone disruptions, screen for cancer, and aid in the diagnosis of obstetrical complications.

Nucleic Acid Amplification Test

Neisseria gonorrhoeae and Chlamydia trachomatis are the most common infections in the United States. Techniques that identify specific regions of DNA are increasingly used to diagnose these sexually transmitted infections using urethral and endocervical swabs or urine samples. Techniques are based on nucleic acid amplification (NAAT), whereby a specific region of DNA is isolated and then amplified (replicated repeatedly) until levels are detectable. Replicated sequences of DNA are attached to chemiluminescent molecules that emit a signal. Results are reported as positive or negative. Reference may be made to **no signal detected** if the test is negative.

Pap Smear

A Papanicolaou smear is performed by obtaining a sample from the squamocolumnar junction using a spatula and from the endocervix using a cotton swab or brush. The samples may also be taken with a cervical sampler that collects cells from the cervical canal and the transition zone and places the cells in suspension. See Table 11-2 on page 357 for an explanation of Pap smear results.

Hormones

Hormone levels play a major role in the diagnosis, monitoring, and treatment of female disorders as well as infertility and pregnancy.

Human Chorionic Gonadotropin

Human chorionic gonadotropin (hCG) levels are primarily used to diagnose pregnancy. The hCG molecule consists of an alpha and beta subunit. The alpha subunit is shared by LH, TSH, FSH, and hCG. The beta subunit of each of these hormones gives each one their specificity, so assays for hCG test specifically for the beta subunit. HCG appears in the blood five to seven days after conception. HCG tests may be qualitative (positive or negative) or quantitative (**Table 11-5**).

Sex Hormones

The majority of testosterone is present in the serum bound to either albumin or to sex hormone binding globulin. Free testosterone is not bound to SHBG or albumin and represents a very small fraction of the

Table 11-5 Beta hCG Levels

Weeks from LMP	Beta hCG Level (Serum) in Units/L
normal, nonpregnant women	<5 units/L
3–4	9–130
4–5	75–2600
5–6	850–20,800
6–7	400–100,200
7–12	11,500–289,000
12–16	18,300–137,000
16–29	1400–54,300
29–41	940–60,000

total testosterone value. **Table 11-6** lists reference ranges for both testosterone and free testosterone.

Table 11-6 Testosterone Levels

Test Name	Reference Range
total testosterone	male: 241–827 ng/mL female: 14–76 ng/mL
free testosterone	male: 9.7 to 54.7 pg/mL female: 0.3 to 3.2 pg/mL

Progesterone is produced by the corpus luteum and by the placenta. Progesterone levels may be drawn to determine if ovulation has occurred and to assess function of the corpus luteum. **Table 11-7** lists progesterone

Table 11-7 Progesterone Levels

Progesterone Values (By Phase of Menstrual Cycle)	Reference Range
follicular	0.5 to 2.4 ng/mL
luteal	2.4 to 20.7 ng/mL
pregnancy	>13 ng/mL

references ranges in the various phases of the menstrual cycle.

Although the body produces three major forms of estrogen (estrone, estradiol, and estriol), estradiol is the most biologically active and therefore the most clinically significant estrogen in premenopausal females (**Table 11-8**). Estradiol levels drop in postmenopausal females due to atrophy of the ovaries. Estrone, produced by the conversion of androstenedione secreted by the adrenal glands, is the most common form of estrogen in postmenopausal women.

Table 11-8 Estradiol Levels

Estradiol Levels	Reference Range
male	10–50 pg/mL
premenopausal female	35–525 pg/mL
postmenopausal female	0–35 pg/mL

Prolactin

Prolactin (**Table 11-9**) is secreted by the pituitary gland and induces lactation. Elevated levels in the absence of pregnancy or lactation may indicate a pituitary lesion. Elevated levels may also cause amenorrhea.

Table 11-9 Prolactin Levels

Gender	Reference Range
male	3–16 ng/mL
female	3–19 ng/mL

Follicle Stimulating Hormone

FSH acts on the ovaries to stimulate maturation of a follicle. In patients with infertility, decreased levels of FSH distinguish primary ovarian failure from pituitary dysfunction. During perimenopause, the ovaries begin to fail and FSH levels rise in an attempt to stimulate the ovaries. FSH levels above 40 milliunits/mL confirms menopause. Males also produce FSH, which stimulates production of sperm.

Table 11-10 lists FSH values in males and in premenopausal and postmenopausal females.

Table 11-10 FSH Levels

FSH Values by Phase of Menstrual Cycle	Reference Range
follicular	1–8 milliunits/mL
ovulatory	4–25 milliunits/mL
luteal	1–5 milliunits/mL
postmenopausal	40–100 milliunits/mL
males	16 milliunits/mL

Luteinizing Hormone

Luteinizing hormone (LH) is released by the pituitary gland under the direction of GnRH secreted by the hypothalamus. LH is secreted in a cyclical pattern in females based on a feedback system with estrogen. The midcycle LH surge precedes ovulation by about 16 hours and is the basis of home **ovulation predictor kits (OPKs)**. Table 11-11 lists LH values in premenopausal and postmenopausal females.

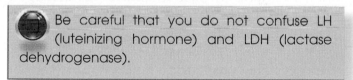
Be careful that you do not confuse LH (luteinizing hormone) and LDH (lactase dehydrogenase).

Table 11-11 LH Levels

LH Values (By Phase of Menstrual Cycle)	Reference Range
prepuberty	<0.2 milliunits/mL
follicular	1–18 milliunits/mL
midcycle	24–105 mIU/mL
luteal	0.4–20 mIU/mL
postmenopausal	15–62 mIU/mL

Antimüllerian Hormone

The müllerian ducts of the embryo develop into the fallopian tubes, uterus, cervix, and upper portion of the vagina. Antimüllerian hormone (**Table 11-12**) plays a role in sexual differentiation of the embryo by preventing the development of the müllerian ducts in the male. In the adult female, AMH controls the formation of primary follicles by inhibiting excessive follicular recruitment. AMH is measured to assess ovarian reserve and is useful in the evaluation of infertility and menopause. AMH is elevated in polycystic ovary syndrome and premature ovarian failure.

Table 11-12 AMH Levels

AMH Levels	Reference Range
elevated	>3.0 ng/mL
normal	0.7 to 2.9 ng/mL
low	<0.3 ng/mL

Alpha Fetoprotein

Alpha fetoprotein (AFP) is produced by the fetus and can be detected in the maternal serum. It serves as a marker for congenital disorders in the developing fetus. The AFP level peaks at approximately 500 ng/mL at about 32 weeks of gestation and then begins to decline. A neural tube defect manifests as spina bifida or anencephaly (no brain). A fetus with a neural tube defect leaks higher levels of AFP into the amniotic fluid, causing the maternal serum levels to be elevated. Women may be screened at 15–20 weeks of pregnancy for elevated levels of AFP for the possible early detection of neural tube defects. Decreased levels of AFP are associated with Down syndrome. The reference range is 0.25 to 2.50 MoM (multiples of the median).

> **(17)** Rh_0 (a subscript zero, not the letter o) is sometimes pronounced $r\bar{o}$ and has given rise to the name of the antiglobulin used to prevent the formation of anti-D antibodies, RhoGAM. This treatment name is derived from <u>Rh</u> zer<u>o</u> and <u>gam</u>maglobulin.

Blood Typing

Blood typing of the ABO and Rh blood group systems is an important step in the prevention of hemolytic disease of the newborn. The ABO system represents two specific antigens: the A antigen and the B antigen. The designation O is actually the absence of both A and B antigens. The Rh antigen is likewise noted to be present (positive) or absent (negative). The Rh blood group system actually consists of over 50 different antigens, but the antigens designated D, C, c, E, and e are the only antigens of real clinical significance. Technically, the term Rh positive refers to the presence of the D antigen. Rh negative indicates the absence of the D antigen, sometimes indicated with a lowercase d. The D antigen is the most immunogenic of the Rh blood group antigens. Two different nomenclature systems were developed for the Rh blood group antigens, but the most common designation for Rh positive is Rh0(D) or Rh_0(D). (17)

The immune system develops antibodies to the A and B antigens even in the absence of direct stimulation by red cells of a different type (ie, individuals with the B antigen form antibodies against the A antigen without ever receiving a transfusion of type A blood). On the other hand, anti-D antibodies are formed by Rh-negative individuals only after exposure to Rh_0(D) blood through blood transfusion or fetomaternal transfusion.

ABO and Rh typing are performed by mixing the patient's red cells with antiserum containing known antibodies against A, B and D. Antibodies directed against red cell antigens will cause the red cells to agglutinate (clump together).

Pharmacology

The two main categories of drugs used in obstetrics and gynecology are hormones and antimicrobial agents.

Antimicrobials

Antibiotics commonly used in the gynecological setting are listed in **Table 11-13**. Details of these medications can be found on the pages indicated.

Prostaglandins

The prostaglandin E2 causes the cervix to soften and induces contractions. It may be used in early pregnancy as an abortifacient or in late pregnancy to induce labor.

Table 11-13 Antimicrobials

Infection	Generic Name or Drug Class
nongonococcal STI	azithromycin, ofloxacin, levofloxacin, erythromycin, or a tetracycline
GC	cephalosporin (ceftriaxone IM or cefixime p.o.)
PID	cephalosporins, probenecid, doxycycline, clindamycin, gentamicin, and metronidazole
trichomonas	metronidazole (Flagyl)
genital herpes	acyclovir (Zovirax), valacyclovir (Valtrex), and famciclovir (Famvir)

A second prostaglandin, designated F2, is also used as an abortifacient or to induce postpartum contractions. Following delivery, the uterus normally contracts in order to stop bleeding by clamping down on blood vessels. Prostaglandin F2 is given to stop postpartum bleeding. **Table 11-14** lists prostaglandins used in obstetrics.

Table 11-14 Prostaglandins

Generic	Brand Name
dinoprostone (prostaglandin E2)	Cervidil Prepidil
carboprost tromethamine (prostaglandin F2)	Hemabate

GnRH Analogs

GnRH (gonadotropin-releasing hormone) was formerly called LHRH (luteinizing hormone releasing hormone). GnRH analogs initially mimic the action of GnRH and cause an initial surge in LH and FSH levels, but after about 10 days, a paradoxical reaction occurs and FSH and LH levels drop, producing a medical castration (hypogonadism). GnRH analogs (**Table 11-15**) induce amenorrhea and are effective in the treatment of DUB and endometriosis. Estrogen may be given as add-back therapy to prevent osteoporosis.

Table 11-15 GnRH Analogs

Generic	Brand Name
leuprolide	Lupron Lupron Depot Eligard
goserelin	Zoladex

Progestins

Progestins (**Table 11-16**) given as a single agent are used to prevent pregnancy and to treat DUB. Progestin alone (without estrogen administration) causes atrophy of the endometrium, allowing the lining to slough off after withdrawal of the drug (withdrawal bleed). Progestins may also be used in the first few weeks of pregnancy to prevent miscarriage.

Table 11-16 Progestins

Generic	Brand Name	Dose
medroxyprogesterone acetate	Provera	2.5 mg, 5 mg, 10 mg
	Depo-Provera	
norethindrone acetate	Aygestin	5 mg
progesterone	Crinone	vaginal gel
	Endometrin	100 mg (vaginal tablet)
	Prometrium	100 mg, 200 mg
levonorgestrel	Plan B	0.75 mg, 1.5 mg
	Mirena	IUD

Estrogens

Estrogen given as a single agent is most commonly used to treat the symptoms of menopause and is recommended for short-term use only due to the increased risk of cancer, blood clots, and stroke. Estrogen given to reverse or prevent osteoporosis may be opposed with progesterone for longer-term use. Single-agent and combination estrogens are listed in **Table 11-17**.

Table 11-17 Estrogens

Generic	Brand Name	Dose
conjugated equine estrogens (CEE)	Premarin	0.3 mg, 0.45 mg, 0.625 mg, 0.9 mg, 1.25 mg
estradiol	Estrace	0.5 mg, 1 mg, 2 mg
	Climara, Estraderm, Vivelle-Dot	Patch
conjugated estrogens and medroxyprogesterone	Prempro	0.3/1.5 mg, 0.45/1.5 mg, 0.625/2.5 mg, 0.625/5 mg
ethinyl estradiol norethindrone	Femhrt	1/5 mg, 0.5/2.5 mg

Contraceptives

Contraceptives may be administered orally, transdermally, as a depot, or in an IUD. They may be classified as single agent (single hormone) or a combination of an estrogen and progestin.

Oral Contraceptives

Combination oral contraceptives (COCPs) contain both an estrogen and a progestin. These combination pills may be monophasic, delivering the same dose of hormones throughout the cycle, or multiphasic (biphasic or triphasic) with varying doses of estrogen, progestin, or both. Most contraceptive pills are taken for 21 days followed by seven days off, for a 28-day cycle. Most pill packs contain either 21 tablets or 28 tablets. The 28-tablet packs contain seven days of inactive tablets that are simply there to maintain a routine of taking one tablet daily.

There are many different combinations of OCPs (too many to list here). Trade names of OCPs often include numbers that indicate the dose, the phases, or the number of pills in the pack. Some preparations also include iron. **Table 11-18** lists examples of OCPs that

Table 11-18 Oral Contraceptives

Brand Name	Contents	Description
Loestrin 21 1.5/30	1.5 mg norethindrone 0.03 mg ethinyl estradiol	21 tablets with combination of estrogen and progestin
Loestrin 24 Fe 1/20	1 mg norethindrone 0.02 mg ethinyl estradiol	24 tablets of combination estrogen and progestin along with four tablets of ferrous fumarate 75 mg
Ortho-Novum 1/35 28	1 mg norethindrone 0.035 mg ethinyl estradiol	21 tablets of combination estrogen and progestin and seven inactive tablets for a total of 28 tablets
Norinyl 1+35	1 mg norethindrone 0.035 mg ethinyl estradiol	21 tablets of combination estrogen and progestin and seven inactive tablets for a total of 28 tablets
Ovcon 35 21-day	0.4 mg norethindrone 0.035 mg ethinyl estradiol	35 mcg of estrogen in a 21-day pack
Ortho-Novum 10/11–28	0.5 mg norethindrone (days 1–10) 1 mg norethindrone (days 11–21) 0.035 mg ethinyl estradiol	pack contains a consistent dose of estrogen with 10 days of 0.5 mg of a progestin followed by 11 days of 1 mg of a progestin with seven days of inactive tablets
Ortho-Novum 7/7/7 28	0.035 mg ethinyl estradiol (days 1–21) 0.5 mg norethindrone (days 1–7) 0.75 mg norethindrone (days 8–14) 1 mg norethindrone (days 15–21)	consistent dose of estrogen for 21 days with seven days each of three different doses of progestin with seven inactive tablets
Ortho Tri-Cyclen	norgestimate and ethinyl estradiol	three doses of progestin in three 7-day phases
Seasonique Seasonale	levonorgestrel and ethinyl estradiol	84 tablets taken continuously followed by seven inactive tablets to produce four menstruations per year (the names reference the four seasons or four cycles per year)

include numbers in the brand name to demonstrate the various ways the preparations are written. Pay close attention to the dictation, as some doses vary only slightly, and consult a pharmaceutical reference to be certain you are transcribing the prescription correctly.

Nonoral Contraceptive Drugs

Hormones to suppress ovulation and prevent pregnancy may be delivered transdermally, by subdermal implant, or by IUD (**Table 11-19**).

Table 11-19 Nonoral Contraceptive Drugs

Generic	Brand Name	Dose
norelgestromin and ethinyl estradiol	Ortho Evra	transdermal patch, replace weekly
etonogestrel and ethinyl estradiol	NuvaRing	vaginal ring, replace monthly
levonorgestrel	Mirena	IUD containing a progestin, lasts up to five years
etonogestrel	Implanon	subdermal implant, lasts up to three years

Ovulatory Drugs

Ovulatory drugs (**Table 11-20**) are used to treat infertility by stimulating the ovaries to release multiple mature ova.

Table 11-20 Ovulatory Drugs

Generic	Brand Name	Dose
urofollitropin (FSH)	Bravelle	75 units
chorionic gonadotropin alfa	Ovidrel	257.5 mcg
clomiphene citrate	Clomid	50 mg
follitropin beta	Follistim	
follitropin alfa	Gonal-f	
menotropin	Menopur Repronex	

Tocolytics

Tocolytics (**Table 11-21**) come from a variety of drug classes—none is used exclusively to reduce contractions and none is highly effective. The main goal of tocolytic administration is to stave off delivery long enough for the infant's lungs to mature following betamethasone administration.

Table 11-21 Tocolytics

Generic	Brand Name
terbutaline (beta 2-agonist)	
indomethacin (NSAID)	Indocin
nifedipine (calcium channel blocker)	Procardia
magnesium sulfate (myosin inhibitor)	

Exercises

Using Context to Make Decisions

Use the sample report on page 384 to answer questions 1–3.

1. Has this patient ever had a vaginal delivery?____

   _____

2. Comments made under the Skin exam support which of the following statements under the Assessment?

   a. Negative for virilization.

   b. Negative for STI.

   c. Probable PCOS.

   d. Tanner stage IV.

3. Under the Ultrasound heading, what word has been transcribed incorrectly? What is the correct term? _____

   _____

Use the following excerpt to answer questions 4–6.

The patient was admitted to the hospital on July 6, 20XX, with complaints of headache and elevated blood pressure. She had been on bedrest at home for ___(1)___. Her laboratory evaluation remained normal, except her proteinuria doubled to greater than 1 g in less than 1 week. She had significant lower extremity edema, with occasional diastolic blood pressure readings in the 90s. Decision was made to proceed with delivery as she was beyond 37 weeks with worsening ___(2)___ on bedrest in the hospital. Cervidil was placed on the evening of July 10, 20XX, and induction was performed on July 11, 20XX. She received the maximum dose of 42 milliunits/min of Pitocin with no cervical change. The decision was made to proceed with ___(3)___. We performed a primary, low-transverse incision without complication.

4. Why was this patient placed on bedrest? (blanks #1 and #2) _____

5. What procedure name goes in blank #3? _____
   _____

6. Why was Cervidil given? _____
   _____

Use the following excerpt to answer questions 7–9.

BRIEF CLINICAL HISTORY

This is a 43-year-old multigravid white female who presents with pelvic pain and heavy irregular bleeding despite a previous NovaSure procedure. She presents for definitive surgical therapy. All risks and benefits, including infection, bleeding, possible injury to bowel, bladder, and major blood vessels, were explained to the patient and accepted.

SUMMARY OF FINDINGS

Upon visualization of the pelvis laparoscopically, the uterus and right side appeared pristine with a normal ovary, although there were obvious ___(1)___ implants high above the pelvic brim on the right side. The left side was completely encased in adhesions, with the left ovary densely adherent to the descending colon as well as the pelvic sidewall. The tube was a ___(2)___ and wrapped into this mass in an indistinguishable fashion.

7. Which of the following goes in blank #1?

   a. fibroid   **c.** molar

   b. endometrial   **d.** ovarian

8. Which of the following goes in blank #2?

   a. corpus luteum   **c.** hydrosalpinx

   b. fourchette   **d.** hematocolpos

9. In this case, definitive treatment refers to:

   a. hysterectomy with BSO

   b. endometrial ablation

   c. conization

   d. laparotomy

10. A patient with a history of HPV and CIN-II would be offered which of the following?

    a. D&C **c.** Hysteroscopy

    b. LEEP **d.** OCPs

11. A patient with $Rh_0(D)$ miscarried at 18 weeks' gestation after a traumatic car accident and was given RhoGAM. Which of the following could be true?

    a. The father is Rh negative.

    b. A Kleihauer-Betke indicated a fetomaternal bleed.

    c. The patient tested positive for hepatitis.

    d. The patient tested positive for the Rh antigen.

12. A 32-year-old patient comes in complaining of menopausal symptoms including hot flashes, vaginal dryness, dyspareunia, and insomnia. In the assessment, the physician dictates an abbreviation as the diagnosis. Which of the following abbreviations would be correct?

    a. POS **c.** TOF

    b. POF **d.** TOS

13. A patient presents to the outpatient clinic with symptoms of an STI for the past 24 hours but with no complaints of pelvic pain. An NAAT is positive for chlamydia. Which of the following could be included in the assessment?

    a. Nongonococcal infection

    b. GC

    c. CIN

    d. PID

14. The physician dictates "seventeen oh ach pee." How would you expand this abbreviation? _____
    _____

Use this excerpt to answer question #15.

ULTRASOUND

She is currently cycle-day 3. The endometrium is 3.6 mm. There is a small area in the posterior wall with a small echogenic focus of unclear significance. The uterus is 7.5 _____ in length, 4.7 _____ in AP diameter, and 5 _____ laterally. The fundus appears to be normal. The right ovary is 24 x 25 _____ with 6 antral follicles. The left ovary is 33 x 27 _____ and has 8–10 small antral follicles. There is no free fluid and no adnexal mass.

15. When dictating the ultrasound findings, the physician dictated the correct measurements but did not dictate the units. Fill in the appropriate metric units.

Terms Checkup

Complete the multiple choice questions for Chapter 11 located at www.myhealthprofessionskit.com. To access the questions, select the discipline "Medical Transcription," then click on the title of this book, *Advanced Medical Transcription*.

Look It Up

Using the guidelines described on page xvii, complete a research project on gestational diabetes.

Transcription Practice

1. Transcribe the key terms and phrases for Chapter 11.

2. Complete the proofing and transcription practice exercises for Chapter 11.

PHYSICAL EXAMINATION

Vital Signs: Height 5 feet 2 inches, weight 114 pounds, blood pressure 125/66, pulse 65.

General: Well-appearing, well-nourished female in no acute distress.

Breasts: Symmetrical without masses. No nipple discharge.

Abdomen: Soft, nontender, no masses. Normal bowel sounds. No surgical incisions. No organomegaly.

Skin: No tattoos, rashes, or abnormal piercings. No excessive hirsutism. No acanthosis nigricans.

Extremities: No edema. No palpable cords or tenderness.

Pelvic: Normal external female genitalia. Normal clear vagina. Normal exocervix with a nulliparous os. Bimanual exam shows an anteverted uterus that is nontender and not enlarged, with no adnexal mass. No nodularities.

ULTRASOUND

She is currently cycle-day 28. The endometrium is mostly homogeneous and measures 7.5 mm. The uterus is anteflexed and measures 7.5 cm in length, 3 cm in AP diameter, and 4.3 cm laterally. The fundus appears to be normal. The right ovary is multifollicular, measuring 32 mm x 22 mm. There are approximately 10–12 annual follicles. The left ovary is 37 mm x 35 mm and is dominated by a complex cyst measuring 19 x 27 mm. This does appear to be a fairly recent corpus luteum cyst, more than an endometrioma. There is no free fluid and no adnexal mass.

Hematology and Oncology

Preview Terms

Before studying this chapter, make sure you understand the following terms. Definitions can be found in the glossary.

adenocarcinoma
blast
clones
cytopenia
cytosis
differentiation
genotype
hematopoiesis
immunophenotype
malignant
metastases
monoclonal
myeloproliferative
pancytopenia
phenotype
primary tumor
stem cell

Learning Objectives

After completing this chapter, you should be able to comprehend and correctly transcribe terminology related to:

▶ anemia of chronic disease, iron deficiency anemia, and sickle cell disease

▶ hemostasis

▶ the diagnosis and treatment of malignancy

▶ breast cancer, colorectal cancer, prostate cancer, and lung cancer

▶ acute and chronic leukemia

▶ Hodgkin lymphoma and non-Hodgkin lymphoma

▶ laboratory and imaging studies used to diagnose and monitor anemia, leukemia, lymphoma, hemostasis, and common forms of cancer

▶ drugs used to treat anemia

▶ chemotherapy regimens used to treat breast, colorectal, prostate, and lung cancer

▶ chemotherapy regimens used to treat leukemia and lymphoma

Introduction

The fields of hematology and oncology have evolved together, and traditionally practitioners have received specialty training in both hematologic disease and cancer. These practitioners are commonly referred to as "Hem/Oncs" (*heme-onks*). Red cell disorders may be genetic or acquired, but the vast majority of red cell disorders are secondary to another disease or condition. Cancer itself and the treatment of malignancies are major causes of both red and white cell deficiencies and dysfunction. Solid tumors and leukemia are leading causes of morbidity and mortality both in the United States and worldwide, and MTs working in almost any environment will encounter some degree of oncology and hematology. The rapidly increasing knowledge in the fields of human genetics, cellular biology, and immunology is having a tremendous impact on the treatment of all forms of cancer and hematologic disorders. For this reason, MTs working in the areas of hematology and oncology should have knowledge of style and nomenclature related to genetic mutations, immunoglobulins, and cell surface antigens.

Hematopoiesis

Red cells originate in the bone marrow from myeloid stem cells, which are pluripotent cells that differentiate to give rise to all the formed elements of the blood except lymphocytes. Once the myeloid stem cell is committed to producing an erythrocyte, it goes through a series of maturation steps including a normoblast (nucleated red blood cell), a polychromatic erythrocyte (reddish purple cell marked by **basophilic stippling**), and finally the mature erythrocyte (■ **Figure 12-1**). Red blood cell (RBC) production (erythropoiesis) is under the control of erythropoietin, which is a hormone produced in the kidneys. Erythropoietin levels rise in response to low oxygen pressure (decreased perfusion or decreased oxygenation) and serve as a feedback mechanism for the bone marrow to maintain or increase red cell mass. RBC production is dependent upon adequate iron stores and sufficient intake of vitamin B_{12} and folate (folic acid).

RBCs are unique in that the nucleus is extruded in the last few steps of red cell maturation. RBCs have a

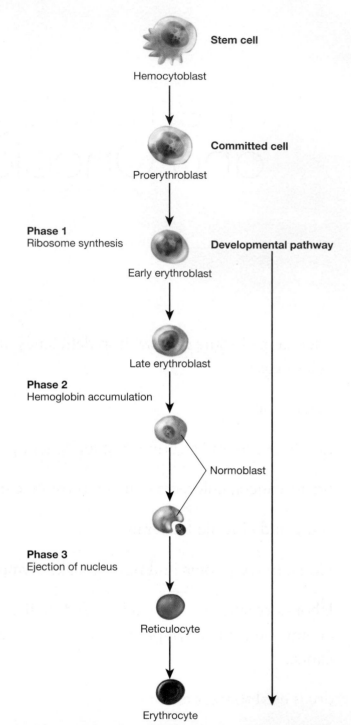

Stem cell
Hemocytoblast

Committed cell
Proerythroblast

Phase 1
Ribosome synthesis

Developmental pathway
Early erythroblast

Late erythroblast

Phase 2
Hemoglobin accumulation

Normoblast

Phase 3
Ejection of nucleus

Reticulocyte

Erythrocyte

FIGURE 12-1 Red cell hematopoiesis.

lifespan of about 120 days. Old and damaged red cells are cleared from the circulation mostly by the spleen but also by the liver and bone marrow. Red cells are dismantled and hemoglobin is broken down into its two

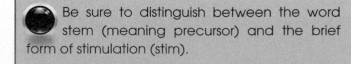

Be sure to distinguish between the word stem (meaning precursor) and the brief form of stimulation (stim).

components—heme and the globin (protein) chains. Heme is immediately converted to bilirubin and the iron is picked up by **transferrin** and transported to the liver and bone marrow.

 Hemoglobin has globin chains (not globulin chains).

The chemical structure of hemoglobin is integral to its function, and hemoglobinopathies result when the structure of the hemoglobin molecule is distorted. Hemoglobin consists of four intertwined polypeptide chains wrapped around a heme component. The four chains are actually two pairs of identical chains designated alpha and beta (■ **Figure 12-2**). Normal hemoglobin is hemoglobin A (Hb A) and consists of two alpha chains and two beta chains. A variant of the beta chain is designated gamma. Fetal hemoglobin (Hb F) contains two alpha chains and two gamma chains (instead of two beta chains). Fetal hemoglobin is present in very high concentrations in newborns, but this form of hemoglobin gradually decreases during the first year of life. Only about 2.5% of the hemoglobin in an adult consists of hemoglobin Hb F, although this form of hemoglobin may become elevated in the presence of a hemoglobinopathy or an aplastic or myeloproliferative disease.

The structure of the hemoglobin chains are under the control of chromosomes. Each person inherits two genes for the alpha chain and two genes for the beta chain (one allele for each type of chain from each parent for a total of four alleles), and all alleles are expressed. People who are homozygous (two identical alleles) for a structural abnormality in one of the two types of chains will be more severely affected than a person that is heterozygous (having two different alleles). Some homozygous changes are so severe they are incompatible with life, resulting in miscarriage or stillbirth.

Each hemoglobin chain is made of a string of amino acids. The sequence and types of amino acids making up the chain change the three-dimensional shape and the chemical properties of the amino acid chain, making a chain lighter, heavier, more positively charged, or more negatively charged. These differences can be detected using **hemoglobin electrophoresis,** a laboratory technique for separating and identifying different hemoglobins. Electrophoretic mobility refers to the distance a molecule moves through this gel when an electric current is applied. Each type of hemoglobin moves a very specific distance across the gel according to its electrical charge and molecular weight.

Hemoglobin variants are determined by their electrophoretic mobility and are named with capital letters (eg, A, B, C, and S). Hemoglobins that have the same results by electrophoresis but still contain some slight structural differences are named according to the city or location where they were discovered (eg, Hb S Memphis, Hb C Harlem).

DIAGNOSIS: Microcytic anemia, lifelong due to being a sickle-cell carrier. Her MCV has ranged in the 70 to low-80 range. Her hematocrit has remained in the upper-20% range to mid-30% range. CBC with differential revealed moderate poikilocytosis with a few teardrop cells and target cells. Mild rouleau was present. Hemoglobin electrophoresis shows 59% hemoglobin A, 5% hemoglobin A2, less than 1% hemoglobin F, and 36% hemoglobin S.

Anemia

Anemia is a deficiency of red blood cells (RBCs). It may also be defined as a decrease in hemoglobin concentration. General diagnostic criteria for anemia are shown in **Table 12-1.** Hematocrit and hemoglobin values for infants and children vary by age, and values are higher in persons living at high altitudes, so local, age-related tables are important for an exact assessment of anemia.

Anemia has two basic causes: diminished RBC production or accelerated RBC loss. Red cell production

Oxyhemoglobin

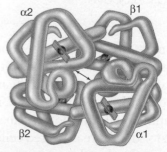

α2 β1

β2 α1

FIGURE 12-2 The hemoglobin molecule with four amino acid chains and four heme groups.

Table 12-1 Diagnostic Criteria for Diagnosing Anemia

Parameter	Men	Women
hemoglobin	<14 g/dL	<12 g/dL
hematocrit	<42%	<37%
RBC	<4.5 million/mcL	<4 million/mcL

may drop because of a lack of dietary resources (eg, iron, B_{12}, folate). Red cell destruction may result from intrinsic or extrinsic causes. Intrinsic causes include red cell membrane defects (eg, hereditary spherocytosis) that allow the cell to break apart easier or sooner than expected. Examples of extrinsic causes of red cell destruction include prosthetic valves (that shred red cell membranes as they pass by) and **microangiopathic (1)** disorders. Anemias are typically divided into three categories based on the red cell size: **microcytic anemia, macrocytic anemia,** or **normocytic anemia.** Microcytic anemias are characterized by small red cell size as indicated by a decreased **mean corpuscular volume (MCV).** They are most often the result of iron deficiency but may be caused by defective or deficient production of the heme component or the globin chains that make up hemoglobin.

Normocytic anemias are often the result of bone marrow exhaustion or marrow failure. The red cells are normal in size (normocytic) and contain normal amounts of hemoglobin (**normochromic**); there are simply too few cells produced. Normocytic anemias have a normal MCV value. A **normocytic, normochromic anemia** may be caused by an inadequate response to erythropoietin, aplastic anemia, myelophthisis, or myelodysplasia. (2) Normocytic anemias are also seen immediately following an excessive hemorrhage due to sudden and dramatic loss of normal red cells.

Pause 12-1 Explain how the term normochromic relates to a normal amount of hemoglobin.

(1) Microangiopathic refers to a disorder affecting or occurring within the small blood vessels.

(2) Myelophthisis is the displacement of normal bone marrow with fibrous or malignant tissue. Myelodysplasia is abnormal development of the bone marrow.

You may hear some physicians dictate "n slash n," meaning normocytic, normochromic. Spell out the terms instead of transcribing the abbreviation.

Macrocytic anemias are characterized by overly large red cells as indicated by an increased MCV. **Macrocytosis** is usually caused by a deficiency of B_{12} or folate. **Megaloblastic anemia** is a macrocytic anemia caused by a deficiency of both B_{12} and folate. Paresthesias in a stocking-and-glove distribution may suggest vitamin B_{12} or folate deficiency. **Pernicious anemia** is a macrocytic anemia caused by poor absorption of B_{12} from a lack of intrinsic factor.

DIAGNOSIS: Macrocytic anemia. Initial hematology evaluation showed a hemoglobin of 11.1, hematocrit 38.8%, MCV 106; with normal TSH, serum folate, and vitamin B_{12} levels; normal serum protein electrophoresis; negative direct Coombs; and normal liver function tests. Reticulocyte count was slightly elevated at 2.4%, with a haptoglobin of 72. Peripheral blood smear was significant for a mild to moderate poikilocytosis with occasional bizarre RBCs and macrocytosis. Bone marrow biopsy and aspirate showed megaloblastic erythroid hyperplasia with no increase in myeloblasts. Megakaryocytes were normal in appearance and number. Iron stain showed marked increase of ringed sideroblasts. Findings felt to be consistent with refractory anemia with ringed sideroblasts (MDS, FAB subtype RARS).

Pause 12-2 Expand the abbreviation "MDS, FAB subtype RARS" taken from the sample dictation above.

Anemias may also be heterogeneous, displaying microcytic, macrocytic, and normocytic cells. This variability in red cell size is reflected in an elevated **red cell distribution width (RDW).** In the recovery stage following a traumatic bleed, the bone marrow attempts to compensate for the decrease in red cells by producing cells quickly and releasing them into the peripheral circulation, some before they are fully mature. Immature red cells are slightly larger than fully mature cells, so the RDW and MCV values are toward the upper limit of normal or above normal. A variation in the size of red cells is described as **anisocytosis** (unequal cells) and corresponds to an increased RDW. Immature red cells also show variation in color from purplish-blue to bluish-red, described as **polychromasia** (many colors). When the bone marrow is extremely stressed, it may even release **nucleated red blood cells (nRBCs),** which are significantly immature cells that still contain a darkly staining nucleus.

Symptoms of anemia, including pallor, easy fatigability, tachycardia, palpitations, and tachypnea on exertion, may be noticed when the hemoglobin level approaches 7 g/dL or less. A severe, chronic deficiency causes skin and mucosal changes, including a smooth tongue (**glossitis**), brittle nails, and **cheilosis** (fissuring of the lips). Anemia is actually a manifestation of another underlying disorder, so the primary cause should always be sought.

Initial laboratory studies include **CBC with differential, reticulocyte count (retic count),** B$_{12}$ and folate levels, and iron studies. A fecal occult blood test (FOBT) is also ordered. Further tests are ordered as indicated. **Bone marrow aspiration and biopsy** may also be needed. Transfusion may be required if the hemoglobin concentration falls below 7 g/dL. This threshold is higher for patients with cardiopulmonary insufficiency.

Anemia of Chronic Disease

Anemia of chronic disease (ACD) is a sequela of a chronic disorder such as infection, inflammation, autoimmune disease, or cancer. It is characterized by low serum iron, low **total iron-binding capacity (TIBC),** and normal or increased serum ferritin. **RBC indices (3)** are often normal. Anemia of chronic disease often begins as a normocytic, normochromic anemia but may advance to a microcytic anemia with iron deficiency.

The exact etiology of ACD is not completely understood, but it is thought that cytokines such as interleukin, interferon, or tumor necrosis factor interfere with iron metabolism and erythrocyte production. Treatment is directed toward the primary disorder. Epoetin alfa (Epogen, Procrit) and iron supplements are given as well.

Iron Deficiency Anemia

Iron deficiency anemia (IDA) is anemia caused by decreased iron stores. The body poorly absorbs iron from dietary sources. To keep up with total-body iron needs, iron is recycled, especially the iron from spent red cells. Because the body relies heavily on the iron recovered from red cells, chronic or severe blood loss leads to iron deficiency. The most common cause of blood loss is a chronic GI bleed. Heavy menstrual bleeding may cause more iron lost than can be compensated by dietary intake; for this reason, premenopausal females with menorrhagia are prone to developing iron deficiency anemia. Iron deficiency may also be caused by decreased absorption from the gastrointestinal lining. The body stores iron in the liver as **ferritin** and as **hemosiderin** in the bone marrow, spleen, and liver. Iron is transported in the blood bound to transferrin. **Transferrin receptors,** located on the cell surface of erythrocyte precursors, receive iron that has been transported to the cell by transferrin. Transferrin receptors may also be detected in the serum as **soluble transferrin receptors (sTfR).**

Symptoms of IDA are the same as those for other anemias. Fatigue also may result from dysfunction of iron-containing cellular enzymes. A classic symptom indicative of iron deficiency is **pica,** which is a craving for items with no nutritional value, such as ice or nonfood items such as dirt or clay. Other symptoms of severe iron deficiency include glossitis, cheilosis, concave nails (**koilonychia**), and, rarely, dysphagia caused by a postcricoid esophageal web (Plummer-Vinson syndrome).

A CBC and iron studies are performed to diagnose IDA and to differentiate IDA from other causes of anemia (see page 426 for a description of iron studies). IDA typically develops in stages. First, iron stores are depleted and then red cells begin to show morphologic changes. RCBs become microcytic and hypochromic (■ Figure 12-3), and later become even more distorted with anisocytosis, **poikilocytosis, target cells,** and **ovalocytes. Table 12-2** lists the results of iron studies and the CBC in the order that the results become abnormal. When iron deficiency is present, serum iron is low and sTfR is elevated due to increased erythrocyte precursors standing ready to create more red cells. Transferrin also becomes elevated when iron is low in an attempt to "scavenge" more iron. Since iron deficiency is a symptom of another disorder, a more extensive search for the cause of iron deficiency (iron loss or poor absorption) should be pursued and treated.

(3) Indices is the plural form of the word index. RBC indices include MCV, MCH, and MCHC (see page 427).

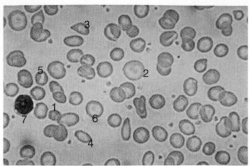

1 Microcyte
2 Target cell
3 Tear drop cell
4 Ovalocyte
5 Stomatocyte
6 Severely hypochromic cell
7 Lymphocyte

FIGURE 12-3 Wright-stained blood smear showing iron deficiency anemia with poikilocytosis and anisocytosis. Normal red cells are about the same size as the nucleus of the lymphocyte. Most of these cells are microcytic and hypochromic (large central pallor). *Source:* Courtesy of Annita B. Watson.

Table 12-2 Abnormalities Detected in IDA (listed in the order that they become abnormal)

Sequence	Abnormality	Change
1	iron stores in the marrow	depleted
2	serum ferritin	drops below 20 ng/mL, eventually drops below 16 ng/mL
3	TIBC	increased
3	transferrin	increased
4	serum iron	decreased (below 50 mcg/dL)
4	percent saturation of transferrin	decreased (below 16%)
4	hemoglobin	decreased
5	sTfR	increased (>8.5 mcg/mL)
7	microcytosis	present
8	hypochromia	present
9	RDW	increased
10	morphologic changes	anisocytosis, poikilocytosis, target cells, ovalocytes

(4) An autosomal disorder is a genetic disorder that is associated with the autosomal chromosomes, (ie, not the sex chromosomes X and Y).

Treatment for IDA is oral **ferrous sulfate** 325 mg three times a day. Iron may also be formulated as **iron gluconate** or **iron fumarate.** Iron absorption is improved with concomitant ingestion of vitamin C in the form of ascorbic acid or in foodstuffs such as orange juice. Anemia should begin to improve within three weeks and return to baseline in approximately two months. Oral iron may cause digestive upset and some patients are noncompliant with the prescribed regimen. In extreme cases, IV **sodium ferric gluconate** can be given in a single dose administered over four to six hours.

LABORATORY DATA: White blood cells 7.9, hemoglobin 10.2, hematocrit 32.2, MCV 76, platelet count 313,000, RDW 15. Peripheral blood smear shows polychromasia, microcytosis, and hypochromasia. No younger white cells noted. Occasional giant platelet noted, otherwise adequate platelets noted. Vitamin B_{12} 183, folate greater than 24, ferritin 1.3, iron saturation 5, total iron-binding capacity 502. Reticulocyte count 2.1, sedimentation rate 23.

Sickle Cell Disease

Sickle cell disease is an autosomal recessive **(4) hemoglobinopathy.** A single change in the DNA that encodes for hemoglobin causes valine to be substituted for glutamine in the sixth position of the beta hemoglobin chain, producing hemoglobin

S (Hb S). This single amino acid substitution causes the shape of the hemoglobin molecule to change when the hemoglobin is deoxygenated (not bound to oxygen). The change in shape distorts the red cell membrane, giving the cell a sickle shape. The membrane is initially able to revert to its normal shape, but repeated distortions of the membrane cause permanent damage. Sickle-shaped cells are inflexible and less able to navigate narrow capillary spaces so they become trapped, creating a blockage. Tissues beyond the jam become ischemic and infarcted. Sickled cells are also more fragile and prone to hemolysis, so they have a much shorter life span. The constant stress on the bone marrow to replace hemolyzed red cells causes hyperplasia of the bone marrow with visible bone deformities, especially in the long bones.

The degree to which patients are affected by sickle cell disease depends on whether they are heterozygous or homozygous. Patients with Hb A (normal hemoglobin) inherited from one parent and Hb S inherited from the other parent are said to have sickle cell trait. These patients typically live normal lives with a normal life span. They may only experience symptoms while under extreme physical distress. Patients homozygous for Hb S have sickle cell disease. Newborns are asymptomatic during the first year of life until Hb F is replaced with Hb S (ie, the gamma chain is replaced by the abnormal beta chain).

Patients with sickle cell disease suffer intermittent episodes of acute pain called a **sickle cell crisis.** A crisis may be brought on by stress (such as a viral infection or trauma), dehydration, or hypoxia. Pain due to ischemia and infarction occurs in the bones of the back, long bones, and chest, and is especially acute in the joints. **Hand-foot syndrome** involves the small joints of the hands and feet. Severe abdominal pain may also occur. Repeated ischemic events in the bones predisposes to osteomyelitis, often caused by Salmonella. Infarction may occur in the heart, spleen, lung, kidney, or retina. An **aplastic crisis** is marked by decreased marrow erythropoiesis occurring during an acute infection, leading to **erythroblastopenia. Acute chest syndrome** is caused by microvascular occlusions in the lungs and may be fatal. Death is often due to infection or organ failure from chronic organ damage. The typical life span of a patient with sickle cell disease is 40–50 years (although this number is rising).

Physical examination reveals a chronically ill-appearing patient. Adolescents show delayed puberty. Jaundice, cardiomegaly, and nonhealing ulcers may be noted. A CBC shows nRBCs in the peripheral blood as well as sickle-shaped cells. The reticulocyte count is also elevated. Patients can be definitively diagnosed by hemoglobin electrophoresis studies identifying the presence of hemoglobin S with no hemoglobin A.

There is no definitive treatment for sickle cell disease. Patients are encouraged to stay well hydrated and avoid high altitudes or situations with low oxygen. Folic acid is prescribed to help maintain red cell production. Administration of hydroxyurea (Hydrea) induces Hb F production, displacing Hb S and reducing

- Red cells originate in the bone marrow from myeloid stem cells. They are dependent upon iron, folic acid, and vitamin B_{12} for adequate production and function.

- Anemia results from either decreased production of red cells or accelerated red cell loss. Anemias are often categorized by the size of the red cell (microcytic, normocytic, or macrocytic) as reflected in the MCV.

- Anemia of chronic disease is a sequela of infection, inflammation, autoimmune disease, or cancer. Treatment is directed at the underlying disorder. Epoetin alfa may be given to increase red cell production.

- Iron deficiency anemia is caused by a lack of iron stores. Iron may be deficient because of excessive loss, decreased consumption, or decreased absorption. Diagnosis relies on laboratory studies of iron and CBC values. Treatment is with iron supplementation.

- Sickle cell disease is an inherited disorder that disrupts the normal structure of the hemoglobin molecule with distortion of the red cell shape, causing mechanical destruction of red cells and obstruction of capillaries. Treatment for sickle cell disease is supportive only; there is no definitive treatment or cure.

the severity of crises. Hydrea is a **teratogen** and cannot be given to women of childbearing age. A sickle cell crisis is managed with **exchange transfusion,** hydration, and antibiotics.

> It is common for dictators to dictate "H & H" for the hematocrit and hemoglobin, but this abbreviation should not be used. For example, "ach en ach were 13 and 39" would be transcribed "hemoglobin was 13 and hematocrit was 39." The lower number is *always* the hemoglobin value.

Hemostasis

Hemostasis is accomplished through a complex series of reactions that begins with the clumping of platelets and culminates in the formation of an insoluble fibrin clot that reinforces the platelet plug. Proteins that participate in clotting are called coagulation factors and are designated with roman numerals I through XIII. A lowercase /a/ is appended to the names to indicate the activated form. **Table 12-3** lists the coagulation factors and their alternative names or function.

Vascular injury exposes tissue factor, a glycoprotein in the endothelial layer of blood vessels, initiating the extrinsic, or tissue-factor, pathway of the coagulation system. Platelets react to the presence of tissue factor and immediately begin to stick together to form a physical barrier over the injured area. The activated platelets then initiate the coagulation cascade, setting off a series of complex proteolytic reactions that activate both procoagulant factors and anticoagulant factors (**■ Figure 12-4**). Procoagulant factors promote the formation of a clot, and anticoagulant factors keep the entire process in check and prevent clots from forming at sites other than the actual site of injury. The process is referred to as a cascade because the activation of one factor subsequently catalyzes the conversion of the next factor into its active form and so on until the final result is the conversion of fibrinogen into fibrin strands. The fibrin strands then become cross-linked within the clot itself, giving the clot stability and strength.

The coagulation cascade may also be provoked by contact with negatively charged foreign substances in the blood (called the contact-activation pathway or the intrinsic pathway). Both the intrinsic and extrinsic pathways join at the common pathway, the point at which prothrombin is converted to thrombin. The integrity of the extrinsic pathway can be assessed by the prothrombin time (PT) test. The integrity of the intrinsic pathway is assessed with the activated partial thromboplastin time (aPTT) test.

Coagulopathies result from either acquired or inherited disorders of hemostasis and may result in bleeding or inappropriate formation of thrombi. All coagulation factors are manufactured by the liver and most are dependent on vitamin K for adequate production. For this reason, many acquired coagulopathies are the result of liver disease. Bleeding may also be caused by thrombocytopenia or acquired platelet disorders (eg, **immune thrombocytopenic purpura [ITP], thrombotic thrombocytopenic purpura [TTP]**).

The most common inherited disorders of hemostasis causing excessive bleeding include **von Willebrand disease** and the hemophilias. Von Willebrand disease is caused by a quantitative or a qualitative deficiency of von Willebrand factor, a protein that plays an integral role in the stickiness of platelets (platelet adhesion). Hemophilia A is an inherited deficiency of factor VIII. Hemophilia B, also called **Christmas disease,** is an inherited deficiency of factor IX. The genes for factor VIII and factor IX are both located on the X chromosome, so hemophilia almost never affects females because a mutation on one X chromosome can be compensated by the other X chromosome.

> The patient is well known to me, as she carries the diagnosis of von Willebrand disease with laboratory results revealing factor VIII activity of 72. She had a slightly low factor VIII antigen at 52% (normal level between 70% and 140%). Von Willebrand activity was only 50%, with normal levels being between 50% and 150%. All of this suggested the possibility of mild von Willebrand disease type 1. The patient did not have any monomers. She delivered 2 children by vaginal delivery without excessive bleeding. She was supported with DDAVP intravenously.

Hypercoagulability may be due to a genetic mutation of factor V, called factor V Leiden. This mutation

Table 12-3 Coagulation Factors

Factor Number or Name	Alternate Name or Function
I	fibrinogen
II	prothrombin
III	tissue factor
IV	calcium
V	proaccelerin, labile factor
VI	unassigned (previously factor Va)
VII	proconvertin
VIII	antihemophilic factor A
IX	antihemophilic factor B or Christmas factor
X	Stuart-Prower factor
XI	plasma thromboplastin antecedent
XII	Hageman factor
XIII	fibrin-stabilizing factor
high-molecular-weight kininogen (HMWK)	Fitzgerald factor
von Willebrand factor	binds to VIII, mediates platelet adhesion
prekallikrein	activates XII and prekallikrein; cleaves HMWK
antithrombin (formerly antithrombin III)	inhibits IIa, Xa, and other proteases
protein C	inactivates Va and VIIIa
protein S	cofactor for activated protein C (APC, inactive when bound to C4b-binding protein)
plasminogen	converts to plasmin, lyses fibrin and other proteins
alpha 2-antiplasmin	inhibits plasmin
tissue plasminogen activator (tPA)	activates plasminogen
urokinase	activates plasminogen
plasminogen activator inhibitor-1 (PAI1)	inactivates tPA and urokinase (endothelial PAI)
plasminogen activator inhibitor-2 (PAI2)	inactivates tPA and urokinase (placental PAI)

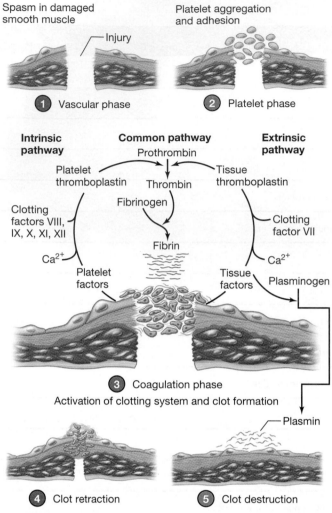

Spasm in damaged smooth muscle

Injury

1 Vascular phase

Platelet aggregation and adhesion

2 Platelet phase

Intrinsic pathway

Common pathway
Prothrombin

Extrinsic pathway

Platelet thromboplastin

Thrombin

Tissue thromboplastin

Fibrinogen

Clotting factors VIII, IX, X, XI, XII

Clotting factor VII

Ca^{2+}

Fibrin

Ca^{2+}

Platelet factors

Tissue factors

Plasminogen

3 Coagulation phase
Activation of clotting system and clot formation

Plasmin

4 Clot retraction

5 Clot destruction

FIGURE 12-4 Phases of hemostasis.

substitutes the amino acid glutamine (abbreviated Q) for arginine (abbreviated R) in the amino acid position 506 (written R506Q). This variant of factor V is resistant to activated protein C (aPC), which normally inactivates factor V and limits the coagulation response. Patients may be heterozygous or homozygous for the mutation. A mutation of methylenetetrahydrofolate reductase (MTHFR) is also associated with hypercoagulability. The most common mutation is designated C677T (thymidine [T] is substituted for cytosine [C] at position 677 of the DNA sequence encoding for MTHFR).

> Rule out hypercoagulable syndrome. Serum homocysteine level elevated to 18.1. Anticardiolipin antibody screen was negative. No evidence of the prothrombin gene mutation. However, the patient was found to be heterozygous for the factor V Leiden, or R506Q, mutation.

Antiphospholipid syndrome (APS) causes an immune-mediated hypercoagulable state. This auto-immune disorder is marked by antibodies directed against phospholipids (anticardiolipin [aCL] antibodies and anti-phosphatidylserine antibodies). The presence of the immune-generated lupus anticoagulant (LA) is also associated with increased risk of DVT and recurrent pregnancy loss. Patients with LA do not necessarily have SLE, but patients with SLE are more likely to have LA. Lupus anticoagulant is so named because of its action *in vitro* (it prolongs the aPTT), but *in vivo* it is actually a procoagulant, increasing the risk of thrombi. Transient elevations of these antibodies are not unusual, so patients must show elevated LA or elevated antiphospholipid antibodies (APAs) on at least two separate occasions for a definitive diagnosis of APS or LA. It is not understood exactly how APS and LA increase the risk of thromboembolic events.

> LABORATORY DATA: INR 0.93, partial thromboplastin time 29.4, fibrinogen 292, fibrin split products negative, D-dimer 368. Lupus anticoagulant negative. Beta 2-glycoprotein negative. Anticardiolipin IgG, IgM, and IgA antibodies are negative. Anti-phosphatidylserine antibody negative. Factor V Leiden mutation negative. Homocysteine level 13.9. MTHFR gene mutation positive for 1 copy of C677T.

Disseminated Intravascular Coagulation

Disseminated intravascular coagulation (DIC) is caused by a systemic activation of the coagulation system. Normally, clots form at a focal point of vascular injury, but DIC is marked by widespread systemic clots. DIC can take two forms: multiple thromboembolisms or severe bleeding. DIC is always the result of an inciting event that causes the release of procoagulant proteins into the systemic circulation, setting off rampant intravascular clotting. Multiorgan failure may occur from thromboses obstructing blood flow to major organs. In some cases, clotting factors and platelets are depleted by ongoing clot activation, which then leads to severe bleeding. Simultaneous clotting and bleeding present a treatment dilemma.

Generally speaking, DIC starts with the exposure of the blood to tissue factors or contactants. Inciting events may include obstetrical complications, trauma, and some forms of cancer (eg, prostate and pancreas) and leukemia (eg, acute promyelocytic leukemia). A leakage of amniotic fluid or release of placental tissue into the maternal bloodstream may activate the coagulation cascade. Sepsis is also known to trigger DIC, especially due to infection with gram-negative bacteria that produce exotoxins capable of triggering the coagulation system.

 Pause 12-3 What is an exotoxin?

DIC may be slowly evolving or acute and fulminant. Slowly evolving DIC typically manifests with thromboembolic events including deep vein thromboses and pulmonary embolism. Rapidly evolving DIC typically results in bleeding due to the rapid depletion of coagulation factors. These patients show **petechiae,** ecchymoses, and oozing at venipuncture sites.

There is no single, definitive test to diagnose DIC. It is suspected in patients with unexplained bleeding or thromboses, especially in a clinical setting of cancer, trauma, or obstetrical complications. The diagnosis is based on symptoms and coagulation studies including platelet count, **prothrombin time (PT), partial thromboplastin time (PTT), fibrinogen,** D-dimer, **antithrombin** levels, and **fibrin degradation products (FDPs),** also called **fibrin split products (FSP).** Platelet counts are reduced due to consumption. The PT and PTT are typically prolonged due to decreased or absent coagulation factors. Fibrinogen, a protein that is cleaved to create the fibrin strands that form the scaffolding of a clot, is also reduced due to consumption. D-dimer and FDPs, breakdown products of a dissolved clot, are elevated.

Because the coagulation factor levels vary with the stage and duration of DIC, serial determinations to establish trends are of more clinical value than single readings.

Treatment of DIC is concentrated first and foremost on correcting the underlying event. Homeostasis may return on its own if the tissue factors are no longer circulating in the blood. Heparin may be useful in the treatment of slowly evolving, thromboembolic DIC. In the case of severe bleeding, coagulation factors may need to be replaced by transfusing **platelet concentrates, cryoprecipitate** (to replace fibrinogen and factor VII), and **fresh frozen plasma (FFP),** which contains both coagulation factors and naturally occurring anticoagulants such as antithrombin, protein C, and protein S.

 Pause 12-4 What are naturally occurring anticoagulants? What is their role?

Oncology

Oncology is the treatment of malignancies. A medical oncologist treats many types of cancer using chemotherapy, hormone therapy, and immunomodulating therapies. A radiation oncologist administers radiotherapy to treat malignancies. Malignant cells are marked by unregulated proliferation and increased replication rates. These cells have lost their normal regulatory mechanisms that control cell growth, including contact inhibition, which normally restrains the growth of a cell when it comes into contact with another cell, as well as programmed cell death (**apoptosis**) that normally occurs after a preset number of cell

- Hemostasis is accomplished through a complex series of enzymatic reactions that creates an insoluble fibrin clot that blocks the outflow of blood from an injured vessel. Components of hemostasis include procoagulants and anticoagulants as well as platelets.
- Coagulopathies may result in bleeding or thromboses and may be acquired or inherited.
- Examples of inherited disorders of hemostasis include the hemophilias, von Willebrand disease, factor V Leiden, and a mutation of the MTHFR gene.

- Examples of acquired disorders of hemostasis include factor deficiencies caused by liver disease, antiphospholipid syndrome, and the immune-mediated thrombocytopenias.
- Disseminated intravascular coagulation is a potentially life-threatening event caused by a systemic activation of the coagulation system leading to uncontrolled bleeding and/or thromboses. Common triggering events include sepsis, cancer, and obstetrical complications. DIC is diagnosed based on clinical symptoms and serial plasma coagulation studies. Treatment involves correcting the underlying event.

divisions. Malignant cells may also fail to differentiate into competent, fully functional cells. Malignant cells are also unique in that they invade distant tissues (metastasize). The immune system is known to play a role in controlling the proliferation of malignant cells, but the reasons why some malignancies escape control of the immune system is not completely understood.

Malignancies may be described as solid tumors, meaning they are distinct masses of cells. This contrasts with the leukemias that do not necessarily produce a mass but create a large number of circulating cells. In the United States, lung, prostate, breast, and colorectal cancer account for the majority of solid malignancies. The single most important risk factor for cancer is age, with the majority of cancers occurring in patients over 75 years.

Genes that play a role in the initiation of cancer are called oncogenes, which are often the result of acquired mutations in somatic cells (5). Mutations may be caused by chemical carcinogens found in the environment, viral infections, or ionizing radiation. Chemicals absolutely known to induce cancer include benzene and asbestos. Mutations include gene amplification (an increased number of copies of a normal gene), a translocation, an **inversion,** or a **point deletion** of genetic material. Some predispositions to cancer are inherited, as in the case of the BRCA1 and BRCA2 genes, which are associated with breast and ovarian cancer.

> **Pause 12-5** What are translocations, inversions, and point deletions? Locate translocations in the *Book of Style* and describe how these genetic mutations are written.

Viruses also contribute to the pathogenesis of neoplasms. Viruses may contribute to malignancy in two ways: through the incorporation of viral genetic material into the host genome that disrupts normal cellular controls or through immune dysfunction caused by an immune response to eradicate the infected cells. Examples of viruses known to increase the risk of cancer include Epstein-Barr virus (Burkitt lymphoma), hepatitis B and C (hepatocarcinoma), and Human papilloma virus (cervical cancer).

(5) Acquired mutations occur in somatic cell lines at some point during the person's life. These mutations are not hereditary.

In addition to genetic mutations that result in malignant cells, some forms of cancer are due to a lack of cellular controls that normally trigger the apoptosis of aberrant cells. Tumor suppressor genes such as p53 may become damaged and nonfunctional, allowing neoplastic cells to proceed unchecked. Overexpression of certain protein products may also block the action of p53.

Cancer is thought to be a chronic, multistep process that usually requires years to manifest as a tumor large enough to be detected by imaging or palpation. It is also believed that many mutations in DNA occur quite frequently throughout the body but various mechanisms are in place to eliminate aberrant cells—either through self-selection (ie, a mutation that renders the cell line nonviable) or by checks and balances within the immune system. Multiple mutations within a single cell line are typically required to manifest as malignancy and these mutations are thought to occur stepwise over many years.

Cancer Prevention

Primary prevention of cancer focuses on lifestyle changes such as smoking cessation, weight control, diet modification to lower fat intake and increase fruits and vegetables, and moderate alcohol consumption. **Chemoprevention** is the use of vitamins, minerals, and essential nutrients to interfere with the multistep process required for a cell to manifest as a malignancy. Chemoprevention may also involve the administration of compounds that interfere with hormones (eg, tamoxifen to interfere with estrogen receptors). Early detection is directly correlated to curability. **Secondary prevention** is the early detection of cancer before the primary lesion invades surrounding tissue and/or metastasizes. **Screening** is the process of looking for cancer in asymptomatic individuals for the purpose of early detection.

Grading and Staging

Grading and **staging** are important components of a cancer diagnosis and treatment plan. Grading is a measure of a tumor's aggressiveness based on histologic studies and provides important prognostic information. Histological studies are performed by a histologist and interpreted by a pathologist (a medical doctor that works in the laboratory setting). Grading is determined by examining a biopsied specimen, noting staining characteristics and cellular morphology. Changes in the cell's morphology, such as the size and shape of the nucleus, the presence of nucleoli, and the amount of cytoplasm relative to the size of the nucleus, relate to the cell's lack of differentiation and aggressiveness. (6) Highly differentiated cells are more mature, less aggressive, and behave more like their normal counterparts. The frequency of mitoses (**proliferation index**) can also be a prognostic indicator and is included in the grading system of some tumors.

The presence of the nuclear antigen **Ki-67** is indicative of cell proliferation. This particular antigen is not detectable in cells that are in the resting phase G_0 (ie, not currently undergoing mitosis). The Ki-67 labeling index denotes the fraction of cells currently going through mitosis. Higher concentrations correlate to a higher proliferative index. The MIB-1 monoclonal antibody is used to detect the Ki-67 antigen.

Tumor cells may also be evaluated for **vascular endothelial growth factor (VEGF).** This protein gives the tumor the ability to stimulate the growth of blood vessels (**angiogenesis**), making the tumor more aggressive because it can foster its own blood supply.

 VEGF may be dictated *vej ef.*

Staging describes the extent of disease based on the patient's clinical findings at the time of diagnosis and is used to make treatment decisions. Staging requires information gathered by physical examination, imaging studies, laboratory tests, biopsies, and **surgical pathology reports**. Staging for most cancers has been standardized according to the **TNM system** used by the American Joint Committee on Cancer (AJCC). The TNM system describes the primary malignancy based on tumor size (T), number of involved lymph nodes (N), and presence of distant metastases (M). Staging is a required component of medical records for all cancer patients. The **World Health Organization (WHO)** is involved in the standardization of the grading and staging of cancers to promote worldwide consistency in reporting incidence and treatment outcomes. The TNM system has been adapted to each type of cancer based on the following general guidelines:

- **T:** size or direct extent of the primary tumor
  - TX: indicates primary tumor cannot be evaluated
  - T0: indicates no evidence of primary tumor
  - Tis: indicates carcinoma in situ (cancer that has not spread beyond its original tissue type)
  - T1 through T4: indicates size or extent of primary tumor

- **N:** degree of spread to regional lymph nodes
  - NX: indicates lymph nodes cannot be evaluated
  - N0: indicates no tumor spread to regional lymph nodes
  - N1-N2: indicates the degree of tumor spread to regional lymph nodes
  - N3: indicates tumor spread to more distant lymph nodes or to numerous regional lymph nodes
- **M:** presence of metastasis
  - M0: indicates no distant metastasis
  - M1: indicates metastasis to distant organs

The lowercase letters a, b, and c may be appended to the T or N values to give more detailed information on the size of the primary tumor or the extent of lymph node involvement. The lowercase letter p may be used to indicate the information was derived from a pathology exam (eg, pT1bN1M0).

 The TNM system is transcribed using uppercase T, N, and M, lowercase a, b, c, and p without any spaces between the characters.

For each type of cancer, the TNM staging is correlated to a stage grouping. Stage groupings are designated with roman numerals and capital letters. An example of stage grouping is shown in **Table 12-4.** Stage groupings and their TNM designations differ slightly among different cancer types.

Response

After a tumor is graded and the patient's disease is staged, treatment is planned based on the prognosis and the patient's desires. Based on statistical data, treatment for a given stage may be **definitive** (aimed at a cure) or **palliative** (aimed at minimizing disease or controlling symptoms). Specific terms are used to describe the response to treatment:

- cure: permanent absence of signs and symptoms of disease
- **partial response:** defined as a 50% or greater reduction in the original tumor mass
- **complete response** or **complete remission:** no clinical evidence of disease

(6) Nucleoli (singular, nucleolus) are specialized areas of the nucleus that transcribe RNA. Nucleoli are visible under the microscope as round, clear areas within the nucleus.

Table 12-4 Breast Cancer Stage Groupings

Stage Group	TNM
Stage 0	TisN0M0
Stage I	T1N0M0
Stage IIA	T0N1M0 T1N1M0 T2N0M0
Stage IIB	T2N1M0 T3N0M0
Stage IIIA	T0N2M0 T1N2M0 T2N2M0 T3N1M0 T3N2M0
Stage IIIB	T4N0M0 T4N1M0 T4N2M0
Stage IIIC	Any T N3M1
Stage IV	Any T Any N M1

- **progression:** an increase of more than 25% in the size of the tumor or the appearance of any new lesions
- **stable disease:** no change—neither improvement nor worsening
- response duration or duration of response: time from response to time of overt progression
- survival time: time from diagnosis to death
- time to progression: the amount of time from treatment until disease begins to worsen
- relapse: a return of symptoms after a period of improvement
- disease-free survival or disease-free interval: the length of time following treatment that the patient survives without signs or symptoms of disease
- **no evidence of disease (NED):** no signs or symptoms of disease to the extent that imaging and laboratory studies can detect

Tumor Markers

Tumor markers may be used to monitor response to treatment and progression of disease. Tumor markers are proteins found in the peripheral blood that are produced by the specific tumor cell. Generally speaking, tumor markers are indicative of the bulk or total volume of tumor cells present (including primary and metastatic cells). Tumor markers are not typically used in the diagnosis of cancer because many tumor markers may be elevated in other conditions. Once a diagnosis is established and the tumor marker is found to be elevated, it can be used as a marker of treatment efficacy. The study of tumor markers is also called **proteomics.** Not all cancer types have tumor markers. The most commonly used markers are listed in **Table 12-5.**

Table 12-5 Common Tumor Markers

Tumor Marker	Associated Tissue
paraproteins (monoclonal immunoglobulins or free light chains)	lymph (eg, leukemia, lymphoma, multiple myeloma)
prostate specific antigen (PSA)	prostate
alpha fetoprotein (AFP)	liver
CA-125	ovary
CEA	colon, lung, breast, and pancreas
CA 15-3, CA 27-29	breast
CA 19-9	pancreas

Performance Status

A patient's overall well-being and comorbidities must be taken into account when planning treatment for malignancies. A patient's ability to function affects both prognosis and treatment. The **performance status** is a measure of how well the patient is able to carry out activities of daily living (ADLs) and is indicative of the impact of treatment. The two scales commonly used include **Karnofsky** and the **Eastern Cooperative Oncology Group (ECOG,** *ē-cäg*). The Karnofsky score is reported as a percent in 10-point increments, with 100% being fully functional and 10% being moribund. ECOG uses a 5-point scale of 0–5 ranging from entirely asymptomatic (0) to bedridden (4). Quality-of-life assessment includes the above scales plus assessment of general well-being including appetite, weight gain, and level of pain.

Sequelae of Cancer

Individual cancer types have unique signs and symptoms, but there are certain sequelae that are common to many types of malignancies. Masses often lead to obstruction of visceral tissues, and death often results from organ failure or multisystem failure. The following sequelae are common to many malignancies, especially in the later stages of disease:

- **cachexia:** wasting of both adipose and skeletal muscle. Patients may lose 10% to 20% of their body weight. Cachexia is not caused by anorexia or lack of calories, but is mediated by certain cytokines (eg, tumor necrosis factor and interleukins). Increasing caloric intake does not improve cachexia. Patients with severe weight loss may be described as **cachectic** and may be noted to have **temporal wasting.**

- effusion: accumulation of fluids in the thoracic or peritoneal cavities, emanating from the pleural membrane or the peritoneal membrane. Need for drainage is common but effusions typically reaccumulate.

- cord compression: encroachment of a mass on the spinal canal leading to **loss of bowel or bladder function** or paralysis. Cord compression should be treated emergently with surgery or radiation therapy.

- coagulopathy: tumors tend to produce tissue factors that promote clotting and increase the risk of thrombus formation with subsequent pulmonary emboli (see also DIC on page 394).

- **tumor lysis syndrome:** caused by release of intracellular components into the bloodstream as a result of massive tumor-cell death. The syndrome is most often seen following treatment of hematologic cancers such as acute leukemia and non-Hodgkin lymphoma. Symptoms include renal failure, hypocalcemia, hyperuricemia, and hyperphosphatemia (see page 191).

- Oncology is the medical specialty involved in the treatment of solid tumors, leukemia, and lymphoma. Cancer is marked by the unregulated proliferation of cells and decreased apoptosis. Malignant cells may or may not be functional.

- Malignancies result from chromosomal changes including translocations, inversions, and point deletions of genetic information. Mutations may be inherited or acquired by a somatic cell line at some point in a person's life. Viruses are known to contribute to the pathogenesis of certain cancers.

- Prevention is an important component of cancer treatment. Primary prevention focuses on lifestyle changes, chemoprevention uses nutrients or hormones to prevent cancer, and secondary prevention focuses on the early detection of cancer. Screening involves testing asymptomatic patients for evidence of cancer.

- Grading is the process of determining the tumor's aggressiveness and is based on histologic studies of malignant cells obtained through biopsy. Staging is the determination of the extent of disease including tumor size as well as the number and location of metastases. Prognosis and treatment are based on the grade and stage of disease.

- The TNM system is a standardized method of expressing the stage of disease at the time of diagnosis and indicates the tumor size, degree of lymph node involvement, and the presence of distant metastases.

- Response describes the results of treatment or the intended result of treatment. Possible responses include cure, partial or complete response (remission), progression, and stable disease.

- Tumor markers are used to monitor response to treatment or detect progression of disease. Tumor markers are found in the peripheral blood and are indicative of the total malignant cell burden (including primary site and metastases).

- Performance status describes the patient's well-being and ability to function while undergoing cancer treatment. Performance status scales include Karnofsky and ECOG.

- Many types of cancer share common symptoms and sequelae including pain, obstruction of organs with organ failure, cachexia, pleural and peritoneal effusions, spinal cord compression, bone lesions with pathological fractures, coagulopathies, superior vena cava syndrome, tumor lysis syndrome, and paraneoplastic syndromes.

- **superior vena cava syndrome:** caused by invasion or compression of the superior vena cava by metastatic tumors. Symptoms include headache, sensation of fullness in the head, facial or upper-extremity swelling, breathlessness while lying down, and plethora. Examination reveals facial and upper-extremity edema and dilated veins in the neck, face, and upper trunk.
- **paraneoplastic syndrome:** caused by the release of physiologically active substances by tumor cells. Substances include hormones, enzymes, and cytokines. Paraneoplastic syndromes have a wide variety of symptoms and presentations depending on the substance produced. Symptoms may include fever, arthritis, arthralgias, myalgias, diarrhea, pruritus, and edema.
- **bone metastases:** invasion of bone tissue by metastatic cells. One of the hallmarks of malignant cells is their ability to thrive outside their normal tissue. Bone metastases typically destroy normal bone, causing severe pain, predisposing long bones to pathological fractures and causing vertebrae to collapse. Bone metastases often cause elevated alkaline phosphatase levels and hypercalcemia.

Overall, pain is the most common symptom of cancer and should be treated aggressively. Pain is typically caused by metastatic disease involving the bones or nerves or by pressure exerted by a tumor mass or effusion. Pain control is an important part of maintaining quality of life and is typically treated quite aggressively using combinations of opioids, fentanyl patches, and tramadol. Pain medications are prescribed around-the-clock with additional doses taken as needed for **breakthrough pain.** Antidepressants may also be given to help with both depression and pain.

Cancer Treatment Modalities

Malignant cells typically have a decreased generation time, which is the time required for a quiescent cell to complete a cycle of cell division. The majority of treatment modalities target these variations in the normal cell cycle in an attempt to selectively kill malignant cells. Cells are most vulnerable to genetic mutations during DNA replication and mitosis so many forms of chemotherapy as well as radiation exploit the increased

proliferation rate of malignant cells by targeting the DNA during replication. Surrounding normal cells are also affected but to a lesser degree because at any given time fewer normal cells are actively replicating their DNA.

Treatment modalities include surgery, chemotherapy in the form of cytotoxic agents and hormonal manipulation, radiation, and the ever-increasing number of modalities using immunotherapy and immunomodulation. Many treatment protocols are standardized, but some patients may present particular challenges determining treatment. Many oncologists participate in a **tumor board,** which is a group of healthcare providers from multiple specialties that meet regularly to discuss difficult cases and collaborate on treatment decisions. Oncologists refer to the intent of treatment using the following terms:

- **curative:** treatment that is intended to cure the disease and is used when there is a reasonable expectation that the cancer can be cured
- **adjuvant:** treatment that is given in addition to the primary treatment to enhance the effectiveness overall. Adjuvant therapy may be in the form of chemotherapy, radiation therapy, hormone therapy, or immunotherapy.
- **neoadjuvant:** treatment that is given prior to the main treatment. Oftentimes, neoadjuvant treatment is given prior to surgery to shrink the size of the tumor and make the tumor more amenable to surgical removal. Neoadjuvant therapy is a form of induction therapy.
- **therapeutic:** treatment that has a positive effect on long-term survival and quality of life.
- palliative: treatment that is given to reduce the symptoms of disease when a cure is not possible.
- **salvage chemotherapy:** treatment that is given after a recurrence in the hope of prolonging life.

Surgery

Local disease is a malignancy confined to the original tissue site. The most common treatment for local disease is surgical resection. Surgery can be both diagnostic and therapeutic. Surgery is often used to remove the bulk of the tumor before the tumor can spread or to relieve pressure, pain, or obstruction. Surgical excision of the tumor is performed primarily with low-stage disease that is potentially curable. Obtaining **clear margins** is paramount for achieving a cure. (7) During the surgical procedure, the excised tumor may be sent to the pathology lab for an immediate **frozen section** tissue examination to determine whether clear margins (also called clean margins) were obtained. This may be performed while the patient is still under anesthesia. If **positive margins** are seen (ie, tumor cells are seen at the cut surfaces of the tissue), a wider excision may be attempted.

Nearby lymph nodes are typically resected and examined for lymph-node involvement. A **sentinel node biopsy** may be performed during surgery or prior to surgery. This procedure injects radioactive colloid or dye into the tissues immediately surrounding the tumor. The injectant is taken up by the lymphatic system and drains into the nearby lymph nodes. Following the path of the injectant with a gamma probe, the surgeon can identify the first few lymph nodes in the drainage path of the tumor. If the tumor has spread, these first lymph nodes are the most likely nodes to contain malignant cells. Removing only the sentinel nodes (ie, the first nodes) for biopsy, as opposed to all regional lymph nodes, eliminates or reduces the severity of lymphedema caused by disruption of lymph node beds.

Generally speaking, metastases are not surgically removed unless a mass is causing debilitating or life-threatening problems. Surgery performed to relieve symptoms or preserve quality of life is referred to as **palliative surgery**. A single metastasis in the lung or liver may be surgically removed depending on tumor size and location. Distant metastases are most commonly treated with radiation, chemotherapy, or hormonal manipulation therapy.

Cytoreductive surgery (cytoreduction), also called **debulking,** may be performed before chemotherapy is initiated. This procedure reduces the size of the tumor, making it more amenable to treatment with systemic therapies.

Radiation

Radiation therapy (XRT) is the use of high-energy rays to destroy cells. Cancer cells are more likely to be damaged and destroyed because they have a higher metabolic rate and are more likely to be irradiated while undergoing DNA replication. Some normal tissue is also destroyed with radiation therapy, but normal tissue is more effective at repairing itself. A well-oxygenated tumor (ie, one with adequate blood supply) is more sensitive to radiation treatment, so surgical debulking is sometimes used to reduce the size of the tumor before radiation therapy begins.

Radiation therapy may be curative, especially when combined with surgery and chemotherapy. It may also be used for adjuvant treatment or palliation. Palliative radiotherapy is commonly used to treat brain tumors, spinal cord compression, superior vena cava syndrome, and painful bone lesions.

External Radiation

Radiation treatment includes several forms of high-energy rays including x-rays and gamma rays. The source of the radiation may be external or internal (relative to the patient). **External beam radiation** originates outside the patient's body and directs radiation toward the tumor. External radiation depends on precise positioning of the patient relative to the source of the beam. Gamma and x-ray radiation using a **linear accelerator** (LINAC) are the most common types of external beam therapy. Gamma rays, commonly used to treat superficial areas such as the extremities, breasts, head, and neck, produce photons with energies of 1.17 and 1.33 **million electron volts (MeV)** that penetrate up to 0.5 cm beneath the skin surface.

X-rays can also be produced by a LINAC with a maximum energy of 4-25 MeV. These **photons** can penetrate 1–6 cm beneath the surface and are used for tumors in deep body cavities. **Orthovoltage** machines produce photons with energies of 0.1 to 0.4 MeV and are used to treat superficial tumors of the skin and subcutaneous tissues. **Proton therapy** is used in areas that overlie highly radiation sensitive tissues because protons can be delivered at an exactly defined tissue depth.

> **Pause 12-6** It is difficult to hear the difference between photon and proton. What contextual clues would help you distinguish these terms?

Before therapy begins, a **simulation** is performed to mark the area to be irradiated, determine optimal patient positioning relative to the external beam, and to create casts or masks to shield surrounding tissue and assure precise patient positioning each time the therapy is administered. **Three-dimensional conformal radiation therapy (3D CRT)** uses a computer to create three-dimensional images of the tumor. Conformal technology helps reduce **scatter** at the **field margins,**

(7) Obtaining clear margins means excising the entire tumor without leaving residual tumor cells at the margins of the excision.

thereby reducing damage to adjacent tissues. Another type of three-dimensional radiation therapy designed to reduce collateral tissue damage is **intensity modulated radiation therapy (IMRT).** This method uses radiation of different intensities aimed at the tumor from more than one angle.

> PLAN: External beam radiation therapy to the laryngeal area employing intensity-modulated radiation therapy (IMRT) at 180 cGy per day to a total localized tumor dose of 7020 cGy. A 6 MeV linear accelerator and an isocentric coplanar technique along with IMRT will be employed. CT will be obtained for 3D treatment planning. Aquaplast will be employed for immobilization.

Radiation may also be used to perform **stereotactic radiosurgery.** This form of therapy uses precise stereotactic localization to deliver a single, high dose of radiation or multiple, smaller doses of radiation to a tumor located in a sensitive area that is otherwise inoperable (eg, the brain or spinal cord). Two trademarked systems are available: **Gamma Knife** and **CyberKnife.**

Gamma Knife radiosurgery is commonly used to treat brain tumors. The device contains over 200 sources of radiation (cobalt 60) arranged in a circular array. Each source is tightly focused on the tumor in order to deliver a single, high dose of radiation that destroys the tumor in one treatment session. The patient wears a helmet surgically attached to the skull to prevent any movement during the procedure.

The CyberKnife is also a radiosurgical device. Unlike the Gamma Knife that only treats intracranial tumors, the CyberKnife is capable of ablating tumors at any site in the body. This device combines robotics with advanced imaging techniques to precisely target the tumor. A **fiducial** is a marker placed within the tumor to help track the tumor.

Internal Radiation

Internal radiation therapy places the radiation source inside the body. **Brachytherapy** is a form of internal radiation that uses radioactive material sealed in needles, seeds, wires, or catheters placed directly into or adjacent to the tumor. Another form of internal

(8) The plural form of Gray is Gray (not Grays).

radiation is **systemic radiation therapy** that uses a radioactive isotope attached to a monoclonal antibody directed against a unique surface protein on the malignant cell. Following IV infusion, the antibody travels throughout the body, attaching directly to the target cell. This approach delivers a damaging dose of irradiation directly to the malignant cells. An example of this is tositumomab attached to iodine 131 (trade name Bexxar) used to treat non-Hodgkin lymphoma. Radioactive isotopes may also be attached to specific molecules that are selectively taken up by a specific organ or cell type. Radioactive iodine is used in this way to treat thyroid cancer. Radioactive **strontium,** selectively taken up by the bone, is commonly used to treat generalized bony metastases, especially in patients with stage IV prostate cancer.

Radiation Dose

Typical courses of radiation consist of large, daily doses given over a period of three weeks for palliative treatment or smaller, daily doses given over six to eight weeks for curative treatment. The radiation oncologist designs a treatment plan specific to the location and size of the tumor to be treated that also takes into account the general well-being of the patient and any concomitant therapy. The radiation **treatment field** (also called a **port**) is designed to encompass the entire tumor volume while excluding as much normal tissue as possible. This is accomplished during the simulation. **Single-field therapy** is typically used for superficial tumors (eg, basal cell carcinoma). **Multiple-field therapy** is used for large or deeply situated tumors. Multiple-field therapy uses two to four treatment fields that converge on the tumor from different directions. **Arc (rotating beam) therapy** is a type of multiple-field therapy that rotates the radiation machine around the patient, essentially producing an infinite number of radiation ports.

Dosimetry is used to calculate the absorbed dose of radiation. The standard unit of radiation is the **gray (Gy).** (8) The **total dose** of radiation for palliative treatment is typically 30–50 Gy delivered over the course of two to three weeks. A total dose of 45–50 Gy is delivered over four to six weeks for eradication of subclinical disease and 60–70 Gy delivered over five to eight weeks for clinically apparent disease. The total dose of radiation prescribed is **fractionated,** that is, administered in smaller doses over a series of therapy sessions that add up to the total dose. The total dose may be **hypofractionated** (fewer doses delivered over a shorter time period) or **hyperfractionated** (more doses delivered over an extended time period). Fractionated doses are usually reported in **centigray (cGy),** which is 1/100 of a gray, and range from 150 to 350 cGy. **(9)**

 Other terms used to describe radiotherapy treatment plans include:

isodose line

isocenter, isocentric

tangential fields

parallel opposed fields

coplanar

PLAN: We are going to start a course of palliative radiation therapy directed to the area around T10. Parallel opposed fields will be employed. CT simulation has been performed today. That area is going to receive a total dose of 3500 rads delivered in 15 fractions at a rate of 235 rads per fraction.

DOSE: The right whole breast was treated with medial and lateral fields using 6 MeV photons prescribed to the 95% isodose line at 180 cGy per fraction x28 fractions. Total dose was 50.4 Gy. A tumor-bed boost was performed with end-phase electrons (10 MeV) prescribed to the 90% isodose line. Dose per fraction was 2 Gy x8 fractions for a total dose of 16 Gy. Total dose given was 66.4 Gy.

Chemotherapy

Because many malignancies metastasize from their primary site, a comprehensive treatment for cancer often includes systemic therapy. **Micrometastases** are focal areas of cancer cells that are too small to detect. Chemotherapy is used to destroy cancer cells that are located at both the primary site and distant sites. Most chemotherapeutic agents act by interfering with the cell cycle, leading to reduced proliferation and cell death.

Chemotherapeutic agents are not selective for malignant cells; chemotherapy is toxic to all cells. But the relative toxicity is reduced for normal cells because of their slower rate of cell turnover (ie, less frequent mitosis).

Chemotherapy agents can be classified according to their mechanism of action. This is a practical way of classifying chemotherapy because drugs with different mechanisms can be combined to increase antitumor effects. The four major classes include:

- **alkylating agents:** bind to DNA and prevent accurate transcription of DNA
- **antimetabolites:** interfere with purine and pyrimidine (molecules that make up DNA) synthesis
- **mitotic inhibitors:** interfere with microtubule assembly, a step required in mitosis
- **antibiotics:** intercalate between DNA base pairs and interfere with normal function. This term is also used to describe antimicrobial therapies, but in the context of oncology, the cells to be destroyed are the malignant cells, not the microbial cells.

Chemotherapy may be administered orally or intravenously. Most chemotherapy protocols are administered every two to three weeks over the course of many months, requiring repeated venous access. Chemotherapy is often toxic to small, peripheral veins, and repeated venipuncture for both phlebotomy and IV access damages these small vessels and precludes their continuous use. Intravenous administration usually requires vascular access in the form of a multilumen external catheter or an implantable central catheter. Brand names of **totally implantable venous access systems (TIVAS)** include **Port-A-Cath, BardPort,** and **PowerPort.** These venous access lines are inserted into the superior vena cava just upstream from the right atrium. The ports are placed under the skin and are accessed using specially designed needles that puncture the skin and pass through the self-healing port membrane. These access systems are less prone to sepsis than percutaneous lines.

(9) Doses may also be measured in sieverts (Sv), which is a way of expressing the dose-equivalent in a biological tissue. Non-SI units may also be used, including rad (1 rad = 1 cGy) and rem (100 rem = 1 Sv). Rem is the acronym for roentgen equivalent in man.

The following terms are used to describe chemotherapy:

- **induction:** initial treatment used to reduce the tumor cell volume. Induction therapy is followed by other treatments such as radiation therapy or hormone therapy to attempt complete eradication. Induction therapy may also be called first-line therapy, primary therapy, or primary treatment. In the treatment of leukemia, induction therapy is intended to obtain complete remission.

- **consolidation:** treatment administered after the initial therapy when evidence of the cancer has disappeared. Consolidation therapy may also be called intensification therapy or postremission therapy. Consolidation attempts to eradicate any cancer cells that may have escaped initial therapy. Induction therapy for leukemia will fail if not followed by consolidation therapy.

- **single-drug therapy:** a protocol that requires only one drug to treat the malignancy.

- **multidrug therapy:** a protocol incorporating drugs with different mechanisms of action and different toxicities.

- **high-dose chemotherapy:** a chemotherapy regimen that results in **myeloablation** (destruction of bone marrow precursors). High-dose therapy must be followed by stem cell transplant to reconstitute the bone marrow.

- **dose-dense chemotherapy:** therapy given in standard doses but administered more frequently and supported with growth factors such as erythropoietin and colony stimulating factors.

- **metronomic chemotherapy:** therapy given in smaller, more frequent doses.

- **regimen:** a treatment plan for administering one or more chemotherapy drugs that specifies the schedule, dose, and number of cycles. Many regimens use standard combinations of chemotherapeutic agents referred to by their acronym (eg, CHOP and FOLFOX). **Table 12-6** lists abbreviations and acronyms for common chemotherapy regimens. Note that the abbreviations and acronyms are based on both generic and trade names. In practice, you may

(10) The ANC is calculated by multiplying the percentage of neutrophils (as determined by the WBC differential) by the total white count (determined by CBC). For example, a patient with a white count of 2000 and a neutrophil (PMN) count on differential of 50% would have an ANC of 1000.

need to cross-reference the names, especially trade names that are commonly used in the generic form.

Pause 12-7 Research the terms regimen, regime, and regiment and use each in a sentence.

Selected cancers may be treated with local or regional administration of chemotherapeutic agents. This approach infuses agents directly into the tumor site or tumor cavity (eg, intravesical therapy for bladder cancer, intraperitoneal therapy for ovarian cancer).

For many regimens, a **nadir white blood cell count** is obtained 7–10 days after a chemotherapy dose to monitor for toxicity. An **absolute neutrophil count (ANC)** (10) of 1000 is typically required before administration of the next dose of chemotherapy.

Hematopoietic Stem Cell Transplant

Hematopoietic stem cell transplantation (HSCT) involves the intravenous infusion of stem cells (also called **progenitor cells**) collected from bone marrow, peripheral blood, or umbilical cord blood to reestablish hematologic and immune function. **Stem cell transplantation (SCT)** is used to treat a variety of neoplastic diseases (cancers and leukemias) as well as nonneoplastic diseases such as hereditary metabolic disorders and severe congenital immunodeficiencies. This form of therapy administers very high doses of chemotherapy and/or **total body irradiation (TBI)** that effectively ablates the bone marrow, resulting in a normally lethal pancytopenia. The patient's red and white cell population is restored by transfusing either autologous or allogeneic bone marrow or stem cells isolated from peripheral blood or umbilical cord blood.

Pause 12-8 Rewrite this sentence in layman's terms. "This form of therapy administers very high doses of chemotherapy and/or total body irradiation (TBI) that effectively ablates the bone marrow, resulting in a normally lethal pancytopenia."

A **syngeneic** SCT utilizes stem cells from an HLA-identical donor (ie, a twin). An **allogeneic** SCT utilizes stem cells harvested from a related or unrelated HLA-matched donor. Related donors are most often siblings. Siblings have a 25% chance of being an identical HLA

Table 12-6 Common Abbreviations and Acronyms for Chemotherapy Regimens

Abbreviation/Acronym	Regimen	Indication
ABVD	Adriamycin, bleomycin, vinblastine, dacarbazine	Hodgkin lymphoma
ABVE DBVE	Adriamycin, bleomycin, vincristine, etoposide DBVE (doxorubicin) Note: etoposide is also known as VP-16, Adriamycin is a trade name for doxorubicin hydrochloride	low-risk, childhood Hodgkin lymphoma
AC	Adriamycin, cyclophosphamide	recurrent and metastatic breast cancer
AC-T	Adriamycin, cyclophosphamide, Taxol	adjuvant treatment for breast cancer
ADE	cytarabine, daunorubicin, etoposide Note: cytarabine is also known as ara-C	childhood acute myeloid leukemia
BEACOPP	bleomycin, etoposide, Adriamycin, cyclophosphamide, Oncovin, procarbazine, prednisone Note: Oncovin is a trade name for vincristine	advanced-stage Hodgkin lymphoma
BEP	bleomycin, etoposide, cisplatin Note: cisplatin is generic for Platinum	adult and childhood ovarian and testicular germ cell tumors
CAF	cyclophosphamide, Adriamycin, fluorouracil	breast cancer
CEOP	cyclophosphamide, epirubicin, Oncovin, prednisone	aggressive non-Hodgkin lymphomas
CP	chlorambucil, prednisone	chronic lymphocytic leukemia
CHOP	cyclophosphamide, hydroxydaunorubicin, Oncovin, prednisone	indolent and aggressive forms of non-Hodgkin lymphoma
CMF	cyclophosphamide, methotrexate, fluorouracil	breast cancer
COPP	cyclophosphamide, Oncovin, procarbazine, prednisone	Hodgkin and non-Hodgkin lymphomas
CVP	cyclophosphamide, vincristine, prednisone	indolent non-Hodgkin lymphoma and chronic lymphocytic leukemia
EPOCH CHEOP	etoposide, prednisone, Oncovin, cyclophosphamide, hydroxydaunorubicin	aggressive B cell and T cell non-Hodgkin lymphomas
FEC CEF	fluorouracil, epirubicin, cyclophosphamide	recurrent and metastatic breast cancer
FOLFIRI	folinic acid, fluorouracil, irinotecan	advanced-stage colorectal cancer
FOLFOX	folinic acid, fluorouracil, oxaliplatin FOLFOX regimens differ in agent dosing and administration schedule and include FOLFOX 4, FOLFOX 6, modified FOLFOX 6 (mFOLFOX 6) and FOLFOX 7	advanced-stage and metastatic colorectal cancer
FL-LV	fluorouracil, leucovorin	colorectal cancer

(Continued)

Table 12-6 Common Abbreviations and Acronyms for Chemotherapy Regimens (*Continued*)

Abbreviation/Acronym	Regimen	Indication
ICE	ifosfamide, carboplatin, etoposide	relapsed and refractory non-Hodgkin and Hodgkin lymphomas
JEB JM8EB	carboplatin, etoposide, bleomycin Note: carboplatin is also known as JM8	childhood extracranial germ cell tumors
R-CHOP	Rituximab, cyclophosphamide, hydroxydaunorubicin, Oncovin, prednisone	immunochemotherapy regimen to treat both indolent and aggressive forms of non-Hodgkin lymphoma
Stanford-V	mechlorethamine, doxorubicin hydrochloride, vinblastine, vincristine, bleomycin, etoposide and prednisone	Hodgkin lymphoma
TAC	Taxotere, Adriamycin, Cytoxan	breast cancer
VAMP	vincristine, Adriamycin, methotrexate, prednisone	low-risk childhood Hodgkin lymphoma
VeIP	Velban, ifosfamide, mesna, cisplatin Note: cisplatin is generic for Platinol, mesna is used to reduce bladder toxicity	advanced-stage extracranial germ cell tumors
XELOX	capecitabine, oxaliplatin Note: capecitabine is generic for Xeloda	advanced stage colorectal cancer

match because the A, B, and DRB1 loci are inherited from each parent as a unit on chromosome 6 and expressed codominantly (equally). Unrelated donors may be used, but it is difficult to locate individuals who are a perfect match for all alleles at the HLA-A, HLA-B, and HLA-DRB1 loci. While it is imperative to use HLA-matched donors, it is not necessary to match ABO blood type. Recipients receiving stem cells from a donor with a different ABO blood type will retain the blood type of their donor, effectively changing their blood type. In addition to restoring the bone marrow, a significant therapeutic effect is achieved by using allogeneic stem cells: the immunocompetent donor immune cells attack occult malignant cells in a **graft-versus-tumor (GVT)** or **graft-versus-leukemia** reaction.

Following myeloablation (indicated by a WBC of less than 0.1), the infusion of stem cells is a relatively simple procedure performed at the bedside. The cells are infused through a central vein over a short period. The stem cells have a homing-like ability to migrate to the bone marrow where they engraft and begin proliferating.

Bone Marrow Transplant

The oldest form of stem cell transplantation is a **bone marrow transplant (BMT).** To perform an autologous BMT, the patient's own bone marrow is harvested prior to administration of chemotherapy or radiation. This allows the patient to receive an extremely high dose of cytotoxic therapy followed by a **bone marrow rescue.** The **harvested marrow** is stored frozen until time to re-infuse the cells. This approach works best when the bone marrow is known to be disease-free, although in some cases neoplastic stem cells can be purged to assure that occult malignant cells are not re-infused. During the **harvesting** procedure, 400–1000 mL of bone marrow is aspirated from the iliac crest and/or the sternum. The harvested marrow is cryopreserved using liquid nitrogen until myeloablation is complete.

Potential allogeneic donors undergo tissue typing to determine HLA phenotypes. When performing an allogeneic BMT, the marrow is harvested from the donor just prior to the infusion so the cells do not need to be cryopreserved.

Patients undergoing BMT require intensive supportive care until the bone marrow fully **engrafts** and pancytopenia resolves. These patients are kept in strict isolation and given antibiotics, antifungals, and blood products. Blood products should be from donors that are seronegative for CMV. Blood products are typically irradiated to prevent T cells in the transfused blood from acting against the host. Blood products used in stem cell transplant patients include irradiated granulocytes, **leukocyte-poor red blood cells** (also called **WBC-depleted RBCs**), and platelet concentrates.

    Primary graft failure occurs when the transplanted stem cells fail to engraft. **Late graft failure** occurs when the graft is initially established but later fails to produce sufficient red and white cells.

Peripheral Blood Stem Cells

The earliest HSCT procedures used stem cells from bone marrow, but the use of peripheral blood as a source of stem cells is becoming more common. Hematopoietic stem cells circulate in the peripheral blood but at far lower concentrations than in the bone marrow, but stem cells can be selectively isolated from peripheral blood. Stem cells express the surface antigen CD34, which can be exploited to preferentially select these cells using monoclonal antibodies combined with flow cytometry or **apheresis. Peripheral stem cell donors** may be given a colony stimulating factor such as filgrastim (Neupogen) to draw the cells out of the bone marrow and into the peripheral blood (ie, mobilize the cells). Four days following administration of the colony stimulating factor, donors undergo apheresis to retrieve the stem cells. Apheresis techniques withdraw donor blood, separate the needed components (in this case CD34$^+$ cells), and return the remainder to the donor. Apheresis is performed in the outpatient setting and requires three to four hours to complete. Donors are attached to apheresis equipment that withdraws blood, passes the blood through the separator mechanism that collects CD34$^+$ cells and immediately returns the remainder of red and white cells to the donor. The dose required for engraftment is 1–2×10^6 CD34$^+$ cells/kg body weight.

 Pause 12-9 What is the difference between apheresis and electrophoresis?

Cord Blood

The first SCT using umbilical cord blood was performed in 1988 to treat a child with Fanconi anemia. The donor was the boy's newborn sister, who was a perfect HLA match. The umbilical cord contains an exceptional number of hematopoietic stem cells with a higher proliferative capacity when compared to adult stem cells. Cord-blood stem cells are relatively immature and are naturally more immune-tolerant since much of a person's immune tolerance is developed in the first few months of life (see page 314). More HLA disparity between the recipient and the cord-blood donor is tolerated because the donor cells will learn "tolerance" to the recipient's cells. Graft versus host disease (see below) is less frequent and less severe in patients receiving cord-blood stem cells.

Mini-transplant

A mini-transplant is a **nonmyeloablative allogeneic peripheral blood stem cell transplant** and involves the infusion of donor hematopoietic cells into a recipient that has *not* undergone a myeloablative regimen. The grafted, immunocompetent cells have a graft-versus-tumor effect that destroys aberrant cells. This technique is used to treat some forms of leukemia. The patient's blood shows evidence of chimerism. (11)

 Pause 12-10 Explain this procedure in layman's terms; nonmyeloablative allogeneic peripheral blood stem cell transplant.

Complications of Stem Cell Transplants

The most significant risk of allogeneic SCT is graft versus host disease (GVHD) in which the immunocompetent cells from the donor attack the host. **Acute GVHD** results from engraftment of allogeneic T lymphocytes that recognize the host's (ie, recipient's) disparate HLA. Symptoms of acute GVHD include erythroderma, voluminous diarrhea, and **immune-mediated hepatitis.** The severity of GVHD is graded in stages I through IV. The prognosis for acute stage III and IV GVHD is grave.

    Chronic GVHD develops 2–12 months after SCT and involves the skin, eyes, mouth, liver, fascia, and almost any organ. Symptoms include chronic **lichenoid** skin changes, dry mouth, and dry eyes. Both forms of GVHD are treated with steroids and cyclosporine.

(11) A chimera expresses genetic material from two different sources. This may also be referred to as mosaicism.

Other complications of myeloablative therapy include infection (bacterial, viral—especially CMV—and fungal); severe, painful mucositis; nonbacterial interstitial pneumonia; hemorrhagic cystitis; and veno-occlusive disease of the liver.

Side Effects of Cytotoxic Treatment

Chemotherapy and radiation therapy are notorious for their high rate of morbidity. Many side effects of chemotherapy are related to its impact on normal cells that have a naturally higher rate of turnover such as the gastrointestinal epithelium, hair, bone, and skin cells. Common side effects include:

- erythema or blistering of the hands and feet
- **myelosuppression** (bone marrow suppression)
- nausea and vomiting
- **stomatitis**
- **alopecia**
- diarrhea or constipation
- allergic reactions
- neurotoxicity

Nausea and Vomiting

The most common side effects of chemotherapy and radiation treatment are **chemotherapy-induced nausea and vomiting (CINV).** Emesis is thought to result from stimulation of the chemoreceptor trigger zone in the vomiting center of the central nervous system. The most effective treatments for chemotherapy-induced nausea are the serotonin-receptor antagonists granisetron (Kytril) and ondansetron (Zofran) administered immediately before and following chemotherapy. These drugs have a very favorable side-effect profile but they are extremely expensive. Patients taking the highly emetogenic drugs such as the platinum complexes are pretreated with both antiemetics and dexamethasone. The antiemetic aprepitant (Emend) is also used to treat chemotherapy-induced nausea. Some patients experience **anticipatory nausea** resulting from the anxiety of treatment, which may be treated with lorazepam (Ativan).

Cytopenias

Cytopenias (anemia, leukopenia, and thrombocytopenia) commonly result from chemotherapy or radiation therapy. Anemia is defined as a hematocrit of less than 30% or hemoglobin less than 10 g/dL. Hematinics in the form of recombinant erythropoietin therapy (eg, Epogen) are used to induce red cell production.

Packed RBC (pRBC) transfusions may also be used, especially if the patient is suffering cardiopulmonary effects of anemia. Some patients require transfusion of **leukocyte-poor RBCs,** which restores red cells without exposing the patient to the platelet-destroying effects of donor T cells. Most white cells are separated from red blood cells by centrifugation (the most common method of separating blood components), but some white cells become trapped in the red blood cell layer. Leukocyte-poor RBCs are treated to remove virtually all white cells. Transfusion products may also be irradiated, especially when given to highly immunocompromised patients, to disable T cells and prevent GVHD. Thrombocytopenia with a platelet count of less than 10,000 is treated with transfusion of platelet concentrates.

Severe neutropenia is defined as an absolute neutrophil count of less than 500. This level of neutropenia places the patient at extremely high risk of infection. Neutropenia may be treated with GM-CSF and G-CSF (colony stimulating factors). Patients should also be treated prophylactically with antiviral medication (e.g., Zovirax) and antibiotics (e.g., Bactrim). Fever greater than 38 degrees Celsius in a neutropenic patient is considered an emergency; patients should be evaluated immediately for the source of infection and treated with broad-spectrum antibiotics such as cefepime (Maxipime), ceftazidime (Fortaz), or ciprofloxacin (Cipro) plus amoxicillin/clavulanate (Augmentin). A persistent fever is treated with antifungal medications such as fluconazole (Diflucan).

Gastrointestinal Effects

Mucositis is a common manifestation of GI toxicity. Epithelial cells in the mouth and throughout the GI tract are affected by chemotherapy because they have a higher turnover rate. Stomatitis (mucositis in the mouth) leads to ulcers and candidiasis that is extremely painful. Treatment is important so that patients can maintain adequate nutrition and hydration. Stomatitis may be treated with oral rinses or nystatin suspension with instructions to **swish and swallow. Viscous lidocaine** given as a mouthwash is prescribed to relieve the pain.

> The patient was given a prescription for Pink Magic (equal parts viscous Xylocaine, Benadryl elixir, and Maalox), 1 pint, to be taken 2 teaspoons before meals, at bedtime, and as needed for stomatitis.

Diarrhea may be treated with kaolin, loperamide (Imodium), or atropine with diphenoxylate (Lomotil).

- Cancer treatment may be described as curative, adjuvant, neoadjuvant, palliative, or salvage.

- Surgery is typically used for local disease and can be curative. Metastases may be treated surgically but typically only for palliation of symptoms. Cytoreductive surgery, also called debulking, may be used to increase the effectiveness of chemotherapy and radiation.

- Radiation therapy may be curative, therapeutic, or palliative. Radiation therapy exploits the higher replication rates of malignant cells by damaging the cell's DNA while the DNA is being replicated.

- The source of the radiation may be positioned externally or internally. Doses of radiation therapy are measured in Gray and centigray. Total doses are fractionated into smaller doses given daily for two to six weeks.

- Chemotherapy is systemic therapy given to treat primary tumors, metastases, and micrometastases. Chemotherapy agents exploit the increased replication rate of malignant cells and interfere with DNA replication and mitosis.

- Oftentimes, multiple chemotherapy agents are administered using a specified protocol over a period of months or years.

- Hematopoietic stem cell transplants are performed to reconstitute the bone marrow following myeloablation. Stem cells may be derived from bone marrow, peripheral blood, or cord blood. Transplants may be autologous or allogeneic. A mini-transplant transfuses donor hematopoietic cells into a donor that has not undergone a myeloablative regimen. The most significant complication of a stem cell transplant is graft versus host disease.

- Side effects of cytotoxic treatments are mostly due to the effect of the therapy on normal cells that also have a high rate of turnover, such as the mucosal lining of the GI tract, hair, bone marrow, and skin.

- Chemotherapy-induced nausea and vomiting is the most common side effect and is treated with antiemetics that act on the vomiting center of the CNS. Cytopenias may be improved by transfusing blood products and administering colony stimulating factors.

Constipation is a common problem in cancer patients due to the use of opioid pain medications. Senna preparations (Senokot) or bisacodyl (Dulcolax) may be helpful. Other laxatives used include milk of magnesia, magnesium citrate, and lactulose.

Anorexia may be due to cancer treatment or from the disease. Appetite stimulants such as Decadron, prednisone, and megestrol (Megace) increase appetite and produce weight gain but have not been shown to improve survival.

Effects on the Hair and Skin

Common effects on the skin include erythema, alopecia, photosensitivity, phlebitis, and tissue necrosis. Hand-foot syndrome causes numbness, tingling, pain, redness, or blistering of the palms of the hands and soles of the feet. This can lead to the disappearance of fingerprints in some patients.

Solid Tumors

The most common cancers in the United States include cancer of the lung, prostate, breast, colon, and rectum.

Breast Cancer

Breast cancer is the most common, although not the most lethal, cancer affecting females. The most common forms involve the glandular tissue of the ducts and lobules. Breast cancer is divided into two major forms: **carcinoma in situ** and **invasive cancer.** Carcinoma in situ is confined to the ducts or lobules. **Ductal carcinoma in situ (DCIS)** may be detected by mammography. At this stage, it has not invaded surrounding tissues but has the potential to do so. **Lobular carcinoma in situ (LCIS)** is usually diagnosed on biopsy and is rarely visualized on mammography. LCIS is often multifocal and bilateral, but is not considered malignant.

The majority of breast cancer cases are **infiltrating ductal carcinoma.** The remainder consists of infiltrating lobular carcinoma, medullary, mucinous, and tubular carcinoma. **Paget disease** (12) is a form of ductal carcinoma that affects the nipple and areola.

(12) Paget disease of the nipple should not be confused with the metabolic bone disease of the same name.

Patients are often diagnosed after **screening mammography** or on palpation of a painless lump in the breast. The location of a lesion is often described in terms of an analog clock superimposed over the breast and read from the perspective of the examiner. For example, a lump in the outer lower quadrant of the left breast would be the 4 o'clock position. Early breast cancer causes few symptoms. Tumors that have advanced may cause breast pain, nipple discharge, erosion, retraction, enlargement or itching of the nipple, redness, generalized hardness, or shrinking of the breast.

Invasive breast cancer is known to metastasize to the lymph nodes and then systemically to other tissues in the body, most commonly the lungs, liver, bone, brain, and skin. Advanced tumors tend to become fixed to the chest wall or overlying skin and produce satellite nodules or ulcers in the skin. Lymphedema causes an exaggeration of the usual skin markings, producing **peau d'orange.** Lymph node involvement may be indicated by matted or fixed axillary nodes, supraclavicular, or infraclavicular lymphadenopathy.

Peau d'orange is pronounced *pō-dŏ-rahnj'.* It means orange peel in French.

Clock positions are transcribed using the word o'clock (eg, 4 o'clock), not colons and digits (4:00).

 Additional imaging revealed multiple osseous lesions on bone scan. Brain MRI showed no evidence of metastatic disease. MRI scan of the thoracic spine showed pathologic compression fracture at T9 with retropulsion but no cord compression. PET-CT scan showed intense uptake of bilateral pulmonary nodules, multiple skeletal lesions, and a few hepatic lesions.

Early detection and treatment of breast cancer vastly improves the prognosis, so a definitive diagnosis of any breast mass or lesion must be made. The evaluation begins with mammography. A screening mammogram is performed on patients with no signs or symptoms of disease. A **diagnostic mammogram** is performed to gain more information about a suspected lesion. Mammography reports include a score on a scale of 0–5 based on the **Breast Imaging and Reporting Data System (BI-RADS).** A zero indicates no suspicion of malignancy and a 5 indicates a high suspicion of malignancy (see Mammography on page 424).

A suspicious lesion on x-ray may be followed by breast MRI, or the physician may have sufficient reason to proceed to biopsy. **Stereotactic biopsy** using mammography or ultrasound improves diagnostic accuracy. **Mammographic localization** uses two views of the breast to place a wire directly into the lesion. The wire is used as a guide for a needle biopsy using **fine-needle aspiration (FNA)** or a large, hollow needle (**core biopsy**). In some cases, an open incision or **excisional biopsy** may be required.

After the lesion is positively identified as malignant, **biomarkers,** proliferation index, and histological studies are performed to grade the malignant cells. The proliferative index is an indication of how quickly the cells replicate and the degree to which the cells are differentiated (matured). The **Bloom-Richardson** grading system is used to assess the aggressiveness of the breast cancer cells and is based on three criteria: how closely the cells resemble nonmalignant breast tissue, the number of mitotic figures (cells in the process of dividing) observed in a single microscopic field, and the morphology of the nuclei. Each of these indicators is assigned a score from 1 to 3. The three scores are added together for a grading scale ranging from 1 to 9 with the following prognoses:

3–5: grade 1, well differentiated, best prognosis

6–7: grade 2, moderately differentiated, medium prognosis

8–9: grade 3, poorly differentiated, worst prognosis

Biomarkers for breast cancer include estrogen and progesterone receptors and epidermal growth factors. Some breast malignancies express **estrogen receptors (ER+)** and/or **progesterone receptors (PR+).** These receptors promote DNA replication and cell division when stimulated by estrogen or progesterone (respectively). Hormonal manipulation can be used to treat these types of tumors, so the presence of ER and PR has become a positive prognostic indicator.

Breast tumors are tested for amplification of human epidermal growth factor receptor 2 (HER2) protein, also called **c-erb B2,** produced by the **HER2/neu** gene. Overexpression of HER2/neu is a poor prognostic indicator. HER2/neu results determined by immunohistochemical studies are reported as 1+ (not overexpressed), 2+, or 3+ (overexpressed). HER2/neu may also be determined using **fluorescent in situ hybridization (FISH),** in which case a result of six or more copies of the HER2/neu gene per nucleus or a FISH ratio greater than 2.2 is considered positive (overexpressed). (13) HER2/neu-positive breast cancer is treated specifically with trastuzumab (Herceptin).

> ▶ Needle biopsy of a right supraclavicular lymph node revealed metastatic carcinoma with immunohistochemistry showing 99% estrogen receptor and 8% progesterone receptor staining; c-erb B2 staining read out as negative. Liver biopsy showed similar pathology with positive ER and PR with borderline-positive HER2 with FISH showing a ratio of approximately 2.15.

> ⏸ **Pause 12-11** Why do you think the terms amplification and overexpression are used to describe epidermal growth factors?

Some breast cancers express the cancer antigens **CA 15-3** or **CA 27-29.** These markers cannot be used to diagnose patients because some people are positive for these antigens in the absence of cancer. When elevated at the time of diagnosis, these cancer antigens correspond to total tumor cell volume. These patients can be followed using CA 15-3 and CA 27-29 cancer markers as an indication of increasing or decreasing cancer burden or recurrence. In addition to receptor studies and marker studies, patients undergo imaging procedures and other diagnostic procedures for staging and treatment planning.

Treatment planning is based on the patient's tumor grade and stage, tumor markers, age, and menopausal status. Patients in all stages of breast cancer are treated with surgery to remove the primary lesion. Most patients receive some form of adjuvant therapy including radiation, chemotherapy, or hormonal therapy. Surgical options include **breast-conserving surgery** (lumpectomy, quadrantectomy, wide excision) or **modified radical mastectomy** (simple mastectomy plus lymph node dissection). A sentinel-node biopsy may be performed prior to surgery or during surgery. Lymph node dissection is performed if the sentinel node is positive.

> ▶ DIAGNOSIS: Stage I, T1cN0MX, right breast carcinoma. Presented as postmenopausal female on hormone replacement therapy with 6-month mammogram showing suspicious area of architectural distortion, mid-outer aspect right breast. Ultrasound confirmed 1.3 cm hyperechoic lesion at the 9-o'clock position. Core biopsy showed infiltrating ductal carcinoma, Bloom-Richardson grade 1, estrogen and progesterone receptor status 98% and 38%, respectively. Right breast lumpectomy showed a 1.3 cm tumor of above histology. Four sentinel lymph nodes were negative for tumor. Minor intraductal component, solid and cribriform, nuclear grade 1. Surgical resection margins clear with closest margin 5 mm. Ki-67 was 25% and HER2/neu staining +1.

> ⏸ **Pause 12-12** Explain the use of the term radical (versus radicle) in the phrase radical mastectomy.

Patients who undergo mastectomy may elect to have reconstructive surgery to replace the breast mound. Options include submuscular or subcutaneous placement of a silicone or saline implant (with or without a **tissue expander**) or creation of a breast mound using a muscle flap. Muscle flaps may be produced from one of several muscles. The **transrectus abdominis muscle flap (TRAM flap)** rotates the rectus abdominis muscle with attached fat and skin in the cephalad direction to create a breast mound. This procedure creates a **pedicle** (ie, leaves one area attached) so the vascular supply is maintained. The **free TRAM flap** is done by completely removing the rectus abdominis (no pedicle) along with overlying fat and skin and using microvascular surgical techniques to reconstruct the vascular supply on the chest wall. A **latissimus dorsi flap (lat flap)** pulls the latissimus muscle pedicle toward the anterior chest to create a breast mound. An implant may be required with this procedure to produce symmetry with the contralateral breast. A free flap may also be created from the gluteus maximus muscle. The **nipple-areola complex** is reconstructed in a

---

(13) Breast cancers that are negative for progesterone and estrogen receptors as well as HER2/neu are called **triple negative breast cancer.**

separate procedure using skin grafts, **nipple sharing** from the contralateral breast, or tattooing.

> Status post right mastectomy and sentinel lymph node surgery with TRAM flap reconstruction.

> Status post right mastectomy, simple, with skin-sparing and sentinel lymph node surgery followed by right-sided breast reconstruction and single-stage silicone implant and AlloDerm. Currently on ovarian suppression with Lupron 7.5 mg intramuscularly monthly and Tamoxifen 10 mg twice daily.

The most common chemotherapy agents used for breast cancer include capecitabine (Xeloda), doxorubicin and daunorubicin (Adriamycin), gemcitabine (Gemzar), the taxanes (Taxol and Taxotere), and vinorelbine (Navelbine). Commonly used regimens include AC (Adriamycin, cyclophosphamide) and CMF (cyclophosphamide, MTX, fluorouracil). Patients with overexpression of HER2/neu are treated with trastuzumab (Herceptin), a monoclonal antibody that binds to HER2/neu receptors.

For the purpose of treatment planning with hormone therapy, women within one year of their last menstrual period are considered premenopausal and women whose menstruation ceased more than a year prior are treated as postmenopausal. Hormonal therapy for premenopausal or postmenopausal breast cancer includes the **selective estrogen receptor modifiers (SERMs)** tamoxifen (Nolvadex) and raloxifene (Evista). Postmenopausal breast cancer is treated with **aromatase inhibitors (AIs),** such as anastrozole (Arimidex), that block the conversion of androgens into estrogen. Patients may also receive hormonal therapy for at least five years following treatment as a form of chemoprevention. Bone metastases may be treated with the bisphosphonate derivative pamidronate (Aredia) administered monthly by IV.

> **Pause 12-13** Why are aromatase inhibitors used in post menopausal women to reduce estrogen levels? (Hint: What is the source of estrogen in women with nonfunctioning or surgically removed ovaries?)

Patients may opt to undergo genetic evaluation for mutations in the **BRCA1** or **BRCA2** gene. These mutations confer a significantly higher lifetime risk of breast cancer. Patients positive for either gene mutation are offered **prophylactic bilateral mastectomies.** Other risk factors, such as family history, age at menarche, age of first parity, age at menopause, exogenous estrogen exposure, and lifestyle can be taken into account to predict lifetime risk of breast cancer. The **Gail model** is a computer program used to calculate breast cancer risk.

> BRCA1 and BRCA2 are pronounced *brăk-ə* one and *brăk-ə* two.

> DIAGNOSIS: Stage IIIA, pT1cN2aMX, invasive lobular carcinoma of the right breast, ER positive, PR positive, HER2/neu negative.
>
> TREATMENT PLAN: Adriamycin 60 mg/m² IV with Cytoxan 600 mg/m² IV day #1; Neulasta 6 mg subcutaneously day #2, every 2 weeks x4 cycles; followed by Taxol 175 mg/m² IV every 2 weeks x4 cycles.

Colorectal Cancer

Colorectal cancer (CRC) is one of the most common forms of adenocarcinoma in the United States. Both environmental and genetic factors have been implicated. Well-characterized forms of hereditary CRC include **hereditary nonpolyposis colon cancer (HNPCC)** and familial adenomatous polyposis (FAP).

CRC most often occurs as a transformation within an adenomatous polyp. For this reason, screening procedures for CRC monitor for polyps and remove all polyps seen. The most common presenting symptoms of rectal cancer include blood in the stool and a change in bowel habits. Patients may also complain of tenesmus, urgency, and perirectal pain. Symptoms of colon cancer depend on the location of the lesion and include abdominal pain, bleeding, constipation, and decreased stool diameter.

Colorectal cancers tend to form bulky, exophytic masses or annular, constricting lesions. CRC spreads in an orderly fashion from a primary lesion to regional lymph nodes and then to distant organs. On barium enema, colon cancer may appear as an **apple core** (a constricting lesion) or a mass with a filling defect. An MRI is useful for determining the depth of penetration into the rectal wall. **Endorectal ultrasound** or **MRI with endorectal coil** is used for staging and preoperative planning. CRC is staged using the TNM system or the **Dukes system:**

Dukes stage A—disease does not extend beyond the muscularis propria

Dukes stage B1—disease extends into muscularis propria

Dukes stage B2—disease extends beyond muscularis propria

Dukes stage C1—stage B1 with positive regional lymph nodes

Dukes stage C2—stage B2 with positive regional lymph nodes

Dukes stage D—distant metastases

Note the spelling of the eponym Dukes (ends with an s)—this is not the possessive form.

 Pause 12-14 On barium enema, colon cancer may appear as an apple core (a constricting lesion) or a mass with a filling defect. What is a filling defect?

Carcinoembryonic antigen (CEA) levels are elevated in the majority of CRC patients. If CEA is high at diagnosis and then falls after treatment, it may be used as a tumor marker. CEA greater than 5 ng/mL prior to resection of the primary tumor is a poor prognostic indicator.

Primary treatment for nonmetastatic disease is wide resection of the tumor and excision of regional lymphatics. The operative procedure depends on the location of the lesion. Options include **abdominoperineal resection** with permanent colostomy, **transanal resection,** and **low anterior resection with colorectal or coloanal anastomosis.** Intraoperative palpation or ultrasound examination of the liver is helpful for detecting liver metastases. Adjuvant therapy may consist of 5-fluorouracil (5-FU) and leucovorin, FOLFOX, or FOLFIRI (see Table 12-6). Hepatic metastases can be treated with local ablative techniques such as cryosurgery, radiofrequency or microwave coagulation, embolization, or **hepatic intraarterial chemotherapy.**

The procedure abdominoperineal resection uses the combining forms of abdominal and *perineal* (not peritoneal).

CRC may be prevented by early detection and resection of colorectal polyps using routine screening by flexible sigmoidoscopy, colonoscopy, or CT colonoscopy (virtual colonoscopy). Patients over age 50 should be screened on a routine basis with fecal occult blood tests (FOBT).

DIAGNOSIS: T3N0M0, stage IIA, poorly differentiated adenocarcinoma of the transverse colon showing high-frequency microsatellite instability (MSI-H). Eleven lymph nodes were removed and free of tumor. There was invasion 2 cm beyond the muscularis propria into the non-peritonealized pericolonic tissue.

TREATMENT: Status post complete resection of the tumor in January, 20XX, and resection of recurrent tumor in July of this year. FOLFOX, leucovorin 400 mg/m², oxaliplatin 85 mg/m², 5-fluorouracil 400 mg/m² bolus, infusional 5-fluorouracil 1200 mg/m² days #1 and #2, cycles #1 and #2. With cycle #3, we decreased the dose of oxaliplatin to 70 mg/m², infusional 5-fluorouracil 1000 mg/m².

DIAGNOSIS: Stage IV, pT3cN2M1, colorectal carcinoma. The patient presented with fever and crampy abdominal pain. Colonoscopy revealed an obstructing tumor at 20–25 cm with biopsies showing invasive adenocarcinoma. Abdominal and pelvic CT scans revealed perforated sigmoid colon cancer, regional adenopathy, as well as a lesion in the right hepatic lobe measuring 6.2 x 4.2 x 4.7 mm. Liver biopsy revealed moderately differentiated adenocarcinoma felt to be consistent with colonic primary, CK20 positive. Initial blood work showed CEA 34.1, CA-125 at 61.6, elevated LDH to 251. The patient went on to have sigmoid resection and primary anastomosis. Pathology confirmed an adenocarcinoma, moderately differentiated, infiltrating and ulcerating, extending through the muscularis propria into the pericolic fat.

Prostate Cancer

Prostate cancer is highly prevalent but the prognosis for most men with localized disease is quite good. Prostate cancer is often very slow growing and more men die *with* prostate cancer (but from other causes) than *from* prostate cancer. Many elderly patients choose **active surveillance** (previously called watchful waiting) as opposed to actively treating the disease. Symptoms of prostate cancer are rare until the tumor is large enough to cause urethral obstruction. Symptoms of advanced disease include hematuria, straining, hesitancy, weak or intermittent stream, a sense of incomplete emptying, and dribbling. Patients may complain of bone pain if metastasis to the bone has occurred.

Diagnosis is suggested by digital rectal examination (DRE) of the prostate and blood levels of prostate specific antigen (PSA). On examination, the prostate may feel hard or nodular. Induration extending to the seminal vesicles and **lateral fixation of the prostate** is highly suggestive of advanced prostate cancer. PSA is a glycoprotein produced by both normal and malignant prostate cells and is indicative of total prostate cell volume. A normal PSA value should be less than 2.0 ng/mL. A slightly elevated value may indicate inflammation, hypertrophy, or infection. A PSA of greater than 4 ng/mL is concerning and should be followed. The PSA velocity is more indicative of cancer than a single, elevated value. Biopsy is indicated for PSA velocities greater than 0.75 ng/mL per year. PSA is also used to monitor patients for cancer recurrence. The PSA value following prostatectomy should be undetectable.

Prostate biopsy may be performed using transrectal ultrasound-guided needle biopsy. Hypoechoic areas are more likely to represent cancer. A sextant biopsy samples six different areas of the prostate. The **Gleason score** is indicative of the tumor's aggressiveness. The Gleason score assigns a grade of 1–5 to the most prevalent cellular pattern seen on the biopsy sample. A second score is assigned to the second-most prevalent cellular pattern. The two scores are added together. A score of 6 or less is considered to be well-differentiated, a score of 7 indicates moderately differentiated, and a score of 8–10 indicates poorly differentiated carcinoma. A lower score indicates a less aggressive and less invasive tumor and portends a better prognosis.

Definitive treatment for prostate cancer confined to the prostate is **radical prostatectomy,** which removes the prostate, seminal vesicles, and ampullae of the vas deferens. Brachytherapy or standard external beam radiation therapy may be used in lieu of prostatectomy. Cryosurgery, which circulates liquid nitrogen through small, hollow-core needles, is also used.

Most cases of prostate cancer are hormone-dependent and respond to **androgen deprivation,** which may be accomplished surgically with bilateral orchiectomies or **medical orchiectomies** using GnRH agonists such as leuprolide (Lupron) or goserelin (Zoladex). Antiandrogens such as flutamide (Eulexin) and bicalutamide (Casodex) may be added to the GnRH agonist for a complete **androgen blockade. Hormone refractory metastatic disease** is treated with docetaxel and palliative radiation therapy for bone metastases. The axial skeleton is the most common site of prostate cancer metastasis.

DIAGNOSIS: Stage pT3b prostate carcinoma. Bilateral biopsies of the prostate gland revealed a Gleason 4 + 4 adenocarcinoma involving the left apex and base with associated focal perineural invasion. Over 95% of 2 cores contained cancer. The patient underwent radical prostatectomy and lymphadenectomy with pathology showing Gleason 4 + 4 adenocarcinoma involving both lobes of the prostate gland. All surgical resection margins were free of tumor. Definite perineural and lymphovascular invasion was identified in the surgical specimen. There was also bilateral seminal vesicle involvement. High-grade prostatic intraepithelial neoplasia was noted in the gland.

Lung Cancer

Worldwide, lung carcinoma is the leading cause of death due to cancer with the vast majority of cases related to cigarette use. Lung cancer is divided into two major categories: **small-cell lung cancer (SCLC)** and **non-small-cell lung cancer (NSCLC).** SCLC is associated with cigarette smoking and is highly aggressive. The majority of patients have metastatic disease at the time of diagnosis. NSCLC has a more variable course than SCLC. Despite many advances in treatment, the prognosis for lung cancer remains extremely poor with only 15% of patients surviving five years or more. Improving survival must be focused on prevention (smoking cessation) and early detection.

Initial symptoms include cough or possibly dyspnea if the airway is obstructed. Some patients complain of vague or localized chest pain. Hemoptysis is less common than might be expected. Anorexia and weight loss are common. If the tumor has spread within the region of the lung, patients may experience superior vena cava syndrome.

Most diagnostic workups begin with the finding of a suspicious lesion on chest x-ray. A solitary pulmonary nodule, called a **coin lesion,** is less than 3 cm and appears as a rounded opacity. X-ray results are reported as **low probability, intermediate probability,** or **high probability** of malignancy. X-ray is typically followed by high-resolution CT scan. A finding of **spiculated margins** and a **peripheral halo** are associated with malignancy.

Biopsy is necessary to confirm the diagnosis. The least invasive procedure that still allows access to the lesion is selected. Sample tissue may be obtained by **transthoracic needle aspiration (TTNA),** bronchoscopy, or **video-assisted thorascopic surgery (VATS).** Bronchoscopy allows the clinician to collect washings, brushings, biopsies, and fine-needle aspirations of visible endobronchial lesions. Lymph nodes, including paratracheal, subcarinal, mediastinal, and hilar, may also be sampled. Open biopsy using VATS is performed if no other less invasive method can be used to access the lesion and if the lesion is felt to be resectable.

SCLC is not divided into numerous stages as in other malignancies. SCLC has only two stages: limited and extensive. **Limited-stage SCLC** is confined to one hemithorax (including ipsilateral lymph nodes) that can be encompassed within a single radiation therapy port. Less than a third of patients present with limited-stage SCLC. Extensive-stage SCLC describes disease that extends beyond one hemithorax, and it is assumed that micrometastases exist. The presence of malignant cells in pleural or pericardial effusions also constitutes extensive disease.

Non-small-cell lung cancer is divided into four stages (I–IV) based on tumor size, location, lymph node involvement, and distant metastases. The TNM system is also applied and grouped into one of the four stages. Whole-body imaging is typically required to assess the patient with NSCLC. CT scans, PET scans, or integrated PET-CT are used for staging.

SCLC is typically responsive to initial chemotherapy treatment but, unfortunately, responses are short-lived. Both chemotherapy and radiotherapy are employed. Surgery is only rarely performed to remove a solitary nodule in patients who otherwise have no evidence of metastases.

Chemotherapy regimens for SCLC may incorporate a variety of drug classes including etoposide, platinum compounds, irinotecan (Camptosar), topotecan (Hycamtin), vinca alkaloids, alkylating agents, taxanes, and gemcitabine (Gemzar). Survival of patients with limited-stage disease is greatly improved with radiation to the hemithorax. Brain micrometastases are common; cranial radiation may be used to prevent brain metastases, especially since chemotherapy has a limited ability to cross the blood-brain barrier.

NSCLC, as opposed to SCLC, is more amenable to surgical resection. Resection may include lobectomy, pneumonectomy, **segmentectomy,** or **wedge resection.** Surgery may be curative for a significant number of patients with stage I or stage II disease. Surgery is followed by adjuvant therapy with chemotherapy and radiation.

DIAGNOSIS: Stage IV, T2N2M1, non-small-cell carcinoma of the lung. Patient presented as a 49-year-old female with acute-onset seizure in mid-July. MRI scan of the brain showed a suspicious lesion near the vertex. Underwent resection with pathology showing adenocarcinoma, immunohistochemistry showing positive TTF1 staining and negative EGFR staining. Further evaluation revealed a right lung mass, pleural-based nodules, as well as mediastinal and subcarinal adenopathy. A PET scan revealed metastatic disease. The evaluation for the ALK rearrangement by Genzyme was positive with 91.5% of cells showing rearrangement by inversion in chromosome 2.

- Breast cancer is the most common cancer in females. Most breast cancers are classified as ductal carcinoma in situ and invasive ductal carcinoma. Mammographic readings are reported using the BI-RADS system. Biomarkers for breast cancer include hormone receptors and epidermal growth factors. Treatment may involve surgery, reconstruction, chemotherapy, radiation therapy, long-term hormonal therapy, and immunotherapy.

- Colorectal cancer most often results from the transformation of an adenomatous polyp. Common presenting symptoms include blood in the stool and a change in bowel habits. An MRI is used to stage the disease using the Dukes classification system. CEA is commonly elevated in colon cancer and is used to monitor disease. Treatment includes resection followed by chemotherapy. FOBT, colonoscopy and polyp removal are important for early detection and CRC prevention.

- Prostate cancer is highly prevalent but not always lethal. Screening for prostate cancer includes digital rectal exam and serum PSA values. Prostate cancer is confirmed on prostate biopsy and is graded using the Gleason score. Treatment includes resection, chemotherapy, and androgen deprivation via medical or surgical orchiectomy.

- Lung cancer is the leading cause of death due to cancer worldwide. Major categories of lung cancer include small-cell carcinoma and non-small-cell carcinoma. Prognosis is generally poor. Diagnosis is confirmed on lung biopsy. Small-cell lung cancer is staged into two groups—limited and extensive. Non-small-cell lung cancer uses the TNM system. Treatment includes resection, chemotherapy, and radiation.

- Secondary lung cancer is metastatic disease caused by a primary tumor in non-lung tissue. Many types of cancer are known to metastasize to the lung including kidney, breast, colon, cervix, and melanoma. Secondary lung cancer causes fewer symptoms than primary lung cancer, and treatment is based on protocols for the primary tumor.

Secondary Lung Cancer

Secondary lung cancer represents metastases from malignancies that originate outside the lungs (non-pulmonary primary). The lungs are common sites of metastases, especially in carcinoma of the kidney, breast, colon, cervix, and melanoma. Multiple nodules are typically found. Symptoms are uncommon and are usually referable to the site of the primary tumor. If metastases to the lungs are discovered before the primary tumor is diagnosed, an extensive workup should be undertaken to discover the primary tumor. At times, biopsy of the lung lesions can help to identify the histological origins of the tumor. Treatment is determined by treatment protocols for the primary tumor.

Leukemia

Leukemia refers to a malignancy involving the hematopoietic cells. The malignant transformation often occurs at the level of the pluripotent stem cell such that the cells have a limited ability to differentiate and thus fail to mature and function normally. Cells show abnormal proliferation, clonal expansion, and diminished apoptosis. The over-proliferation of abnormal, nonfunctioning cells in the bone marrow outcompetes normal cells for space and resources, leading to a functional immunoincompetence. Extramedullary infiltration (14) of leukemic cells causes hepatomegaly, splenomegaly, and lymph node enlargement. Meningeal infiltration causes increasing intracranial pressure with cranial nerve palsies.

Pause 12-15 Explain functional immunoincompetence.

The leukemias are divided into acute and chronic categories. Acute leukemia includes **acute lymphocytic leukemia (ALL)** and **acute myelocytic leukemia (AML).** Chronic leukemias include **chronic lymphocytic leukemia (CLL)** and **chronic myelocytic leukemia (CML).** The maturation stages of white and red cells are shown in ■ **Figure 12-5.**

(14) Extramedullary infiltration refers to cells migrating into tissues other than the bone marrow.

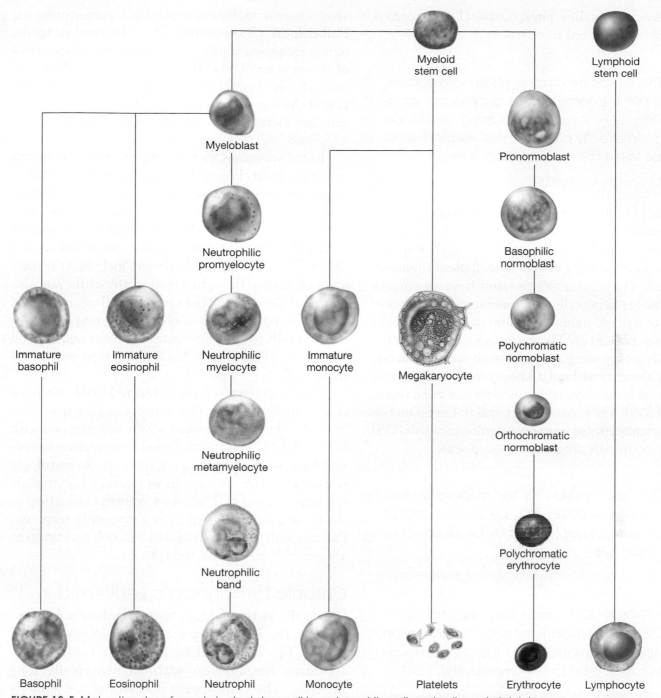

Myeloid
stem cell

Lymphoid
stem cell

Myeloblast

Pronormoblast

Neutrophilic
promyelocyte

Basophilic
normoblast

Immature
basophil

Immature
eosinophil

Neutrophilic
myelocyte

Immature
monocyte

Megakaryocyte

Polychromatic
normoblast

Neutrophilic
metamyelocyte

Orthochromatic
normoblast

Neutrophilic
band

Polychromatic
erythrocyte

Basophil

Eosinophil

Neutrophil

Monocyte

Platelets

Erythrocyte

Lymphocyte

FIGURE 12-5 Maturation steps from pluripotent stem cell to mature white cells, red cells, and platelets.

Study Figure 12-5 and take special note of the following:

- the two types of precursors are lymphoid and myeloid
- immature forms are larger and contain more nuclear material
- granulocytes (cells containing granules) consist of basophils, eosinophils, and neutrophils and are named according to the way the granules stain (see also Figure 10-1 on page 310)
- platelets are cytoplasmic fragments of megakaryocytes

Pause 12-16 Look at Figure 12-5. Why do you think the leukemias are sorted into lymphocytic and myelocytic categories?

A **leukemoid reaction** may mimic leukemia. Leukemoid reactions are marked by granulocytic leukocytosis (WBC greater than 30,000) and usually occur in response to infection or cancer. A leukemoid reaction may appear similar to CML but it is not a malignancy.

The **leukocyte alkaline phosphatase (LAP) score** is increased in leukemoid reactions.

> The leukocyte alkaline phosphatase score is not the same test as alkaline phosphatase. The LAP score is a staining technique performed directly on leukocytes. Alkaline phosphatase levels are measured in the serum.

Some patients with lymphoproliferative disorders have elevated levels of **paraproteins,** which are monoclonal immunoglobulins (a single antibody) or simply kappa or lambda light chains (incomplete immunoglobulins). These paraproteins result from an unregulated clone of plasma cells that manufacture an excessive amount of a single immunoglobulin or one of the light chains (see page 312). These proteins can be detected in the laboratory using **serum protein electrophoresis (SPEP).** Patients without a known myeloproliferative disease may have detectable amounts of a paraprotein in their blood. These patients are said to have a **monoclonal gammopathy of unknown significance (MGUS)** and may eventually progress to overt disease.

> The abbreviation for serum protein electrophoresis (SPEP) may be pronounced as an acronym (es-pep) or it may be dictated as the initialism SPE.

> LABORATORY: Total iron 94, transferrin 222.8, iron-binding capacity 313, saturation 30, ferritin 65. Hemoglobin A_{1c} 8.3. SPE previously negative for monoclonal gammopathy.

Chronic Myelogenous Leukemia

CML is a myeloproliferative disorder in which myeloid cells are overproduced but typically retain their capacity to differentiate function. The disease may remain stable for years without the manifestations of malignancy and then suddenly convert to an overt malignancy with the appearance of a **blast crisis.** Average

(15) The fusion gene bcr/abl may be dictated b-c-r able.

age of onset is 55. Patients with CML demonstrate the **Philadelphia chromosome.** This abnormality results from a reciprocal translocation between the long arms of chromosome 9 and chromosome 22. A fusion gene occurs (called bcr/abl) **(15)** at the point where the section of chromosome 9 joins with chromosome 22. This gene has increased tyrosine kinase activity, leading to a leukemic reaction.

Initial symptoms include fatigue, night sweats, and low-grade fever. Physical examination shows splenomegaly and possibly sternal tenderness (due to marrow expansion). The hallmark of the disease is an elevated WBC, which may be modest to extremely high (greater than 150,000). A peripheral blood smear will show a shift to the left in the myeloid series including the presence of blasts. Basophils and eosinophils are also increased. Patients in blast crisis typically show anemia and thrombocytopenia caused by overexpansion of myeloid cells to the detriment of platelet and red cell precursors. The Philadelphia chromosome is detected using PCR.

The emergence of the tyrosine-kinase inhibitor drug imatinib (Gleevec) has transformed the treatment of CML. This drug produces a 98% response rate with few intolerable side effects. Blood counts return to normal after several weeks of treatment (**hematologic response**). After six months of treatment, cytogenic assessment using PCR shows a dramatic reduction in the bcr/abl gene, referred to as a **cytogenic response.** Patients with a poor response to imatinib may undergo allogeneic bone marrow transplant.

Chronic Lymphocytic Leukemia

CLL is the most common type of leukemia encountered in the US with a median age of onset of 65 years. CLL is marked by proliferation of mature-appearing lymphocytes with an abnormally long life span. The cells appear normal but are actually incompetent. The majority of CLL cases involve proliferation of CD5[+] B cells. Initially, lymphocytes accumulate in the bone marrow but eventually increase in the peripheral blood and then infiltrate extramedullary organs, resulting in splenomegaly and hepatomegaly. Anemia, neutropenia, and thrombocytopenia result from abnormal hematopoiesis. Disrupted B-cell and T-cell interactions result in decreased immunoglobulin production (hypogammaglobulinemia) and an increased propensity toward autoimmune diseases directed at red cells and platelets. Often patients have a positive

Coombs test with autoimmune hemolytic anemia and autoimmune thrombocytopenia.

 Pause 12-17 What is autoimmune hemolytic anemia?

Onset of CLL is usually insidious and many patients are incidentally noted to have lymphocytosis on routine CBC. The CBC report may note the presence of **smudge cells,** which are lymphocytes that appear as if they were ruptured and smashed when viewed on a peripheral blood smear. Symptoms include nonspecific complaints such as fatigue, anorexia, weight loss, and dyspnea on exertion. Physical exam may reveal lymphadenopathy and hepatosplenomegaly. Staging is based on either the **Rai** (stage 0 through IV) or **Binet** (stage A through C) staging criteria.

Standard of care for early, indolent CLL is observation only. Chemotherapy is instituted with symptomatic organomegaly or the advent of **constitutional symptoms** such as fever, night sweats, extreme fatigue, and weight loss. Lymphocytosis greater than 100,000 or infection may also prompt treatment. CLL is treated with fludarabine (Fludara) combined with rituximab (Rituxan) or the three-drug regimen of fludarabine, rituximab, and cyclophosphamide. Alemtuzumab (Campath) is used for refractory CLL and to reduce **minimal residual disease.**

> Patient presented to this office with 10-year history of mild leukocytosis, lymphocyte predominant. White blood cell count was 15,000 with 66% lymphocytes and 32% neutrophils, hemoglobin 13, and normal platelet count. Peripheral blood smear showed an increased percentage of mature-appearing lymphocytes with an occasional smudge cell. Peripheral blood immunophenotypic studies confirmed a monoclonal lambda, CD5+ B-cell neoplasm consistent with chronic lymphocytic leukemia. However, CD23 was negative. LDH was 158 and SPEP was normal.

Acute Leukemia

Acute leukemia is marked by sudden onset with symptoms occurring only days or weeks before diagnosis.

The most common acute leukemia is acute lymphocytic leukemia (ALL) with a peak incidence between three and seven years of age. Although ALL does occur in adults as well, it is the most common cancer in the pediatric population. Acute-onset leukemia may also be classified as acute myelocytic leukemia (AML). You may also hear it dictated as **acute myelogenous leukemia.**

Symptoms of acute leukemia include anemia, pallor, fatigue, fever, malaise, infection, and weight loss. Easy bruising and bleeding may manifest as epistaxis, bleeding gums, petechiae, and menorrhagia. Examination may reveal lymphadenopathy, splenomegaly, hepatomegaly, and **leukemia cutis** (a raised, nonpruritic rash). CBC shows **hyperleukocytosis** with an elevated circulating blast count up to 200,000 or more. Extremely high white counts cause **hyperviscosity** of the peripheral blood that impairs circulation, causing headache, confusion, and dyspnea.

Diagnosis is based on CBC and peripheral blood smear, bone marrow biopsy and aspiration, and cellular studies to differentiate specific forms of acute leukemia. The hallmark of acute leukemia is pancytopenia with blasts in the peripheral blood. In rare cases, blasts are not present in the peripheral blood and this is referred to as **aleukemic leukemia.**

Once acute leukemia is recognized, it is imperative to classify the predominant cell as either lymphoid (ALL) or myeloid (AML). Histochemical studies, **cytogenetics,** and **immunophenotyping** are used to differentiate the two major cell lines. The **Auer rod,** seen on Wright stain as an eosinophilic (red), needle-like inclusion in the cytoplasm, is pathognomonic for AML. Histochemical studies to differentiate AML and ALL include **myeloperoxidase (Sudan black stain)** for AML and **nonspecific esterase stain** which identifies monocytic cells of AML. If AML has been ruled out, ALL is presumed and is confirmed using flow cytometry to identify lymphoid surface antigens, including CD2, CD5, CD7, CD10, and CD19. ALL is usually positive for **terminal deoxynucleotidyl transferase (TdT).**

Both types of acute leukemia require similar supportive care, including transfusions, antibiotics, antifungal and antiviral drugs, hydration, and alkalinization of the urine. Patients may need to be transfused with red blood cells, granulocytes, or platelets. Patients with a hemoglobin value of less than 8 g/dL receive pRBCs. Platelet transfusions are given when the platelet count falls below 10,000. Granulocytes may be transfused to help fight an ongoing infection.

Initial treatment with chemotherapy causes massive lysis of cells with release of intracellular components that need to be flushed rapidly, so hydration at twice the normal daily volume is required to prevent hyperuricemia, hyperphosphatemia, and hyperkalemia due to tumor lysis syndrome. Allopurinol or rasburicase (Elitek) may be given before starting chemotherapy to prevent hyperuricemia. Maintaining alkaline urine prevents crystal formation and helps flush these metabolites.

Patients with acute leukemia, despite the high peripheral white count, are neutropenic and immunosuppressed. Patients with an ANC below 500 should be treated with broad-spectrum antibiotics, antifungal, and antiviral medications along with granulocyte infusions.

 Pause 12-18 How can you have a high peripheral white count and still be neutropenic?

Acute Lymphocytic Leukemia

ALL is classified using the **French-American-British (FAB)** classification, which is based on morphology:

L1 lymphoblasts with uniform, round nuclei and scant cytoplasm

L2 more variability in lymphoblasts

L3 lymphoblasts with finer nuclear chromatin and blue cytoplasms with vacuoles

Prognosis varies according to karyotype (determined by cytogenetic studies) and presenting symptoms. The following are good prognostic indicators:

- young age (three to five years)
- hyperdiploid states
- WBC less than 25,000 at initial presentation
- no CNS disease at diagnosis
- FAB L1 classification
- t(12;21) karyotype

ALL may also be associated with the Philadelphia chromosome (**Ph+ALL**). The presence of the chromosome translocations t(9;22) and t(4;11) are poor prognostic indicators. Other unfavorable factors include abnormal chromosomal morphology, increasing age (over 45), and B-cell immunophenotype.

As with CML, imatinib (Gleevec) has been shown to be very efficacious in Philadelphia-positive ALL. Patients without the Philadelphia chromosome are treated with chemotherapy and possibly stem cell transplant. Chemotherapy is divided into four phases:

phase 1: remission induction

phase 2: CNS prophylaxis

phase 3: postremission consolidation or intensification

phase 4: maintenance

Induction therapy often includes daily prednisone with weekly vincristine plus anthracycline or asparaginase. Other regimens combine cytarabine (Cytosar-U), etoposide, and cyclophosphamide (Cytoxan). Yet other regimens might include **high-dose methotrexate with leucovorin rescue** (see page 433). ALL is known to infiltrate the meninges, producing symptoms within the central nervous system. CNS prophylaxis uses **intrathecal** methotrexate, cytosine arabinoside, and corticosteroids.

Consolidation therapy follows induction therapy and uses a different regimen than the induction stage. Maintenance therapy is typically with methotrexate and mercaptopurine (Purinethol). Duration of therapy is typically two and a half to three years. Many patients are cured, but relapse occurs in about 20% of patients. A bone marrow transplant with an HLA-matched sibling offers the best hope of cure.

Acute Myelocytic Leukemia

AML is characterized by proliferation of immature cells that can be traced back to a point somewhere along the myeloid stem cell line. AML is a diverse and heterogeneous group of leukemias, and this diversity stems from the fact that genetic mutations (and hence leukemic transformation) can occur at a number of steps along the differentiation pathway from the progenitor myeloid stem cell to a fully mature white cell, red cell, or platelet (Figure 12-5). Risk of AML increases with age with a median onset of 50 years. AML also occurs as a secondary cancer 20–30 years after treatment of a previous cancer.

The FAB classification system divides AML into eight categories, many of which have specific chromosomal abnormalities. The chromosomal translocations create abnormal fusion proteins that contribute to maturation arrest (ie, the point at which differentiation is halted and clones are produced). The FAB categories along with associated chromosomal translocations are as follows:

M0: minimally differentiated acute myeloblastic leukemia

M1: acute myeloblastic leukemia without maturation

M2: acute myeloblastic leukemia with granulocytic maturation [t(8;21)(q22;q22), t(6;9)]

M3: acute promyelocytic leukemia [t(15;17)]

M4: acute myelomonocytic leukemia [inv(16) (p13;q22), del(16q)]

M4eo: M4 with eosinophilia [inv(16), t(16;16)]

M5: acute monoblastic leukemia [del(11q), t(9;11), t(11;19)]

M6: acute erythroid leukemia

M7: acute megakaryoblastic leukemia [t(1;22)]

M8: acute basophilic leukemia

Prognostic factors are important for determining the treatment protocol. Patients with more negative prognostic indicators are typically given more intense therapy. The karyotype is the most important prognostic indicator. Karyotypes t(8;21), t(15;17), and inv(16) (p13;q22) are associated with favorable outcomes. Patients with no karyotypic abnormality have an intermediate prognosis. Poor outcomes are associated with deletion of chromosome 5 or 7, trisomy 8, or a karyotype with more than three abnormalities.

The most common induction therapy is known as **7 + 3.** Cytarabine is given as a continuous IV infusion for seven consecutive days with an anthracycline given for three consecutive days as an IV push. Induction therapy is followed by consolidation using the same regimen or one similar. Stem cell transplant may be an option for some patients, especially those diagnosed at a younger age or at high risk of relapse.

Acute promyelocytic leukemia (APL) is an important subgroup of AML and is treated differently than

- Leukemia is a malignancy of the hematopoietic cells. Cells fail to fully differentiate and do not function normally. Leukemia is marked by abnormal proliferation, clonal expansion, and diminished apoptosis.

- CML is a chronic myeloproliferative disorder marked by overproduction of mostly functional white cells of the myeloid cell line caused by a translocation called the Philadelphia chromosome. CML is treated with Gleevec.

- CLL is the most common leukemia in the U.S. and is marked by proliferation of mature-appearing yet incompetent lymphocytes. CLL may be accompanied by anemia, neutropenia, and thrombocytopenia as well as antiplatelet antibodies and a positive Coombs test. Treatment is started with the onset of constitutional symptoms or symptomatic organomegaly and includes chemotherapy and immunotherapy.

- The acute leukemias are marked by the sudden onset of symptoms, including fatigue, fever, infection, and bleeding. The hallmark of acute leukemia is increased numbers of blasts

and immature cells in the peripheral blood. Immunophenotyping and histology studies are used to distinguish lymphoid and myeloid acute leukemia.

- ALL is classified according to the FAB classification system. Prognosis varies depending on the karyotype. Treatment includes chemotherapy and imatinib if positive for the Philadelphia chromosome. Intrathecal chemotherapy is given for CNS disease. Treatment protocols may span two and a half to three years and include four phases: induction, CNS prophylaxis, consolidation, and maintenance.

- AML is a diverse group of leukemias affecting the myeloid cell line. AML is classified using the FAB classification. Many forms of AML are due to chromosomal translocations that create fusion proteins, leading to maturation arrest. Treatment and prognosis vary greatly among the various types of AML. Most forms of AML are treated with chemotherapy except for APL, which is treated with all-trans-retinoic acid.

the other classifications. In this form of AML, the t(15;17) translocation produces a fusion protein that binds to the retinoic acid receptor and inhibits myeloid differentiation. These patients are treated with **all-trans-retinoic acid (ATRA)** and daunorubicin with a good outcome. These patients often present with disseminated intravascular coagulation because promyelocytes contain procoagulant substances within their intracytoplasmic granules, and degranulation sets off a cascade of clotting events. Care must be taken to prevent DIC in this patient population, especially during treatment.

Lymphoma

Lymphomas represent a group of malignant diseases that originate in the lymphatic system and primarily involve the lymph nodes, spleen, liver, and bone marrow. Lymphomas are divided into two major categories: Hodgkin lymphoma and non-Hodgkin lymphoma.

Hodgkin Lymphoma

Hodgkin lymphoma (HL), also called **Hodgkin disease (HD),** is distinguished from non-Hodgkin lymphoma by the presence of binucleated **Reed-Sternberg cells.** Hodgkin lymphoma also extends in an orderly fashion to nearby lymph node clusters as opposed to non-Hodgkin lymphoma that disseminates randomly. The malignancy affects lymphocytes of B-cell origin. The cause of the malignant transformation is not known but certain occupations and some infections (eg, EBV, TB, HSV, and HIV) increase the risk for Hodgkin lymphoma.

Patients often present with painless cervical lymphadenopathy. They may also experience constitutional symptoms such as fever, night sweats, and unintentional weight loss (greater than 10% of their body weight over the previous six months). **Pel-Ebstein fever (PE fever),** which is characterized by a few days of high fever alternating with a few days or weeks of normal or below-normal temperature, may also be noted. Systemic symptoms are sometimes called **B symptoms** (see staging information below).

Physical examination may show splenomegaly and hepatomegaly. Bone involvement may cause vertebral osteoblastic lesions called **ivory vertebrae.** On palpation, lymph nodes feel rubbery or swollen. Enlarged lymph nodes may compress nearby structures causing jaundice (liver compression), dyspnea (bronchopulmonary compression), peripheral edema, neuralgias, or

paraplegia (cord compression). As the disease progresses, lymphocytes become defective and humoral immunity is depressed. Patients are susceptible to bacterial, fungal, viral, and protozoal infection. Death is often the result of sepsis.

Diagnosis requires lymph node or bone marrow biopsy. Mediastinal nodes are accessed by mediastinoscopy or by **Chamberlain procedure** (a limited left anterior thoracostomy). Biopsy reveals the pathognomonic Reed-Sternberg cells in a characteristically heterogeneous cellular infiltrate consisting of histiocytes, lymphocytes, monocytes, plasma cells, and eosinophils. Classic Hodgkin lymphoma is separated into four histological subtypes based on the appearance of the Reed-Sternberg cells and the surrounding cells:

- nodular sclerosis
- mixed cellularity
- lymphocyte-rich
- lymphocyte-depleted

All four classic subtypes are associated with the immunophenotype CD15$^+$, CD30$^+$, and CD20$^-$, which help distinguish Hodgkin and non-Hodgkin lymphomas. A fifth (nonclassical) type is **nodular lymphocyte-predominant** and shows a different immunophenotype: CD15$^-$, CD30$^-$, CD20$^+$, EMA$^+$ (epithelial membrane antigen).

CT scans and PET scans are performed to stage the disease. Hodgkin lymphoma is staged according to the **Ann Arbor** staging criteria:

- stage I: involvement of a single lymph node region (I) (mostly the cervical region) or single extralymphatic site (Ie)
- stage II: involvement of two or more lymph node regions on the same side of the diaphragm (II) or of one lymph node region and a contiguous extralymphatic site (IIe)
- stage III: involvement of lymph node regions on both sides of the diaphragm, which may include the spleen (IIIs) and/or limited contiguous extralymphatic organ or site (IIIe, IIIes)
- stage IV: disseminated involvement of one or more extralymphatic organs

The letter A appended to the stage means there are no systemic symptoms. The letter B indicates at least one systemic symptom is present. Symptomatology correlates to treatment response—patients with fewer symptoms respond better to treatment than patients with constitutional symptoms. Elevated levels of **beta 2-microglobulin** are associated with a less favorable prognosis and an increased chance of relapse. The beta 2-microglobulin is a component of the MHC proteins and can be detected in the urine.

Treatment of HL is based on the stage. The most common regimen used for Hodgkin lymphoma is **ABVD (Adriamycin, bleomycin, vinblastine, dacarbazine)** and ABVD with irradiation. **Involved-field radiation** may be used for moderate- or advanced-stage disease. XRT directed above the diaphragm is called **mantle-field radiation. (16)** Radiation below the diaphragm to the abdomen, spleen, and/or pelvis is called **inverted Y-field radiation.** Patients with relapsed or refractory Hodgkin's may be treated with autologous peripheral stem cell transplant. The overall survival rate for HL is good.

Non-Hodgkin Lymphoma

The non-Hodgkin lymphomas make up the remainder of the lymphomas (ie, those not classified as Hodgkin lymphoma). **Non-Hodgkin lymphoma (NHL)** is more common than HL and is the sixth most common cancer in the US. The majority of cases are malignancies of the B-cell line but T-cell lymphomas are also seen. There is some overlap with NHL and leukemia, as both involve proliferation of immature lymphocytes. Generally, NHL is distinguished from leukemia by more nodal involvement with fewer abnormal cells in the peripheral circulation and fewer blasts seen in the bone marrow.

Classification of NHL continues to evolve. Currently, the WHO separates NHL into four broad categories (mature B or T cells and precursor B or T cells) with 43 subcategories. It also recognizes a newer category called **mucosa-associated lymphoid tumors (MALTomas). (17)** Lymphomas may be described as indolent or aggressive. Indolent lymphomas are slowly progressive and treatable but not currently curable. Aggressive lymphomas progress rapidly but are curable.

Often patients present with peripheral lymphadenopathy. Most patients have disseminated disease at the time of diagnosis. Lymphadenopathy, especially mediastinal and retroperitoneal lymphadenopathy, often causes compression on nearby organs and structures that may cause noticeable symptoms.

As with HL, a lymph node biopsy is performed to determine the specific diagnosis. NHL is characterized by destruction of normal lymph-node architecture and invasion of the lymph-node capsule and adjacent fat. Immunophenotyping helps to further define the disease and plan the course of treatment. As with Hodgkin lymphoma, elevated levels of beta 2-microglobulin are associated with a less favorable prognosis and an increased chance of relapse. The **International Prognostic Index (IPI)** is used to predict survival and is based on five criteria:

- age greater than 60
- poor performance status
- elevated LDH
- more than 1 extranodal site involved
- stage III or IV disease

Treatment includes chemotherapy, radiation therapy, and the addition of the anti-CD20 monoclonal antibody rituximab (Rituxan). Two other monoclonal antibodies developed for NHL include ibritumomab tiuxetan (Zevalin) and ^{131}I tositumomab (Bexxar). There are numerous chemotherapy protocols for NHL, some of which are listed in Table 12-6. Patients may also undergo stem cell transplantation.

DIAGNOSIS: Stage IVA non-Hodgkin lymphoma. Patient presented with increasing pelvic fullness and left lower quadrant discomfort. Pelvic ultrasound revealed an approximately 6 x 4 x 3 cm left adnexal fullness. Followup abdominal and pelvic CT scan revealed extensive retroperitoneal, mesenteric, and abdominal adenopathy. Pathology showed follicular center cell lymphoma, grade 1, with monotonous infiltration of lymphocytes. Immunohistochemistry showed positive staining for CD10, CD45, CD19, CD20, CD23, FMC7, HLA-DR. The cells were restricted to lambda chain immunoglobulin staining of intermediate intensity.

(16) Mantle field refers to the chest and shoulders (the area of the body covered by a cloak or mantle). This spelling should not be confused with mantel, which surrounds a fireplace.

(17) The term MALToma is derived from the acronym MALT combined with a suffix -oma (meaning tumor) and is pronounced *mält-ō-ma.*

- Lymphomas are a group of malignant diseases that originate in the lymphatic system and primarily involve the lymph nodes, spleen, liver, and bone marrow. Lymphoma has two classifications: Hodgkin and non-Hodgkin lymphoma.

- Hodgkin lymphoma is distinguished by the presence of Reed-Sternberg cells and affects lymphocytes of B-cell origin. Presenting symptoms include painless lymphadenopathy, splenomegaly, and hepatomegaly. Due to B-cell involvement, patients are prone to bacterial,

fungal, viral, and protozoal infections. Treatment includes ABVD chemotherapy and irradiation.

- Non-Hodgkin lymphoma represents the group of lymphomas that do not qualify as Hodgkin lymphoma and may be difficult to distinguish from leukemia. NHL is classified into more than 40 subcategories, including MALT lymphomas. Treatment involves chemotherapy, radiation therapy, and immunotherapy with monoclonal antibodies.

Imaging Studies

All forms of imaging tests have a role in the screening, diagnosis, and management of malignancies. CT scans are especially useful for assessing lymphadenopathy. MRI with gadolinium is used to evaluate both primary and metastatic brain tumors. Positron emission tomography (PET) scans show metabolic activity more so than structure and are helpful for locating areas of increased metabolic activity, a characteristic of both tumors and focal areas of infection. The PET scan uses **fluorodeoxyglucose (FDG),** a glucose analog attached to the radioisotope fluorine 18. FDG is taken up in higher concentrations by tissues that are actively using glucose, indicating higher metabolic activity. PET images are taken after injecting the patient with FDG. Tissues with high metabolic activity are described as **FDG avid.** Integrated PET-CT is especially valuable in the evaluation of the lung and breast, head and neck tumors, and in lymphoma.

PET-CT scan showed intense FDG uptake in a 13 x 22 mm supraclavicular lymph node along the left side. There is a new area of FDG uptake in the manubrium measuring approximately 9 mm with a small lytic lesion to the left. No change in the moderately intense FDG uptake along the enlarged lymph nodes in the left periaortic region. The left lung nodule appears markedly reduced in size with no residual FDG uptake.

Mammography

Mammography is commonly used to screen for breast cancer. The most common finding associated with breast cancer is **clustered polymorphic microcalcifications** with or without a nearby mass. Findings on mammography may be described using the following terms:

- **circumscribed:** a lesion with well-defined margins with an abrupt demarcation of the abnormal lesion and the surrounding tissue.

- **indistinct:** a lesion with poorly defined margins, concerning for infiltration into the surrounding tissue.

- spiculated margins: lines radiating outward from the mass.

- **architectural distortion:** distortion of normal breast architecture but no visible mass. Examples include spicules without a distinct mass, focal retraction, or a change in the appearance of the parenchyma.

- **asymmetric density:** a lesion with no specific shape or other characteristics described above. The tissue may be visibly different but there is no true mass.

- **calcifications:** deposits of calcium, which may be described as **amorphous** (no specific shape), **pleomorphic** (many shapes), fine, linear, and/or branching (**casting**). Calcifications may be associated with malignancy but not always.

A screening mammogram may raise suspicion, requiring further studies to characterize the abnormality. Comparison to previous studies is also important whenever possible. Additional studies may include a **spot compression,** magnification, special mammographic views, ultrasound, or breast MRI. All mammogram reports should include a BI-RADS category based on the following criteria:

0-Need Additional Imaging Evaluation

1-Negative (no masses, architectural distortions, or suspicious calcifications)

2-Benign Finding (no mammographic evidence of malignancy but benign abnormalities noted)

3-Probable Benign Finding—Short Interval Followup Suggested (most likely a benign lesion but suspicious enough to warrant followup to establish stability of the lesion)

4-Suspicious Abnormality—Biopsy Should Be Considered (a lesion that is not distinctly malignant but is suspicious enough to warrant biopsy)

5-Highly Suggestive of Malignancy—Appropriate Action Should Be Taken

Laboratory Studies

All the major laboratory studies (CBC, BMP, CMP, electrolytes, liver function tests) are used in the diagnosis and management of hematologic and oncologic disorders. Elevated liver enzymes (alkaline phosphatase, LDH, ALT, AST) may indicate liver metastases. LDH is elevated in some anemias and leukemias. Elevated alkaline phosphatase along with elevated serum calcium is highly suspicious for metastases to the bones. Elevated uric acid levels are common in myeloproliferative and lymphoproliferative disorders. In addition to these general laboratory evaluations, a variety of tests has specific roles in the management of leukemia, lymphoma, anemia, and cancer.

Coombs Test

The Coombs test is used to detect the presence of anti-RBC antibodies. Two versions of the Coombs test are available: indirect Coombs and **direct Coombs.** To perform the indirect Coombs test, reagent RBCs (ie, RBCs provided in the test kit) are mixed with the patient's serum. If antibodies directed against RBCs are present in the patient's serum, they will bind to the reagent RBCs. An antiglobulin antibody is then added to the test. This antibody cross-links antibodies that have been bound to the reagent RBCs and causes the red cells to become clumped, which is visible to the naked eye. This test is a helpful screening test for the presence of antibodies directed against red cells. Once antibodies are known to exist, additional tests can be run to determine their specificity.

The direct Coombs test is used to determine if antibodies have already coated the patient's RBCs in vivo. The patient's RBCs are mixed with antihuman globulin. If antibodies are present on the surface of the red cells, the antihuman globulin will cross-link the red cells, causing them to clump.

> The direct Coombs test is also called the direct antibody test (DAT). The indirect Coombs is also called the indirect antibody test.

Blood Typing

The blood bank is tasked with typing a patient's blood and assuring that the unit of blood issued for the patient is sufficiently matched for ABO and Rh compatibility and unlikely to cause a transfusion reaction. A **type and screen** is requested when blood *may* be needed, as in the case of elective surgery. The patient's blood is typed for ABO and Rh antigens as well as screened for antibodies using the indirect Coombs test. If no antibodies are detected, a compatible unit of blood may be issued (if and when actually needed) without further testing. If the patient is found to have an antibody on the screening test, a crossmatch procedure will be required using the actual unit of blood to be given.

A **type and crossmatch** (also called a **type and cross**) is ordered when the patient is very likely or will definitely require a transfusion. This procedure tests the patient's blood for ABO and Rh type and also crosses (mixes) the patient's plasma with donor red cells pulled from the actual unit of red cells to be transfused. The crossmatch procedure assures that the patient does not already have antibodies that would react against the red cells to be transfused. These antibodies are typically from the Duffy, Kell, and Lewis antigen systems, which are also located on RBC surfaces (just like ABO and Rh). Patients who have received multiple transfusions or patients with hemolytic anemias are more likely to have antibodies directed against these other antigens located on the red blood cell surface.

Cancer Markers

Cancer markers (**Table 12-7**) can be used to follow a patient that has already been diagnosed. In general, cancer markers are not used to establish a diagnosis because some markers are elevated in the absence of cancer.

Table 12-7 Serum Cancer Markers

Test Name	Associated Cancer	Normal Range
PSA (prostate specific antigen)	prostate	<4 ng/mL
CEA (carcinoembryonic antigen)	lung, digestive tract, and pancreas	<5.0 ng/mL
AFP (alpha-fetoprotein)	hepatocellular carcinoma and embryonal cancers	<15 ng/mL
CA-125	ovary	<35 units/mL
CA 19-9	digestive tract carcinomas	<37 units/mL

Iron Studies

Iron studies include ferritin, transferrin, soluble transferrin receptor, total iron-binding capacity, and serum iron (**Table 12-8**). **Transferrin saturation** is the ratio of serum iron to **total iron-binding capacity (TIBC)** and represents the amount of transferrin molecules that are carrying the maximum amount of iron. Transferrin saturation decreases (ie, less iron occupying the iron-binding sites) in iron deficiency. Transferrin saturation is elevated (usually over 60%) in patients with **iron overload.**

Table 12-8 Iron Studies

Test Name	Reference Range
serum iron	male: 65–177 mcg/dL female: 50–170 mcg/dL
TIBC (total iron-binding capacity)	240–450 mcg/dL
transferrin saturation	male: 20% to 50% female: 15% to 50%
serum ferritin	male: 20–250 mcg/L female: 15–150 mcg/L
soluble transferrin receptor (sTfR)	3.0 to 8.5 mcg/mL

Transferrin receptor (TfR) is a protein on the surface of all cells, but is found in higher concentrations on erythroid precursors. Soluble transferrin receptor (sTfR) is the same protein as TfR, but it is not bound to cell surfaces. This protein becomes detectable in the serum when iron stores have been depleted and during periods of increased erythropoiesis. On the other hand, sTfR decreases with iron overload and with decreased erythropoiesis.

Ferritin is the storage form of iron. Iron is a strong oxidizing agent and is toxic when not stored within the body properly. Ferritin molecules consist of several protein strands wrapped around a core of iron and is designed to safely store iron in the tissues, especially in the liver, spleen, skeletal muscle, and bone marrow. Serum levels of ferritin parallel ferritin levels in the tissues, so in most cases, serum ferritin is a reliable indicator of iron stores. Ferritin may be increased (independent of iron stores) in inflammatory reactions, cancer, and following transfusion therapy. Elevated ferritin is seen in hereditary hemochromatosis. Accumulations of intracellular ferritin are broken down by lysosomes to form hemosiderin, which can be seen under the microscope with cell-staining techniques. Cells containing large amounts of hemosiderin are called **siderocytes. Hemosiderosis** may be seen in patients who have received multiple transfusions.

Folate and B_{12} Levels

Measuring serum folate and B_{12} levels (**Table 12-9**) can be helpful in the diagnosis of anemias because red cell production is dependent on these nutritional factors.

Table 12-9 Folate and B_{12}

Test Name	Reference Range
folate (folic acid)	3–20 ng/mL
B_{12}	110–800 pg/mL

Complete Blood Count

Table 12-10 outlines components of a complete blood count (CBC).

> Unless the patient is anemic, the hematocrit value should be equal to approximately three times the hemoglobin value.

A CBC with differential (**CBC with diff**) includes the percentage of each type of white cell (**Table 12-11**).

Table 12-10 Complete Blood Count

Test Name	Abbreviation	Reference Range
white blood cell count	WBC	4000–11,000/mcL
red blood cell count	RBC	males: 4.31 to 5.84 million/mcL females: 4.00 to 5.00 million/mcL
hemoglobin	Hgb or Hb	males: 13.0 to 17.0 g/dL females: 12.0 to 15.0 g/dL
hematocrit	Hct	males: 40% to 50% females: 36% to 45%
mean corpuscular volume	MCV	80–99 fL (femtoliter)
mean corpuscular hemoglobin (average amount of hemoglobin per red cell)	MCH	24–34 pg (picogram)
mean corpuscular hemoglobin concentration (a measure of the hemoglobin level in individual RBCs)	MCHC	32% to 36%
red cell distribution width	RDW	<14.5%
platelets	Plt	140,000–400,000/mcL
mean platelet volume (average size of platelets)	MPV	9.4 to 12.3 fL

Table 12-11 White Cell Differential

Cell Type	Reference Range (Percent and Absolute Counts)	Comment
lymphocytes (lymphs)	25% to 40% 1000–4400 cells/mcL	
monocytes (monos)	5% to 8% 200–880 cells/mcL	
neutrophils, also called segmented neutrophils or "segs"	40% to 70% 1600–7700 cells/mcL	
bands, also called stabs	0–8% 0–880 cells/mcL	a slightly immature neutrophil with a band-shaped nucleus (not yet segmented), seen in acute infection and during parturition
basophils (basos)	0–1% 0–110 cells/mcL	
eosinophils (eos)	0–5% 0–550 cells/mcL	
polymorphonuclear leukocytes (PMNs)	40% to 76% 1600–8360 cells/mcL	the total of neutrophils, basophils, and eosinophils
promyelocytes, metamyelocytes (youngs)	0	immature myelocytic cells, indicative of leukemia
blasts	0	indicative of leukemia

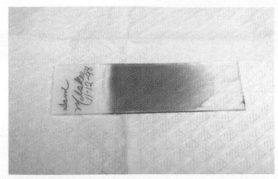

FIGURE 12-6 Peripheral blood smear before staining with Wright stain. Blood smears are used to assess red cell morphology and to perform a manual differential count.

An **automated diff** reports the percentage of each type of white cell as calculated by automated equipment. The differential count should always equal 100 because the differential reports the number of each type of white cell per 100 cells (ie, the percent). An automated count may report the differential with decimals that may add up to 100 +/-1.

A manual differential (**manual diff**) may be performed by a technologist using a microscope to examine a smear of blood (■ **Figure 12-6**) stained with Wright stain. Patients with cancer, leukemia, and other critical illnesses typically have abnormal cells that cannot be characterized by automated equipment and require a manual differential and review of RBC and WBC morphology.

Red cell morphology can be indicative and sometimes diagnostic for certain diseases (eg, sickle cells are only seen in patients with sickle cell disease, ■ **Figure 12-7**). The

presence of red cell variants is reported using a grading system of 1+ (approximately 10% of cells affected) through 4+ (greater than 75% of cells affected). Characteristics that may be reported on an examination of a peripheral blood smear are described in **Table 12-12.** See also Figure 12-3.

Table 12-13 lists white cell and platelet characteristics that may be reported on a Wright-stained smear of peripheral blood.

Reticulocyte Count

Reticulocytes are immature red cells. They are typically released from the bone marrow into the peripheral blood when the marrow is attempting to compensate for a decreased red cell count. The presence of reticulocytes following a large, traumatic bleed is a good sign that the marrow is compensating for the loss of cells. Reticulocytosis can also be a pathologic sign, indicating excessive or chronic red cell destruction. A decreased reticulocyte count in the setting of anemia indicates decreased red cell production. A reticulocyte count (**Table 12-14**) is reported as the percentage of red cells that stain with a reticular (web-like) pattern using methylene blue.

> LABORATORY DATA: WBC 7.2, hemoglobin 11.9, hematocrit 35, MCV 86, platelet count 452,000. Peripheral blood smear showed basophilic stippling and polychromasia. Normal WBCs with no young forms seen. Adequate platelets. Reticulocyte count 1.5%. Iron saturation 10% and ferritin 5.3. Vitamin B_{12} 517, folate greater than 24, TSH 2.06. Protein electrophoresis with no paraprotein detected. IgA 466, IgG 1442, IgM 156.

Bone Marrow Aspiration and Biopsy

A bone marrow aspiration and biopsy are typically performed to characterize myeloproliferative diseases as well as myelodysplastic and aplastic disorders. Hematopoietic stem cells differentiate and replicate in the bone marrow, producing the cellular components of the peripheral blood, so examining the number and characteristics of the immature cells in the marrow provides valuable diagnostic information. The biopsy is performed by a physician in either an outpatient or inpatient setting using mild sedatives

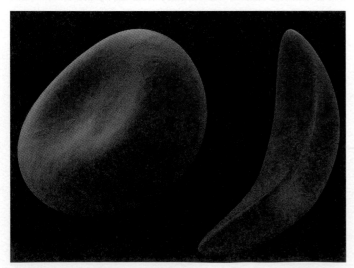

FIGURE 12-7 A normal red cell (left) and a sickle cell (right).
Source: © Sebastian Kaulitzki/fotolia.

Table 12-12 Red Cell Morphology

RBC Changes Seen on Peripheral Blood Smear	Corresponding Indices on CBC	Description
normocytic, normochromic	normal Hct and Hb	normal, biconcave, disk-shaped red cells with the typical central pallor
hypochromia	decreased MCH and MCHC	red cells with an enlarged central pallor
microcytes	decreased MCV (<80 fL)	small red cells
macrocytes	increased MCV (>100 fL)	large red cells
polychromasia	possibly increased MCV	slightly immature red cells that appear purplish blue or purplish red
acanthocytes (spur cells)		red cells with spurs projecting from the cell surface indicating cell membrane damage
helmet cells		damaged red cells shaped like a helmet
ovalocytes (elliptocytes)		oval-shaped red cells
spherocytes		red cells without a central pallor, seen in a variety of illnesses, especially hereditary spherocytosis
sickle cells (drepanocytes)		red cells shaped like a sickle (a curved blade) seen in patients in sickle cell crisis
target cells (codocytes)		red cells with a central dark spot in place of the normal central pallor
schistocytes		fragments of red cells due to red cell destruction, seen in DIC, hemolytic anemia, microangiopathic hemolytic anemia (MAHA), and possibly patients with prosthetic valves
tear drops		red cells shaped like a tear drop
stomatocytes		red cells with a more oval shape and a flat, bar-shaped central zone
rouleaux ($r\bar{u}\text{-}l\bar{o}'$)		red cells stuck together like a stack of coins due to abnormal plasma protein concentrations
anisocytosis	increased RDW	red cells of various sizes (microcytes, normocytes, and macrocytes)
poikilocytosis		red cells of various shapes and sizes (tear drops, ovalocytes, etc)
basophilic stippling	possibly increased MCV	immature red cells with a purplish-blue, grainy appearance
Howell-Jolly bodies		RBC inclusions consisting of DNA fragments, seen in asplenic or hyposplenic patients (these DNA fragments are normally plucked from the red cell as it passes through the spleen)
nucleated red blood cells (nRBC), also called **normoblasts**		red blood cells that have not yet extruded their nucleus, indicative of bone marrow stress

Table 12-13 White Cell and Platelet Changes

WBC and Platelet Changes on Peripheral Smear	Description
atypical lymphocytes	large lymphocytes with irregular shapes and increased cytoplasm, seen in acute viral infections
toxic granulation	increased granulation seen in PMNs, indicative of acute infection and during parturition
Dohle bodies (dō'-lē)	round, small, sky-blue inclusions noted in the cytoplasm of PMNs, seen in patients with acute infection, cancer, and burns
hypersegmented neutrophils	neutrophils with greater than five nuclear segments, seen in patients with folate and B_{12} deficiencies
giant platelets	a preponderance of overly large platelets
vacuoles	"holes" in the cytoplasm of PMNs caused by engulfing and then extruding bacteria

Table 12-14 Reticulocyte Count

Test Name	Reference Range
reticulocyte count	0.5% to 1.5% 50,000–150,000 cells/mcL

and analgesics or possibly conscious sedation. The biopsy removes a small core of bone from the posterior iliac crest, using a trephine such as a **Jamshidi needle.** The aspiration uses a large-bore needle and syringe to withdraw approximately 0.3 mL of bone marrow from either the posterior superior iliac crest or the sternum. Due to the risk of puncturing a major blood vessel, biopsies are not performed on the sternum. Bone marrow appears similar to blood but is normally highly cellular so it is much thicker and has small clumps called spicules.

Various cellular staining techniques are used to examine the aspirated cells. A typical pathology report of the bone marrow aspirate describes the **myeloid-to-erythroid ratio.** Cytogenetic and molecular analyses are also performed and iron stores are evaluated. Cultures may be performed, especially to evaluate **fever of unknown origin (FUO).**

Coagulation Studies

Coagulation studies (**Table 12-15**) are used to diagnose coagulopathies, monitor anticoagulation therapy, and diagnose DIC. Most tests are performed on serum drawn into a blue-top blood-sample tube containing the anticoagulant sodium citrate. Fibrinogen is converted to fibrin in the last stage of coagulation and is integral to the formation of a fibrin clot. Patients with low fibrinogen (hypofibrinogenemia) or structurally abnormal fibrinogen (dysfibrinogenemia) are at risk of bleeding. Decreased levels of fibrinogen may be due to overconsumption (as in DIC) or to decreased production (due to liver disease). Levels below 70 mg/dL interfere with coagulation. Fibrinogen is also an acute-phase protein and is elevated by infection or inflammation.

The **prothrombin time (PT or pro time)** tests for factor deficiencies in the extrinsic and common clotting pathways (see Figure 12-4) as well as the presence of coagulation inhibitors such as lupus anticoagulant. The PT is also used to monitor warfarin (Coumadin) therapy. The test reports the time (in seconds) required for a clot to form. Longer clotting times are indicative of factor deficiencies or the presence of coagulation inhibitors.

Laboratory measurements of the PT can vary slightly because the potency of thromboplastin used to perform the test varies from one batch (lot) to another, so laboratories have adopted the **international normalized ratio (INR)** as a standardized method of reporting the prothrombin time. The INR takes into account the unavoidable variability in the testing reagents, so PT values measured can be accurately compared to one another over several days or weeks and between different labs.

> PT values reported with the INR may be dictated as PT INR, PT/INR or PT-INR. There does not seem to be a consensus on how to transcribe this test name.

The partial thromboplastin time (PTT) **(18)** is a measure of the integrity of the intrinsic pathway (also called the contact pathway) as well as the common coagulation pathway. The PTT is the time (in seconds) required for the patient's sample to clot after adding a contact activator.

After a clot forms, the clot must be dismantled (dissolved). This process involves activation of the fibrinolytic pathway that lyses the fibrin stands holding the clot together. Fibrinolysis breaks the fibrin strands of a clot into various fragments; one of which is designated the D fragment. D-dimer gets its name from the fact that it consists of two cross-linked D fragments. **(19)** Elevated levels of D-dimer indicate that a fibrin clot was formed and then subsequently degraded. The D-dimer assay is a highly sensitive test for the presence of a degraded clot, but it is not specific as to the cause or location of a clot. Results are reported in **fibrin equivalent units (FEU).** Other breakdown products of clot formation are called fibrin degradation products (FDPs), also called fibrin split products (FSPs).

Protein S and protein C (**Table 12-15**) are naturally occurring anticoagulants. These proteins work together to degrade coagulation factors and enhance fibrinolysis. Decreased activity of protein C and protein S predispose the patient to thrombosis.

> Dictators may dictate the phrase protein C and S, which sounds like CNS or C&S. These are distinct proteins and should be transcribed separately (not as protein CNS or protein C&S).

Antithrombin (formerly antithrombin III) is a naturally occurring anticoagulant that inactivates several factors in the coagulation pathway to prevent runaway clotting. Levels may be decreased due to consumption (as in DIC and PE), increased loss (as in nephrotic syndrome) or due to decreased production (as in liver disease). Decreased levels predispose patients to thrombosis. Heparin interacts with antithrombin as part of its anticoagulant mechanism, and antithrombin levels (**Table 12-15**) may be evaluated to assess resistance to heparin therapy.

Table 12-15 Coagulation Studies

Test name	Normal Range
PT (prothrombin time or pro time)	11–13 seconds
PTT (partial thromboplastin time)	21–35 seconds
INR	Normal ratio is 1. Target ranges for INR vary according to the underlying disease: DVT prophylaxis 1 to 1.5 recurrent DVT 3–4 atrial fibrillation 2–3
D-dimer	<0.5 mcg/mL FEU
FSP (fibrin split products)	<5 mcg/mL
fibrinogen	200–400 mg/dL
antithrombin	80% to 130%
protein C activity	70% to 140%
protein S activity	57% to 140%

Factor V Leiden

Factor V Leiden is a point mutation in the gene that encodes coagulation factor V. Factor V Leiden is resistant to the proteolytic activity of activated protein C, resulting in a hypercoagulable state. The presence of factor V Leiden accounts for a significant number of deep venous thromboses. It is also implicated in recurrent pregnancy loss. The mutation is detected using PCR technology. Results are reported as not present, present-heterozygous, or present-homozygous.

Transfusion Therapy

Components that may be transfused include:

- packed RBCs: used to increase hemoglobin (1 unit typically increases the hemoglobin value by 1 g/dL)

(18) The PTT may also be referred to as the activated partial thromboplastin time (aPTT).

(19) A dimer is a compound molecule made of two identical molecules.

- washed RBCs (saline-washed RBCs): RBCs without plasma or platelets
- WBC-depleted RBCs (leukocyte-poor RBCs): RBCs that have been filtered to remove all WBCs
- fresh frozen plasma (FFP): a source of clotting factors (without platelets) for correction of bleeding due to factor deficiencies
- cryoprecipitate: a concentrate prepared from FFP for replacement of coagulation factors
- platelets: concentrated platelets used in severe thrombocytopenia and patients with bleeding due to platelet dysfunction (one unit raises the platelet count by approximately 10,000)
- platelets by cytapheresis: uses a single donor and apheresis techniques to create a unit of platelets equal to about six random platelet units; reduces exposure to multiple donors and preferred for platelet transfusion when available
- autologous donation: a patient's own blood collected and stored prior to elective surgery
- directed donation: blood collected for transfusion to a specific person, typically a relative or friend of the recipient

Pharmacology

Hematology and oncology use an extensive set of pharmaceuticals to treat patients and to improve quality of life. The chemotherapy arsenal contains cytotoxic agents, immunomodulating agents, targeted antibodies, hormones, and growth factors. Quality of life is improved with hematinics, antiemetics, and pain medicines.

Hematinics

Pharmacologic agents that stimulate the body to produce red cells or white cells are hematinics. These include colony stimulating factors, erythropoietin, iron, B_{12}, and folate.

Colony Stimulating Factors

Colony stimulating factors (**Table 12-16**) are used most often in conjunction with chemotherapy to stimulate white-cell production. Two forms include granulocyte colony-stimulating factor (G-CSF) or granulocyte-macrophage colony-stimulating factor (GM-CSF).

Table 12-16 Colony Stimulating Factors

Generic	Brand Name
pegfilgrastim	Neulasta
filgrastim	Neupogen
romiplostim (for platelets)	Nplate
darbepoetin alfa	Aranesp
epoetin alfa (EPO)	Procrit Epogen
sargramostim	Leukine

Iron

Iron may be given in the form of iron salts such as ferrous sulfate, ferrous gluconate, or ferrous fumarate (**Table 12-17**). A dose of 325 mg of ferrous sulfate provides 60 mg of elemental iron (the remainder of the 325 mg dose represents the "sulfate" portion of the molecule).

Table 12-17 Iron Supplements

Generic	Brand Name	Dose
ferrous sulfate	Feosol	325 mg
ferrous fumarate	Femiron	324 mg
ferrous gluconate	Fergon	240 mg

Chemotherapeutic Agents

The chemotherapy dose is often based on the patient's body surface area (BSA), which is calculated using the patient's height and weight and administered in milligrams per meter squared. The dose is also calculated so that a range of blood concentration is achieved, called the **area under the curve (AUC).** The dose is based on the patient's glomerular filtration rate and is intended to balance the therapeutic dose with toxicity.

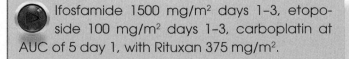

Ifosfamide 1500 mg/m² days 1–3, etoposide 100 mg/m² days 1–3, carboplatin at AUC of 5 day 1, with Rituxan 375 mg/m².

Antimetabolites

DNA consists of four base nucleotides (adenine, guanine, thymidine, and cytosine). RNA uses the same nucleotides, except thymidine is replaced by uracil. The antimetabolite class of chemotherapy drugs (**Table 12-18**) includes nucleotide analogs and folic acid blockers. The analogs are incorporated into the DNA and RNA base molecules, but their structure varies slightly so that the modified molecules disrupt normal DNA and RNA synthesis and halt normal cellular processes.

Table 12-18 Antimetabolites

Generic	Brand Name
fludarabine	Fludara
mercaptopurine	Purinethol
capecitabine	Xeloda
cytarabine	Cytosar
fluorouracil (5-FU)	Adrucil
gemcitabine	Gemzar

Folic acid is required for pyrimidine to be converted to cytosine and thymine. Antimetabolites such as methotrexate block the synthesis of folic acid, therefore interfering with DNA synthesis. Fast-growing cells, including T cells and B cells, are particularly affected by the inhibition of nucleotide synthesis, thereby suppressing the autoimmune response. Patients being treated with high doses of methotrexate may be "rescued" using leucovorin (folinic acid), listed in **Table 12-19**. Folinic acid is one metabolic step closer to the active form of folic acid and its conversion to folic acid is not affected by methotrexate. Leucovorin allows GI cells and other rapidly dividing cells to resume normal metabolism.

Table 12-19 Methotrexate and Leucovorin

Generic	Brand Name
methotrexate (MTX)	
pemetrexed	Alimta
leucovorin (for rescue)	

Anthracyclines

Anthracyclines (**Table 12-20**) are antibiotics derived from bacteria of the genus Streptomyces. This class of chemotherapeutic agent acts by damaging DNA and is used against a wide variety of cancers. It is one of the most effective chemotherapeutic agents. The anthracyclines are known for their cardiotoxicity. Patients are typically evaluated with a **multigated acquisition (MUGA) scan** before receiving an anthracycline-based therapy.

Table 12-20 Anthracyclines

Generic	Brand Name
doxorubicin	Adriamycin
daunorubicin	Cerubidine
daunorubicin (liposomal)	DaunoXome
doxorubicin (liposomal)	Doxil
epirubicin	Ellence

Alkylating Agents

The alkylating agents (**Table 12-21**) act by attaching alkyl groups to DNA that interfere with DNA replication and transcription. In low doses, the alkylating agents are commonly used to treat autoimmune disorders. In higher doses, they are effective against cancer.

Table 12-21 Alkylating Agents

Generic	Brand Name
cyclophosphamide	Cytoxan
melphalan	Alkeran
chlorambucil	Leukeran
ifosfamide	Ifex
busulfan	Myleran
carmustine (BCNU)	Gliadel
lomustine	CeeNU
dacarbazine (DTIC)	DTIC-Dome

Mitosis Inhibitors

Mitosis inhibitors include several classes of drugs that interfere with cell division (mitosis).

The taxanes (**Table 12-22**) are a class of chemotherapeutic drugs derived from the yew tree (genus Taxus). The taxanes' primary mode of action is to disrupt microtubule function, thereby interfering with mitosis. Microtubules form the cytoskeleton and are required for cell division.

Table 12-22 Taxanes

Generic	Brand Name
paclitaxel	Taxol
paclitaxel (protein bound)	Abraxane
docetaxel	Taxotere

The vinca alkaloids (**Table 12-23**) are alkylating agents derived from the periwinkle plant (genus Vinca).

Table 12-23 Vinca Alkaloids

Generic	Brand Name
vinblastine	Velban
vincristine	Oncovin
vinorelbine	Navelbine

Podophyllotoxin and topoisomerase inhibitors (**Table 12-24**) both interfere with DNA replication.

Table 12-24 Mitosis Inhibitors

Generic	Brand Name
etoposide	VePesid
irinotecan	Camptosar
mitoxantrone	Novantrone
topotecan	Hycamtin

Platinum Drugs

As their name suggests, the platinum drugs (**Table 12-25**) contain the metal platinum. This class of drug cross-links DNA, interfering with replication and transcription.

Table 12-25 Platinum Drugs

Generic	Brand Name
carboplatin	Paraplatin
cisplatin (cisplatinum)	
oxaliplatin	Eloxatin

Hormone Therapies

Hormonal therapies used in the treatment of cancer either block the action of hormones on cells or reduce the amount of circulating hormone. Both of these effectively starve hormone-responsive cells from the stimulative effects of hormones. Drugs that act against both male and female hormones are used.

Antiandrogen drugs (**Table 12-26**) block the action of testosterone and are used to treat advanced prostate cancer.

Table 12-26 Antiandrogens

Generic	Brand Name	Dose
bicalutamide	Casodex	50 mg
flutamide	Eulexin	125 mg
nilutamide	Nilandron	150 mg

Antiestrogen drugs (**Table 12-27**) block the action of estrogen. Tamoxifen and toremifene are selective estrogen receptor modulators (SERMs, pronounced as the acronym) because they do not affect all estrogen receptors in the same way. Tamoxifen acts as an agonist on estrogen receptors located on the uterus and bone but as an antagonist on breast tissue. Fulvestrant is not a SERM; it is antagonistic in all tissues.

Table 12-27 Antiestrogens

Generic	Brand Name	Dose
fulvestrant	Faslodex	150 mg, 300 mg
tamoxifen	Nolvadex	10 mg, 20 mg
toremifene	Fareston	60 mg

The GnRH analogs (**Table 12-28**) initially mimic the action of GnRH on the pituitary gland, but after an initial flare, result in a dramatic decrease in LH and FSH, ultimately reducing the production of testosterone, estrogen, and progesterone.

Table 12-28 GnRH Analogs

Generic	Brand Name
goserelin	Zoladex
leuprolide	Eligard Lupron

Aromatase is an enzyme that converts androgens to estrogens. Aromatase inhibitors (**Table 12-29**) block the action of aromatase, thereby reducing the levels of estrogens. Aromatase inhibitors are effective in postmenopausal women who no longer produce estrogen in the ovaries but rather in the adrenal glands through the conversion of androgens.

Table 12-29 Aromatase Inhibitors

Generic	Brand Name	Dose
anastrozole	Arimidex	1 mg
exemestane	Aromasin	25 mg
letrozole	Femara	2.5 mg

Monoclonal Antibodies

Monoclonal antibodies (**Table 12-30**) are used to identify or tag a specific cell by binding to antigens on the cell's surface. Once tagged with the antibody, the body's own immune mechanisms destroy the antibody-tagged cell. Two of these drugs (Bexxar and Zevalin) are combined with radioactive isotopes to deliver radiation therapy directly to the targeted cell.

Table 12-30 Monoclonal Antibodies

Generic	Brand Name
alemtuzumab	Campath
bevacizumab	Avastin
cetuximab	Erbitux
rituximab	Rituxan
trastuzumab	Herceptin
tositumomab and iodine 131	Bexxar
ibritumomab with indium 111 and yttrium 90	Zevalin

Tyrosine Kinase Inhibitors

Tyrosine kinase is an enzyme that plays an important role in regulating cellular activity. Some cancers are characterized by increased tyrosine kinase activity. Tyrosine kinase inhibitors (**Table 12-31**) block the action of this enzyme.

Table 12-31 Tyrosine Kinase Inhibitors

Generic	Brand Name	Dose
imatinib	Gleevec	100 mg, 400 mg
dasatinib	Sprycel	20 mg, 50 mg, 70 mg, 100 mg
nilotinib	Tasigna	200 mg

Epidermal Growth Factor Inhibitors

Epidermal growth factors stimulate cells to proliferate, differentiate, and grow. All cells have growth factor receptors, but neoplastic cells tend to have more receptors, making them more sensitive to growth factor inhibitors (**Table 12-32**).

Table 12-32 Epidermal Growth Factor Inhibitors

Generic	Brand Name	Dose
erlotinib	Tarceva	25 mg, 100 mg, 150 mg
gefitinib	Iressa	250 mg

Pain Medications

Controlling pain is an important part of a cancer patient's treatment. Cancer typically requires a combination of pain medications (**Table 12-33**) including narcotics. Morphine and opioid medications should be given around-the-clock with codeine-based pain relievers given for breakthrough pain. Fentanyl patches may also be given for continuous pain relief. Gabapentin helps relieve neuropathic pain.

Table 12-33 Pain Medications

Generic	Brand Name	Dose
fentanyl	Actiq	(transmucosal) 200 mcg, 400 mcg, 600 mcg, 800 mcg, 1200 mcg, 1600 mcg
	Duragesic	transdermal patch
	Sublimaze	IV
oxycodone	OxyContin	10 mg, 15 mg, 20 mg, 30 mg, 40 mg, 60 mg, 80 mg
	Roxicodone	5 mg, 15 mg, 30 mg
morphine	MS Contin	15 mg, 30 mg, 60 mg, 100 mg, 200 mg
	Roxanol	(oral) 20 mg/mL, 100 mg/5 mL
gabapentin	Neurontin	100 mg, 300 mg, 400 mg, 600 mg, 800 mg

Antiemetics

Chemotherapy-induced nausea and vomiting can be severe and interfere with treatment and quality of life. **Table 12-34** lists antiemetics that are given orally or intravenously to treat CINV. See also page 86.

Table 12-34 Antiemetics for CINV

Generic	Brand Name	Dose
dronabinol (THC)	Marinol	2.5 mg, 5 mg, 10 mg
aprepitant	Emend	
palonosetron	Aloxi	0.5 mg

Exercises

Using Context to Make Decisions

Use the following excerpt to answer questions 1–5.

> By mammogram and ultrasound, the patient has a lesion located in her right upper quadrant measuring 8 x 7 x 6 mm. The biopsy revealed invasive ductal carcinoma, grade 2, ER and ___(1)___ negative, ___(2)___/neu 3+ positive. The patient underwent lumpectomy with ___(3)___ lymph node biopsy. The pathology results did not reveal presence of residual invasive carcinoma. There was ductal carcinoma in situ. All of the margins were clear. Three lymph nodes were negative for metastatic disease. FISH was positive for HER2/neu, which was amplified. The patient was started on chemotherapy with Taxotere 75 mg/m², carboplatin ___(4)___ of 6, and ___(5)___ 8 mg/kg and then 6 mg/kg given every 3 weeks.

1. Which of the following would complete blank #1?

   a. GR   **c.** BR

   b. PR   **d.** DR

2. How would you complete blank #2? _____

   _____

3. What word completes the phrase containing blank #3? _____

4. Which of the following would complete blank #4?

   a. BUD   **c.** VEGF

   b. AUC   **d.** LAP

5. Which of the following would complete blank #5?

   a. Bexxar   **c.** Herceptin

   b. Rituxan   **d.** Gleevec

Use the following excerpt to answer questions 6–8.

> The patient returns today for followup for ___(1)___ anemia. In May, 20XX, her hemoglobin was 10.6, ___(2)___ 31.5, and MCV 82. The patient complained of fatigue and frequent stomachaches. Her diet is very poor in red meat. She was evaluated by Dr. Linn with a barium swallow and endoscopy that revealed strictures and an ulcer. The patient states she is feeling much better after endoscopy. I gave her ferrous gluconate over the summer. In September, 20XX, her hemoglobin was 12.2, hematocrit 36.1. Her red blood cells were getting bigger, up to 75. Today she states she is feeling better and is less tired.

6. What type of anemia does this patient have (blank #1)? _____

   _____

7. What term goes in blank #2? _____

   _____

8. What is incongruous in this excerpt? _____

   _____

Use this excerpt to answer question #9.

> Patient returns for follow up of anemia. At her last visit, hematocrit was 35 with an MCV of 101.5. WBC and platelet count are normal. TSH is normal. Serum folate and vitamin B_{12} are slightly decreased. Iron studies are completely normal.

9. What type of anemia does this patient have?

   a. microcytic   **c.** IDA

   b. macrocytic   **d.** sickle cell

10. Punctuate the following excerpt. Add periods, commas, decimals, and capitalization as needed. Assume there are no spelling or transcription errors.

    evaluation by dr rossi in october showed a hemoglobin of 111 hematocrit 388 mcv 106 and normal serum tsh level serum folate and vitamin b12 levels serum protein electrophoresis direct agglutination test liver function tests reticulocyte count was slightly elevated to 24 with a haptoglobin of 72 bone marrow biopsy and aspirate showed megaloblastic erythroid hyperplasia with no increase in myeloblasts megakaryocytes were normal in appearance and number iron stain showed marked increase in ringed sideroblasts findings felt to be consistent with refractory anemia with ringed sideroblasts

11. Match the following values with the correct component of a CBC. Assume the values are all within the normal range. The eosinophil value is 4%.

    _____ 7.2   a. WBC
    _____ 12.2   b. RBC
    _____ 92   c. Hb
    _____ 56%   d. Hct
    _____ 28%   e. MCV
    _____ 4.5   f. Plt
    _____ 37.1   g. segs
    _____ 142,000   h. lymphs
    _____ 10%   i. monos
    _____ 2%   j. basos

Use the following excerpt to answer question #12.

    The treatment consisted of a total of 4500 _____ delivered to the region of the pancreatic involvement and adjacent areas utilizing an IMRT technique with 6 MV photons.

12. What term would complete the blank?

    _____

Use the following excerpt to answer questions #13 and #14.

    The patient presents today for followup evaluation of diffuse large B-cell ____(1)____ involving the left inguinal area. The patient received chemotherapy with vincristine, cyclophosphamide, and Adriamycin. He also received Rituxan. He achieved a complete response. In February, the patient was started on a course of ____(2)____-field radiation therapy to the left inguinal region.

13. What term completes blank #1?

    _____

14. Which term completes blank #2?

    a. involved   c. devolved
    b. resolved   d. evolved

Use this excerpt to answer question #15.

    Patient presented with 9-year history of mild lymphocytosis in the setting of a normal total white blood cell count. Current laboratory data shows a WBC count of 31,000, hemoglobin 12, hematocrit 36.7%, MCV 91, platelet count 153,000, with 80% lymphocytes and 13% neutrophils. Peripheral blood smear continues to show an increased population of mature-appearing lymphocytes, otherwise unremarkable. Immunophenotypic studies revealed a monoclonal B-cell population that was positive for CD5, CD19, and CD20 and negative for CD38. Normal LDH and erythrocyte sedimentation rate. No peripheral lymphadenopathy or organomegaly.

15. Which of the following diagnoses fits with the above data?

    a. acute myelogenous leukemia
    b. chronic lymphocytic leukemia
    c. non-Hodgkin lymphoma
    d. acute lymphocytic leukemia

Terms Checkup

Complete the multiple choice questions for Chapter 12 located at www.myhealthprofessionskit.com. To access the questions, select the discipline "Medical Transcription," then click on the title of this book, *Advanced Medical Transcription*.

Look It Up

Using the guidelines described on page xvii, complete a research project on hemochromatosis and multiple myeloma.

Transcription Practice

1. Transcribe the key terms and phrases for Chapter 12.
2. Complete the proofing and transcription practice exercises for Chapter 12.

PEARSON
myhealthprofessionskit™

To access the transcription practice exercises for this chapter, go to www.myhealthprofessionskit.com. Select the discipline "Medical Transcription," then click on the title of this book, *Advanced Medical Transcription*.

Appendix A: Terms Bank

Chapter 2

5.07 Semmes-Weinstein monofilament
abdominal aortic aneurysms (AAA)
abdominal circumference
abdominal-visceral obesity
Accu-Chek
ACE inhibitors
Acetest
acidosis
ADA diet
albuminuria
angiotensin converting enzyme inhibitors (ACE inhibitors)
angiotensin II receptor blockers (ARBs)
anion gap
anorexiants
antihypertensive agent
bariatric surgery
basic metabolic panel (BMP)
below-knee amputation (BKA)
beta-blockers
bile acid binding resins
bile acids
blood pressure diary
blood urea nitrogen (BUN)
body mass index (BMI)
bolus
brittle diabetics
calcium channel blockers
candidal vaginitis
capillary blood glucose (CBG)
cardiac output
Charcot arthropathy
choked disc
cholesterol ratio
concomitant
continuous subcutaneous insulin infusion (CSII)
coronary heart disease (CHD)
creatinine
diabetes mellitus (DM)
diabetic coma
diabetic ketoacidosis (DKA)
diabetic nephropathy
dumping syndrome
dyslipidemia

early satiety
EBCT (electron beam CT scan)
efficacy of treatment
essential hypertension
euglycemia
familial hypertriglyceridemia
fasting blood glucose
fasting blood sugar (FBS)
fasting lipid panel
fibrates
foot care
free T3 (FT3)
free T4 (FT4)
FreeStyle
fructosamine
gastroparesis
Glucometer Elite
glycosylated hemoglobin
Hashimoto thyroiditis
hydrochlorothiazide (HCT, HCTZ)
HDL-C
health maintenance
hemoglobin A_{1c}
high-density lipoproteins (HDL)
high waist-to-hip ratio
high-dose niacin
hypercholesterolemia
hyperosmolality
hypertensive emergency
hypertensive heart disease
hypertensive urgency
hypoalbuminemia
independent risk factor
insulin-dependent diabetes mellitus (IDDM)
insulin resistance
juvenile-onset diabetes
ketone bodies (ketonemia)
ketones
ketonuria
Ketostix
labile diabetics
labile hypertension
laparoscopic gastric banding
laparoscopic Roux-en-Y gastric bypass
LDL particles (LDL-P)
LDL-C

lifestyle modifications
low-density lipoproteins (LDL)
low-dose aspirin
malignant hypertension
metabolic acidosis
microalbuminuria
milliequivalents (mEq)
modifiable risk factor
morbid obesity
myositis
myxedema
neuropathy
NMR LipoProfile
nocturnal enuresis
noncompliance
non-insulin-dependent diabetes mellitus (NIDDM)
obstructive sleep apnea (OSA)
omega-3 oils
OneTouch
oral glucose tolerance test (OGTT or GTT)
oral hypoglycemic agents
osmolality
osmotic diuresis
peripheral neuropathy
peripheral paresthesia
peripheral vascular disease (PVD)
plaques
polydipsia
polyphagia
polyuria
psyllium
refractory
renal function studies
sequestrants
serial blood pressure readings
serum osmolality
sliding scale
statins
stocking-glove distribution
syndrome X
systolic ejection murmur (SEM)
target-organ damage
thyroid function tests (TFTs)
thyroid stimulating hormone (TSH)
thyroxine binding globulin (TBG)

tight metabolic control
titrated
transaminitis
urine osmolality
very low calorie diet
very low density lipoproteins (VLDL)
vibratory sensation
white coat syndrome

Chapter 3

abdominal series
absorbable sutures
accordion sign
achalasia
achlorhydria
acute abdomen
adenomatous polyps
advanced under direct visualization
adynamic ileus
aerobic and anaerobic culture
air-fluid levels
ambulatory pH monitoring test
antibiotic-associated colitis
antigliadin antibodies (AGA)
antimesenteric anastomosis
antineutrophil cytoplasmic antibodies with perinuclear staining (pANCA)
anti-Saccharomyces cerevisiae antibodies (ASCA)
antral nipple sign
appendicitis
appendicolith
apple-core sign
approximate
ascites
Ashkenazi Jews
aught
autoimmune metaplastic atrophic gastritis (AMAG)
bacterial peritonitis
Barrett esophagus
Billroth I
Billroth II
bird-beak sign
bird-beak deformity
blunt and sharp dissection
blunting of intestinal villi
bolus of food
borborygmi
bougie dilator

bright red blood on the toilet paper
bright red blood per rectum
Brooke ileostomy
celiac disease
celiac sprue
celiac trunk
chemical peritonitis
clean-based ulcer
cobblestone
coffee grounds emesis
coffee bean sign
currant-jelly stool
dentate line
Dermabond
dermatitis herpetiformis
Dieulafoy lesion
digital rectal exam (DRE)
disordered motility
diverticulitis
diverticulosis
Dor fundoplication
double-balloon enteroscopy
double-contrast study
duodenal ulcer with a clean base
dysmotility
dysphagia for solids
empirically
Endoclip
endoscopic banding
endotracheal intubation
end-to-end anastomoses
enterotomy
eosinophilic esophagitis
Escherichia coli O157:H7
esophageal dysphagia
esophageal function studies
esophageal manometry
esophageal motility studies
esophagogastroduodenoscopy (EGD)
estimated blood loss
exploratory laparoscopy
exploratory laparotomy
extraintestinal manifestations
familial adenomatous polyposis (FAP)
fascial
fat halo sign
fecal antigen test
fecal occult blood test (FOBT)
field block
figure-of-eight

fired and reloaded
flat and upright abdominal x-rays
flexible weighted bougies
fluid resuscitation
fluid-filled, dilated small-bowel loops
free intraperitoneal air
functional abdominal pain syndrome (FAPS)
gastric outlet obstruction
gastroesophageal reflux disease (GERD)
gastrointestinal string sign
globus hystericus
globus sensation
gluten enteropathy
guaiac-negative stool
guaiac-positive stool
H_2-blockers
H_2-receptor antagonists
harmonic scalpel
Hasson trocar
haustral folds
held in apposition
Helicobacter pylori (H pylori)
Heller myotomy
heme-negative stool
heme-positive stool
Hemoccult-positive stool
Hemoccult-negative stool
hemodynamically significant
hemolytic uremic syndrome
hepatic flexure
hiatal hernia
hiatus hernia
high-resolution manometry (HRM)
high-pitched peristalsis with rushes
HLA-B27 antigen
hydrochloric acid (HCl)
hypertrophy of intestinal crypts
ileocecal Crohn's
ileus
incomplete evacuation
increasing abdominal girth
inferior mesenteric artery (IMA)
infiltration of lamina propria with lymphocytes and plasma cells
inflammatory bowel disease (IBD)
inflammatory phlegmon
infraumbilical
insufflate
interrupted

intrinsic factor
intussusception
intussusceptum
intussuscipiens
irritable bowel syndrome (IBS)
J maneuver
kept n.p.o.
lead-pipe appearance of colon
left lateral recumbent x-rays
Levin sump
ligament of Treitz
loss of haustral markings
loss of haustration
lower esophageal sphincter (LES)
lower GI bleed (LGIB)
Mallory-Weiss syndrome
maroon-colored stools
mattress
McBurney point
megacolon
mesenteric ischemia
mesoappendix
minimally invasive surgery
Morison pouch
multidetector CT (MDCT)
muscularis mucosae
napkin-ring sign
nasogastric tube (NG tube)
needle, instrument, and sponge
  counts
negative FOBT, positive FOBT
Nissen fundoplication
nocturnal regurgitation
noncardiac chest pain
nonerosive esophageal reflux disease
  (NERD)
nonsteroidal antiinflammatory drugs
  (NSAIDs)
nontropical sprue
nonulcer (functional) dyspepsia
normal flora
nuclear bleeding scans
nutcracker esophagus
obturator sign
oropharyngeal dysphasia
ova and parasites (O&P)
pancolitis
paraesophageal hiatal hernia
pedunculated
peptic stricture
peptic ulcer disease (PUD)
pericolic stranding

peristalsis
peritoneal reflection
peritoneal signs
periumbilical
pneumaturia
pneumoperitoneum
pouchitis
postanesthesia care unit (PACU)
probiotics
prokinetic
prone jackknife position
proton pump inhibitors (PPIs)
pseudomembranous colitis
psoas sign
pursestring
push endoscopy
push enteroscopy
pyrosis
quiet abdomen
rebleeding
rebound tenderness
rectal vault
reflux esophagitis
retractors
retrocecal
retroileal
retroperitoneal
Rome criteria
rugae
running
Salem sump
saline leak test
scalloping and atrophy of duodenal
  folds
Schatzki ring
sclerotherapy
selective COX-2 inhibitors
serum-ascites-albumin-gradient
  (SAAG)
sessile polyp
side-to-side anastomoses
side-to-side isoperistaltic
  strictureplasty (SSIS)
silent abdomen
sitz baths
skip lesions
sliding hiatal hernia
small bowel obstruction (SBO)
small-bowel meal
snare cautery
sphincter of Oddi
splenic flexure

spot films of the terminal ileum
squamocolumnar junction
stool for culture and sensitivity
straining at stool
Stretta procedure
strictureplasty
stricturoplasty
subcuticular
subtotal colectomy with ileostomy
superior mesenteric artery (SMA)
supraumbilical
surgically reduced
technically adequate study
tense ascites
the triangle of Calot
third spacing
thrombosed external hemorrhoids
thumbprinting
transient lower esophageal sphincter
  relaxations (tLESRs)
transvenous intrahepatic
  portosystemic shunt (TIPS)
trocar sites
tubular adenoma
tubulovillous
tympanitic abdomen
upper GI series with small bowel
  followthrough
urea breath test
valvulae conniventes (mucosal folds
  of the small intestine)
Veress needle
video capsule endoscopy
villoglandular polyps
villous adenoma
volvulus
white line of Toldt
wireless capsule endoscopy (WCE)
Zenker diverticulum
Z line

Chapter 4

2-log reduction in viral load
acalculous cholecystitis
acholic stools
acoustic shadowing
acute liver failure (ALF)
alcoholic hyaline bodies
alkaline phosphatase
alpha fetoprotein
aminotransferase levels
ampulla of Vater

anicteric hepatitis
antidote
anti-HAV IgG
anti-HAV IgM
anti-HBc
anti-HBc IgG
anti-HBc IgM
anti-HBs
APACHE II
atypical lymphocytes
Bacteroides
Balthazar grading system
biliary sludge
blood culture bottles
blunted sensorium
branched DNA (bDNA)
brush cytology
Budd-Chiari syndrome
CA 19-9
CAGE questionnaire
carcinoembryonic antigen (CEA)
cavernous hemangiomas
Charcot triad
Child-Pugh scale
cholangiography
cholangitis
cholecystectomy
cholecystitis
choledocholithiasis
cholelithiasis
cholescintigraphy
cholestasis
cholestatic jaundice
chronic calcifying pancreatitis
chronic carrier state
chronic inflammatory pancreatitis
chronic obstructive pancreatitis
chymotrypsin
cirrhosis
clay-colored stools
Clostridia
collateral veins
colon cutoff sign
common bile duct
common hepatic duct
conjugated bilirubin
core antigen (c)
coronary-to-gastroesophageal
  collateral veins
creatorrhea
Cullen sign
culture and sensitivity (C&S)

cystic duct
defervescence
direct bilirubin
distal pancreatectomy
drug-induced liver injury (DILI)
easy fatigability
echogenic lesion suspicious for
  tumor
emphysematous cholecystitis
empyema
endoscopic retrograde cholangiopancreatography (ERCP)
Enterobacter
Enterococcus
envelope antigen (e)
exsanguination
extradural sensors
fatty liver disease
fibrosis
filling defect
fulminant hepatic failure
fulminant hepatitis
gallstone pancreatitis
genotype 1
genotype 2
Glasgow
Grey Turner sign
HBcAb
HBsAb
hemorrhagic pancreatitis
hepatic artery
hepatic encephalopathy
hepatic failure
hepatic portal vein
hepatitis
hepatitis A virus (HAV)
hepatitis B immune globulin
  (HBIG)
hepatitis B surface antigen (HBsAg)
hepatitis B virus (HBV)
hepatitis C virus (HCV)
hepatitis D virus (HDV)
hepatobiliary iminodiacetic acid
  (HIDA scan)
hepatocarcinoma
hepatocellular carcinoma
hepatopulmonary syndrome
hepatorenal syndrome
hyperbilirubinemia
icteric phase
idiosyncratic drug reactions
immune globulin

Imrie
incubation period
indirect bilirubin
indolent
insidious
intense echoes with distal acoustic
  shadowing that move with gravity
interferon
intrahepatic cholestasis
intraoperative cholangiography
intrapulmonary right-to-left
  shunting
jaundice (icterus)
Klebsiella
Korsakoff psychosis
lactate dehydrogenase
lactulose
Laennec cirrhosis
lap choley (laparoscopic
  cholecystectomy)
lateral pancreaticojejunostomy
limited diaphragmatic excursion
liver function tests (LFTs)
lower esophageal and gastric varices
magnetic resonance cholangiopancreatography (MRCP)
main pancreatic duct (MPD)
Mallory bodies
mannitol
medium-chain triglycerides (MCTs)
MELD score
microlithiasis
mixed anaerobes
model for end-stage liver disease
  (MELD score)
N-acetylcysteine (NAC)
necrotizing pancreatitis
nonalcoholic fatty liver disease
  (NAFLD)
nonalcoholic steatohepatitis
  (NASH)
nucleoside analog
nucleotide analog
obstructive jaundice
open cholecystectomy
pancreatic amylase
pancreatic duct
pancreatic lipase
pancreatoduodenectomy
pearl-necklace sign
pegylated interferon
percutaneous liver biopsy

percutaneous transhepatic cholangiography (PTC)

pericholecystic fluid

phlegmon

plasma

pneumobilia

polymerase chain reaction (PCR)

porcelain gallbladder

portacaval shunts

portal hypertension (PH)

portal thrombus

portosystemic encephalopathy

portosystemic shunting

preicteric phase

pressure gradient

primary sclerosing cholangitis

pseudocalculus sign

pseudocysts

Puestow procedure

Ranson score

recombinant immunoblot assay (RIBA)

recrudescent hepatitis

refractory steatorrhea

retrograde ascent

Reynold pentad

Rokitansky disease

sentinel loop

sequestered

seroconversion

shift to the left

sludge in the gallbladder

sonographic Murphy sign

steatohepatitis

stigmata of liver disease

subclinical

subfulminant disease

superinfection

superior and inferior mesenteric veins

surface antigen (s)

Swan-Ganz catheter

thickened gallbladder wall

thrombocytopenia

titer

total parenteral nutrition (TPN)

transabdominal ultrasound

transaminases

transcription mediated amplification (TMA)

treatment naïve

trypsin

tumor necrosis factor alpha (TNF alpha)

ultrasound elastography

unconjugated bilirubin

urobilinogen

viral hepatitis

viral load

viremia

Wernicke encephalopathy

Whipple procedure

Chapter 5

2-point discrimination

3.5 mm compression plate

3-phase bone scan

active range of motion (AROM)

adhesive capsulitis

Aircast ankle brace

angulation

anterior cruciate ligament (ACL)

anterior drawer sign

acetaminophen (APAP)

Apley test

apprehension sign

arthrodesis

arthroscopic lavage

artifact

avascular necrosis (AVN)

avulsion

axial loading

axillary view

Baker cyst

ballottable patella

birefringent

bisphosphonates

bivalved

boggy

bony remodeling

both-bone forearm fracture

botulinum toxin injections

Bouchard nodes

Buck traction

bucket handle

buckle

bursitis

calcium oxalate

calcium phosphate

calcium pyrophosphate

callus

Cam Walker

cannulated lag screws

capsaicin

carpal tunnel release (CTR)

cemented

cementless

cephalomedullary (gamma type) nail

cerclage wires

Charcot joint

chip fracture

chondromalacia patella

chronic venous insufficiency

clenched fist views

closed fracture

closed reduction

coagulase-negative staphylococci

cock-up wrist splints

Colles fracture

comminuted fracture

comminuted pilon

comminuted segmental fracture

compound fracture

condylar screw-plate

coned views

contrast venography

cortical lucency

counterforce brace

creatine phosphokinase (CPK)

crepitus

crescent sign

CT scan with bone windows

decreased radiodensity

degenerative joint disease (DJD)

delayed primary closure

delayed union

displaced fracture

distal median nerve latency

distraction

doughnut sign

dowager's hump

draining sinuses

drugs of abuse

dual-energy x-ray absorptiometry (DEXA)

dynamic compression plates

dynamic hip compression screw

effusion

electromyelography (EMG)

enthesopathy

epiphyseal

Evans classification

external fixation

external fixator

extracapsular

falls from standing height

fat embolization syndrome

fat suppression

femoral shaft fractures

flattening of the lordotic curve

flexion tendon bowstringing

fluid-attenuated inversion-recovery (FLAIR)

full weightbearing

full-thickness tears

functional magnetic resonance imaging (fMRI)

Galeazzi fracture

Garden classification

gated (MRI)

geode

glucosamine and chondroitin sulfate

gonococcal

graduated compression stockings

greenstick

Heberden nodes

hemarthrosis

hemiarthroplasty

high signal intensity

Homans sign

home exercise program

hot spots

hyaluronan

hyperuricemia

Ilizarov fixator

impacted

impedance plethysmography

inferior vena cava filter (IVCF)

interfragmentary screw fixation

intermittent pneumatic compression (IPC)

intraarticular

intracapsular

intramedullary rod

inversion (varus) sprains

iontophoresis

ipsilateral

irrigation and debridement (I&D)

joint-space narrowing

Jones fracture

Kirschner wire fixation (K-wire)

kyphoplasty

Lachman test

lateral epicondylitis

lipping of the marginal bone

loose bodies

low signal intensity

low-molecular-weight heparin

Maisonneuve fracture

malunion

march fractures

maximal equinus

methylene diphosphonate (MDP)

millicuries (mCi)

McMurray test

medial collateral ligament (MCL)

medial epicondylitis

medial joint line

medical synovectomy

medullary lucency

Merchant views

metaphysial

methyl methacrylate

monoarticular arthritis

monolateral fixator

monosodium urate (MSU) crystals

Monteggia fracture

mop ends

mortise views

motor strength

nail plate

narrowing of the joint space

needle trephination

Neer staging

negatively birefringent crystals

nerve conduction velocity (NCV)

neuroarthropathy

neurogenic arthropathy

nondisplaced fracture

nongonococcal arthritis

nonselective chocolate agar

nonunion

nonweightbearing

oblique fracture

open fracture

open reduction

open reduction and internal fixation (ORIF)

osteophytes

overhanging rim of cortical bone

paraspinal muscle spasm

paratenon

paratenonitis

paravertebral muscle spasm

parrot beak

partial meniscectomy

partial weightbearing

passive range of motion (PROM)

patella alta

patella baja

patellar fracture

patellar tilt test

patellar tracking

patellectomy

patellofemoral syndrome (PS)

pathologic fractures

pendulum exercises

periosteal elevation

Phalen sign

phonophoresis

pin tract infection

plafond fractures

plantar fasciitis

plica

plyometrics

podagra

point tenderness

postphlebitic syndrome

progressive resistive exercises (PREs)

proprioception

proximal tibiofibular syndesmosis

Q angle

quinolone antibiotics

radiocapitellar view

radiolucent line

rat bites

reamed intramedullary nail

recommend clinical correlation

reduced

remodeling

resistance

rest, ice, compression, and elevation (RICE)

retrocalcaneal bursa injection

risk factor modification

ruptures

sail sign

Salter-Harris classification

Schatzker classification

senile osteoporosis

septic arthritis

sequential compression devices (SCDs)

sharpened articular margins

short-T1 inversion-recovery (STIR)

snuffbox

spica cast

spin-lattice relaxation time

spin-spin relaxation time

spiral fracture
stellate fracture
stepoff
sterile synovitis
stress fractures
subacromial decompression
sugar-tong splint
sunrise views
supraspinatus outlet view
surgical release
T scores
T1-weighted images
T2-weighted images
TED hose
tendinopathy
tense effusion
tension band wires
tension-band technique
tetanus prophylaxis
Thayer-Martin agar
theater sign
thenar muscle strength
Thera-Bands
Thompson test
thumb spica cast
tibial plateau fracture
tidal irrigation lavage
Tinel sign
toe touch
tophaceous gout
tophi
torus
total hip replacement (THR)
total joint arthroplasty
total knee arthroplasty (TKA)
touch down
transverse
triphasic bone scan
unfractionated heparin
unicompartmental
unicondylar knee replacement
unload the plantar enthesis
uricosuric drugs
varus deformity
vertebral fracture analysis
vertebroplasty
water signal
Weber system
weightbearing as tolerated
wet reading
white zone
Z scores

Chapter 6

2-beat clonus
ACD with fusion (ACDF)
activities of daily living (ADLs)
Adams forward-bending test
allogeneic bone
anal wink
annulus
anterior arch
anterior cervical diskectomy (ACD)
anterior cervical diskectomy and
    fusion (ACDF)
anterior cervical plate
anterior longitudinal ligament
anterior lumbar interbody fusion
    (ALIF)
anterior wedge fracture
anteroposterior subluxation
artificial disk replacement (ADR)
atlantoaxial joint
atlas
axial lumbar interbody fusion
    (Axial LIF)
axis
Babinski reflex
BAK cage
bone morphogenetic protein (BMP)
bone tamp
bowel or bladder dysfunction
bridging osteophytes
bulging
burst fractures
cadaveric bone
café au lait spots
cauda equina
cauda equina syndrome
caudal ESI
central canal stenosis
central herniation
cervical collar
cervical epidural steroid injection
    (CESI)
cervical spondylosis
construct
corpectomy
costal facets
crossed straight leg test
CT myelogram
degenerative arthritis
degenerative disk disease (DDD)
degenerative spondylolisthesis

dens
desiccation
diathermy
disk space narrowing
diskogenic pain
diskogram
diskography
dura mater
dural sac
endplate destruction
epidural steroid injections (ESI)
extreme lateral interbody fusion
    (XLIF)
extruded
facet hypertrophy
facet joint arthropathy
facetectomy
facets
flexion and extension views
fluoroscopic localization
foot drop
foraminotomy
Fortin finger sign
fusion with instrumentation
hemilaminectomy
herniated nucleus pulposus (HNP)
hip flexor contractures
Hoffmann reflex
hypertrophied ligamentum flavum
hypertrophy of the facet joints
idiopathic scoliosis
iliopsoas shortening
interbody cages
interlaminar ESI
internal disk degeneration (IDD)
intervertebral disk
intervertebral disk arthroplasty
intervertebral foramina
intradiskal electrothermal
    annuloplasty (IDEA)
intradiskal electrothermal therapy
    (IDET)
jumped facets
lamina
laminectomy
laminoplasty
laminotomy
lateral bending
lateral herniation
lateral recess stenosis
ligamenta flava
ligamentous hypertrophy

load bearing
long-tract signs
loss-of-resistance
lumbar epidural steroid injection (LESI)
lumbar spondylosis
medial branch blocks
medial branch nerve
microdiskectomy
Milwaukee brace
myofascial release
nerve decompression
neural arch
neural foramina
neurogenic claudication
neuropathic pain
nucleus pulposus
odontoid fractures
on a scale of 1–10
open-mouth view
osteophytosis
pars interarticularis
pedicle screws
pedicles
PEEK cage
pelvic rocking
pituitary rongeurs
point tenderness
polymethylmethacrylate (PMMA)
posterior lumbar interbody fusion (PLIF)
posterior superior iliac spine (PSIS)
primary stenosis
protruding
radicular pain
radiofrequency ablation (RFA)
radiofrequency rhizotomy
recurrent laryngeal nerve
retrolisthesis
rib slope
Risser stage
Romberg test
sacral hiatus
sacral sulcus
saddle anesthesia
sciatica
scoliometer
Scottie dog
secondary stenosis
segmental neurologic deficits
semi-Fowler position
SI joint dysfunction

sidebending
somatosensory evoked potentials (SEPs)
spinal stenosis
spondylolisthesis
spondylolysis
spondylolytic
spondylosis
spot lateral views
Spurling test
straight leg raise test
strut graft
superior and inferior articular processes
swan-neck deformity
thecal sac
thoracic epidural steroid injection (TESI)
thoracolumbosacral orthosis (TLSO)
Torg ratio
total disk replacement (TDR)
transforaminal ESI
transforaminal lumbar interbody fusion (TLIF)
transpedicular approach
uncovertebral joint hypertrophy
Valsalva maneuver
vertebral foramina
Visual Analog Scale (VAS)
watchful waiting
zygapophyseal joints (Z joints)

Chapter 7

5-alpha-reductase inhibitors
abacterial prostatodynia (nonbacterial prostatitis)
abdominal leak point pressure (ALPP)
acute glomerulonephritis
acute pyelonephritis
acute renal failure (ARF)
acute renal injury
acute tubular necrosis (ATN)
alkalinizing agents
anal wink reflex
anasarca
anechoic
appendicolith
arteriovenous fistula (AV fistula)
arteriovenous graft (AV graft)
arteriovenous shunt

atrophic urethritis
AUA score
basket-extraction technique
basketing technique
benign prostatic hypertrophy (BPH)
bimanual exam
bladder outlet obstruction
bladder sling suspension
Bosniak classification
broad, waxy casts
bruit
bulbocavernosus reflex
bulbous
cadaveric donors
catheter exit site
catheter tract
Chlamydia trachomatis
Christmas-tree shape
chronic kidney disease (CKD)
clean-catch voided urine
colony forming units (CFU)/mL
colpocystourethropexy
community-acquired UTIs
conjugated estrogens
continuous ambulatory peritoneal dialysis (CAPD)
continuous cyclic peritoneal dialysis (CCPD)
continuous hemofiltration
continuous renal replacement therapy
costovertebral angle (CVA)
cough test
Credé method
crescentic glomerulonephritis
CT urography
CVA tenderness
cystine
cystometrogram (CMG)
cystometry
cystourethroscopy
defervescence
detrusor activity
detrusor hyperactivity with impaired contractility (DHIC)
detrusor muscles
detrusor sphincter dyssynergia (DSD)
direct visualization
diuresis
diuretic renography
double voiding
double-J ureteral stent

dysgeusia
echogenic
echogenic kidneys
effacement of the corticomedullary boundaries
electromyography (EMG)
emphysematous cystitis
emphysematous pyelonephritis
endoscopic lithotripsy
end-stage renal disease (ESRD)
excretory urography (EXU)
exquisitely tender
extracorporeal shockwave lithotripsy (ESWL)
fascia lata
fatty cast
flexible ureteropyeloscopy
fractional excretion of sodium (FENa)
fractional excretion of urea (FEUrea)
functional incontinence
gated lithotripsy
gent peak (gentamicin peak)
gent trough (gentamicin trough)
glomerular basement membrane (GBM)
glomerular filtrate
glomerular filtration rate (GFR)
glomerulonephritis (GN)
Gore-Tex
gouty diathesis
granular cast
group A beta-hemolytic streptococci
herpes simplex virus (HSV)
high anion gap acidosis
high-power field
high-intensity focused ultrasound (HIFU)
HLA typing
holmium laser
holmium:YAG (yttrium-aluminum-garnet)
honeymoon cystitis
hospital-acquired infections
hyaline casts
hydrochlorothiazide (HCTZ)
hydronephrosis
hydroureter
hydroureteronephrosis
hypercalciuria

hypermobile
hyperphosphatemia
hypertensive nephroangiosclerosis
hyperuricosuria
hypocitruria
hyposthenuria
inflammatory chronic pelvic pain syndrome (CPPS)
instrumentation
intake and output (I's & O's)
intermittent catheterization
intermittent hemodialysis
intermittent self-catheterization
intracorporeal lithotripsy
intramural ureter
intravenous pyelogram (IVP)
intrinsic sphincter deficiency
ionized calcium
isosthenuria
Kegel exercises
KUB study
Kussmaul respirations
lead pipe urethra
left ventricular hypertrophy
leukocyte esterase
leukocytosis with a left shift
lipiduria
lithotrites
long dwell
loop diuretics
low-power field
Malecot stent
Maltese cross
mature graft
MDRD equation
medical expulsive therapy (MET)
midstream clean-catch urine
Muehrcke lines
multichannel
multicystic kidney
multiple organ dysfunction syndrome (MODS)
nanograms per milliliter
natriuresis
Neisseria gonorrhoeae
neodymium:yttrium-aluminum-garnet (Nd:YAG)
nephritic
nephrolithiasis
nephromegaly
nephrostomy
nephrostomy tubes

nephrotic
nephrotic syndrome
neurogenic bladder
nidus
noncontrast CT scans
nongonococcal urethritis (NGU)
noninfectious glomerulonephritis
obstructive nephropathy
obstructive ureterolithiasis
obstructive uropathy
open simple prostatectomy
osteitis fibrosa cystica
overactive bladder dry
overactive bladder syndrome (OAB)
overflow incontinence (OI)
peak and trough levels
pelvic organ prolapse
pelvocaliectasis
pendulous urethra
percutaneous endourology
percutaneous nephrolithotomy
percutaneous nephrolithotripsy (PCNL)
percutaneous nephrostolithotomy
percutaneous nephrostomy
percutaneous nephrostomy tube
percutaneous suprapubic tube
perinephric stranding
peritoneal dialysis
pessaries
phleboliths
photovaporization of the prostate (PVP)
picograms per milliliter
pigtail (locking-loop or Cope loop) catheters
postinfectious glomerulonephritis
postvoid residual volume
potassium sparing
pressure flow study
prostate specific antigen (PSA)
prostatodynia
PSA velocity
pubovaginal slings
pyelonephritis
pyonephrosis
Q-Tip test
rapidly progressive glomerulonephritis (RPG)
RBC casts
rectus fascia
renal artery stenosis

renal colic
renal ectopia
renal encephalopathy
renal insufficiency
renal osteodystrophy
renal perfusion
renal replacement therapy (RRT)
renal vein thrombosis
renovascular disorders
retrograde pyelogram
retrograde ureteral stent placement
rim sign
rugae
sandwich therapy
scintigraphy
scout film
scout reconstruction
second-look procedure
Seldinger technique
sensorimotor polyneuropathy
sextant prostate biopsy
sodium polystyrene sulfonate (PSP)
specific gravity
spiral (helical) CT scan
spot urine
staghorn calculus
steinstrasse
stone burden
stone pushback
streaking in the perinephric fatty tissue
stress incontinence (SI)
struvite
subtracted cystometrogram (CMG)
Sudan staining
tension-free vaginal tape (TVT)
thiazide diuretics
thrill
too numerous to count (TNTC)
trabeculation
transurethral incision of the prostate (TUIP)
transurethral laser-induced prostatectomy (TULIP)
transurethral microwave thermotherapy (TUMT)
transurethral needle ablation of the prostate (TUNA)
transurethral resection of the prostate (TURP)
Trichomonas vaginalis
trigone

UA with micro
UA with reflex to micro
uninhibited contractions
uremic fetor
uremic frost
ureteral stent
ureterocolic
ureterolithiasis
ureteropelvic junction (UPJ)
ureteroscopic lithotripsy
ureterovesical junction (UVJ)
ureterovesical valves
urethral bulking
urethroscopy
urethrovesical junction
urge incontinence (UI)
urine dipstick
urinomas
urodynamic study (UDS)
uroflow
urosepsis
urothelium
vascular access
vascular steal syndrome
vesicoenteric
vesicoureteral reflux (VUR)
vesicovaginal fistula
videourodynamic studies
voiding cystourethrogram (VCUG)
voiding diary
voiding dysfunction
volitional anal sphincter contraction
washout
waxy casts
WBC casts
xanthine

Chapter 8

99mTc-MAA
absent tactile fremitus
accessory muscles
accessory muscles of respiration
acid-fast bacilli (AFB)
activated partial thromboplastin time (aPTT)
actuations
acute respiratory distress syndrome (ARDS)
acute respiratory failure (ARF)
adventitious breath sounds
air bronchograms

alpha-1-antitrypsin (ATT) deficiency
anterior axillary line
anteroposterior (AP) view
anticardiolipin antibodies
antiphospholipid antibodies
antithrombin
apnea-hypopnea index (AHI)
arterial blood gas analysis (ABGs)
arytenoepiglottic folds
atmospheres
atopic dermatitis
atopy
atrial septal defect (ASD)
azygous lymph nodes
barotrauma
barrel chest
bed-to-chair limitations
bibasilar increase in peribronchial and perivascular markings
bilevel positive airway pressure (BiPAP)
blue bloaters
blunting of the lateral costophrenic angle
blunting of the posterior costophrenic angle
BODE index
bronchoalveolar lavage (BAL)
bronchopneumonia
bronchoprovocation testing
bull neck
bullae
carbon monoxide (DL_{CO})
cardiac silhouette
carina
cavitation
central (hilar) pulmonary arteries
chest physiotherapy
Cheyne-Stokes respiration
chronic obstructive pulmonary disease (COPD)
chylous effusion
community-acquired pneumonia (CAP)
compliance
consolidation
costophrenic angles
Coumadin clinic
cruciferous vegetables
D-dimer
decortication

deep sulcus sign
diffusing capacity for carbon monoxide (DLCO)
directly observed therapy (DOT)
dullness to percussion
egophony (E-to-A change)
elevated central venous pressure
endobronchial biopsy
endobronchial ultrasound (EBUS)
excursion
exercise-induced asthma (EIA)
exercise-induced bronchospasm (EIB)
extrapulmonary signs
exudate
$FEV_1\%$
FEV_1-FVC ratio
flattening of the diaphragm
flow-volume loops (FVL)
focal pneumonia
forced expiratory volume in one second (FEV_1)
forced vital capacity (FVC)
hairline shadows
Heimlich valve
helical (spiral) CT
hemothorax
heparin-induced thrombocytopenia
high flow rates
high-resolution CT (HRCT)
hilar lymphadenopathy
Hoover sign
hospital-acquired pneumonia (HAP)
hypermetabolic
hyperresonant
hypersomnolence
hyperventilation
hypnotics
hypometabolic
idiopathic pulmonary arterial hypertension (IPAH)
intercostal retractions
interstitial pneumonia
jugular venous pressure (JVP)
Kerley A lines
Kerley B lines
Kussmaul breathing
lateral costophrenic angle
lateral decubitus view
lateral views
lobar pneumonia

loculated effusions
long-acting beta 2-agonists (LABA)
lordotic
loud second heart sound (S2)
low-flow O_2
lung volume reduction surgery (LVRS)
lupus anticoagulant
macroglossia
malignant pleural effusion
Mantoux
mast cell stabilizers
mast cells
MDI with a spacer
mean pulmonary arterial pressure
mechanical ventilatory support
mediastinal shift
metered-dose inhalers (MDI)
methacholine
micrognathia
midaxillary line
midclavicular line
miliary disease
multiple-drug resistant (MDR) organisms
multiple-drug resistant TB (MDR-TB)
nasal cannula
nasal continuous positive airway pressure (nasal CPAP)
nasal flaring
nebulizer
New York Heart Association class IV (NYHA class IV)
nicotine agonists
nighttime appliances
noninvasive positive pressure ventilation (NIPPV)
nonrebreather face mask
nonsegmental pneumonia
O_2 saturation
obtundation
orthodeoxia
PA pressures
parapneumonic pleural effusions
paratracheal lymph nodes
partial pressure
peak expiratory flow (PEF)
peak-flow monitoring
pendulous uvula
peribronchial cuffing
peribronchial thickening

perihilar bat-wing distribution of infiltrates
phosphodiesterase inhibitors
pink puffers
platypnea
pleural effusion
pleural fluid
pleural friction rub
pleural sclerosis
pleural space
pleuritic chest pain
pleurocentesis
pleurodesis
pneumococcal pneumonia
Pneumocystis pneumonia (PCP)
pneumothorax
positive pressure ventilation
posteroanterior (PA)
poudrage
protein C
protein S
prothrombin gene mutation
pulmonary arteriography
pulmonary artery wedge pressure
pulmonary embolism (PE)
pulmonary function tests (PFTs)
pulmonary hypertension (PH)
pulmonary thromboendarterectomy
pulmonic component (P2)
pulse oximetry
purified protein derivative (PPD)
pursed-lip breathing
R-to-S wave ratio greater than 1
rapid tapering of hilar vessels
rescue medications
respiratory alkalosis
restless leg syndrome
ribosomal DNA probes
right-sided heart catheterization
secondary pulmonary hypertension
segmental bronchioles
short-acting beta 2-agonists (SABA)
shunt
single-breath diffusing capacity of carbon monoxide (DL_{CO})
somnolence
splinting
splitting of the first and second heart sounds (split S1 and S2)
standardized uptake value (SUV)
status asthmaticus
subcarinal lymph nodes

subsegmental bronchioles
superinfection
surfactant
sympathomimetics
technetium DTPA
tension pneumothorax
thoracentesis
thrombolytic therapy
tidal volume
tracheal deviation
tracheobronchial lymph nodes
transbronchial biopsy
transbronchial needle aspiration
    (TBNA)
transudate
tricuspid regurgitant jet
tube thoracostomy
tuberculin skin testing (TST)
tuberculosis (TB)
upright chest radiographs
uvulopalatopharyngoplasty
    (UPPP)
V/Q mismatch
V/Q scan
vancomycin-resistant Enterococcus
    (VRE)
ventilation-perfusion ratio (V/Q
    ratio)
ventilator-associated pneumonia
    (VAP)
Venturi mask
vesicular breath sounds
visceral-pleural line
vocal cord dysfunction
work of breathing
xenon

Chapter 9

1 mm ST-segment depression
12-lead EKG
2-vessel
3-vessel
acute coronary syndromes (ACS)
akinesis
ambulatory EKG
angina pectoris
angiography
ankle-brachial index (ABI)
anterior wall
anterior wall akinesis
anterolateral severe hypokinesis
antiplatelet therapy

aortic stenosis (AS)
aortobifemoral bypass
atrial fibrillation (AF)
atrial septal defect (ASD)
atrial-paced (A-paced)
atrioventricular blocks (AV
    blocks)
atrioventricular node (AV node)
augmented limb leads
automatic implantable cardioverter-
    defibrillator (AICD)
balloon angioplasty
battery life
bovine
bradyarrhythmia
bradycardia
brain natriuretic peptide (BNP)
Bruce protocol
bruit
bundle of His
cardiac arrest
cardiac catheterization
cardiac output
carotid angioplasty and stenting
    (CAS)
carotid artery disease
carotid bifurcation
carotid duplex ultrasound
carotid endarterectomy (CEA)
cath lab
cerebrovascular accident (CVA)
chordae
chronically anticoagulated
CK-MB
coarctation of the aorta
color flow Doppler
commissurotomy
common carotid artery (CCA)
concentric left ventricular
    hypertrophy
concentric plaques
congestive heart failure (CHF)
coronary artery bypass grafting
    (CABG)
coronary calcium score
crescendo-decrescendo murmur
Cypher
decrescendo diastolic murmur
defibrillation
dependent edema
depolarization
diastolic filling

direct current cardioversion (DC
    cardioversion)
door-to-balloon time
downsloping ST segment
drug-eluting stent
dyspnea at rest
dyspnea on exertion
early systolic
eccentric plaques
echocardiogram
ectopic beats
ejection fraction
electrocardiogram (EKG or ECG)
electron-beam computed tomogra-
    phy (EBCT)
electrophysiology studies (EP
    studies)
Endeavor (stent)
enteric-coated aspirin
event recorder
external carotid artery (ECA)
fascicles
fascicular blocks
femoropopliteal bypass (fem-pop
    bypass)
fraction flow reserve (FFR)
global hypokinesis
Graham Steell murmur
harvested vein
hepatojugular reflux
holosystolic
Holter monitor
hypokinesis
impedance
in the upper interscapular area
inducible myocardial ischemia
innominate artery
in-stent restenosis
intermittent claudication
internal carotid artery (ICA)
intima
intravascular ultrasound (IVUS)
inverted T wave
irregularly irregular
jugular venous pressure (JVP)
jugular venous pulsations
leaflets
left internal mammary artery
    (LIMA)
left sternal border
left ventricular ejection fraction
    (LVEF)

left ventricular hypertrophy
left axis deviation
left-sided heart disease
left-to-right shunts
limb leads
long-QT syndrome
magnetic resonance angiography
    (MRA)
middiastolic
midsystolic click
mitral annular calcification
mitral annulus
mitral insufficiency
mitral regurgitation (MR)
mitral valve stenosis
Mobitz type I, II or III
mode
mode switches
modifiable risk factors
monocular blindness
multi-vessel bypasses
murmur best heard at the apex
murmur best heard over the aorta
murmur best heard over the infra-
    scapular area
murmur best heard parasternally
murmur heard best in the 3rd or 4th
    intercostal space
myocardial infarction
myocardial perfusion
myocardial perfusion study
near syncope
negative for inducible myocardial
    ischemia
New York Heart Association
    (NYHA)
no intracardiac masses
no intramural thrombi
no regional wall motion
    abnormalities
no valvular vegetations seen
noncardiogenic
noninvasive tests
nonspecific ST (segment) and
    T-wave changes
non-ST-segment elevation
    myocardial infarction (NSTEMI)
normal sinus rhythm (NSR)
nuclear stress test
outflow tract
pacemaker interrogation
pansystolic

paroxysmal supraventricular
    tachycardia (PSVT)
patent ductus arteriosus
patent foramen ovale (PFO)
peak systolic velocity (PSV)
percutaneous coronary intervention
    (PCI)
percutaneous transluminal balloon
    valvuloplasty
perfused
perfusion
perfusion defects
peripheral artery disease (PAD)
peripheral artery occlusive disease
    (PAOD)
peripheral vascular disease (PVD)
pharmacological stress test
pitting edema
plain old balloon angioplasty
    (POBA)
poor R-wave progression over the
    precordium
porcine
precordial leads
premature family history
pulmonary stenosis
pulse deficit
radiating to the base
radiofrequency catheter ablation
    (RFCA)
regional wall motion abnormalities
repolarization
retrograde flow
right bundle branch block (RBBB)
right sternal border
right ventricular systolic pressure
    (RVSP)
right axis deviation
right-to-left shunt
rule out myocardial infarction
    (ROMI)
saphenous vein
sclerotic valve
segmental wall motion
    abnormalities
serial enzymes
short-QT syndrome
sick sinus syndrome
sinoatrial node
sinus node
smoking cessation
split heart sound

stress echocardiogram
stress test
ST-segment depression
ST-segment elevation
ST-segment elevation myocardial
    infarction (STEMI)
subendocardial MI
sudden cardiac death
Swan-Ganz catheter
tachyarrhythmia
tachycardia
Taxus
technetium 99c sestamibi
Tetralogy of Fallot
thallium 201
Thrombolysis in Myocardial
    Infarction (TIMI)
TIMI grade flow
TIMI score
to a therapeutic INR of 2–3
transesophageal echocardiogram
    (TEE)
transient ischemic attacks (TIA)
transmural
transposition of the great arteries
transvalvular gradient
troponin I
turbulence
unstable angina
valve area
valvuloplasty
vegetations
ventricular fibrillation (VF)
ventricular sensed (v-sensed)
ventricular septal defect
ventricular tachycardia (VT)
ventriculography
well-healed sternal scar
Wolff-Parkinson-White syndrome
    (WPW)
Xience V stent

Chapter 10

abnormal bone signals
ABO (blood group) antigens
accessory salivary glands
acquired immunodeficiency
    syndrome (AIDS)
acute-phase reactants
allograft
anaphylactic shock
anemia of chronic disease

angioedema
anticardiolipin IgG or IgM
anticyclic citrullinated peptide (anti-CCP)
anti-dsDNA
antinuclear antibodies (ANA)
antiproliferative agents
anti-Smith (anti-Sm)
atlantoaxial subluxation
atopy
autograft
autoimmune hemolytic anemia
Bence Jones proteins
bone marrow edema
boutonniere deformities
bridging therapy
bronchiolitis obliterans
bronchiolitis obliterans-organizing pneumonia (BOOP)
Burkitt lymphoma
calcineurin inhibitors
centromere
chronic allograft nephropathy
clusters of differentiation (CD)
colony stimulating factor (CSF)
complement
complement fixation
Coumadin with a target INR of 3
crossmatching
cytopenias
disease modifying antirheumatic drugs (DMARDs)
disseminated lupus erythematosus
double-stranded DNA (anti-dsDNA, also called anti-native DNA)
envenomization
EpiPen
Felty syndrome
flexion contractures
genotyping
graft vs host disease (GVHD)
hammertoes
hematopoietic stem cells (HSC)
heterotopic transplant
highly active antiretroviral therapy (HAART)
histocompatibility
HLA typing
homogeneous
Human immunodeficiency virus (HIV)
human leukocyte antigens (HLA)

hyperglobulinemia
hypocomplementemia
idiopathic thrombocytopenic purpura (ITP)
immunodeficiency
immunofluorescence antibody (IFA)
immunoglobulin therapy
immunosuppression
injection
interferons
interleukins
isograft
Jaccoud arthritis
juxtaarticular demineralization
Kaposi sarcoma
kappa
keratitis filiformis
keratoconjunctivitis sicca
lactated Ringers
lambda
LE cell prep
living related donors
living unrelated donors
lymphocytotoxicity assay
major histocompatibility complex (MHC)
malar rash
marginal erosions
mixed connective tissue disease (MCTD)
nosocomial
nucleic acid sequence-based amplification (NASBA)
nucleolar
nucleolar/cytoplasmic
orthotopic transplant
panel-reactive antibody (PRA)
pannus formation
parotid glands
periprocedural ischemia
periungual erythema
plasma cells
plasma expanders
plasma HIV RNA level
positive direct Coombs
presensitization antibodies
primary biliary cirrhosis
prodromal symptoms
radioallergosorbent testing (RAST)
rapamycins
Raynaud phenomenon

rejection
reperfusion injury
retroviruses
reverse transcriptase
reverse transcription-PCR (RT-PCR)
rheumatoid arthritis (RA)
rheumatoid factor (RF)
rheumatoid nodules
ribonucleoprotein (RNP)
Schirmer test
sed rate
selective IgA deficiency
seropositive
severe combined immunodeficiency (SCID)
Sjögren syndrome (SS)
small nuclear ribonucleoprotein (snRNP)
speckled
SS-A (Sjögren syndrome antigen A)
SS-B (Sjögren syndrome antigen B)
systemic lupus erythematosus (SLE)
tissue typing
TNF blockers
ulnar deviation
ulnar drift
vanishing bile duct syndrome
wasting syndrome
Western blot assay
xenografts
xerostomia

Chapter 11

17-hydroxyprogesterone
5% acetic acid
abnormal placentation
abortion (Ab)
abortus
acanthosis nigricans
Actinomycete
add-back therapy
adhesiolysis
adrenarche
amenorrhea
amniotomy
ampulla
android
androstenedione
aneuploidy
anteflexed

anteverted

anthropoid

antimüllerian hormone (AMH)

anti-Rh$_0$(D) antibody titers

anti-Rh$_0$(D) IgG injections (RhoGAM)

antral follicles

Apgar score

arrest of descent

arrest of dilation

arrest of labor

Asherman syndrome

assisted reproductive techniques (ART)

asynclitism

atypical squamous cells of undetermined significance (ASC-US)

back labor

balanced translocation

Ballard score

Bartholin

beta unit of human chorionic gonadotropin hormone (beta hCG)

Bethesda system

bilateral salpingo-oophorectomies (BSO)

biparietal diameter (BPD)

bladder reflection

blastocyst

blighted ovum

bloody show

breech presentation

Canavan disease

categories A, B, C, D, and X

cephalic presentation

cephalohematoma

cephalopelvic disproportion (CPD)

cervical cerclage

cervical intraepithelial neoplasia (CIN)

cervical motion tenderness

cervical ripening

cervicitis

cesarean delivery

cesarean hysterectomy

Chadwick sign

chocolate cysts

chorioamnionitis

choriocarcinomas

chorionic villus sampling (CVS)

climacteric

clitoral index (CI)

clitoromegaly

clomiphene challenge test

clue cells

colposcopy

combination oral contraceptive pills (COCPs)

complete Ab

complete and partial moles

complete breech

condylomata acuminata

cone biopsy (conization)

contraction stress test

controlled ovarian hyperstimulation (COH)

corpus luteum

crown-rump length

cul-de-sac

Cushing disease

cytoreduction

decelerations

decreased ovarian reserve

defeminization

dehydroepiandrosterone sulfate (DHEA-S)

demise

depilation

dilation and curettage (D&C)

diploidy

disseminated intravascular coagulation

DNA probes

double footling

Down syndrome (trisomy 21)

Duffy

dysfunctional uterine bleeding (DUB)

dyssynchronous endometrium

dystocia

E2

eclampsia

ectopic pregnancy

effacement

egg retrieval

elective (induced) abortion

elective induction

empty sella syndrome

endometrial ablation

endometrial biopsy

endometrial stripe

endometriosis

endometriotic tissue

endometritis

engaged

enter the myometrium

episiotomy

erythroblastosis

erythroblastosis fetalis

escutcheon

estimated date of confinement (EDC)

estradiol

estradiol valerate

estriol

estrogen breakthrough bleeding

estrogen withdrawal bleeding

estrone

external cephalic version

externalized

factor V Leiden

failure to progress

ferning

Ferriman-Gallwey score

fetal heart motion

fetal heart tones

fetal lie

fetal pole

fetal status monitoring

fetomaternal hemorrhage

fetopelvic disproportion

fetus papyraceus

fill and spill

fimbriae

fimbriated end

Fitz-Hugh-Curtis syndrome

fixed uterus

folate (folic acid)

follicle stimulating hormone (FSH)

follicular recruitment

forceps

fourchette

frank breech

free pelvic fluid

free testosterone

functional hypothalamic amenorrhea

fundal height

galactorrhea

Gardasil

Gardnerella vaginalis

genetic amniocentesis

gestational age

gestational diabetes

gestational sac
gestational trophoblastic disease
glans of clitoris
GnRH analogs
gonadotropin-releasing hormone (GnRH)
gonococcal (GC) infection
graafian follicle
gravid
gravid uterus
gravidity
group B streptococci (GBS)
gynecoid
head circumference
head is delivered onto the perineum
Hegar sign
HELLP syndrome
helmet cells
hematocolpos
hematometra
hemoglobin S, C, or F; alpha or beta thalassemia
hemolytic disease of the newborn (HDN)
herpes simplex virus type 2 (HSV-2)
heterotopic pregnancy
hirsutism
homogeneous
human chorionic gonadotropin
Human papilloma virus (HPV)
hydatid moles
hydatidiform moles
hydrops fetalis
hydrosalpinx
hyperemesis gravidarum
hypergonadotropic hypogonadism
hyperprolactinemia
hypertrichosis
hypogonadotropic hypogonadism
hysterosalpingogram (HSG)
hysteroscopy
hysterotomy
imperforate hymen
in vitro fertilization (IVF)
incision-to-delivery time
incompetent cervix
incomplete Ab
increased parity
indirect Coombs
inevitable Ab
infundibulum
inhibin A

intact perineum
intracavitary
intracytoplasmic sperm injection (ICSI)
intraligamentous
intramural
intrauterine device (IUD)
intrauterine fetal resuscitation
intrauterine insemination (IUI)
intravaginal pessary
introitus
invasive moles
isthmus
Joel Cohen
Kallmann syndrome
Kell
Kidd
Kleihauer-Betke test
KOH preparation (KOH prep)
L/S ratio
labor, delivery, recovery, and post-partum (LDRP)
laminaria
lanugo
lateral disease
leiomyomas
Leopold maneuver
Lewis
LH surge
linea alba
linea nigra
lithotomy position
lochia
lochia alba
lochia rubra
lochia serosa
loop electrical excision procedure (LEEP)
lower uterine transverse incision
Lugol solution
lumbar epidural
luteinizing hormone (LH)
macroadenomas
macrosomia
magnesium sulfate ($MgSO_4$)
male factor
malpresentation
mask of pregnancy
Maylard
McDonald
McRobert maneuver
meconium aspiration

meconium staining
mediolateral episiotomy
melasma
methylenetetrahydrofolate reductase (MTHFR)
MICRhoGAM
microadenomas
microangiopathic
middle cerebral artery flow
midline episiotomy
missed Ab
molar pregnancy
mole
Montevideo units (MVU)
müllerian dysgenesis
multifetal pregnancy
multigravida
multiparous
Mycoplasma genitalium
myomectomy
neural tube defects
no signal detected
nongonococcal infections
nonreassuring
nonreassuring fetal status
nonstress test
normal singleton pregnancy
normal spontaneous vaginal delivery (NSVD)
nuchal cord
nuchal fold test
nuchal translucency testing
nucleic acid amplification tests (NAAT)
nulligravida
nulliparous
nulliparous cervix
occipitoanterior (OA)
occipitoposterior (OP)
occult prolapsed cord
off-label use
oligohydramnios
oophoritis
operative vaginal delivery
opposing progesterone
oral contraceptive pills (OCPs)
organogenesis
outflow tract obstruction
ovarian torsion
overt prolapsed cord
ovulation induction (OI)
ovulation predictor kits (OPKs)

oxytocics
panhypopituitarism
Papanicolaou (Pap) test
paracervical block
parametrial
parity
parturition
pedunculated fibroid
pelvic inflammatory disease (PID)
pelvimetry
percutaneous umbilical blood sampling (PUBS)
perineal infiltration
peritubal and periovarian adhesions
Pfannenstiel
placenta accreta
placenta increta
placenta percreta
placenta previa
placental abruption
platypelloid
polycystic ovary syndrome (PCOS)
polyhydramnios
position
posterior vaginal fornix
postterm pregnancy
powder-burn lesions
preeclampsia
pregnancy-associated plasma protein A (PAPP-A)
premature ovarian failure (POF)
premature rupture of membranes (PROM)
presentation
preterm birth
preterm labor
primary ovarian insufficiency (POI)
primigravida
primiparous
products of conception (POC)
progesterone challenge test
progestin withdrawal bleed
progestins
prolactinomas
pudendal block
puerperium
pyosalpinx
quad test
quantitative serum hCG
quickening
rapid protein reagin (RPR)

reassuring
rectovaginal septum
recurrent pregnancy loss
reflex antibody screening
resting follicles
resuscitation bassinet
retroflexed
retroverted
$Rh_0(D)$
right sacrum posterior (RSP)
rosette test
ruptured endometriotic cyst
saline wet mount
salpingectomy
salpingitis
salpingo-oophorectomy
salpingostomy
Schiller test
schistocytes
secundigravida
semiconservative therapy
sex hormone binding globulin (SHBG)
sexually transmitted diseases (STDs)
sexually transmitted infections (STIs)
Shirodkar
sickle cell trait
single footling
Skene glands
sonographic age
sonohysterogram (saline-instilled sonogram)
spinnbarkeit
spontaneous abortion (SAb)
station
stillbirth
subfertility
submucosal
subserosal
suction curettage
superovulation
surgical menopause
Tanner staging
Tay-Sachs
teratogenesis
thelarche
therapeutic abortion (TAb)
thin PCOS
threatened Ab
tocolytics

total abdominal hysterectomy and bilateral oophorectomies (TAH-BSO)
translocation
transmural incision
transvaginal ultrasound (TVUS)
transverse vaginal septum
trilaminar
triple screen
triploidy
tuboovarian abscess (TOA)
Turner syndrome
two-embryo transfer
umbilical cord prolapse
unbalanced translocation
unopposed estrogen
Ureaplasma urealyticum
uterine artery embolization
uteroplacental vascular insufficiency
uterosacral ligaments
vacuum extractor
vaginal agenesis
vaginal birth after cesarean delivery (VBAC)
vanishing twin
vasa previa
vertex
vertex, left occipitoanterior [LOA]
vesicouterine peritoneal reflection
viable intrauterine pregnancy
virilization
visual field cuts
well-woman exam
whiff test
Woods screw maneuver
yolk sac
Zavanelli maneuver

Chapter 12

7 + 3
abdominoperineal resection
absolute neutrophil count (ANC)
ABVD (Adriamycin, bleomycin, vinblastine, dacarbazine)
acanthocytes (spur cells)
active surveillance
acute chest syndrome
acute GVHD
acute lymphocytic leukemia (ALL)
acute myelocytic leukemia (AML)
acute myelogenous leukemia
acute promyelocytic leukemia (APL)

adjuvant
aleukemic leukemia
alkylating agents
allogeneic
all-trans-retinoic acid (ATRA)
alopecia
amorphous
androgen blockade
androgen deprivation
angiogenesis
anisocytosis
Ann Arbor
antibiotics
anticipatory nausea
antimetabolites
antiphospholipid syndrome (APS)
antithrombin
apheresis
aplastic crisis
apoptosis
apple core
arc (rotating beam) therapy
architectural distortion
area under the curve (AUC)
aromatase inhibitors (AIs)
asymmetric density
atypical lymphocytes
Auer rod
automated diff
B symptoms
BardPort
basophilic stippling
beta 2-microglobulin
Binet
biomarkers
blast crisis
Bloom-Richardson
bone marrow aspiration and biopsy
bone marrow rescue
bone marrow transplant (BMT)
bone metastases
brachytherapy
BRCA1
BRCA2
breakthrough pain
Breast Imaging and Reporting Data System (BI-RADS)
breast-conserving surgery
CA 15-3
CA 27-29
cachectic
cachexia

calcifications
carcinoma in situ
casting
CBC with differential (CBC with diff)
centigray (cGy)
c-erb B2
Chamberlain procedure
cheilosis
chemoprevention
chemotherapy-induced nausea and vomiting (CINV)
Christmas disease
chronic GVHD
chronic lymphocytic leukemia (CLL)
chronic myelocytic leukemia (CML)
circumscribed
clear margins
clustered polymorphic microcalcifications
coin lesion
colorectal cancer (CRC)
complete remission
complete response
consolidation
constitutional symptoms
Coombs test
coplanar
core biopsy
cryoprecipitate
curative
CyberKnife
cytogenetics
cytogenic response
cytoreductive surgery (cytoreduction)
debulking
definitive
diagnostic mammogram
direct Coombs
Dohle bodies
dose-dense chemotherapy
dosimetry
ductal carcinoma in situ (DCIS)
Dukes system
Eastern Cooperative Oncology Group (ECOG)
endorectal ultrasound
engrafts
erythroblastopenia

estrogen receptors (ER+)
exchange transfusion
excisional biopsy
external beam radiation
FDG avid
ferritin
ferrous sulfate
fever of unknown origin (FUO)
fibrin degradation products (FDPs)
fibrin equivalent units (FEU)
fibrin split products (FSP)
fibrinogen
fiducial
field margins
fine-needle aspiration (FNA)
fluorescent in situ hybridization (FISH)
fluorodeoxyglucose (FDG)
fractionated
free TRAM flap
French-American-British (FAB)
fresh frozen plasma (FFP)
frozen section
Gail model
Gamma Knife
giant platelets
Gleason score
glossitis
grading
graft-versus-leukemia
graft-versus-tumor (GVT)
gray (Gy)
hand-foot syndrome
harvested marrow
harvesting
helmet cells
hematologic response
hematopoietic stem cell transplantation (HSCT)
hemoglobin electrophoresis
hemoglobinopathy
hemosiderin
hemosiderosis
hepatic intraarterial chemotherapy
HER2/neu
hereditary nonpolyposis colon cancer (HNPCC)
high probability
high-dose chemotherapy
high-dose methotrexate with leucovorin rescue
Hodgkin disease (HD)

reticulocyte count (retic count)
rouleaux
salvage chemotherapy
scatter
schistocytes
screening mammography
secondary prevention
segmentectomy
selective estrogen receptor modifiers (SERMs)
sentinel node biopsy
serum protein electrophoresis (SPEP)
sickle cell crisis
sickle cell disease
sickle cells (drepanocytes)
siderocytes
simulation
single-drug therapy
single-field therapy
small-cell lung cancer (SCLC)
smudge cells
sodium ferric gluconate
soluble transferrin receptors (sTfR)
spherocytes
spiculated margins
spot compression
stable disease
staging
stem cell transplantation (SCT)

stereotactic biopsy
stereotactic radiosurgery
stomatitis
stomatocytes
strontium
Sudan black stain
superior vena cava syndrome
surgical pathology
swish and swallow
syngeneic
systemic radiation therapy
tangential fields
target cells
target cells (codocytes)
tear drops
temporal wasting
teratogen
terminal deoxynucleotidyl transferase (TdT)
therapeutic
three-dimensional conformal radiation therapy (3D CRT)
thrombotic thrombocytopenic purpura [TTP]
tissue expander
TNM system
total body irradiation (TBI)
total dose
total iron-binding capacity (TIBC)

totally implantable venous access systems (TIVAS)
toxic granulation
transanal resection
transferrin
transferrin receptors
transferrin saturation
transrectus abdominis muscle flap (TRAM flap)
transthoracic needle aspiration (TTNA)
treatment field
triple negative breast cancer
tumor board
tumor lysis syndrome
tumor markers
type and cross
type and crossmatch
type and screen
vacuoles
vascular endothelial growth factor (VEGF)
video-assisted thorascopic surgery (VATS)
viscous lidocaine
von Willebrand disease
WBC-depleted RBCs
wedge resection
World Health Organization (WHO)

Sample Report 2A

Consultation

REASON FOR CONSULTATION
Postoperative medical management.

HISTORY OF PRESENT ILLNESS
Patient is status post laparoscopic gastric banding and has failed multiple medical interventions for weight loss. At the current time, she is extubated on room air with oxygen saturations in the mid-90s. Intraoperatively she received about 2L of Ringer lactate and has put out about 250 mL of urine.

Her medical course has been complicated by morbid obesity and its complications thereof including diabetes, hypertension, obstructive sleep apnea, and fatty liver. These will be described in greater detail in the past medical history.

She has undergone an upper GI, which showed a properly positioned gastric band without any leak or obstruction.

PAST MEDICAL HISTORY
1. Type 2 diabetes since 2007, treated with metformin. Last hemoglobin A_{1c} in July 20XX was 6%.
2. Hypertension for the last 6 years, controlled on lisinopril.
3. Obstructive sleep apnea diagnosed in the last 3 years. Patient does not wear a CPAP mask due to claustrophobia. The last study was in April 20XX.
4. Multiple episodes of pericarditis, last in January 20XX. She subsequently mentions that lupus was ruled out; however, she reports using prednisone and colchicine during these bouts. She has had 6–7 bouts of pericarditis to date.
5. Gastroesophageal reflux disease.
6. Dyslipidemia, controlled.
7. Fatty liver.
8. Iron deficiency anemia, presumed secondary to heavy menstrual losses.
9. Thyroid nodules. Last thyroid sonogram in February 20XX indicated these were stable.
10. Polycystic ovarian disease. Patient reports heavy periods occurring every 4 weeks.

PAST SURGICAL HISTORY
Appendectomy, cholecystectomy, C-section, and wedge resection of ovarian cysts.

MEDICATIONS
Lisinopril 10 mg daily, metformin 500 mg daily, colchicine 600 mg b.i.d.

ALLERGIES
Iodine causes skin rash with hives and "throat closes up."

FAMILY HISTORY
Dad died of prostate cancer at age 68. Mom is 71 years old and has diabetes and hypertension.

SOCIAL HISTORY
Patient is married. She teaches computer classes to 8th graders. She has a 12-year-old daughter who is healthy. Denies alcohol, tobacco, or illicit drug use.

REVIEW OF SYSTEMS
A detailed, 11-point review of systems was done and is negative except for mild abdominal pain.

PHYSICAL EXAMINATION
Pleasant, morbidly obese female in no acute distress.
VITAL SIGNS: Afebrile, pulse 95, respirations about 20 per minute, blood pressure 104/57, O_2 saturation 95% on room air.
HEENT: Normocephalic, atraumatic. Pupils equal, round and reactive to light and accommodation.
NECK: Supple. No jugular venous distention.
RESPIRATORY: Clear to auscultation.
CARDIOVASCULAR: Normal heart sounds.
ABDOMEN: Surgical laparoscopic wounds are seen with no oozing. Mild tenderness around the surgical wounds. Bowel sounds are heard. No masses are felt.
NEUROLOGICAL: Nonfocal.
EXTREMITIES: No pedal edema. Good peripheral pulses.

LABORATORY
BMP shows sodium 138, potassium 4.0, chloride 103. Hemoglobin A_{1c} 6%. Urinalysis shows 6–8 white blood cells. Cholesterol shows LDL of 87, HDL at 60.

Chest x-ray was reportedly negative. Pulmonary function tests indicate mild restriction.

ASSESSMENT AND PLAN
1. Status post laparoscopic gastric banding, currently extubated on room air.
2. Nonnarcotic analgesia p.r.n. We will order SCDs and TED hose for deep venous thrombosis prophylaxis.
3. Diabetes. Will hold metformin for the time she is n.p.o. and institute NovoLog sliding scale.
4. Hypertension. At the current time, her blood pressure is about 104/57. When she is on a p.o. diet, I will restart her ACE inhibitor.
5. Obstructive sleep apnea. She has never used a CPAP mask. We will monitor her closely in step-down ICU setting. Will institute a CPAP at the lowest pressures. If this is an issue, will need pulmonary consult.
6. Fatty liver/dyslipidemia. Will hold any statin therapy for now.
7. Iron deficiency anemia. This was mild to begin with. We will check a complete blood count tomorrow and see how she is doing on this.

Thank you for this consult. We will continue to follow along with you.

Sample Report 3A

Consultation

REASON FOR CONSULTATION
Chronic abdominal pain and diarrhea.

HISTORY OF PRESENT ILLNESS
The patient is a very pleasant 20-year-old male who is referred by Dr. Harvey for GI consultation. The patient complains of a chronic history of upper abdominal discomfort with concurrent bloating and severe gastroesophageal reflux disease. In addition, he often has postprandial diarrhea with an average of 3-5 loose stools per day.

Due to his clinical presentation, the patient was previously seen by Dr. Umi who recommended that he proceed with a diagnostic upper endoscopy and colonoscopy. However, due to personal reasons, the studies were not performed. However, he had instituted PPI therapy, which typically controlled reflux symptoms. However, if acid-reduction therapy is discontinued, there is recurrent burning, retrosternal discomfort. In addition, he voices profound weight gain over the last year despite no significant change in nutritional intake, but his lifestyle has been somewhat more sedentary than in the past.

He voices no prior history of peptic ulcer disease, pancreatitis, or colitis. He denies a previous endoscopic inspection of the gastrointestinal tract.

MEDICATIONS
None at this time.

ALLERGIES
No known drug allergies.

FAMILY HISTORY
Negative for intestinal malignancies or intrinsic liver disease.

SOCIAL HISTORY
Nonsmoker, nondrinker; denies previous history of tattoos, illicit drug usage, or blood transfusions.

PHYSICAL EXAM
VITAL SIGNS: Blood pressure 179/111, temperature 98.3, current weight 280 pounds.
SKIN: No jaundice, petechiae, spider angiomata, or rashes.
HEENT: Pupils are equal, reactive to light and accommodation. Extraocular movements are intact, without nystagmus. There is no scleral icterus. The fundi are not visualized.
LUNGS: Clear to auscultation and percussion.
CARDIOVASCULAR: S1 and S2 within normal limits, without gallops or murmurs.
ABDOMEN: Bowel sounds are present in all 4 quadrants without organomegaly, mass, or ascites.
RECTAL: Hemoccult-negative stools. No evidence of mass within the rectal vault.
NEUROLOGIC: No focal findings.
EXTREMITIES: No cyanosis, clubbing, or edema.

ASSESSMENT
1. Refractory abdominal pain with concurrent bloating favors irritable bowel and/or intestinal gas syndrome.
2. Refractory gastroesophageal reflux disease, presently not well controlled since discontinuation of PPI acid-reduction therapy, although the patient often remains symptomatic with acid reduction.
3. Chronic refractory diarrhea concerning for inflammatory bowel disease or irritable bowel syndrome.

PLAN
The patient will be scheduled for a diagnostic upper endoscopy and colonoscopy with possible tissue biopsy. During the interim, he will reinstitute PPI acid-reduction therapy and avoid food and/or beverages which may exacerbate symptoms, specifically dairy products and caffeine. Today we will obtain a copy of the patient's abdominal ultrasound report for review. He will follow up after procedures are complete to discuss results. Further recommendations will follow.

Sample Report 3B

Consultation

REASON FOR CONSULTATION
Gastroesophageal reflux disease, vomiting.

HISTORY OF PRESENT ILLNESS
The patient is a very pleasant 42-year-old female referred for GI consultation. The patient states she was in her usual state of health until approximately 3 years ago when she began having vague abdominal discomfort best described as bloating, for which she underwent a colonoscopy at St. Paul Hospital. Per the patient, this study was normal, but we do not have the endoscopic report available for review.

In addition, she developed GE reflux disease that has been managed with PPI acid-reduction therapy. However, despite acid reduction, recently she has had breakthrough symptoms at night, complaining of burning, retrosternal discomfort with concurrent nausea and vomiting. There has been some dyspepsia but no active gastrointestinal bleeding.

Lastly, she complains of occasional difficulty with swallowing in the distal esophageal region, predominantly with solids. She consumes liquids without difficulty. As a result of her symptoms, an upper GI series was performed, documenting a small hiatal hernia, severe GE reflux, and esophageal motility disorder with lack of primary peristaltic wave and multiple tertiary contractions throughout the esophagus. The patient voices no previous diagnostic endoscopic inspection of the upper GI tract.

PAST MEDICAL HISTORY
1. Asthma.
2. Hiatal hernia.
3. High blood pressure.
4. Migraine headaches.
5. Depression.

SURGICAL PROCEDURES
Appendectomy in 1998.

MEDICATIONS
Exforge, Nexium, Singulair, and Advil.

ALLERGIES
VERAPAMIL.

FAMILY HISTORY
The patient voices that her mother had colon polyps, but there are no other family members with known intestinal neoplastic disease.

SOCIAL HISTORY
The patient currently smokes half a pack of cigarettes per day and has been using tobacco products for approximately 20 years, but she is a nondrinker. There has been no previous requirement for transfusion of packed red blood cells.

PHYSICAL EXAM
VITAL SIGNS: Blood pressure is 167/103, temperature is 98.3, current weight is 274 pounds.
SKIN: There is no jaundice, petechiae, spider angiomata, or rashes.
HEENT: Pupils are equal, reactive to light and accommodation. Extraocular muscles are intact. There is no scleral icterus. The fundi are not visualized.
LUNGS: Clear to auscultation and percussion.
CARDIOVASCULAR: S1 and S2 within normal limits, without gallops or murmurs.
ABDOMEN: Moderately distended abdomen with slight discomfort in the epigastrium, but no guarding or rebound. Bowel sounds are present in all 4 quadrants without organomegaly, mass, or ascites.
RECTAL: Hemoccult-negative stools. No evidence of mass within the rectal vault.
NEUROLOGIC: No focal findings.
EXTREMITIES: No cyanosis, clubbing, or edema.

ASSESSMENT
1. Refractory gastroesophageal reflux despite PPI acid-reduction therapy.
2. Distal esophageal dysphagia. Rule out underlying obstructive process. Upper GI findings are concerning for possible primary dysmotility disorder.
3. Hiatal hernia documented via imaging.
4. Average colon cancer risk based on age criteria, status post colonoscopy 3 years ago without evidence of neoplastic disease, per patient history.
5. Obesity.
6. Intestinal gas syndrome.

PLAN
The patient will be scheduled for a diagnostic upper endoscopy with possible Savary-guided dilatation and tissue biopsy. During the interim she will continue PPI therapy. Also, add Reglan 10 mg 1 pill p.o. at bedtime. Follow up after test is complete to discuss endoscopic findings and reassess clinical progress after addition of gastroprokinetic therapy. Lastly, I have asked her to avoid food and/or beverages that may exacerbate symptoms.

Sample Report 4A

Discharge Summary

ADMITTING DIAGNOSES
1. Jaundice, with weight loss.
2. Distended gallbladder.
3. History of prostate cancer.
4. Abnormal liver function tests.

SUMMARY OF HOSPITALIZATION

The patient is a 76-year-old male who was admitted with a complaint of nausea and early satiety. The patient also has been having difficulty swallowing. The patient appeared jaundiced. He had undergone a CT of the abdomen that revealed common bile duct dilatation and a distended gallbladder. His white blood cell count was elevated at 19,000. He had a bilirubin of 10 and liver function tests were all abnormal.

EGD and ERCP were recommended. Dr. Bariga attempted an ERCP, but the common bile duct could not be cannulated. The patient is status post remote Billroth II gastrectomy. He recommended repeating ERCP in 48 hours. The patient spiked a temperature of 103. He was placed on IV antibiotics. It was decided to change the procedure to percutaneous transhepatic cholangiography. Balloon dilatation of the ampulla and stone extraction was performed with internal-external biliary stenting. The patient's condition improved. His bilirubin began to decrease. The patient was continued on IV antibiotics. His white blood cell count came back to normal at 6.8. It was noted that the patient's blood culture was positive for E coli.

The patient's status continued to improve. He was tolerating his diet well. He completed 8 days of IV Zosyn. He had a repeat cholangiogram on 3/11/20XX with extraction of another stone. He was continued with the stent placement. On 3/11/20XX, we decided to continue the stent and a repeat cholangiogram will be done as an outpatient. He was placed on Augmentin, and he was discharged to be followed up by the home health nurse. He will return to our office in 1 week. He was dismissed in stable condition on 3/13/20XX.

FINAL DIAGNOSES
1. Obstructive jaundice secondary to common bile duct stones.
2. Status post percutaneous transhepatic cholangiography with extraction of stones.
3. Escherichia coli bacteremia.
4. Status post remote Billroth II gastrectomy secondary to gastric ulcers.
5. Prostate cancer by history.

DISCHARGE MEDICATIONS

Augmentin 875 mg 1 p.o. b.i.d., Nexium 40 mg 1 daily, and hydrocodone 5/500 mg 1 q.6 h. p.r.n.

Sample Report 5A

CHIEF COMPLAINT
Right hip pain.

HISTORY OF PRESENT ILLNESS
The patient is a 73 year-old white female complaining of right hip pain. This has been ongoing and has been worse over the last couple of months. She had an MRI of the hip that showed bilateral avascular necrosis. She states that her pain is now to the point that it is significantly affecting her activities of daily living, and she is ready for definitive management.

PAST HISTORY
Remarkable for rheumatoid arthritis, liver disease, cancer, and hypertension.

PAST SURGICAL HISTORY
Remarkable for appendectomy, hysterectomy, hand and foot surgery.

MEDICATIONS
1. Prednisone 5 mg 1 p.o. daily.
2. Nadalol 10 mg 1 p.o. every night.
3. Hydrocodone p.r.n. for pain.

ALLERGIES
No known drug allergies.

FAMILY HISTORY
Remarkable for CVA.

SOCIAL HISTORY
The patient does not smoke; drinks alcohol once or twice a week.

REVIEW OF SYSTEMS
Noncontributory.

PHYSICAL EXAMINATION
HEENT: Normocephalic and atraumatic.
CHEST: Clear to auscultation.
HEART: Regular rate and rhythm.
ABDOMEN: Soft and nontender to palpation. Bowel sounds x4.
EXTREMITIES: Right lower extremity has marked reproduction of pain with internal rotation of her right hip. Neurovascularly intact.

X-RAYS
AP pelvis and frogleg lateral of the right hip shows severe osteopenia. Difficult to see but shows some possible early collapse of the femoral head. MRI shows avascular necrosis of both femoral heads, more marked on the right than the left.

ASSESSMENT
Avascular necrosis of the right hip.

PLAN
The plan is to have the patient taken to the operating room for right total hip arthroplasty. The patient understands the risks, benefits, and complications, and she consents to the procedure. The patient has been seen and given preoperative clearance by Internal Medicine.

Sample Report 5B

Operative Note

PREOPERATIVE DIAGNOSIS
Left knee medial meniscal tear with possible lateral meniscal tear.

POSTOPERATIVE DIAGNOSIS
Left knee medial meniscal tear with lateral meniscal tear and medial plica.

PROCEDURE
Left knee arthroscopy with partial medial meniscal resection, partial lateral meniscal resection, and resection of medial plica.

ANESTHESIA
General endotracheal.

COMPLICATIONS
None.

INDICATIONS
The patient is a 67-year-old female who has had left knee pain that has been recalcitrant to conservative management. She was evaluated with an MRI that revealed the possibility of a medial and/or lateral meniscal tear. She is scheduled for a left knee arthroscopy. The risks and benefits of surgery were discussed with her preoperatively, and all questions were answered prior to surgery. She wished to proceed with left knee arthroscopy in an effort to ameliorate her left knee pain.

PROCEDURAL DETAILS
Once the patient was properly identified and consented, she was brought into the operating room theater. She was placed in a supine position and successfully anesthetized. Her left lower extremity then was wrapped with a nonsterile tourniquet high upon her left thigh, and the distal third of her thigh was placed into a well-padded arthroscopic leg holder and prepped and draped in the usual sterile fashion.

The surgical portion of the procedure began with the establishment of an inferolateral portal followed by an inferomedial portal through which the camera was utilized, along with a working inferomedial portal to systematically review the knee. Beginning with the anterior compartment, the distal pole of the patella was found to have grade 2 cartilaginous changes, the lateral facet with grade 3 changes. The medial facet was found to have mild to grade 1 changes only. The femoral trochlear groove along the lateral femoral condyle superiorly was found to have grade 1 changes covering an area of approximately 25 x 25 mm. Following this, the medial gutter was examined after some difficulty due to the large medial plica which was evident upon entry of the medial gutter. No loose bodies were found; however, there was significant synovitis noted in the medial gutter. The medial joint line was then examined, and although there was no frank radial or horizontal tearing, the posterior third of the medial meniscus was found to be macerated and degenerated. Also, the tibial plateau along the medial joint line was found to have grade 4 cartilaginous changes throughout with the exception of a 5–6 mm lip of cartilage that remained along the anterior margin only.

With approximately 40% of the posterior third of the medial meniscus resected using a combination of baskets and shaver, attention was then turned to the trochlear notch, and the ACL was found to be viable and patent with anterior drawer testing. The lateral joint line was then entered, and the lateral meniscus at the middle of the lateral third was found to have a near full-thickness radial tear which required resection of approximately 80% of the meniscus at the apex of the lateral tear. This was then tapered both anteriorly and posteriorly and shaved to a smooth and stable meniscal base. No other meniscal tears or injury about the lateral compartment were identified, including the femoral condyle and/or tibial plateau. The lateral gutter was likewise found to be free of any loose bodies and did not contain any significant synovitis. With the medial and lateral menisci addressed, attention was then turned with the knee in full extension to the medial plica which was resected using the same 4.5 mm incisor plus shaver utilized for the meniscal resections. With this also accomplished and well documented photographically, the knee was then drained of excess arthroscopic fluid. The arthroscopic equipment was removed from the knee and the knee portals were then sutured with 4-0 nylon using a simple interrupted suture, dressed with Silvadene, Telfa, fluffy gauze, and overwrapped with a sterile Ace wrap from the foot to midthigh. The patient was then awakened from anesthesia, taken to the postanesthesia recovery room in excellent condition, having tolerated the procedure well with no complications.

ESTIMATED BLOOD LOSS
Minimal.

TOURNIQUET TIME
15 minutes.

DRAINS
None.

DISPOSITION
The patient will be taken to the postanesthesia recovery room and transferred home once criteria are met. She will be asked to elevate and ice her left lower extremity and use Ibuprofen and Vicodin as necessary to control her pain. She will also be asked to follow up in approximately 5-7 days at the office for an early wound check and was advised that should she experience any significant nausea and/or vomiting, chest pain, shortness of breath, dizziness, loss of consciousness, or have any other questions, to call the office for immediate further instructions.

Sample Report 6A

Lumbar Spine—2 Views

INDICATION
Status post fall.

FINDINGS
Grade I anterolisthesis at L4-5. Grade I retrolisthesis at L3-4. Mild wedging of L1. Mild loss of vertebral body height at L2, L3, and L4. Mild to moderate wedging of T12. Moderate anterior osteophytosis. Degenerative facet disease at L4-5 and L5-S1. Mild levoscoliosis.

IMPRESSION
1. Moderate wedging of T12. Mild wedging of L1. Mild loss of vertebral body height at L2, L3, and L4. Uncertain chronicity.
2. Degenerative changes, as above.

Sample Report 6B

Progress Note

SUBJECTIVE
This is a lady who has had anterior lumbar interbody fusion, which did not heal, and then she had a secondary procedure by me 2½ years ago for a posterior fusion at L4-5. She has had an excellent result and has had no problems with her back until recently. She has had no recent history of trauma, but she has severe back pain. She has no true radicular pain. She has pain in the medial aspect of the right knee.

OBJECTIVE
On physical exam, she has limited lumbar motion with reproduction of back pain and pain over the anserine bursa, indicating a bursitis.

IMAGING
Her x-rays today show good position of her construct with no evidence of any adjacent disk disease of any significance.

PLAN
I would like to get an MRI to rule out herniated nucleus pulposus. We will see her in 10 days. I am going to put her on Naprosyn for her anserine bursitis.

Sample Report 6C

History and Physical

CHIEF COMPLAINT
Right-sided low back pain radiating down the right buttock, down the outside of his thigh, down the outside of his calf, and down the inside of his thigh.

PRESENT ILLNESS
This is a 31-year-old right-hand dominant male who had the above symptoms with onset in November 20XX. He states initially it started kind of low in his back and over the next several months worsened to include his leg. He states his pain now is 100% in his leg with a 7 out of 10 on the pain scale. He states his symptoms are worse with straining, sitting, driving, bending forward, lying on his right or left side, walking, twisting and bending forward, and lifting. He states that sitting is the worst, whereas standing is the best. He has numbness in the right leg and calf. He denies weakness. He has morning pain and pain throughout the day but denies fever, chills, night sweats, and has no new bowel or bladder problems. He has undergone physical therapy throughout this ordeal and he initially had gotten better. He was recently placed on a Medrol Dosepak. He did improve somewhat with the first 2 days of treatment but developed symptoms again in the latter days of the treatment. He is actually here for a second opinion. He was told he needed an interbody fusion.

IMAGING
He presents with an MRI performed on 04/01/20XX that shows an L2-3 posterior disk bulge impinging on the central spinal canal that is superimposed on bilateral facet arthritis. There is slight bilateral foraminal narrowing without nerve root impingement. At L3-4, there is a circumferential disk bulge that is superimposed on a posterior disk protrusion lateralizing toward the right with inferior extension behind L4.

Flexion and extension views of the lumbar spine show a degenerative disk at L3-4. There is no spondylolisthesis noted. There are no fractures noted.

IMPRESSION
1. Degenerative disk L3-4.
2. Herniated nucleus pulposus, right far lateral L3-4.

PLAN
At this time, I have recommended microdiskectomy far lateral on the right at L3-4. His neurosurgeon has suggested an XLIF. At this time, I do not think that is an avenue he should explore. He has not really ever had symptoms prior to the herniation. He will make his decision and schedule a far lateral right microdiskectomy should he so desire.

Sample Report 7A

Urodynamics

The patient was placed in the dorsal lithotomy position. A 7-French double-lumen catheter was placed per urethra into the bladder. The rectal probe was inserted as a 7-French abdominal sensor. External EMG patches were placed in the perineum. Prior to the procedure, a uroflow was performed with a postvoid residual urine. The patient was filled with sterile water at a fill rate of 60 mL/min. The patient was filled to capacity, and voiding pressure studies were performed. Following that, the flow rate was performed for the pressure-flow phase of the study. This is a 7-channel output and the findings are as follows: Uroflow was 93 mL. A peak flow of 13 mL/s with a postvoid residual urine of only 30. Her cystometrogram was carried out. Her first sensation was at 41 and her maximum capacity was 60. She had a detrusor contraction of 49 cmH$_2$O. She did have overactivity with leak, and she was unable to inhibit her contractions. Her capacity was small at only 60. She had no detrusor-sphincter dyssynergia. She had urinary urge incontinence, and the compliance was difficult to measure because of the minimal amount of capacity.

ASSESSMENT
Hyperreflexic bladder with stress urinary incontinence.

Sample Report 8A

Consultation

REASON FOR CONSULTATION
Possible pneumonia.

HISTORY OF PRESENT ILLNESS
The patient is a 95-year-old white male with a history of congestive heart failure who was admitted to Presbyterian Hospital on July 12, 20XX, with evidence of an acute myocardial infarction with congestive heart failure. His chest x-ray on admission showed bilateral pulmonary infiltrates compatible with edema. He had an elevated white blood cell count. Blood cultures were obtained and have remained negative. The patient was treated conservatively initially. A couple of days later, because of increased pulmonary infiltrates, a quinolone antibiotic was added for possible pneumonia. He continued to have leukocytosis, although he did not have any significant fever. In the last 24 hours, the patient has developed progressive hypotension and was started on vasopressors. He subsequently developed runs of ventricular tachycardia and was transferred to the ICU setting. His chest x-ray shows significant worsening of his pulmonary infiltrates. He also has developed progressive elevation of his creatinine. The Levaquin was switched to moxifloxacin. An infectious disease consultation is requested in regard to management of antimicrobial therapy in this case.

PAST MEDICAL HISTORY
Remarkable for a history of cholelithiasis, recent history of cholecystitis, status post percutaneous placement of a drain in his gallbladder. A recent culture from the bile draining from his gallbladder grew Klebsiella pneumoniae. Patient has a history of significant congestive heart failure. He has a history of gastroesophageal reflux disease. He has a history of hypothyroidism. He is status post an ERCP and gallbladder drain placement as above.

FAMILY HISTORY
Noncontributory.

SOCIAL HISTORY
He lives at Presbyterian Village North and is widowed. There is no history of alcohol use or smoking cigarettes.

REVIEW OF SYSTEMS
Difficult to obtain as the patient is currently short of breath on nonrebreather mask, with runs of ventricular tachycardia.

PHYSICAL EXAMINATION
He is alert. His vital signs show a blood pressure of 98/64, a pulse of 108, and on the monitor he has runs of ventricular tachycardia. Respiratory rate 34. O_2 saturation 97% on nonrebreather mask with oxygen at 15 L/min. HEENT: Pupils equal and reactive to light. There is no pallor or jaundice. Oral cavity without thrush. Neck is supple. Chest with bilateral rales. Heart with tachycardia, off and on, irregular. I did not auscultate any murmurs. No rubs were appreciated. Abdomen is soft and does not appear to be tender. I did not elicit any guarding or rebound.

There is a drain in the right upper quadrant draining bile. Bowel sounds are present and somewhat hyperactive. Skin with no rashes. Lower extremities show no edema or cyanosis. There is no clubbing.

LABORATORY DATA
CBC shows a white blood cell count of 14.2, hemoglobin 12.5, hematocrit 37%, and platelet count 425,000. His sodium is 141, potassium 4.7, chloride 106, CO_2 22, glucose 222, BUN 65, and creatinine 2.1. His BNP remains elevated at 2563. Blood cultures x2 on admission were negative. A culture from the bile from the drain in his gallbladder grew a pansensitive Klebsiella pneumoniae. Urine culture from admission showed no growth. Chest x-ray shows extensive bilateral upper lung zone pulmonary infiltrates, slightly worse within the perihilar regions, consistent with pulmonary edema versus pulmonary infiltrates.

IMPRESSION
This is a very elderly man with known history of congestive heart failure who presented with shortness of breath and an acute myocardial infarction. Certainly, his leukocytosis and abnormal chest x-ray could be compatible with his presentation of acute myocardial infarction. However, within the last 24 hours, he has significantly worsened his clinical condition with hypotension requiring vasopressors and also the development of runs of ventricular tachycardia. Worsening of his pulmonary infiltrates could be due exclusively to his cardiac problems, but I cannot completely rule out the possibility of the development of a lower respiratory tract infection.

RECOMMENDATIONS
Will continue moxifloxacin as ordered and will add cefepime 1 g IV piggyback every 12 hours. If the creatinine continues to rise, we may need to adjust the cefepime dose. If he is able to produce any sputum, we will order a sputum for culture and sensitivity. Also would like to obtain 2 additional blood cultures 15–30 minutes apart today.

Sample Report 9A

New Patient Consult

HISTORY OF PRESENT ILLNESS

The patient is a 56-year-old female with multiple cardiovascular risk factors who is scheduled to undergo hip replacement surgery tomorrow. An EKG done as part of her preoperative evaluation revealed questionable previous anterior infarct and questionable inferior ischemia. Cardiac evaluation was subsequently requested. The patient has no symptoms of angina or shortness of breath on mild exertion, orthopnea, or paroxysmal nocturnal dyspnea. She has no palpitations.

PAST MEDICAL HISTORY

1. Type 2 diabetes mellitus, known for about 1 year.
2. Hypertension, known for 3 years.
3. Dyslipidemia with elevated triglycerides.
4. History of deep venous thrombosis and pulmonary embolism twice in 20XX and 20XX.
5. Osteoarthritis.
6. Hypothyroidism.
7. Edema.

CURRENT MEDICATIONS

Triamterene HCTZ 75/50 mg daily; Mobic 7.5 mg b.i.d.; atenolol 50 mg daily; Synthroid 0.088 mg daily; TriCor 145 mg daily; Januvia 100 mg daily; Coumadin daily, which was stopped on 10/11/20XX as part of her plan for surgery as described above; hydrocodone p.r.n.; aspirin 81 mg daily (discontinued 1 week ago).

ALLERGIES

PENICILLIN

SOCIAL HISTORY

Married with no children. She lives with her husband who is present today. She continues to work. She has no history of smoking or alcohol abuse. She follows a diabetic diet. No regular exercise activity. Her mobility has been limited because of her severe hip arthralgia. She is using a cane.

FAMILY HISTORY

Her father died at age 57 of metastatic kidney cancer. He had a myocardial infarction at the age of 49. Her mother died at age 77 of breast cancer. One brother has a known history of coronary artery disease and had several percutaneous interventions at age 47 and 49. Another brother, who is 58 years old, has no heart disease.

REVIEW OF SYSTEMS

She has been overweight for a few years. No recent fever or chills. She has been complaining of easy fatigability and lack of energy. No recent visual disturbance. No chronic headache.

No symptoms of lightheadedness, dizziness, or syncope. No history of stroke or seizure disorder. She does have occasional ankle edema. No complaints of palpitations. No chronic cough or sputum. No wheezing. No nausea, vomiting, abdominal pain. No history of GI bleed, melena, or hematuria. No history of gout. She does have severe arthralgia in her hips. No symptoms of claudication. She does complain of easy bruising.

PHYSICAL EXAMINATION
This is a pleasant, moderately overweight female in no acute distress. Her weight is 213 pounds. Blood pressure is 112/74. Heart rate is 67 beats per minute. Mucosae are moist. There is no conjunctival icterus. Neck: There is no jugular venous distention. Carotid upstrokes are symmetrical with no carotid bruits. There is no cervical lymphadenopathy and no thyroid mass or goiter. Chest is clear with no rales or wheezing. Breath sounds are symmetrical. Heart: The PMI is not discernible. Cardiac rhythm is regular. There is no murmur, rub, or gallop. Abdomen is soft, obese, and nontender. Extremities: Trace edema seen around her ankles. Distal pulses are present and symmetrical. No clubbing or cyanosis. No motor deficits in the upper or lower extremities.

ELECTROCARDIOGRAM: The EKG done today showed sinus rhythm with a rate of 67 beats per minute and mild ST-segment depression in the inferior lead with nonspecific Q-wave abnormalities in the precordial leads.

ECHOCARDIOGRAM: The echocardiogram done today showed normal left ventricular systolic function with no segmental wall motion abnormalities. No significant valvular abnormalities seen.

NUCLEAR STRESS TEST: An adenosine nuclear stress test was performed today. It showed normal myocardial perfusion with no evidence of myocardial ischemia or prior infarct. Her left ventricular ejection fraction was normal at 70%.

ASSESSMENT AND PLAN
1. Cardiac preoperative evaluation before hip replacement surgery with evidence of abnormal EKG and multiple cardiovascular risk factors with strong family history of premature coronary artery disease. Her nuclear stress test is normal, which indicates low likelihood of inducible myocardial ischemia or obstructive coronary artery disease. I reassured her about her heart condition. I explained to her that her cardiac risk to her upcoming surgery is low.
2. Hypertension, well controlled on her current regimen.
3. Previous history of pulmonary embolism, on Coumadin therapy. An IVC filter was placed 2 weeks ago.
4. Dyslipidemia, on TriCor. Optimal lipid control is indicated in this patient with numerous cardiovascular risk factors.

Sample Report 10A

Consultation

HISTORY OF PRESENT ILLNESS
This is a 38-year-old lady who is being referred for joint pain and apparently increased inflammatory markers. She claims that about 3–4 months ago she had been having intermittent pain, initially in the foot and subsequently in the knee, hands, and the shoulder. She said that she has pain in the knee whenever she is walking, standing, and climbing up the stairs, and she takes ibuprofen p.r.n. for pain. Likewise, she has been having a lot of pain in the hands, the wrists, with a morning stiffness of about 30 minutes. Recently she has also been complaining of shoulder pain, more on the right compared to the left, and has difficulty elevating the shoulder, for which she was actually prescribed ibuprofen. Subsequently she saw Dr. Smith who did an inflammatory marker, which was high (the result of which we do not know). She likewise had an x-ray, which we also do not know the results. For about 3 months, she claims that she had some mild dry mouth, and about a year ago started complaining of intermittent hair loss. Likewise, the patient has a history of PE. She was diagnosed 10 years ago and was admitted to the hospital. She had an initial thoracentesis and subsequently was seen by a pulmonary doctor. She was put on Coumadin for 1 year and since then has not been on any Coumadin. She denies any history of birth control pill use at that time. The patient was not sure whether she had a full workup for this or not.

PAST MEDICAL HISTORY
1. Negative for diabetes.
2. Negative for hypertension.
3. Negative for depression.

PAST SURGICAL HISTORY
She has had a thoracentesis but no previous surgery.

MEDICATIONS
1. Calcium with vitamin D 600 twice a day.
2. Ibuprofen 800 mg 3 times a day.

ALLERGIES
None.

FAMILY HISTORY
Diabetes (father). Negative for hypertension. Negative for cardiac disease. Negative for arthritis.

SOCIAL HISTORY
Nonsmoker. No alcohol. No use of drugs.

REVIEW OF SYSTEMS
She denies any oral ulcers. No malar rash. No Raynaud's. No dyspareunia. No recurrent candida infection. She denies any pleurisy though she does complain of intermittent shortness of breath. No chest pain. No melena. No hematochezia. No seizure, loss of consciousness, DVT. No recent pulmonary embolism. She is gravida 2, para 2-0-0-2. The children are now ages 4 and 7.

PHYSICAL EXAMINATION

VITAL SIGNS: Blood pressure 134/90, pulse rate 100, respiratory rate 20, temperature 98.2, weight 158, height 5 feet 1 inch.

HEENT: There is definitely thinning of the hair with alopecia on the vertex as well as on the temporal area. No malar rash. No Raynaud's. No oral ulcers.

NECK: JVP is normal.

HEART: Regular rate and rhythm.

LUNGS: No crackles. No wheezes.

ABDOMEN: Soft, nontender. No hepatosplenomegaly.

MUSCULOSKELETAL: There is mild limitation in range of motion of the left shoulder compared to the right. Elbow, wrists: No synovitis. MCPs, PIPs: Tender but no frank synovitis. Minimal synovitis, 2nd and 3rd PIP. Hip range of motion is normal. Crepitation in both knees. Positive for squeeze sign. Ankle and MTP: No synovitis.

DIAGNOSTIC DATA

No laboratories, though the patient claims that she had a previous HIV test during pregnancy that was negative.

ASSESSMENT

1. Polyarthralgia with alopecia.
2. History of spontaneous pulmonary embolism.
3. Dry mouth. Rule out systemic lupus erythematosus, rule out Sjögren's, rule out rheumatoid arthritis.

PLAN

I would like to get a shoulder x-ray, bilateral knees, bilateral hands with Norgaard view, bilateral knees with weightbearing view, bilateral feet, and a chest x-ray. I would like to get a lupus anticoagulant, beta 2-glycoprotein, anticardiolipin antibodies, and antiphospholipid antibodies. Recheck CBC, CMP, ESR, CRP, ANA, specific antibodies, hepatitis B and C, C3, C4, UA, B_{12}, folate, CPK, aldolase, and vitamin D. Return visit in 6–8 weeks.

Sample Report 10B

Progress Note

HISTORY OF PRESENT ILLNESS
The patient says that she has been doing fine. No significant joint pain. A few Raynaud's with the changes in the weather, but at the present time she said Raynaud's seems to not bother her. No reflux recently. She has been watching what she is eating.

MEDICATIONS
1. Diovan 80 mg daily.
2. Plaquenil 200 mg twice a day.
3. Calcium twice a day.

REVIEW OF SYSTEMS
She denies any fever. No chills. No cough. No chest pain. No PND. No melena or hematochezia.

PHYSICAL EXAMINATION
VITAL SIGNS: Blood pressure 120/80, pulse rate 72, respiratory rate 18, weight 147.
HEENT: A few telangiectasias on the face. Dilated capillary folds. No Raynaud's. No oral ulcers. No malar rash.
HEART: Regular rate, rhythm.
ABDOMEN: Soft, nontender. No hepatosplenomegaly.
MUSCULOSKELETAL: Shoulder, elbow, wrist: No synovitis. MCPs, PIPs: No synovitis. Crepitation in both knees. Ankle and MTP: No synovitis.
NEUROLOGIC: No localizing sign.

DIAGNOSTIC DATA
Pulmonary function test did show normal lung volumes except for a slight decrease in the residual volume. Airway resistance normal. Diffusing capacity is normal; however, compared to previous study there is a slight drop in the residual volume and mild drop in the diffusing capacity.

Echocardiogram shows a pulmonary systolic pressure of 28, mild TR, mild MR.

ASSESSMENT
1. Systemic lupus erythematosus, Sjögren's overlap, biopsy-proven with scleroderma antibody positive, dilated capillary fold, and Raynaud's.
2. Mild mitral regurgitation, tricuspid regurgitation.

PLAN
Discussed with the patient the results of the echo as well as pulmonary function tests. I would like to repeat the chest x-ray including high resolution CT and DL_{CO}. Recheck the CBC, CMP, and the urinalysis. Patient is planning to go to Mexico in the next few months. I would like to see the patient in 2 weeks and continue present medication.

Sample Report 11A

New Patient History and Physical

HISTORY OF PRESENT ILLNESS

Lindsey is a 17 year-old nulligravida who is here for evaluation of primary amenorrhea. She turned 17 in January. Despite a history of normal pubertal development (breast development, adrenarche), she has never had a menses. She is the youngest of 3 girls. Her mother Elizabeth notes that her second daughter (age 22) also had late onset of menses (age 16½). Testing to date has included FSH 5.3 and estradiol 10, negative pregnancy test, and normal prolactin (7.2), and TSH level (1.9). Because of hypoestrogenism, she underwent an MRI of the brain that was reportedly normal. The report is not available today. This was apparently complicated by contrast allergy. She reports that she had a transabdominal pelvic sonogram that showed no signs of obstruction and a normal uterus. Lindsey said that breast development began at approximately age 12. She has experienced completely normal, full adult growth. Likewise, pubic and axillary hair began developing at age 11 or 12. She is not sexually active and has never tried to insert a tampon. She admits that she has been experiencing some increased hair growth, specifically on the upper lip and chin area (sparse to few terminal hairs) over the last 4 years. She is using waxing for this on a regular basis.

MEDICATIONS
None.

ALLERGIES
Contrast.

PAST MEDICAL HISTORY
1. Mild asthma, mostly related to seasonal allergies (not on any regular medications).
2. Depression, which she feels is related to stress, and she has occasional panic attacks (not currently on medication).

SURGICAL HISTORY
Tonsillectomy and adenoidectomy in 20XX.

SOCIAL HISTORY
Lindsey is an upcoming senior in high school. She does not smoke or use alcohol. Caffeine use is minimal.

FAMILY HISTORY
Negative for any known genetic or congenital abnormalities. Her mother, Elizabeth, notes that she has a diagnosis of protein S deficiency, which was diagnosed during her sister's evaluation for history of recurrent DVTs. Her sister's testing showed protein S deficiency, and therefore, Elizabeth was tested before she underwent laparoscopy for TAH/BSO for diagnosis of granulosa cell tumor.

Interestingly, Elizabeth had 3 uneventful pregnancies, although she believes she may have had a postpartum DVT after her 2nd pregnancy. Lindsey's oldest sister (age 24) had genetic testing showing a normal protein S level. Lindsey and her middle sister have never undergone testing. Family history is positive for heart disease, hypertension, and diabetes. She is of mixed European ancestry.

PHYSICAL EXAMINATION:
VITAL SIGNS: Height 5 feet 4 inches   Weight 172 pounds   BMI 29.5   BP 130/68   Pulse 90
GENERAL: Well-appearing, well-nourished female in no acute distress.
HEENT: Neck supple, normal thyroid, no lymphadenopathy.
LUNGS: Clear throughout and symmetric.
CARDIAC: Normal rate and rhythm. No rubs, murmurs, or gallops.
BREASTS: Symmetrical without masses. Tanner stage 4. No nipple discharge.
ABDOMEN: Soft, nontender, no masses. Normal bowel sounds. No surgical incisions. No organomegaly.
SKIN: Minimal facial acne. Moderate hair growth along the upper lip and chin area. The lower back has a moderate to large amount of excess terminal hairs that extend into the upper buttock area. There is a small amount of terminal hair on the midline to the level of the umbilicus. There are a few strands of hair around the nipples bilaterally. No tattoos, rashes, or abnormal piercings. No acanthosis nigricans.
EXTREMITIES: No edema. No palpable cords or tenderness.
PELVIC: Normal external female genitalia. Hymen is intact. Pelvic exam deferred.

ULTRASOUND

Transabdominal sonogram is done with the bladder moderately filled. The uterus is seen and is anteverted and nonenlarged. The uterus is 5 cm in length, 2.5 cm in AP diameter. The ovaries can be seen and appear to be fairly multifollicular. The right ovary is 45 x 32 mm. The left ovary is 30 x 28 mm. There appears to be greater than 20 antral follicles on her ovaries. There does not appear to be a pelvic mass.

ASSESSMENT
1. 17-year-old with primary amenorrhea (normal gonadotropic hyperandrogenism).
2. History of normal cranial imaging and reported normal pelvic sonography showing normal, unobstructed anatomy. Today's sonogram demonstrates multifollicular ovaries.
3. Contrast allergy.
4. Family history of protein S deficiency (mother and maternal aunt).

PLAN: A 17-OHP and DHEAS, total and free testosterone, and protein S activity were drawn today. Interestingly, we started discussing possible options for cycle control before Lindsey's mother started discussing the possible family thrombotic disorder. I think that if Lindsey's testing is negative, she may still be a good candidate for low-dose OCPs. I briefly explained to her that the default diagnosis was that of hyperandrogenic anovulation or PCOS. However, other conditions need to be ruled out. With her low serum estrogen levels, she would be a good candidate for oral contraceptive pills, mainly for bone protection. However, if she has concurrent thrombotic disorder, the risks would probably outweigh the benefit. In that case, if she is profoundly hypoestrogenic, bone density measurements would probably be reasonable sometime soon. We will have them schedule a phone consultation or return visit after the above testing. If this is normal, I will suggest that she undergo a progestin withdrawal; although, with her low estrogen level and thin endometrium (6 mm today) she may not have a withdrawal bleed. If her protein S testing is normal, then we will discuss the use of oral contraceptive pills.

Sample Report 11B

History and Physical Report

HISTORY OF PRESENT ILLNESS
This is a 21-year-old Caucasian female, now G2, P1, SAB 1.

Prenatal care initiated on December 14, 20XX, and proceeded for 6 visits. Blood type is O positive, negative serology, rubella immune, with negative HBsAg, HIV, HSV, GC and chlamydia, with a normal Pap smear. Her MSAFP was normal. Her Glucola was negative and her group B strep is pending. She was taking prenatal vitamins and had no known drug allergies. Her problems and risks were associated with some malnutrition prior to her presenting for obstetrical care. Ultrasound at 21 weeks and 5 days confirmed a pregnancy at 20 weeks and 4 days. Her prenatal course was essentially negative.

Tricia had called the hospital at approximately 8 o'clock or 8:30 on the evening of May 3, 20XX, stating that she felt like she had started contractions. She was told to come in for evaluation and did not arrive until approximately 11:30 secondary to inability to get a ride. Upon her arrival, nursing staff found her to have a cervix at 7.5 cm, 90% effaced, and bulging membranes. I was contacted at home. I proceeded to the clinic to obtain her records, which had not yet been forwarded to the hospital. Her records were copied and placed within her chart, and ampicillin was ordered for unknown group-B status. It was also requested that Respiratory Therapy and CRNA be contacted for the possibility of respiratory dysfunction in the newborn.

Fetal heart tones were noted to be in the 130s with some accelerations into the 150s and contractions every 2 to 3 minutes. No remarkable or consistent decelerations were noted. After spontaneous rupture of membranes just prior to delivery, the infant continued to progress quite rapidly. Delivery of the head occurred at approximately 10 minutes after midnight on the morning of May 4. Because of mom's high position in the bed, the baby could not be suctioned prior to delivering the shoulders. Once the baby was completely delivered, bulb suction was performed of the mouth and nares. Then clamping of the umbilical cord was performed and the cord was severed. It should be noted that mom received 50 mcg of fentanyl prior to delivery for analgesia secondary to our inability to get an epidural placed quickly enough. In actuality, she had progressed so rapidly that it was deemed more complicating and distracting than beneficial to perform the epidural.

Upon delivery of the infant over a secondary perineal laceration, the infant was noted to be somewhat cyanotic and floppy. Weak respiratory efforts were noted. The infant was quickly passed to nursing staff who took him to the warmer and proceeded with routine stimulation, drying, and blow-by oxygen. Heart rate was reported in the 150s but began to decline. Positive-pressure ventilations were provided for approximately 1 minute, during which Narcan 0.3 mg was administered for a total of 3. The infant quickly began to resolve his symptoms and Apgar scores were reported as 5 and 8. He has had some mild grunting, mild retraction, but is holding his O_2 sats in the high 90s with blow-by. He currently has been placed under an Oxy-Hood at 40% oxygen and is maintaining his O_2 sats in the high 90s as well.

Attention was turned to mom's perineal laceration. The area was anesthetized with 1% lidocaine without epinephrine and 2-0 chromic was used to close the laceration. Fundal massage resulted in brisk clamping down of the uterus without the assistance of Pitocin. Mom is currently resting at baby's warmer in a wheelchair in good spirits.

OBJECTIVE
VITAL SIGNS: Pulse 84, respirations 18, temperature is 97.7, blood pressure 121/76.
GENERAL: She is alert and oriented, talkative but relaxed, in no acute distress.
LUNGS: Clear.
HEART: Regular.
ABDOMEN: Rotund. Uterus firming.
EXTREMITIES: Spontaneously moving all 4 extremities.

IMPRESSION
1. A 21-year-old Caucasian female now gravida 2, para 1, with 1 SAB, status post normal spontaneous vaginal delivery at 35 weeks' gestation.
2. Status post repair of a second-degree perineal laceration.

PLAN
Routine observation and postpartum orders are anticipated.

Sample Report 12A

Consultation

I had the pleasure of seeing James Ford today for ongoing followup and management of his newly defined lymphoproliferative disorder. Please see below a summary of my evaluation.

HISTORY OF PRESENT ILLNESS
1. Stage IIB Hodgkin disease, diagnosed November 19XX. Patient presented with right supraclavicular adenopathy and bilateral hilar adenopathy. Biopsy confirmed Hodgkin disease, subtype unknown. CT scanning and gallium scanning confirmed disease only above the diaphragm. Treated at Massachusetts General Hospital with Adriamycin, bleomycin, Velban, and DTIC with 6 cycles completed May 19XX, complete response. Total nodal or mantel irradiation given in consolidation.
2. Evolving pancytopenia, 20XX. The patient underwent evaluation in September due to white blood cell count in the 4 range, hemoglobin 12, hematocrit mid-30% range, and platelet count in the 110,000 to 120,000 range. Peripheral blood revealed slightly increased percentage of mature-appearing lymphocytes. Blood work revealed erythrocyte sedimentation rate 16, beta 2-microglobulin 4.1, negative direct agglutination test, haptoglobin less than 6, no microangiopathic changes on smear, normal LDH at 179. Reticulocyte count 2%. Peripheral blood immunophenotypic studies, September 14, 20XX, revealed a CD5-positive co-expressing B-cell population suspicious for a lymphoproliferative disorder; this comprising less than 10% of the total cells evaluated. Bone marrow biopsy and aspirate revealed a mature B-cell lymphoma consistent with chronic lymphocytic leukemia or small lymphocytic lymphoma. Lymphocytes appear to comprise approximately 50% of nucleated cells. No dysplastic change in the red blood cells or platelets were noted. Bone marrow immunophenotypic studies revealed an abnormal CD5 population of lymphocytes that appeared to stain positive for CD45, CD19, CD20, CD5, CD22, CD23, and HLA-DR. Negative staining for CD10, CD38. Chest and abdominal CT scanning, September 20XX, revealed no evidence of lymphadenopathy. Mild splenomegaly was noted. Clinical picture felt most suggestive for stage IVA non-Hodgkin lymphoma or Rai stage IV chronic lymphocytic leukemia based on anemia and thrombocytopenia. FISH analysis on lymphocytes pending.
3. Chronic lymphocytic leukemia/small lymphocytic lymphoma, diagnosed October 20XX. See above.

TREATMENT: Hodgkin disease treated with Adriamycin, bleomycin, Velban, and DTIC for 6 cycles, completed May 19XX, followed by total nodal irradiation, management at Massachusetts General Hospital. ABVD reportedly well tolerated.

PAST MEDICAL HISTORY
1. Hypertension.
2. Hypothyroidism.
3. Adult-onset diabetes mellitus diagnosed April 20XX.
4. Status post cholecystectomy.
5. Renal insufficiency, diagnosed 20XX.
6. Hypercholesterolemia.
7. Hypothyroidism.
8. Erectile dysfunction.

MEDICATIONS
1. Synthroid.
2. Hydrochlorothiazide.
3. Avapro.
4. Metformin.
5. Atenolol.
6. Prilosec.
7. Lisinopril.
8. Multivitamin.
9. Gemfibrozil.
10. Cialis as needed.

ALLERGIES
No known drug allergies.

SOCIAL HISTORY
He continues to work full-time as a police officer. He completed his master's degree this summer. He had a son who died of relapsed acute lymphoblastic leukemia at age 9 during the time that he was undergoing treatment for his Hodgkin disease. He does not smoke and drinks alcohol occasionally.

FAMILY HISTORY
No history of blood dyscrasias.

INTERVAL HISTORY
Jim returns to the office today for a scheduled visit. He is here largely to discuss his newly diagnosed lymphoproliferative disorder. He is following up about 2 weeks after the confirmatory bone marrow biopsy and aspirate. Today, he reports feeling reasonably well. His fatigue is slightly improved. He has no new fevers, chills, sweats, bruising, or bleeding. He has no new headache or dizziness. He has not experienced any new anorexia or weight loss. He is still working as usual.

REVIEW OF SYSTEMS
GENERAL: Negative for fatigue, weight loss, weight gain.
SKIN: Negative for rash, bruising.
ENT: Negative for change in hearing, tinnitus, sinus pain, hoarseness, sore throat, mouth sores.
EYES: Negative for change in vision, blurred vision, double vision.
HEART: Negative for chest pain, palpitations, ankle swelling.
LUNGS: Negative for cough, shortness of breath, hemoptysis, wheezing.
GASTROINTESTINAL: Negative for nausea, vomiting, dysphagia, abdominal pain, constipation, diarrhea, blood in stool, jaundice.
GENITOURINARY: Negative for hematuria, dysuria, incontinence.
MUSCULOSKELETAL: Negative for bone pain, joint pain.
NEUROLOGICAL: Negative for headache, weakness, numbness, tingling.
PSYCHOLOGICAL: Negative for anxiety, depression.
IMMUNE: Negative for fever, adenopathy.
ENDOCRINE: Negative for increased thirst, sweats, tremor.

PHYSICAL EXAMINATION: Shows an overall comfortable-appearing gentleman. Vital signs show a temperature of 98, heart rate 80 and regular, respiratory rate 18, blood pressure 122/70, weight 257 pounds. HEENT exam shows anicteric sclerae, no oral lesions or thrush. Neck supple without cervical or supraclavicular adenopathy. There is no thyromegaly. Lungs are clear. Good bilateral breath sounds. Cardiac exam shows regular rate and rhythm, no extra heart sounds or murmurs. Chest wall exam is unremarkable. Abdominal exam reveals no organomegaly or masses and is nontender; no abdominal wall tenderness or nodularity. There is no peripheral adenopathy. Extremity exam reveals no cyanosis, clubbing, edema. Back reveals no spinal or paraspinal tenderness. Neurologic exam is nonfocal. Patient is alert, oriented, appropriate. Skin exam reveals no petechia or purpura.

IMPRESSION

1. Prior history stage IIB Hodgkin disease. No evidence of recurrence.
2. Chronic lymphocytic leukemia/small lymphocytic lymphoma. Today, I spent about an hour with Jim discussing the newly diagnosed lymphoproliferative disorder. We discussed the incidence of seeing a non-Hodgkin lymphoma present years out from being treated successfully for Hodgkin disease. Technically speaking, the patient would be considered to have a stage IVA non-Hodgkin lymphoma or chronic lymphocytic leukemia. It is likely that the slightly reduced blood count is related to the bone marrow disease as well as perhaps the mild splenomegaly. We are at least pleased that the patient has no systemic symptoms outside of mild fatigue. I mentioned to Jim that the mechanism of a possible hemolytic component is less clear, as typically we will find patients to have a Coombs-positive hemolytic process in this setting. In any case, I reviewed with Jim the typical management of a patient with his disorder. We will typically consider an observation or surveillance strategy until complications demand active therapy. In terms of treatment options, I reviewed everything from oral chlorambucil, Rituxan, to newer regimens consisting of bendamustine or fludarabine. Jim understands the paradox of having a typically low-grade or indolent process yet incurable disease. We are clearly hoping that the new molecular therapies will come through with more durable responses. We also discussed the possibility of participating in a clinical research trial. Importantly, I still await the set of genetic and molecular studies on the bone marrow. I made Jim aware of the ability to use molecular analysis to better prognosticate and even help refine treatment options. He is aware that in his case it is likely the blood counts that may be the parameter most closely followed for indication for therapy. We also discussed complications related to this disorder, including an increased risk for infection and even solid tumors over time.
3. Pancytopenia. Mild, stable.
4. Fatigue. Likely multifactorial. At least potentially related to lymphoproliferative disorder.
5. Disposition: The patient's spirits and attitude remain hopeful.

RECOMMENDATIONS

Jim was provided extensive reading materials on non-Hodgkin lymphoma as well as chronic lymphocytic leukemia. He was given a copy of the National Comprehensive Cancer Network guidelines on overall management. At this time, we are holding off on active therapy based on the lack of complications from his disease and manageable fatigue. His blood counts will be closely followed. I await the set of genetic studies and FISH analysis on his bone marrow.

I have offered to have Jim see colleagues, either at Massachusetts General Hospital or Dana Farber for a second opinion. He will give this consideration. We discussed the importance of undergoing a flu shot. I asked him to practice good health habits given his increased risk for infection. He will be following up with you in the near future. He apparently will finish a course of prednisone for reactive airway disease. By the end of our lengthy meeting, I had spent over 50% of the time on counselling and discussing the above issues.

Sample Report 12B

Consultation

I saw Eleanor today in consultation with her daughter Carol for ongoing management of MALT lymphoma, history of breast cancer, and lung cancer. Eleanor reports chronic constipation with typically small bowel movements every 2–3 days. She reports no change in her chronic neuropathy. She denies nausea, vomiting, abdominal pain, blood in stool, fever, night sweats, lymphadenopathy, or change in her breasts or chest wall. She plans to move out of her condominium into a small apartment soon. She does not smoke and typically has 3–4 alcoholic beverages per week.

HISTORY OF PRESENT ILLNESS

1. Stage IIA, T2N0M0, well-differentiated infiltrating ductal carcinoma of the left breast, diagnosed in 19XX when the patient was found to have multiple, new, well-defined nodules in the axillary tail of the left breast by mammography. Total tumor size was 3.2 x 2 x 1 cm. There was extensive grade I cribriform intraductal carcinoma and focal lymphatic space invasion. Eight axillary nodes were negative for metastases. Final surgical margins were clear. Estrogen receptor 90%, progesterone receptor 70%, Ki-67 10% by immunohistochemistry. Treatment included left wire-localization biopsy, left modified radical mastectomy, and tamoxifen 20 mg daily for 5 years.

2. Stage IIAe extranodal, marginal zone B-cell lymphoma of mucosa-associated lymphoid tissue (MALT lymphoma) of the transverse colon and appendix, diagnosed May 4, 20XX, when patient underwent colonoscopy to evaluate an abnormal PET scan. The tumor extended through the muscularis propria to the serosal surface. The tumor size was 10 x 6 x 2 cm with an exophytic and focally ulcerating configuration. The proximal ileal resection margin was equivocal for involvement by lymphoma; the distal margin was clear, and the radial and mesenteric margins were positive for lymphoma. Vascular margin was involved by tumor. There was lymphatic invasion but no venous or perineural invasion. Twelve of 12 pericolonic lymph nodes were involved with tumor. There was equivocal involvement of the omentum. The tumor was positive for CD20, CD79a IgM, and negative for CD23, CD21, CD10, and cyclin-D1. PET scan, 04/04/XX, demonstrated a large focus of intense FDG uptake in the right midabdomen, anterior and inferior to the kidney, corresponding to the transverse colon. Complete blood count, LDH, albumin, were normal. Beta 2-microglobulin level was 2.51. Sedimentation rate 45. Helicobacter pylori was negative. The patient has an associated IgG kappa monoclonal gammopathy with a total IgG level of 1280 mg/dL with normal IgA and IgM levels. Treatment included laparoscopic right and transverse colectomy, Rituxan 375 mg/m^2 intravenously weekly x4 weeks, and maintenance Rituxan 375 mg/m^2 intravenously every 3 months x2 years.

3. T1N0M0, moderately differentiated squamous cell carcinoma of the right upper lobe diagnosed in July 20XX when patient presented with a slowly enlarging, PET-positive, right upper lobe nodule. The tumor measured 2 cm in diameter. Three peribronchial nodes and 1 right paratracheal node were free of tumor. Treatment included wedge resection of the right upper lobe of the lung.

PAST MEDICAL HISTORY
1. Hypertension.
2. Guillain-Barré with essentially a full recovery.
3. Cholecystectomy in 19XX.
4. Right hand surgery recently.
5. Gravida 6, para 6.
6. Left chest wall cellulitis, 05/19XX.
7. Fibroadenoma, mildly proliferative fibrocystic change without atypia by right breast biopsy, 9/21/20XX, for evaluation of cluster of microcalcifications by screening mammogram.
8. Colonic adenoma by colonoscopy, 05/04/20XX. Polyp and inflammation by colonoscopy, 06/13/20XX, with inadequate preparation. Serrated adenoma at the anastomosis, hyperplastic polyp, and mild active colitis of the sigmoid colon by colonoscopy, 09/23/20XX.
9. Punctate acute or subacute infarction within the posterior limb of the internal capsule with associated left facial droop and dysarthria following VATS procedure, 07/24/20XX.
10. Mohs surgery for skin cancer of the nose, 20XX.
11. Right cataract surgery, 01/20XX.

MEDICATIONS
Verapamil 240 mg daily, triamterene and hydrochlorothiazide daily, calcium daily, multivitamins daily, Spiriva daily as needed, aspirin 81 mg daily, Benefiber daily, milk of magnesia as needed.

ALLERGIES
No known drug allergies.

FAMILY HISTORY
There is no family history of breast, uterine, colon or ovarian carcinoma. A son was diagnosed with squamous cell carcinoma of the throat at the age of 51.

REVIEW OF SYSTEMS
GENERAL: Negative for fatigue, weight loss, weight gain.
SKIN: Negative for rash, bruising.
ENT: Positive for diminished hearing bilaterally. Negative for sinus pain, hoarseness, sore throat, mouth sores.
EYES: Negative for change in vision.
HEART: Negative for chest pain, palpitations, ankle swelling.
LUNGS: Negative for recurrent cough, shortness of breath, wheezing. Positive for mild dyspnea on exertion.
UROLOGICAL: Negative for hematuria, dysuria, incontinence.
GYNECOLOGIC: Negative for vaginal bleeding, significant vaginal discharge, pelvic pain.
MUSCULOSKELETAL: Negative for bone pain, joint pain.
NEUROLOGICAL: Positive for chronic poor balance, decreased sensation in the hands, and weakness of the hands.
IMMUNOLOGIC: Negative for fever, adenopathy.

PHYSICAL EXAMINATION

Weight 122.6 pounds, temperature 98.4, pulse 90, blood pressure 122/70, oxygen saturation 94% on room air. Performance status 0, pain 0. Well-developed, well-nourished elderly woman in no acute distress. HEENT: Normal hair, anicteric sclerae, no oral lesions or thrush. Sinuses nontender. Neck supple without thyromegaly. Nodes: No significant lymphadenopathy. Lungs are clear to auscultation and percussion. Breath sounds are normal bilaterally. There are well-healed chest-wall scars postthoracotomy. Left mastectomy scar is well healed without evidence of locally recurrent disease. Right breast has a well-healed periareolar scar but is without dominant mass, nipple discharge, or suspicious skin changes. Cardiac exam: Regular rate and rhythm without murmurs, rubs, or gallops. Abdomen has well-healed surgical scars, is soft, nontender, without hepatosplenomegaly or abdominal mass. Extremities without cyanosis, clubbing, or edema. Spine is nontender. Neurologic exam: The patient is awake, alert, oriented x3. Gait is mildly ataxic.

LABORATORY DATA

Hemoglobin 14.2, hematocrit 41.1, white blood cell count 7.4, platelet count 252,000, absolute neutrophil count 4800.

IMPRESSION

1. Stage IIA left breast carcinoma, clinically without evidence of recurrent disease, now 13 years since diagnosis.
2. Stage II MALT lymphoma of the transverse colon and appendix, clinically without evidence of recurrent disease, now 18 months since completion of maintenance Rituxan therapy.
3. Stage I right upper lobe squamous cell carcinoma of the lung, clinically without evidence of recurrent disease, now more than 2 years since diagnosis.

RECOMMENDATIONS

I reassured Eleanor that she remains clinically without evidence of recurrent carcinoma and lymphoma. I ordered chemistries today and will be in contact with Eleanor by phone regarding any significant abnormalities. She was advised to proceed with followup colonoscopy this winter and CT scan in April 20XX or sooner as clinically indicated. In addition, she will proceed with screening mammogram in January. I advised the patient not to receive an influenza vaccine due to her prior history of Guillain-Barré. I plan to see Eleanor in followup in 3 months or sooner as needed.

Appendix C: Resources

Reference and Tools

Stedman's (Lippincott Williams and Wilkins) electronic medical dictionary, electronic word lists, Quick Look Drug Reference, printed reference materials
  http://www.Stedmans.com and
  http://www.StedmansOnline.com

MTWerks (author's personal website)
  http://www.MTWerks.com

Instant Text by Textware Solutions (text expansion software)
  http://www.Textware.com

SpeedType (text expansion software)
  http://www.SpeedType.com

Transcription Gear (transcription equipment, supplies, and software)
  http://www.TranscriptionGear.com

People and Places

For a list of all cities in a given state, search Google using phrase "All cities in <state name>" Wikipedia. This gives you a list of links to Wikipedia pages with census information and a list of all cities and towns in that state. See also http://www.usacitylink.com/.

American Hospital Directory
  http://www.ahd.com/freesearch.php3

Veteran's Administration (list of VA hospitals)
  http://www.va.gov/

AMA Doctor Finder (nationwide resource for locating doctors)
  http://ama-assn.org

Direct link to AMA DoctorFinder
  http://dbapps.ama-assn.org/iwcf/iwcfmgr206/
  aps?seed=1510

Anatomy and Diseases References

Interactive anatomy site
  http://www.innerbody.com/htm/body.html

Merck Manual Professional Edition
  http://www.merckmanuals.com/professional/
  index.html

MEDLINE and PubMed
  http://www.nlm.nih.gov

Medline Plus Surgical Procedures on Video
  http://www.nlm.nih.gov/medlineplus/surgeryvideos
  .html

eMedicine (clinical reference site with up-to-date, searchable, peer-reviewed medical articles organized by specialty)
  http://emedicine.medscape.com/

Drugs, Tests, and Terminology

National Cancer Institute Dictionary of Cancer Terms
  http://www.cancer.gov/dictionary

RxList Pharmaceutical Information (drug monographs and drug search)
  http://www.RxList.com

Lexicomp (medications recently approved by the FDA or those likely to be FDA approved within the next year)
  http://www.lexi.com/web/newdrugs.jsp

FDA (database for newly approved drugs and devices)
  http://www.fda.gov/search/databases.html

ClinLab Navigator Laboratory Reference
  http://www.clinlabnavigator.com/

Lab Handbook (extensive list of laboratory and pathology tests)
  http://www.healthsystem.virginia.edu/pub/medlabs/
  lab-handbook-test-directory

Merriam-Webster's Collegiate Dictionary
  http://www.m-w.com/home.htm

OneLook Dictionary Search (compilation of online dictionaries with wildcard searches and reverse searches)
  http://www.OneLook.com

Grammar Reference
  http://www.dailygrammar.com

Common Errors in English (list of sound-alike terms and commonly confused English words and phrases)
  http://www.wsu.edu/~brians/errors/errors.html#errors

Chicago Manual of Style Online
  http://www.ChicagoManualofStyle.org/contents.html

Gregg Reference Manual Online
  http://www.mhhe.com/business/buscom/gregg/
  resources.htm

Professional Associations and Industry Resources

Association for Healthcare Documentation Integrity (AHDI, formerly American Association for Medical Transcription)
http://www.AHDIonline.org

Clinical Documentation Industry Association (CDIA, formerly Medical Transcription Industry Association)
http://www.CDIAweb.org

American Health Information Management Association (AHIMA)
www.ahima.org

For the Record (industry trade magazine)
http://www.ForTheRecordMag.com/

Advance for Health Information Management (industry trade magazine)
http://health-information.advanceweb.com/

Health Level Seven (standards setting body for health information)
www.hl7.org

Office of the National Coordinator for Health Information Technology (ONCHIT)
http://healthit.hhs.gov/portal/server.pt/community/healthit_hhs_gov__home/1204

ASTM International
www.ASTM.org

The Health Story Project
www.HealthStory.com

Appendix D: Preview Terms Glossary

Chapter 1

acronym: An abbreviation formed by the first letters of several words and pronounced as a single word (eg, GERD).

blank: A notation within a transcribed document, either a line, an asterisk or other symbol, to indicate a word or words are missing due to incomprehensible or obscured dictation.

bookmarking: Saving a website's address in a list of frequently used sites.

browse: To move through a list.

combining form: A single word created from two words such as anteromedial (anterior and medial) and posterolateral (posterior and lateral).

compound modifier: Two or more descriptive words preceding a noun.

context: Words, phrases, and paragraphs surrounding any given word that help explain the full meaning of the word.

definition: In the context of an electronic reference, the definition is the description of the currently selected word in the indexed list.

deletions: Dropping sounds (letters) when pronouncing a word, usually caused by the inability to articulate the sound.

devoicing: Pronouncing a sound without vibrating the vocal cords; the same sound when spoken by a native speaker would produce vibration.

English as a second language (ESL): A term used to describe an English-speaking individual whose first language was not English.

entry: In the context of an electronic reference, the term associated with a definition or with related words and phrases.

filter: To hide information or eliminate specific information in order to narrow the search results and make it easier to locate the needed information.

Find: A command used to locate specific words or a phrase on the current web page or in the current document.

flag: To mark a report, either physically with a sticky note or ink marking, or electronically with a programmed marker, to indicate there is a problem with the report that must be addressed by quality assurance staff or the provider before the report is added to the patient's record.

headword: The primary entry in an electronic word list or electronic dictionary.

homophones: Words that are pronounced the same yet have different meanings and may have different spellings (eg, bear and bare).

index: In the context of an electronic reference, the index is the alphabetical list of words defined or described within the reference.

indications: In the context of an electronic reference, a list of words divided by topic, especially lists of drugs categorized by diagnosis or reason for prescribing.

initialisms: Abbreviations that use the first letter of each word in the abbreviated phrase (eg, CBC, CMP) and that are pronounced as successive letters (cf acronym).

keywords: In the context of an electronic reference, a list of words divided by topic, especially lists of drugs categorized by indication or reason for prescribing.

phoneme: The smallest sound of speech that has meaning.

query: In the context of electronic search, a query is a request for a specific type of information; a way of describing the information you are looking for.

s/l: A notation meaning "sounds like" often used by transcriptionists to indicate the sounds they heard at the point of a blank. A sounds-like notation can be helpful to the quality assurance staff or to the provider in deciphering the blank.

search on definition/subentry: To search for a word in an electronic reference using words or concepts contained within the definition or within the associated words or phrases in a word list.

search on index: To search the index using a partial word and wild cards (asterisks and question marks to represent missing letters), also referred to as partial word searches.

search operators: Words or symbols used as part of a query to help describe the information needed.

sound-alikes: Words and phrases that are pronounced so similarly that they may be indistinguishable without context (Lasik and Lasix).

subentry: In the context of an electronic reference, the subentry includes the terms and phrases associated with an indexed word in a word list.

substitutions: Replacing a letter/sound with a different letter/sound when pronouncing a word, usually caused by the inability to articulate the sound.

Universal Resource Locator (URL): The unique address that lists the website name, domain name, and page name.

vowel insertions: Pronouncing a word with more vowel sounds than actually contained within the word.

vowel shortening: Pronouncing a word with the correct vowel sound but with less time spent pronouncing the vowel sound.

wild cards: Symbols such as asterisks and question marks that represent missing characters in a word or phrase search.

Chapter 2

atherosclerosis: A pathologic process causing hardening of the vascular walls and partial or complete occlusion of the vessel lumen.

cell receptors: Molecules, often consisting of glycoproteins (sugars and amino acids) that are embedded in the surface of cell membranes. Receptors are essential to the body's overall communication system. Each receptor is very specific to a given hormone or other "messenger" molecule. Receptors are only expressed on the cell surface of cells that are intended to respond to the given messenger molecule. Molecules circulating in the blood stream bind to cell receptors, signaling the cell to respond in a defined way.

electrolytes: Sodium (Na^+), potassium (K^+), chloride (Cl^-) and bicarbonate ions (HCO_3^-) (positively and negatively charged molecules).

extracellular: Outside of a cell or the space surrounding a cell.

intracellular: Within a cell or cells.

intravascular: Within the blood vessels.

metabolism: The combined chemical and physical actions of catabolism and anabolism. Catabolism is the process of breaking down larger molecules into smaller molecules. Anabolism is the process of changing smaller molecules into larger ones.

mole: A unit of measure equal to Avogadro's number, 6.023×10^{23}. A way of expressing the number of atoms or molecules where a mole is always the same number of atoms or molecules. Just as a dozen is always 12 of any item, a mole always contains 6.023×10^{23} items. Concentrations of molecules are often expressed in moles or millimoles per liter (mol/L or mmol/L).

morbidity and mortality: The degree of disease, disability, and death associated with a given condition.

osmosis: The diffusion of water across a cellular membrane toward the side of higher solute concentration. For example, water will diffuse into the intracellular space if the concentration of sodium (and other solutes) is higher in the intracellular space compared to the extracellular space.

solute: The dissolved substance in a solution.

transport (carrier) proteins: Molecules consisting predominantly of protein that are designed to carry other molecules through the bloodstream. Many molecules needed for metabolism are not water soluble and therefor would not stay in solution in the blood. Transport proteins are essential for regulating the proper levels of metabolic components and distributing them throughout the body. Albumin is one of the most important nonspecific transport proteins, but there are many other highly specialized transport proteins.

Chapter 3

anorexia: Diminished appetite.

constipation: Irregular or infrequent pattern of bowel movements or stools that are hard and difficult to pass; may be accompanied by a sense of incomplete evacuation.

diarrhea: Frequent stools that are semisolid or fluid.

distal: A point situated away from the center of the body or the point of origin (compare proximal).

dyspepsia: Acute, chronic, or recurrent pain or discomfort centered in the upper abdomen. Symptoms include upper abdominal fullness, early satiety, burning, bloating, belching, nausea, retching or vomiting.

hematemesis: Vomiting blood.

hematochezia: Passage of bloody stools.

melena: Passage of dark, tarry stools containing digested blood.

nausea: A vague, intensely disagreeable feeling that may or may not be accompanied by retching and vomiting. The feeling of nausea originates in the medullary vomiting center in response to conditions in either the gastrointestinal tract or the central nervous system.

proximal: A point situated closer to the trunk or the point of origin (compare distal).

regurgitation: Spitting up of gastric contents without accompanying nausea or forceful contractions of the abdominal muscles.

vomiting: The forceful expulsion of stomach contents caused by the involuntary contraction of the abdominal muscles and the gastric fundus with concomitant relaxation of the esophageal sphincter.

Chapter 4

abdominal quadrants: Four areas of the abdomen demarcated by imaginary lines that cross perpendicularly through the umbilicus. Quadrants are referred to as right upper quadrant (RUQ), left upper quadrant (LUQ), right lower quadrant (RLQ), and left lower quadrant (LLQ).

abdominal regions: The abdomen is divided into nine regions: umbilical, epigastric (central above the stomach), hypogastric (central area below the stomach), left and right lumbar, left and right iliac, and left and right hypochondriac (just below the ribs).

carrier proteins: Protein molecules used to bind substances and transport those substances through the blood stream and/or across cellular membranes. Carrier proteins help to maintain metabolically active concentrations of substances in the blood and keep substances that are not normally water soluble dissolved in the blood. Examples include transferrin (iron), ceruloplasmin (copper), and albumin.

colic: Spasmodic abdominal pain.

deoxyribonucleic acid (DNA): The building blocks of chromosomes that encodes for proteins, enzymes and other structural and functional components of cells. DNA consists of rows of nucleotides (adenine, guanine, cytosine, and thymine). DNA is found universally in plants, animals, microbes, and some viruses.

extrahepatic: Occurring outside the liver.

hepatocyte: A liver cell.

hepatomegaly: Enlargement of the liver.

hepatotoxic: Toxic to the parenchymal cells of the liver.

hepatotropic: A substance or organism with an affinity for liver tissue.

intrahepatic: Occurring within the liver.

parenchyma: The functional cells of a gland or organ that are supported by a framework of connective tissue.

remote: In reference to an infection, a time period preceding the current time period; in the distant past.

ribonucleic acid (RNA): A molecule with a chemical structure similar to DNA that plays a central role in the translation and transcription of DNA into protein.

splenomegaly: Enlargement of the spleen.

Chapter 5

appendicular skeleton: The extremities (appendages).

articulation: Movement about two objects that are connected or joined loosely.

chondral: Pertaining to cartilage.

condyle: A round, knob-like structure that articulates with another bone. An enlarged area of a condyle is called an epicondyle.

immobilization: To prevent the movement around a joint or to hold a fractured bone in a static position.

Chapter 6

axial skeleton: Bones of the head and spine, as opposed to appendicular skeleton, which includes the bones of the extremities.

foramen, pl. foramina: An opening through a bone allowing the passage of another anatomical structure.

myelopathy: Nerve disorder due to compression or damage to the spinal cord.

paraspinal muscles: Muscles of the back that lie on either side of the spine.

process: A prominent projection on the surface of a bone used to attach tendons or ligaments. A knob-like projection is referred to as a tubercle, and a sharp projection is called a spine or spinous process.

radiculopathy: Nerve disorder originating at the nerve root (radicle).

Chapter 7

anuria: Urinary output of < 50 mL per day.

bacteriuria: Bacteria present in the urine.

dysuria: Difficulty or pain with urination.

frequency: Urinating more than eight times in a 24-hour period that does not result in a larger total volume of urine.

gross hematuria: A visible amount of blood in the urine.

hesitancy: Difficulty starting or maintaining a urinary stream.

incontinence: Involuntary release of urine.

irritative voiding: Urination accompanied by frequency, urgency, dysuria, sense of incomplete bladder emptying and/or nocturia.

lower urinary tract: The area of the urinary tract that includes the bladder and urethra.

microhematuria (microscopic hematuria): Small amounts of blood in the urine that cannot be seen with the naked eye.

nocturia: An urge to urinate that wakes the person from sleep.

oliguria: Urinary output of < 400 mL per day.

osmolality: A measure of the total number of dissolved particles in a solution.

osmosis: Movement of water across a membrane from an area of higher water concentration to an area of lower water concentration.

percutaneous: A surgical approach that inserts instruments or ports through the skin without making a surgical incision. The most common percutaneous technique is the Seldinger technique.

upper urinary tract: The area of the urinary tract that includes the kidneys and ureters.

urgency: A sudden, compelling need to urinate.

vesical: Another term to reference a bladder, typically the urinary bladder (cf vesicle).

Chapter 8

atelectasis: Literal meaning is incomplete (ateles) expansion (ectasis). In reference to the lung, atelectasis is a diminished volume of air in part or all of the lung.

CO: Abbreviation for carbon monoxide, representing one carbon atom and one oxygen atom.

CO_2: Abbreviation for carbon dioxide, representing one carbon atom and two oxygen atoms.

cor pulmonale: Right ventricular hypertrophy or right-sided cardiac failure as a direct result of a lung disorder.

cyanosis: A bluish color of the skin and mucous membranes caused by a decreased ratio of oxygenated to deoxygenated hemoglobin. Cyanosis in and of itself is not a reliable indicator of hypoxemia because the bluish color is dependent upon the hemoglobin concentration. Anemia may obscure cyanosis and polycythemia may cause cyanosis even in the presence of adequate oxygen.

dyspnea: A subjective feeling of being unable to breathe or obtain enough oxygen.

hemoptysis: Spitting up of blood originating in the respiratory tree.

hypercapnia: Elevated levels of carbon dioxide in the blood with symptoms of somnolence and decreased level of consciousness.

hypoventilation: Decreased gas entering the alveoli per unit of time.

hypoxemia: Decreased oxygen concentration in the blood (cf hypoxia).

hypoxia: Decreased oxygen concentration (cf hypoxemia) causing dyspnea, use of accessory muscles of respiration, tachypnea, tachycardia, diaphoresis, cyanosis, confusion, and somnolence.

O: (the letter O) Abbreviation for oxygen.

perfusion: In reference to the lung, perfusion is the flow of blood through the lung tissue.

ventilation: Exchange of air.

Chapter 9

atherosclerosis: A pathologic process characterized by lipids and inflammatory cells deposited in the intimal layer of arterial vessels leading to hardening of the vascular walls and partial or complete occlusion of the vessel lumen.

bruit: An abnormal sound detected on auscultation of an artery, indicative of disrupted or altered blood flow due to stenosis.

congestion: Increase in the volume of fluid contained in a vessel or chamber, causing increased pressure on the surrounding tissues.

diastole: The dilation phase of the cardiac cycle that allows the ventricles to fill with blood.

hypertrophy: Increase in the bulk of an organ or part of an organ due to an increase in cell size and not an increase in the number of cells.

infarction: Localized area of tissue receiving no oxygen.

ischemia: Localized area of tissue receiving decreased oxygen.

perfuse: To force blood into the vascular bed to supply oxygen and nutrients to the tissues.

sclerosis: Hardening of tissue, often due to scarring.

stenosis: Narrowing of a lumen or passageway.

systole: The contraction phase of the cardiac cycle.

Chapter 10

allergy: Any exaggerated immune response to a foreign antigen.

antibody: A protein produced by the immune system that specifically recognizes a single antigen and is capable of binding to that antigen. The shape of an antibody matches exactly to the shape of its corresponding antigen, much like a lock and key, so there is a one-to-one relationship between antigens and antibodies.

antigen: Molecules capable of eliciting a response from the immune system. Most antigens are made of protein or combinations of proteins (eg, glycoproteins).

autoimmune: An immune reaction directed against the person's own tissues.

differentiation: The maturation process that changes the cell's morphology and function from that of its precursor cell to a specialized cell with a specific function.

immune complex: An antibody bound to its antigen.

mediators (cell mediators): Substances that act as a form of chemical communication system. Mediators are released by one cell and cause a reaction in another cell.

Chapter 11

adrenarche: The development of hair growth under the arms and in the pubic area.

amenorrhea: No menses for at least six months.

aneuploid: Having an abnormal number of chromosomes. Humans have two sets of 23 chromosomes, so the haploid number is 23, the diploid number is 46. Aneuploid is 45, 47, or any number other than 46.

dysmenorrhea: Painful menses.

dyspareunia: Pain with intercourse.

hirsutism: (in females) Excess hair on the upper lip, chin, and between the breasts.

karyotype: The characterization of a cell's chromosomes, including the total number of chromosomes, the number of each chromosome, the presence of abnormal chromosomes, or abnormal numbers of any one chromosome.

menarche: The time of the first menstrual period.

menometrorrhagia: Prolonged or excessive bleeding at irregular intervals.

menorrhagia: Prolonged or excessive bleeding occurring at regular intervals.

menstruation: The cyclic, orderly sloughing of the uterine lining due to the interactions of hormones produced by the hypothalamus, pituitary, and ovaries.

metrorrhagia: Irregular, frequent uterine bleeding of varying amounts but not excessive.

oligomenorrhea: Periods occurring at intervals greater than 35 days resulting in less than nine menstrual periods per year.

puberty: The development of secondary sexual characteristics.

thelarche: The development of breasts at puberty.

Chapter 12

adenocarcinoma: A neoplasm arising from epithelial tissue that has glandular or secretory-like properties (cf sarcoma, which is a neoplasm arising from connective tissue).

blast: An extremely immature cell.

clones: Cells derived from the same precursor cell that are genetically identical.

cytopenia: A reduced number of cells in the peripheral blood. May also be used as a combining form with a specific cell type (eg, pancytopenia).

cytosis: An increased number of cells in the peripheral blood. May also be used as a combining form (eg, granulocytosis).

differentiation: The maturation process that changes the cell's morphology and function from that of its precursor cell to a specialized cell with a specific function.

genotype: The specific DNA sequencing that constitutes a gene or group of genes, usually used in reference to a particular attribute or character trait encoded by a single gene or a collection of genes (see also phenotype).

hematopoiesis: The formation and maturation of red cells, white cells, and platelets.

immunophenotype: The characteristic of a cell as determined by immunologic techniques (ie, using antibodies to identify a cell type by the presence of surface proteins). It is most commonly used to identify cells using cluster of differentiation (CD) proteins.

malignant: Capable of invading other types of tissue and spreading beyond its normal location.

metastases: Malignant cells thriving in a location other than their point of origin.

monoclonal: Produced by a single clone of cells; often used to describe a particular antibody produced in very large quantities, either in the laboratory for diagnostic and therapeutic uses or by the body caused by a myeloproliferative disorder.

myeloproliferative: Characterized by abnormal growth and reproduction of myelogenous (bone marrow) cells.

pancytopenia: A decrease in all cell types.

phenotype: An observable characteristic of an organism or biochemical molecule. A phenotype may describe a physical characteristic such as eye color or hair color or a biochemical characteristic such as a protein molecule's structure. A genotype may be modified by environmental or developmental factors to produce different phenotypes.

primary tumor: The initial location or cell type that gives rise to metastatic tumors.

stem cell: A precursor cell capable of creating daughter cells that differentiate into specialized cells.

Index

Note: terms with *f* indicate figures; those with *t* indicate tables.